TEXTBOOK OF
DIABETES

TEXTBOOK OF
DIABETES

EDITED BY

JOHN C. PICKUP MA, BM, DPhil, MRCPath
DIVISION OF CHEMICAL PATHOLOGY
UNITED MEDICAL AND DENTAL SCHOOLS OF
GUY'S AND ST THOMAS'S HOSPITALS
GUY'S HOSPITAL, LONDON
AND
GARETH WILLIAMS MA, MD, MRCP
DEPARTMENT OF MEDICINE
THE UNIVERSITY OF LIVERPOOL
ROYAL LIVERPOOL HOSPITAL, LIVERPOOL

IN TWO VOLUMES
VOLUME TWO

OXFORD

BLACKWELL SCIENTIFIC PUBLICATIONS

LONDON EDINBURGH BOSTON

MELBOURNE PARIS BERLIN VIENNA

© 1991 by
Blackwell Scientific Publications
Editorial Offices:
Osney Mead, Oxford OX2 0EL
25 John Street, London WC1N 2BL
23 Ainslie Place, Edinburgh EH3 6AJ
3 Cambridge Center, Cambridge,
    Massachusetts 02142, USA
54 University Street, Carlton
    Victoria 3053, Australia

Other Editorial Offices:
Librairie Arnette SA
2, rue Casimir-Delavigne
75006 Paris
France

Blackwell Wissenschaft-Verlag
Meinekestrasse 4
D-1000 Berlin 15
Germany

Blackwell MZV
Feldgasse 13
A-1238 Wien
Austria

First published 1991
Reprinted 1991

Set in Palatino by Setrite Typesetters, Hong Kong
Printed and bound in Hong Kong by
China Translation & Printing Services

DISTRIBUTORS

Marston Book Services Ltd
PO Box 87
Oxford OX2 0DT
(*Orders*: Tel: 0865 791155
        Fax: 0865 791927
        Telex: 837515)

USA
Blackwell Scientific Publications, Inc.
3 Cambridge Center
Cambridge, MA 02142
(*Orders*: Tel: 800 759−6102)

Canada
Times Mirror Professional Publishing, Ltd
5240 Finch Avenue East
Scarborough, Ontario M1S 5A2
(*Orders*: Tel: 416 298−1588)

Australia
Blackwell Scientific Publications
(Australia) Pty Ltd
54 University Street
Carlton, Victoria 3053
(*Orders*: (03) 347−0300)

British Library
Cataloguing in Publication Data

Textbook of diabetes.
    1. Man. Diabetes
    I. Pickup, John C. (John Christopher).
    II. Williams, Gareth
    616.462

ISBNs
    Vol. 1   0−632−03056−9
    Vol. 2   0−632−03058−5
    The set   0−632−025948−1

Contents

List of Contributors

A. MICHAEL ALBISSER, BEng, MA, PhD, *Director, Loyal True Blue and Orange Research Institute, P.O. Box 209, Richmond Hill, Ontario, L4C 4YZ, Canada*

CLIFFORD J. BAILEY, BSc, PhD, *Senior Lecturer, Department of Pharmaceutical Sciences, Aston University, Aston Triangle, Birmingham B4 7ET, UK*

PETER J. BARRY, FRCS, FCOphth, *Consultant Ophthalmic Surgeon, Royal Victoria Eye and Ear Hospital and St Vincent's Hospital, Dublin, Ireland*

PETER H. BENNETT, MB, FRCP, FFCM, *Chief, Phoenix Epidemiology and Clinical Research Branch, National Institute of Diabetes and Digestive and Kidney Diseases, 1550 East Indian School Road, Phoenix, Arizona 85014, USA*

D. JOHN BETTERIDGE, BSc, MD, PhD, FRCP, *Reader in Medicine and Honorary Consultant Physician, Department of Medicine, University College and Middlesex School of Medicine, The Rayne Institute, 5 University Street, London WC1E 6JJ, UK*

RUDOLF W. BILOUS, MD, MRCP, *Senior Registrar in Diabetes and Endocrinology, Department of Medicine, The Medical School, Framlington Place, Newcastle upon Tyne NE2 4HH, UK*

CHRISTIAN BINDER, MD, *Chairman, Steno Memorial and Hvidøre Hospital, Niels Steensensvej 2, DK-2820 Gentofte, Denmark*

ANNE E. BISHOP, PhD, *Principal Research Officer, Department of Histochemistry, Royal Postgraduate Medical School, Hammersmith Hospital, London W12 0HS, UK*

MICHAEL BLISS, MA, PhD, FRSC, *Professor of History, History Department, University of Toronto, Toronto, Ontario, Canada M5S 1AI*

STEPHEN R. BLOOM, DSc, MD, FRCP, *Professor of Endocrinology, Department of Medicine, Royal Postgraduate Medical School, Du Cane Road, London W12 0NN, UK*

GEREMIA B. BOLLI, MD, *Associate Professor of Diabetology, Istituto Patologica Medica, Via E Dal Pozzo, 06100 Perugia, Italy*

ADRIAN J. BONE, BSc, DPhil, *Lecturer in Molecular Endocrinology, Professorial Medical Unit, Room LD 68, Level D, South Laboratory and Pathology Block, Southampton General Hospital, Tremona Road, Southampton SO9 4XY, UK*

EZIO BONIFACIO, BSc, PhD, *Research Fellow, Department of Immunology, University College and Middlesex School of Medicine, Arthur Stanley House, 40−50 Tottenham Street, London W1P 9PG, UK*

KNUT BORCH-JOHNSEN, MD, *Senior Research Assistant, Steno Diabetes Centre, Niels Steensenvej 2, DK-280, Gentofte, Denmark*

GIAN FRANCO BOTTAZZO, MD, FRCP, *Professor of Clinical Immunology, Department of Immunology, University College and Middlesex School of Medicine, Arthur Stanley House, 40−50 Tottenham Street, London W1P 9PG, UK*

MICHAEL BROWNLEE, MD, *Anita and Jack Salts Chair of Diabetes Research, Professor of Medicine and Pathology, Albert Einstein College of Medicine, 1300 Morris Park Avenue, The Bronx, New York, NY 10461, USA*

RAYMOND BRUCE, MB, ChB, *Clinical Research Fellow, Wynn Institute for Metabolic Research, 21 Wellington Road, London NW8 9SQ, UK*

TERENCE CHADWICK, BSc, MB, ChB, MRCP, MFPP, *Head of Medical Affairs, Fisons PLC, Bakewell Road, Loughborough, Leicestershire LE11 0RH, UK (Former Programme Director for New Insulins, NOVO Industrials)*

AH WAH CHAN, MB, BCh, MRCP (UK), *Registrar, Professorial Medical Unit, Royal Liverpool Hospital, Prescot Street, Liverpool L7 8XP, UK*

CHI KONG CHING, MB, ChB, MRCP, *Senior Registrar, Derbyshire Royal Infirmary, London Road, Derby, DE1 2QY, UK*

DONALD J. CHISHOLM, MB, BS, FRACP, *Assistant Director, Garvan Institute of Medical Research, St Vincent's Hospital, Sydney 2010, Australia*

PENELOPE M. S. CLARK, PhD, MRCPath, *Principal Biochemist, Department of Clinical Biochemistry, Addenbrooke's Hospital, Hills Road, Cambridge CB2 2QR, UK*

BASIL F. CLARKE, MB, FRCPE, *Consultant Physician and Senior Lecturer, The Royal Infirmary, Edinburgh EH3 9YW, UK*

PHILIP COHEN, BSc, PhD, *Royal Society Research Professor, Department of Biochemistry, University of Dundee, Medical Sciences Institute, Dundee DD1 4HN, UK*

CAROLINE J. CRACE, PhD, *Formerly Research Assistant, Clinical Sciences Centre, University of Sheffield, Department of Paediatrics, Northern General Hospital, Sheffield S5 7AU, UK*

ADRIAN J. CRISP, MA, MD, MRCP (UK), *Consultant Rheumatologist, Addenbrooke's Hospital, Hills Road, Cambridge CB2 2QQ, UK*

JOHN L. DAY, MD, FRCP, *Consultant Physician, Department of Medicine, The Ipswich Hospital, Heath Road Wing, Ipswich, Suffolk IP4 5PD, UK*

TORSTEN DECKERT, MD, DMSc, *Chief Physician, Steno Memorial Hospital, Niels Steensensvej 2, DK-2820, Gentofte, Denmark*

JOHN DUPRÉ, FRCP (Lond.), FRCP (C), *Chief of Endocrinology and Metabolism, University Hospital London, Ontario N6A 5A5, Canada*

MICHAEL E. EDMONDS, MD, MRCP, *Senior Lecturer, Diabetic Department, King's College Hospital, Denmark Hill, London SE5 9RS, UK*

JEAN-MARIE EKOÉ, MD, *Visiting Professor of Medicine, Department of Medicine and Epidemiology Research Unit, Hôtel-Dieu de Montréal, University of Montréal, 3840 Rue St-Urbain, Montréal, Québec H2W 1T8, Canada*

DAVID J. EWING, MD, FRCP, *Wellcome Trust Senior Lecturer, Department of Medicine, The Royal Infirmary, Edinburgh EH3 9YW, UK*

PETER R. FLATT, BSc, PhD, *Professor of Biological and Biomedical Sciences, Biomedical Sciences Research Centre, Department of Biological & Biomedical Sciences, University of Ulster, Coleraine, Co. Londonderry BT52 1SA, Northern Ireland, UK*

ALI V. M. FOSTER, BA (Hons), DPodM, SRCh, *Chief Chiropodist, Diabetic Clinic, King's College Hospital, Denmark Hill, London SE5 9RS, UK*

ALAN K. FOULIS, BSc, MD, MRCPath, *Consultant Pathologist, Department of Pathology, Royal Infirmary, Glasgow G4 0SF, UK*

BRIAN M. FRIER, BSc, MD, FRCP, *Consultant Physician and Senior Lecturer, The Royal Infirmary, Edinburgh EH3 9YW, UK*

GEOFFREY V. GILL, MSc, MD, FRCP, DTM & H, *Consultant Physician, Arrowe Park Hospital, Arrowe Park Road, Upton, Wirral, Merseyside L49 5PE, UK*

BARRY J. GOLDSTEIN, MD, PhD, *Assistant Professor of Medicine, Harvard Medical School, and Investigator, Research Division, Joslin Diabetes Center, One Joslin Place, Boston, Massachusetts 02215, USA*

DEREK W. R. GRAY, DPhil, FRCS, MRCP, *Clinical Reader and Consultant Surgeon, Nuffield Department of Surgery, John Radcliffe Hospital, Headington, Oxford OX3 9DU, UK*

STEPHEN A. GREENE, MB, BS, MRCP, *Consultant Paediatrician and Paediatric Endocrinologist, Department of Child Health, Ninewells Hospital & Medical School, Dundee DD1 9SY, UK*

ANASUYA GRENFELL, MA, MD, MRCP, *Senior Medical Registrar, Ipswich Hospital, Heath Road Wing, Ipswich, Suffolk IP4 5PD, UK*

C. NICK HALES, MA, MD, PhD, FRCPath FRCP, *Professor of Clinical Biochemistry, Department of Clinical Biochemistry, Addenbrooke's Hospital, Hills Road, Cambridge CB2 2QR, UK*

KRISTIAN F. HANSSEN, MD, *Consultant Physician, University Department of Medicine, Aker Hospital, 0514 Oslo 5, Norway*

D. GRAHAME HARDIE, MA, PhD, *Reader, Department of Biochemistry, University of Dundee, Medical Sciences Institute, Dundee DD1 4HN, UK*

SUSAN HALL, *Department of Dermatology, Toronto General Hospital, 101 College Street, Toronto, Ontario M5G 1L7, Canada*

GRAHAM A. HITMAN, MB, FRCP, *Senior Lecturer and Honorary Consultant Physician, Department of Medicine, The Royal London Hospital, Whitechapel, London E1 1BB, UK*

RURY R. HOLMAN, MB, ChB, MRCP (UK), *Honorary Consultant Physician, Diabetes Research Laboratories, Radcliffe Infirmary, Woodstock Road, Oxford OX2 6HE, UK*

PHILIP D. HOME, MA, DPhil, FRCP, *Senior Lecturer and Consultant Physician, University of Newcastle upon Tyne, Freeman Diabetes Unit, Freeman Hospital, Newcastle upon Tyne NE7 7DN, UK*

SIMON L. HOWELL, BSc, PhD, DSc, *Professor of Endocrine Physiology, Biomedical Sciences Division, King's College, Campden Hill Road, London W8 7AH, UK*

STEPHEN L. HYER, MD, MRCP, *Senior Registrar (Diabetes and Endocrinology), St George's Hospital, Blackshaw Road, London SW17 0QT, UK*

KARL IRSIGLER, MD, *Professor of Medicine, 3rd Medical Department with Metabolic Diseases and Luolwig Boltzmann Research Institute for Metabolic Diseases and Nutrition, City Hospital Vienna-Lainz, Wolkerbergenstraße 1, A-1130 Vienna, Austria*

JAMES G. L. JACKSON, MD, (h.c.) *Formerly Executive Director, European Association for the Study of Diabetes, 'Cobbles', 10 Fam Court, Longcross Road, Chertsey, Surrey KT16 0DJ, UK*

R. JOHN JARRETT, MD, FFCM, *Professor of Clinical Epidemiology, Department of Public Health Medicine, United Medical and Dental Schools, Guy's Campus, London SE1 9RT, UK*

ROGER H. JAY, MA, MB, BS, MRCP, *Associate Research Fellow and Honorary Clinical Lecturer, Department of Medicine, University College and Middlesex School of Medicine, The Rayne Institute, 5 University Street, London WC1E 6JJ, UK*

PATRICIA M. JOHNS, RN, RM, *Dip Nursing, Diabetes Nurse Specialist, Maidstone Hospital, Hermitage Lane, Barming, Maidstone, Kent ME16 9QQ, UK*

DESMOND G. JOHNSTON, FRCP, PhD, *Professor of Clinical Endocrinology, Alexander Simpson Laboratory for Metabolic Research, St. Mary's Hospital Medical School, London W2, UK*

JACQUELINE N. JONES, BSc, SRN, *Research Nurse, Diabetic Day Care Centre, Greenwich District Hospital, Vanbrugh Hill, London SE10 9HE, UK*

RICHARD H. JONES, MA, MB, FRCP, *Senior Lecturer, Department of Medicine, United Medical and Dental Schools of Guy's and St Thomas's Hospitals, Medway Hospital, Gillingham, Kent ME7 5NY, UK*

C. RONALD KAHN, MD, *Mary K. Iacocca Professor of Medicine, Harvard Medical School, Chief, Division of Diabetes and Metabolism, Brigham and Women's Hospital, and Director, Research Laboratory, Joslin Diabetes Center, One Joslin Place, Boston, Massachusetts 02215, USA*

HARRY KEEN, MD, FRCP, *Professor of Human Metabolism, Unit for Metabolic Medicine, United Medical and Dental Schools (Guy's Campus), London SE1 9RT, UK*

LAURENCE KENNEDY, MD, FRCP, *Consultant Physician, Sir George E. Clark Metabolic Unit, Royal Victoria Hospital, Belfast BT12 6BA, Northern Ireland, UK*

RONALD KLEIN, MD, MPH, *Professor of Ophthalmology, Department of Ophthalmology, University of Wisconsin—Madison, F4/334 Clinical Sciences Center, 600 Highland Avenue, Madison, Wisconsin 53792, USA*

ANTHONY H. KNIGHT, FRCP, *Consultant Physician, Stoke Mandeville Hospital, Aylesbury, Bucks HP21 8AL, UK*

EVA M. KOHNER, MD, FRCP, *Professor of Medical Ophthalmology and Consultant Physician, Royal Postgraduate Medical School, Hammersmith Hospital, Du Cane Road, London W12 0HS, and Moorfields Eye Hospital, City Road, London EC1V 2PD, UK*

VEIKKO A. KOIVISTO, MD, *Senior Lecturer, Department of Medicine, Helsinki University Second Hospital, 00290 Helsinki Central, Finland*

EDWARD W. KRAEGEN, BSc, PhD, *Head, Diabetes Research Group, Garvan Institute of Medical Research, St Vincents Hospital, Sydney 2010, Australia*

BERNHARD KREYMANN, MD, *ii. Medizinische Klinik und Poliklinik Der Technischen Universität München, Ismaninger Strasse 22, 8000 München 80, Germany*

A. J. KRENTZ, MB, ChB, MRCP, *Senior Registrar, The General Hospital, Steelhouse Lane, Birmingham B4 6NH, UK*

ANTONY KURTZ, PhD, FRCP, *Reader, University College and Middlesex School of Medicine, London W1N 8AA, UK*

MIKE E. J. LEAN, MA, MD, FRCP, *Senior Lecturer, University of Glasgow Department of Human Nutrition, Royal Infirmary, Queen Elizabeth Building, Alexandra Parade, Glasgow G12 2ER, UK*

DAVID LESLIE, MD, FRCP, *Senior Lecturer, Department of Medicine, Charing Cross and Westminster Medical School, Westminster Hospital, 17 Horseferry Road, London SW1P 2AR, UK*

BIRGITTA LINDE, MD, PhD, *Assistant Professor and Consultant Physician, Department of Clinical Physiology, Karolinska Hospital, Box 60500, 104 01 Stockholm, Sweden*

WILLIAM D. LOUGHEED, PEng, *Biomedical Engineer, Loyal True Blue and Orange Research Institute, PO Box 209, Richmond Hill, Ontario, L4C 4YZ Canada*

CLARA LOWY, MB, MSc, FRCP, *Reader in Medicine, Division of Medicine, St Thomas's Campus, United Medical and Dental Schools, Unit of Endocrinology and Diabetes, Diabetic Day Center, St Thomas's Hospital, Lambeth Palace Road, London SE1 7EH, UK*

DAVID R. MCCANCE, BSc, MD, MRCP, *Senior Registrar, Sir George E. Clark Metabolic Unit, Royal Victoria Hospital, Belfast BT12 6BA, Northern Ireland, UK*

IAN A. MACFARLANE, MD, MRCP, *Consultant Physician, The Diabetes Centre, Walton Hospital, Rice Lane, Liverpool L9 1AE, UK*

TERESA MCLEAN, MA (Oxon), *Writer and Cricket Journalist, 31 Newmarket Road, Cambridge CB5 8EG, UK*

ANDREW MACLEOD, MA, MRCP, *Lecturer, Department of Medicine, United Medical and Dental Schools, St Thomas's Hospital, London SE1 7EH, UK*

ALASDAIR MCLEOD, BSc, BDS, *Research Fellow, Laboratory of Molecular Biology, Department of Crystallography, Malet Street, London WC1E 7HX, UK*

J. L. MAHON, MD, FRCP (C), *Research Fellow, Endocrinology and Metabolism, University Hospital London, Ontario N6A 5A5, Canada*

JIM I. MANN, MA, DM, PhD, *Professor of Human Nutrition, University of Otago, and Consultant Physician, Dunedin Hospital, Dunedin, New Zealand*

BRENDAN MARSHALL, PhD, *Postdoctoral Fellow, Department of Medicine, The London Hospital, Whitechapel, London E1 1BB, UK*

HUGH M. MATHER, MD, FRCP, *Consultant Physician, Ealing Hospital, Uxbridge Road, Southall, Middlesex UB1 3HW, UK*

V. MOHAN, MD, MNAMS, PhD, *Deputy Director, Diabetes Research Centre, 4 Main Road, Royapuram, Madras 600–013, India*

PETER J. MORRIS, PhD, FRCS, FRACS, FACS (Hon.), *Nuffield Professor of Surgery, University of Oxford, John Radcliffe Hospital, Headington, Oxford OX3 9DU, UK*

CATHLEEN J. MULLARKEY, MD, *Instructor, Department of Medicine, Albert Einstein College of Medicine, 1300 Morris Park Avenue, The Bronx, New York 10461, USA*

MALCOLM NATTRASS, MB, ChB, PhD, FRCP, *Consultant Physician, The General Hospital, Steelhouse Lane, Birmingham B4 6NH, UK*

JOHN C. PICKUP, MA, BM, DPhil, MRCPath, *Reader and Honorary Consultant Physician, Division of Chemical Pathology, United Medical and Dental Schools of Guy's and St Thomas's Hospitals, Guy's Hospital, London SE1 9RT, UK*

JULIA M. POLAK, DSc, MD, FRCPath, *Professor of Endocrine Pathology; Head, Histochemistry Unit and Deputy Director, Department of Histopathology, Royal Postgraduate Medical School, Du Cane Road, London W12 0NN, UK*

MASSIMO PORTA, MD, PhD, *Associate Professor of Medicine, University of Sassari, Italy, and Honorary Clinical Assistant, Diabetic Retinopathy Unit, Hammersmith Hospital, Du Cane Road, London W12 0NN, UK*

A. RAMACHANDRAN, MD, MNAMS, PhD, *Deputy Director, Diabetes Research Centre, 4 Main Road, Royapuram, Madras 600–013, India*

LUIS C. RAMIREZ, MD, *Assistant Professor of Medicine, Department of Internal Medicine, University of Texas Southwestern Medical Center at Dallas, 5323 Harry Hines Boulevard, Dallas, Texas 75235, USA*

PHILIP RASKIN, MD, *Professor of Medicine, Department of Internal Medicine, University of Texas Southwestern Medical Center at Dallas, 5323 Harry Hines Boulevard, Dallas, Texas 75235, USA*

S. SETHU K. REDDY, MD, FRCPC, *Department of Medicine, 5303 Morris Street, Gerard Hall, Camp Hill Medicine Centre, Dalhousie University, Halifax Nova Scotia, Canada*

JONATHAN M. RHODES, MA, MD, FRCP, *Senior Lecturer in Medicine and Gastroenterology, Royal Liverpool Hospital, Prescot Street, Liverpool L7 8XP, UK*

PATRICK SHARP, MD, MRCP, *Lecturer in Endocrinology, St. Mary's Hospital Medical School, Norfolk Place, Paddington, London W2 1PG, UK*

GARY R. SIBBALD, BSc, MD, FRCP (C), ABIM, DAAD, *Acting Head, Division of Dermatology, Department of Medicine, Women's College Hospital, University of Toronto, 76 Grenville Street, Toronto, Ontario M5S 1B2, Canada*

ANGELA C. SHORE, BSc, PhD, *Research Fellow, Diabetes Research (Microvascular Studies), Postgraduate Medical School, Royal Devon & Exeter Hospital, Exeter, Devon EX2 5DW, UK*

JUDITH M. STEEL, MB ChB, FRCPEd, *Associate Specialist, Department of Diabetes, Edinburgh Royal Infirmary, Lauriston Place, Edinburgh EH3 9YW, UK*

JOHN C. STEVENSON, MB, MRCP, *Consultant Endocrinologist, Wynn Institute for Metabolic Research, 21 Wellington Road, London NW8 9SQ, UK*

C. R. STILLER, MD, FRCP (C), *Professor of Medicine, University of Western Ontario; Director of Immunology, Robarts Research Institute; Chief, Multi-organ Transplant Service, University Hospital, 339 Windermere Road, London, Ontario N6A 5A5, Canada*

ROBERT W. STOUT, MD, DSc, FRCP, FRCPEd, FRCPI, *Professor of Geriatric Medicine, Department of Geriatric Medicine, The Queen's University of Belfast, Whitla Medical Building, 97 Lisburn Road, Belfast BT9 7BL, Northern Ireland, UK*

ROBERT SUTTON, MB, BS, FRCS, DPhil (Oxon), *Lecturer in Surgery, Nuffield Department of Surgery, John Radcliffe Hospital, Headington, Oxford OX3 9DU, UK*

TERESA M. SZOPA, BSc, PhD, *Research Fellow, Medical Unit, London Hospital, Whitechapel, London E1 1BB, UK*

HOWARD S. TAGER, PhD, *Louis Block Professor, Department of Biochemistry and Molecular Biology, The University of Chicago, 920 East 58th Street, Chicago, Illinois 60637, USA*

PETER R. W. TASKER, MB, BS, DCH, FRCGP, *General Practitioner, Doomsday House, Hall Lane, South Wootton, King's Lynn, Norfolk PE30 3LQ, UK*

ROBERT B. TATTERSALL, MD, FRCP, *Professor of Clinical Diabetes, University Hospital, Queen's Medical Centre, Nottingham NG7 2UH, UK*

KEITH W. TAYLOR, MA, PhD, MRCP, *Emeritus Professor of Biochemistry, Medical Unit, London Hospital, Whitechapel, London E1 1BB, UK*

ROY TAYLOR, BSc, MD, FRCP, *Consultant Physician and Senior Lecturer, Royal Victoria Infirmary, Queen Victoria Road, Newcastle upon Tyne NE1 4LP, UK*

P. K. THOMAS, DSc, MD, FRCP, FRCPath, *Professor of Neurological Science, Royal Free Hospital School of Medicine, Rowland Hill Street, London NW3 2PF, UK*

JOHN E. TOOKE, MA, MSc, DM, MRCP, *Consultant Physician and Senior Lecturer, Diabetes Research (Microvascular Studies), Postgraduate Medical School, Royal Devon and Exeter Hospital, Exeter, Devon EX2 5DW, UK*

ROBERT C. TURNER, MD, FRCP, *Clinical Reader, Diabetes Research Laboratories, Radcliffe Infirmary, Woodstock Road, Oxford OX2 6HE, UK*

GIAN CARLO VIBERTI, MD, FRCP, *Professor of Diabetic Medicine, Unit for Metabolic Medicine, 4th Floor, Hunts House, United Medical and Dental Schools, Guy's Hospital Campus, London SE1 9RT, UK*

M. VISWANATHAN, MD, FAMS, *Director, Diabetes Research Centre, 5 Main Road, Royapuram, Madras 600–013, India*

JAMES D. WALKER, BSc, MRCP, *Senior Medical Registrar, 4th Floor, King George V Block, St Bartholomew's Hospital, West Smithfield, London EC1, UK*

JOHN D. WARD, BSc, MD, FRCP, *Consultant Physician, Royal Hallamshire Hospital, Glossop Road, Sheffield S10 2JF, UK*

PER WESTERMARK, MD, *Professor of Pathology, University of Uppsala, Department of Pathology, University Hospital, S–751 85 Uppsala, Sweden*

GREG WILKINSON, FRCP (Edin.), MRCPsych, *Director, Academic Sub-Department of Psychological Medicine, University of Wales College of Medicine, North Wales Hospital, Denbigh, Clwyd LL16 5SS, UK*

D.R.R. WILLIAMS, MA, PhD, MFPHM, *University Lecturer in Community Medicine, Level 5, Addenbrooke's Hospital, Hills Road, Cambridge CB2 2QQ, UK*

GARETH WILLIAMS, MA, MD, MRCP, *Senior Lecturer, Department of Medicine, University of Liverpool, PO Box 147, Liverpool L69 3BX, and Honorary Consultant Physician, Royal Liverpool Hospital, Prescot Street, Liverpool L7 8XP, UK*

R. MALCOLM WILSON, DM, MRCP, *Senior Lecturer, Department of Medicine, Royal Hallamshire Hospital, Glossop Road, Sheffield S10 2JF, UK*

PETER H. WISE, MB, BS, PhD, FRCP, FRACP, *Consultant Physician, Charing Cross Hospital, Fulham Palace Road, London W6 8RF, UK*

STEVEN P. WOOD, BSc, DPhil, *Senior Research Fellow, Laboratory of Molecular Biology, Department of Crystallography, Birkbeck College, Malet Street, London WC1E 7HX, UK*

Foreword

The diabetic state commands more attention now than ever before. At a time when in all branches of medicine, indeed in all branches of science, the engagement generally with the problem becomes increasingly demanding and technologically complex, understanding diabetes occupies a continuingly prominent place. Diabetes has always stood out in the history of medicine and science. The graphic descriptions by ancient observers must put the severe, insulin-deficient diabetic state among the earliest of the readily recognized clinical conditions, the paradigm of the 'clinical syndrome'. Exploration of the nature of diabetes claimed the attention of the father of experimental medicine, the great Claude Bernard, so much of whose thought and perception remains with us today. He understood the importance of the balance between glucose production and glucose consumption in determining the level of glucose concentration though he had little conception of the factors which regulated them. He saw diabetes essentially as the outcome of a disturbance of relationships, a distortion of a homeostatic system, a disorder of adaptation.

Bernard shared the scientific stage with the other giant of 19th century biomedical science, Louis Pasteur, whose discoveries promoted a quite different model of disease, one that was more direct and simple. The disease process resulted from a single, well-defined causal agency — a germ. If the germ was not present, the disease could not occur, though having the germ did not guarantee the appearance of the disease. The Pasteurian notion of disease in the present day context can be extended to include the abnormal gene or a toxic substance as the causal agency of disease. Had Pasteur ever pronounced upon diabetes, he might well have wondered about some specific enzymatic abnormality in the pathways of glucose metabolism, an area not unfamiliar to him.

In the contemporary world of diabetes, the Bernardian and the Pasteurian views contend. A pure Bernardian would regard the diabetic state as a disorder of adaptation, a breakdown in the interrelation and regulation of the balance of factors determining glucose production and disposal. It is perhaps best exemplified in the debates in the 1990s by the Reaven concept of glucose intolerance and non-insulin-dependent diabetes mellitus (NIDDM). His construct of the conditions resulting in the diabetic state introduces the interaction of regulatory mechanisms unknown in their nature to Bernard and Pasteur. This construct is compatible with the observed 'continuous distribution' of glucose tolerance/intolerance in most populations, showing no clear break between the normal and the abnormal.

The scientific advances of recent decades might seem to promote the Pasteurian view of the diabetic state. We have witnessed an explosive expansion of knowledge and understanding of the genetic control of cell structure and function, and its role in the causation of disease. The search for a diabetes (susceptibility) gene has excited much research interest and is best established in the insulin-dependent variety of diabetes. An environmental trigger which initiates a process culminating in the destruction of the pancreatic B cell is also sought and fulfils the Pasteurian expectation of a single causal factor of major effect operating in a genetically susceptible setting.

It becomes likely that these two major views of the causation of the diabetic state are not mutually incompatible and indeed both operate to explain the occurrence of diabetes in man. Thus, genetic factors contribute to the adaptive disorder of NIDDM (though their nature remains far from clear) while the process affecting the B cell in the insulin-dependent variety of the disease may fall far short of complete destruction of insulin-producing cells in many of the people it affects and is itself presumably modulated by other genetic and environmental factors.

The diabetic state impacts upon mankind in many ways. At the 'macro' level, it throws up the question of the adequacy of provision of medical services, the question of prescriptive screening, and the social and emotional predicament of the diabetic individual. For the individual, it carries a variety of clinical and therapeutic problems, often complicated in the long course of the disease by damage to the eye, the kidney, the peripheral nerves, and the arterial wall. It is these delayed 'complications' which provide most of the burden of diabetes upon the individual and upon society. While the diabetic state appears to be the *sine qua non* of their appearance, other individual factors, some probably genetic, will also determine their time of onset, their rate of progression and their ultimate severity.

For clinical and basic scientists, diabetes is the point of departure for research enquiries in many fields. The history of the discovery of insulin, its characterization, structure and synthesis have contributed much to broaden understanding of biochemistry and genetics. Research into the insulin receptor is telling us about the mechanisms of hormonal signals. Immunological mechanisms are bound up with some forms of the diabetic state; their understanding and control may well lead to the prevention of insulin-dependent diabetes in the foreseeable future.

These and many other aspects of the diabetic state are dealt with in the chapters that follow. Clear answers as to 'the cause' of diabetes and its complications are not yet available. However, the growing pace of research and its increasingly prompt application to the patient make the lot of the person with diabetes progressively easier to bear. The comprehensive account of our knowledge of the disease in this book will make a substantial contribution to improving both our understanding of the disease and the care of patients suffering from it.

HARRY KEEN
London, July 1990

Preface

Our main intention in producing this book was to disseminate information about diabetes mellitus amongst the many different people involved in tackling the scientific, medical and social problems of the disease. The ramifications of diabetes extend into so many areas that it demands a truly multidisciplinary approach. Its clinical management depends on an integrated team of specialists as diverse as physicians, chiropodists, nurses, psychiatrists and general practitioners, and research into the disease and its treatment requires the combined skills of immunologists, physiologists, pathologists, chemists and many others. The problems of diabetes will only be identified and solved if there is understanding and effective communication between these various groups.

We therefore set out to summarize the key clinical and scientific topics of diabetes in a form which would be useful to the specialist in a given area and yet readily accessible to the non-specialist who wishes to learn about the main principles and challenges of disciplines beyond his or her own. The 'clinical' chapters are intended to provide a clear and up-to-date guide to the features, diagnosis and treatment of diabetes and its complications, which will be of real practical value to those concerned with the everyday management of the disease. In the 'scientific' (non-clinical) sections, we have aimed to cover the major aspects of metabolism and what is known of the disease processes which result in diabetes; we hope that these are both comprehensive and, for the most part, interesting and intelligible to those who are not career scientists. Throughout the book, we have attempted to highlight recent clinical and scientific advances and their impact on the understanding and treatment of diabetes, as well as the questions which remain unanswered.

Overall, we have tried to cater for a wide range of interests and requirements. The book should also be useful for those preparing for postgraduate examinations.

Each chapter is constructed as a self-contained essay prepared by an expert in the field and, as such, should stand alone; we therefore make no apologies for the reiteration of important concepts in more than one chapter. At the same time, the book is designed as an integrated text and we have tried to avoid unnecessary repetition through extensive cross-referencing. We have edited each chapter according to a common format, beginning with a summary of its major points, and have made extensive use of figures, flow-charts and tables where these usefully illustrate important points in the text. If we have managed to produce an integrated book, we hope that this has been achieved without stifling the individuality of the contributors.

Every textbook runs the risk of various criticisms, some of which we have tried to anticipate. The first is that any book of this size will inevitably be out of date by the time it appears. We have tried to incorporate new and important material at all stages up to the final proofs, and can only hope that the great distress which this has caused our publishers has been justified. Secondly, every textbook is parochial to some extent. We have aimed to encompass a wider view of diabetes than that encountered in our own practice by including contributions from authors in a dozen or so countries, which cover topics such as diabetes in the Third World, malnutrition-related diabetes and diabetes in ethnic groups in the UK. Finally, the scope of a book such as this is sometimes questioned. We hope that our choice of chapters reflects both the breadth and the excitement of diabetes and that, for example, those dealing with the historical background of diabetes and the short but thought-provoking personal view of the disease will not be neglected.

This book's gestation slightly exceeded that of the blue whale and, at times, the book seemed likely to join the whale on the list of endangered species. Fortunately, several groups of people have fought to ensure its survival. We are profoundly grateful for their contributions to the book, which range from the obvious to the invisible. The first, of course, is the 120 authors who have provided the substance of the book with skill and authority. We would like to thank them, not only for the quality of their contributions, but also for their stoical and (mostly) gallant tolerance of editorial interference with their work. We are particularly indebted to those who, through efficiency or intimidation, managed to meet or even beat our deadlines. The second group is the team at Blackwell Scientific Publications, who have distinguished themselves by their endless support, enthusiasm and ability to apply firm but generally painless pressure at crucial moments. Karen Anthony and Rachel Nalumoso deserve special mention for having served so nobly (and indeed survived) in the front-line skirmishes between publishers, authors and editors. Peter Saugman initiated the project and provided constant support and encouragement throughout. Thirdly, many friends and colleagues have helped in various ways, particularly by providing clinical photographs and other material, hounding elusive references and making suggestions — sometimes kind but always constructive — about the content of the book. We have especially valued the help of Ian MacFarlane, Geoff Gill and Paul Drury in this respect, and also acknowledge the assistance of Charles Bodmer and Alan Patrick in struggling through the proofs, and of Jackie Williams and Adrian Brown in drawing up the tables for Chapter 79. The fourth group is our secretariat, namely Caroline Williams, Luine Weir and Denise Janson, whose skills in typing, organization and cryptography are fortunately underpinned by the rare virtues of patience and good humour.

Finally, we are indebted to our families for having tolerated the book's relentless invasion of evenings, weekends and holidays, and for having accepted so many times our increasingly flimsy assurances that it would be finished one day.

JOHN C. PICKUP
GARETH WILLIAMS
London and Liverpool, July 1990

SECTION 13
CHRONIC DIABETIC COMPLICATIONS

PART 13.1
GENERAL MECHANISMS OF DIABETIC COMPLICATIONS

52   The Determinants of Microvascular Complications in Diabetes: An Overview

Summary

● The 'microvascular' ('microangiopathic' or 'small-vessel') complications of diabetes include retinopathy, nephropathy and neuropathy, even though the contribution of microangiopathy to neuropathy is unknown.

● Microvascular complications are specific to diabetes and do not occur without long-standing hyperglycaemia. Other metabolic, environmental and genetic factors are undoubtedly involved in their pathogenesis.

● Both IDDM and NIDDM are susceptible to microvascular complications, although patients with NIDDM are older at presentation and may die of macrovascular disease before microvascular disease is advanced.

● The duration of diabetes and the quality of diabetic control are important determinants of microvascular disease but, because of other individual factors, do not necessarily predict their development in individual patients.

● Different microvascular complications are commonly associated in individual patients, but their prevalence as a function of the duration or severity of diabetes may differ markedly.

● In IDDM, background retinopathy is rare before 5 years of diabetes but its prevalence increases steadily thereafter to affect over 90% of patients after 20 years. After several years of diabetes, the risk of proliferative changes is about 3% of patients per year, with a cumulative total of over 60% after 40 years.

● Diabetic nephropathy affects 20–40% of patients with IDDM, particularly those presenting before puberty and possibly those with an inherited tendency to hypertension. NIDDM patients are also susceptible to nephropathy.

● Over 40% of subjects with IDDM survive for more than 40 years, half of them without developing significant microvascular complications.

The terms 'microvascular' or 'microangiopathic' complications commonly embrace diabetic retinopathy, nephropathy and neuropathy, even though the classification of the latter as a true microvascular complication remains controversial (see Chapter 61). The purpose of this chapter is to outline in general the factors thought to contribute to the development of these complications. The possible pathophysiological mechanisms are reviewed later in this section (Chapters 53–55) and the specific complications themselves in Chapters 56–68.

Most investigators now agree that diabetic microvascular complications result from the interaction of multiple metabolic, genetic and other factors, of which chronic hyperglycaemia is the most significant. Microvascular complications are common to both IDDM and NIDDM (in which severe complications may occur) and do not develop in the absence of long-standing hyperglycaemia. Epidemiological and long-term clinical studies strongly suggest that hyperglycaemia, or closely associated factors, is of major importance in both the initiation and progression of microvascular disease. Moreover, there is evidence that the various microvascular complications have a common cause. Diabetic patients with incipient nephropathy (persistent microalbuminuria) have 5–10 times the risk of developing proliferative retinopathy than those free from albuminuria; moreover, diabetic nephropathy is almost invariably accompanied by retinopathy. The evolution of the various complications therefore seems to be interrelated.

However, there is immense variability in susceptibility to microvascular disease, which in individual patients cannot be predicted from their glycaemic behaviour. Other factors must therefore be involved. Some of the putative determinants of microvascular disease will now be discussed in more detail.

Age

IDDM patients whose disease appears before puberty have an increased risk of developing diabetic nephropathy, which is associated with premature death [1], but apparently not with retinopathy in these cases [2].

Many NIDDM patients are relatively old when diabetes appears and some do not survive long enough to develop severe microvascular complications. However, some studies suggest that the frequency of retinopathy in NIDDM is similar to that in IDDM of equivalent duration [3]. There may be qualitative differences in retinopathy between NIDDM and IDDM, in that proliferative retinopathy is rarer and visual loss due to maculopathy is commoner in NIDDM as compared with IDDM. NIDDM patients are by no means 'protected' against nephropathy, even though this is commonly viewed as a complication predominantly of IDDM. About 40% of North American diabetic patients requiring renal dialysis have NIDDM, and nephropathy is particularly common in those ethnic groups (e.g. Asian and Afro-Caribbean populations) in which NIDDM appears at earlier ages [4].

Sex

Both sexes are vulnerable to diabetic microvascular disease, although there is an unexplained male preponderance of diabetic nephropathy and proliferative retinopathy [5]; there are no systematic glycaemic differences between males and females.

Duration of diabetes

This is an important determinant of microvascular disease although, as discussed below, the relationship between duration of diabetes and the evolution of the complications is not simple. The issue is further complicated in NIDDM, whose insidious onset may follow several years of subclinical disease; clinically important microvascular complications may be present at diagnosis.

Diabetic treatment can prevent acute metabolic deterioration but does not achieve biochemical normality, resulting in a novel condition including various combinations of hyperglycaemia, hyperketonaemia, hyperlipidaemia and other alterations (see Chapter 32). These 'components of diabetic exposure' are interdependent to a certain degree and their levels are generally reflected by the integrated plasma glucose and HbA_1 concentrations, the most convenient measures in clinical use.

Each component can be characterized by its intensity, duration and cumulative dose (= mean intensity × duration). Epidemiological studies suggest that specific microvascular complications, although generally interrelated, may be determined by different aspects of exposure to these metabolic abnormalities. Various dose−response curves are theoretically possible. With a linear response, for example, the *incidence* of a complication would rise in proportion to the duration of diabetes, and the *cumulative risk* of the complication would rise considerably faster, in proportion to the square of the duration [6]. Other possible dose−response profiles include an incidence rate which rises to a plateau after a certain cumulative dose, or even one which decreases. In each of these cases, the cumulative risk increases with time, but the relationships between the incidence rate and the duration of diabetes differ markedly. Such divergences are illustrated by reference to diabetic retinopathy and nephropathy in IDDM.

Risk profiles of retinopathy in IDDM

Figures 52.1 and 52.2 respectively show the incidence rate and cumulative risk of background and proliferative retinopathy in IDDM patients. The first conclusion is that the prevalence of both increases with increasing duration of the disease; indeed, after 20 years, over 95% of IDDM patients have demonstrable retinopathy, although mostly without visual impairment [2]. Background retinopathy is rare before 5 years of diabetes, suggesting that duration is more important than intensity, although the latter presumably must exceed some threshold (Fig. 52.3) [6].

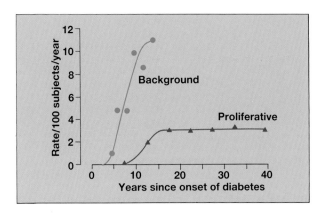

Fig. 52.1. Incidence rates of background and of proliferative retinopathy in subjects with IDDM, as a function of the duration of diabetes. (Redrawn from Krolewski *et al.* 1987 [6] with permission from *The New England Journal of Medicine*.) See text for explanation.

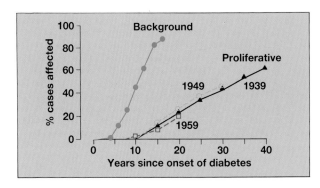

Fig. 52.2. Prevalence of background retinopathy and cumulative incidence of proliferative retinopathy in IDDM as a function of the duration of the disease. The data for proliferative retinopathy have been calculated for three cohorts of patients, diagnosed in 1939, 1949 and 1959. (Redrawn from Krolewski *et al.* 1987 [6] with permission from *The New England Journal of Medicine*.)

The risk profile for proliferative retinopathy, the principal cause of blindness in IDDM, is strikingly different. Patients become vulnerable after several years of diabetes and the incidence increases rapidly between 10 and 15 years (Fig 52.1), at a time when background retinopathy has already developed in virtually all patients. Thereafter, the incidence rate remains remarkably constant at about 3% of previously unaffected patients per year, regardless of whether they have been diabetic for 20 or 40 years. The cumulative risk of proliferative retinopathy after 40 years of diabetes is about 62% (Fig. 52.2). The fact that the incidence rate of proliferative retinopathy does not decline even after many years of diabetes suggests that almost all IDDM patients are susceptible to this complication, just as they are to background lesions. However, the constant risk of proliferative retinopathy after 15 years duration implies a different pathophysiological process. As noted before, a constant risk cannot be explained by dependence on the cumulative exposure to diabetes, as the incidence would increase steadily with duration. A more likely cause is some acute effect of the intensity of the exposure, such as the haemodynamic alterations which accompany severe hyperglycaemia [7]. These may contribute to retinal ischaemia and neovascularization in the presence of damaged retinal vessels which are unable to autoregulate blood flow. This hypothesis is consistent with the observation that the risk of proliferative retinopathy is related to the intensity of exposure to diabetes during the several years preceding the onset of this complication.

A final observation is that the risk curves for the development of proliferative retinopathy in cohorts of patients diagnosed in 1939, 1949 and 1959 are virtually superimposable (Fig. 52.2). This implies that any improvements in diabetic management during these decades have not affected the natural history of the complication; fortunately, however, the advent of photocoagulation has revolutionized its prognosis (Chapter 59).

Nephropathy

The pattern is quite different for diabetic nephropathy. After 40 years of diabetes, the cumulative incidence of nephropathy in IDDM patients was 45% of those who developed diabetes in 1939 (Fig. 52.4), but was substantially lower in those diagnosed 20 years later, showing that improved health care or other environmental factors can influence the prevalence of diabetic nephropathy [1, 6]. The frequency rises steeply to a maximum of 21% after 20 years and thereafter falls slowly (Fig. 52.5). This suggests that only a subset of patients are susceptible to diabetic nephropathy. The scarcity of new cases of nephropathy among patients who have had diabetes for many years is due to the fact that this complication has occurred in most of the susceptible persons earlier in the course of diabetes.

Genetic factors

Little is known about the possible genetic factors which determine microvascular complications,

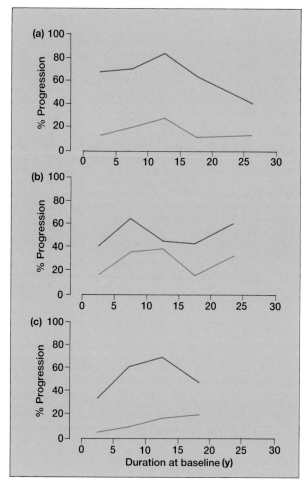

Fig. 52.3. 4-year progression of retinopathy by quartiles of glycosylated haemoglobin and duration of diabetes as measured at baseline examination in persons with (a) younger-onset diabetes; (b) older-onset diabetes, taking insulin; and (c) older-onset diabetes, not taking insulin. Red line = lowest quartile HbA$_1$. Blue line = highest quartile HbA$_1$. Note that retinopathy progresses more in the patients in the highest quartile than in the lowest, in each group, although the relationship with the duration of diabetes is variable. (Redrawn from Krolewski *et al*. 1987 [6] with permission from *The New England Journal of Medicine*.)

although their role may differ between the various complications and between IDDM and NIDDM. Genetic factors seem unimportant in determining retinopathy in IDDM, in that many co-twins with IDDM of similar duration show marked differences in the extent of retinopathy [8].

Susceptibility to nephropathy has recently been attributed to a genetic predisposition to hypertension, as indicated by a parental history of high blood pressure [10] or abnormally high sodium—lithium countertransport activity in red blood cells [11]; the latter is a marker for essential hypertension which aggregates in affected families. Young adults with 14–18 years of IDDM had a threefold higher

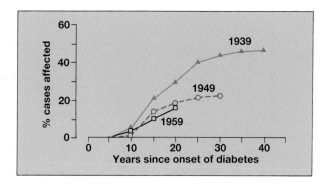

Fig. 52.4. Cumulative incidence of nephropathy (persistent proteinuria) according to the duration of IDDM, in separate cohorts of patients diagnosed in 1939, 1949 and 1959. (Redrawn from Krolewski *et al*. 1987 [6] with permission from *The New England Journal of Medicine*.)

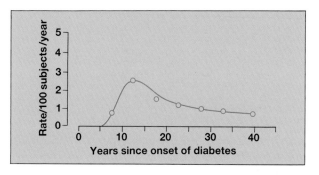

Fig. 52.5. Incidence rate of nephropathy (defined as persistent proteinuria) according to the duration of IDDM (Redrawn from Krolewski *et al*. 1987 [6] with permission from *The New England Journal of Medicine*.)

risk of nephropathy if one or both parents were hypertensive and the risk increased still further if their glycaemic control was poor [10]. However, this does not appear to be a universal finding and further study is required to clarify the possible role of an inherited tendency to hypertension.

Genetic (and/or social) factors may contribute to extended survival of IDDM patients, as the parents of long-term surviving IDDM subjects also tend to live longer than expected [12].

There is no firm evidence concerning the possible role of HLA types in microvascular disease, for example, in patients with neuropathy [9]. This area is particularly difficult to investigate in IDDM patients, a high proportion of whom (over 90% in some populations) possess DR3 and/or DR4 genotypes.

Hypertension

Hypertension is inextricably linked with the advanced (macroalbuminuric) stage of diabetic nephropathy, but its involvement in the earlier evolution of microalbuminuria is controversial (see Chapter 65). As retinopathy and nephropathy often develop together, it is difficult to ascribe a definite role for hypertension in the pathogenesis of diabetic retinopathy.

Glycaemic control

As mentioned above, hyperglycaemia is now implicated in the genesis and progression of microvascular complications, although the relationship may be complex and may differ from one complication to another [13].

Epidemiological studies show that the risk of developing microvascular complications is very low when the blood glucose value 2 h after an oral glucose tolerance test is less than about 11 mmol/l [14] (Fig. 52.6). Pirart [15] followed 2795 diabetic subjects — both IDDM and NIDDM — for up to 25 years and concluded that poor long-term glycaemic control was clearly related to a higher prevalence and incidence of neuropathy, nephropathy and particularly severe retinopathy (Fig. 52.7). More recently, a strong correlation between previous HbA_1 levels and the development of background and proliferative retinopathy has been shown by Klein et al: the risk of developing proliferative retinopathy is 22 times higher in those patients with HbA_1 values during the previous 4 years in the highest quartile as compared

with those in the lowest quartile of the population [16]. Microalbuminuria, thought to precede overt diabetic nephropathy and a powerful independent predictor of excess cardiovascular mortality [17–20], is associated with higher HbA_1 levels than in patients without microalbuminuria (Bangstad HJ et al. unpublished observations).

There is therefore convincing evidence that blood glucose levels are important in the evolution of microangiopathy in the diabetic population at large. Nonetheless, not all patients with chronic, severe hyperglycaemia develop severe microangiopathy and, conversely, a few with seemingly good control may develop severe complications. Hyperglycaemia and its associated metabolic abnormalities therefore seem to be necessary but not always sufficient for the development of severe diabetic complications. As mentioned above, the genetic and environmental factors responsible for individual susceptibility remain unknown and, at present, high-risk patients cannot be identified before they develop indications of microangiopathy. There is evidence, however, that patients with microalbuminuria (urinary albumin excretion 30–300 mg/day; see Chapter 64) are at greatly increased risk of developing overt nephropathy and of dying prematurely from macrovascular disease [17–20]. Microalbuminuria presumably reflects widespread damage through the entire vascular bed.

Apart from the adverse effect of sustained hyperglycaemia, large variations in blood glucose

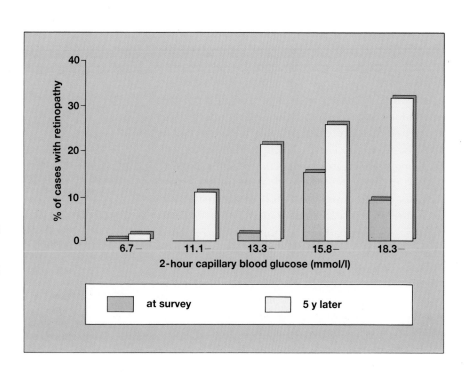

Fig. 52.6. Frequency of diabetic retinopathy in diabetic patients and those with impaired glucose tolerance in the Bedford survey, as a function of the 2-h capillary blood glucose value after a 50-g oral glucose load. Histograms show frequency at survey and 5 years later. (Data from Jarrett and Keen 1976 [14] with permission from *The Lancet.*)

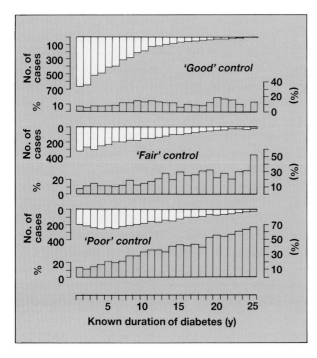

Fig. 52.7. Prevalence of diabetic neuropathy (pink) as a function of duration of diabetes (yellow) in patients with 'good', 'fair' and 'poor' control. Clinical and biochemical data were collected annually from 4398 cases, over a 25-year period. (Redrawn from Pirart 1978 [15].)

levels over extended periods may also contribute to microangiopathy. Recent studies have convincingly shown that rapid improvement in blood glucose control from previously high levels may cause transient deterioration in diabetic retinopathy [21], and may even provoke proliferative changes [22] (see Chapter 42). An older clinical observation is that imposition of good glycaemic control, especially with insulin treatment, may temporarily aggravate or precipitate diabetic neuropathy (Chapter 62). However, the possible role of *hyper*glycaemia must not be forgotten: large glycaemic falls are only possible if the preceding levels were high. The available evidence suggests that long-term improvements in glycaemic control, which are now feasible with continuous subcutaneous insulin infusion (CSII) or intensified injection regimens, can ameliorate the course of *early* diabetic nephropathy, retinopathy and neuropathy [23–25], and that any worsening in these is only a temporary phenomenon. Indeed, animal studies suggest that by establishing tight metabolic control from the onset of diabetes, it may be possible to prevent the development of microvascular complications [26].

The biochemical mechanisms through which high blood glucose levels might damage the microvasculature are unknown. Theoretical possibilities are dealt with later in this section (Chapter 54) and include a direct toxic effect of glucose itself or of some unidentified associated metabolite; glycation of structural proteins and enzymes; abnormalities of the polyol pathway; and haemodynamic factors, including the hyperperfusion and loss of autoregulation caused by hyperglycaemia in many tissues [7].

Health care implications

In view of the huge effort expended on diabetic management, it is clearly important to ask whether there is any evidence that the quality of care in any way modifies the course of diabetic microvascular disease. There are encouraging signs that this is so, such as the finding that patients attending a specialized hospital diabetic clinic live significantly longer than those who do not [27], and the recent demonstration of a fall in mortality in IDDM [1]. Furthermore, the optimistic message to our patients is that 42% of IDDM subjects survive for more than 40 years, half of them without developing late diabetic complications [5].

The last few years have therefore witnessed both a great increase in our understanding of microvascular disease and a decline in relative mortality, indicating that improved diabetes care may be rewarded by reducing the terrible impact of the microvascular complications of the disease.

KRISTIAN F. HANSSEN

References

1 Kofoed-Enevoldsen A, Borch-Johnsen K, Kreiner S *et al.* Declining incidence of persistent proteinuria in type 1 (insulin-dependent) diabetic patients in Denmark. *Diabetes* 1987; **36**: 205–9.
2 Klein R, Klein BEK, Moss SE, Davis MD, De Mets DL. The Wisconsin epidemiologic study of diabetic retinopathy. II Prevalence and risk of diabetic retinopathy when age at diagnosis is less than 30 years. *Arch Ophthalmol* 1984; **102**: 520–6.
3 Nathan DM, Singer DE, Godine JE *et al.* Retinopathy in older type II diabetics. Association with glucose control. *Diabetes* 1986; **35**: 797–901.
4 Grenfell A, Watkins PJ. Diabetic nephropathy: Epidemiology, natural history. In: Watkins PJ, ed. *Long Term Complications of Diabetes. Clinics in Endocrinology and Metabolism.* Vol. 15. London: Saunders, 1986: 783–805.
5 Borch-Johnsen K, Nissen H, Salling N *et al.* The natural history of insulin-dependent diabetes in Denmark: 2. Long-term survival — who and why. *Diabetic Med* 1987; **4**: 211–16.

6 Krolewski AS, Warram JH, Rand LI, Kahn CR. Epidemiologic approach to the etiology of type 1 diabetes mellitus and its complications. *N Engl J Med* 1987; **317**: 1390–8.

7 Zatz R, Brenner BM. Pathogenesis of diabetic microangiopathy; the hemodynamic view. *Am J Med* 1986; **80**: 443–53.

8 Leslie RDG, Pyke DA. Genetics of diabetes. In: Alberti KGMM, Krall LP, eds. *The Diabetes Annual 3*. Amsterdam: Elsevier, 1987.

9 Boulton AJM, Worth RC, Drury J. Genetic and metabolic studies in diabetic neuropathy. *Diabetologia* 1984; **26**: 15–19.

10 Krolewski AS, Caressa N, Warram JH, Laffe LMB, Christlieb AR, Knowler WC, Rand LI. Predisposition to hypertension and susceptibility to renal disease in insulin-dependent diabetes. *N Engl J Med* 1988; **318**: 140–5.

11 Mangili R, Bending JJ, Scott G, Gupta A, Viberti GC. Increased sodium–lithium counter-transport in red blood cells in patients with insulin-dependent diabetes and nephropathy. *N Engl J Med* 1988; **318**: 146–50.

12 Nissen H, Borch-Johnsen K, Nerup J. Long term survival with Type 1 diabetes mellitus — a familial trait? *Diabetologia* 1986; **29**: 576A.

13 Hanssen KF, Dahl-Jørgensen K, Lauritzen T *et al*. Diabetic control and microvascular complications: the near-normoglycemic experience. *Diabetologia* 1986; **29**: 677–84.

14 Jarrett RJ, Keen H. Hyperglycaemia and diabetes mellitus. *Lancet* 1976; ii: 1009–12.

15 Pirart J. Diabetes mellitus and its degenerative complications: A prospective study of 4400 patients observed between 1947 and 1973. *Diabetes Care* 1978; **1**: 168–88.

16 Klein R, Klein BEK, Moss S. Glycosylated hemoglobin predicts the incidence and progression of diabetic retinopathy. *Diabetes* 1988; **37** (suppl 1): 51A.

17 Viberti GC, Jarrett RJ, Mahmud U *et al*. Microalbuminuria as a predictor of clinical diabetic nephropathy in insulin dependent diabetes mellitus. *Lancet* 1982; ii: 1430–2.

18 Parving H-H, Oxenbøll B, Svendsen PA, Christiansen JS, Andersen AR. Early detection of patients at risk of developing diabetic nephropathy: A longitudinal study of urinary albumin excretion. *Acta Endocrinol* 1982; **100**: 550–5.

19 Borch-Johnsen K, Andersen PK, Deckert T. The effect of proteinuria on relative mortality in Type 1 (insulin-dependent) diabetes mellitus. *Diabetologia* 1985; **28**: 590–6.

20 Borch-Johnsen K, Kreiner S. Proteinuria: value as predictor of cardiovascular mortality in insulin-dependent diabetes mellitus. *Br Med J* 1987; **294**: 1651–4.

21 Dahl-Jørgensen K, Brinchmann-Hansen O, Hanssen KF *et al*. Rapid tightening of blood glucose control leads to transient deterioration of retinopathy in insulin dependent diabetes mellitus. The Oslo Study. *Br Med J* 1985; **290**: 811–15.

22 Rosenlund E, Haakens K, Brinchmann-Hansen *et al*. Transient proliferative retinopathy during intensified insulin treatment. *Am J Ophthalmol* 1988; **105**: 618–25.

23 Dahl-Jørgensen K, Brinchmann-Hansen O, Hanssen KF *et al*. Effect of near-normoglycaemia for two years on progression of early diabetic retinopathy, nephropathy and neuropathy. *Br Med J* 1986; **293**: 1195–9.

24 Feldt-Rasmussen B, Mathiesen ER, Deckert T. Effect of two years of strict metabolic control on progression of incipient nephropathy in insulin-dependent diabetes. *Lancet* 1986; ii: 1300–4.

25 Deckert T, Feldt-Rasmussen B, Borch-Johnsen K *et al*. Proteinuria, an indicator of malignant angiopathy. In: Andreani D, Crepaldi G, Di Mario U, Pozza G, eds. *Diabetic Complications: Early Diagnosis and Treatment*. Chichester: John Wiley, 1987: 257–61.

26 Engermann RL, Kern TS. Progression of incipient diabetic retinopathy during good glycemic control. *Diabetes* 1987; **36**: 808–12.

27 Borch-Johnsen K, Nissen H, Salling N, Henriksen E, Kreiner S, Deckert T, Nerup J. The natural history of insulin-dependent diabetes mellitus in Denmark: Long term survival with and without late diabetic complications. *Diabetic Med* 1987; **4**: 201–10.

53 Pathophysiology of Microvascular Disease: An Overview

Summary

• In diabetes, the microvasculature shows both functional and structural abnormalities.
• The structural hallmark of diabetic micro-angiopathy is thickening of the capillary basement membrane. The main functional abnormalities include increased capillary permeability, blood flow and viscosity, and disturbed platelet function. These changes occur early in the course of diabetes and precede organ failure by many years.
• Many chemical changes in basement membrane composition have been identified in diabetes, including increased Type IV collagen and its glycosylation products, decreased heparan sulphate proteoglycan and increased binding of plasma proteins.
• In patients with poorly controlled diabetes, even of short duration, blood flow is increased in many tissues including skin, retina and kidney; in the latter, this is reflected by an elevated glomerular filtration rate.
• Increased capillary permeability is manifested in the retina by leakage of fluorescein and in the kidney by increased urinary losses of albumin which predict eventual renal failure. Both defects probably reflect a generalized vascular abnormality which may also involve the intima of large vessels.
• Platelets from diabetic patients show an exaggerated tendency to aggregate, perhaps mediated by altered prostaglandin metabolism. Plasma and whole blood viscosity are increased whereas red blood cell deformability is decreased in diabetes. These rheological defects, together with the platelet abnormalities, may cause stasis in the microvasculature, leading to increased intravascular pressure and to tissue hypoxia.
• The production by endothelium cells of von Willebrand factor and endothelial-derived relaxing factor and other substances may also be abnormal in diabetes and could contribute to microthrombus formation.

Microvascular disease, notably retinopathy and nephropathy, is frequently seen in patients with long-standing IDDM and may affect NIDDM subjects of shorter disease duration. Indeed, microvascular damage is so characteristic of the veteran diabetic patient that it could almost be considered as part of the natural history of the condition.

The abnormalities associated with diabetic microangiopathy are both structural and functional. Structural changes include thickening of the capillary basement membranes throughout the body together with mesangial expansion in the glomerulus, whereas functional, haemodynamic alterations include increased blood flow, raised intravascular pressure and enhanced vascular leakiness. The relationship between the structural and functional abnormalities, and whether either or both are the cause or consequence of diabetic microangiopathy, are still matters for investigation and debate.

This chapter will review the various pathophysiological mechanisms suggested to play a role in diabetic microvascular disease. The biochemical defects identified are discussed in detail in Chapter 54 and the functional changes of the microcirculation in general in Chapter 55. Specific aspects relating to the causes of retinopathy and nephropathy are described in Chapters 57, 65 and 66.

Structural changes

The light microscopic appearances of 'hyaliniz-ation' (thickening) of the retinal capillaries in diabetic patients were first reported in 1949 [1]. This is now recognized as a characteristic feature of diabetic retinopathy [2, 3]. Subsequently, electron microscopic studies have revealed thickening of the capillary basement membrane (CBM) to be the ultrastructural hallmark of diabetes-induced damage in a wide variety of tissues [4−6].

The structure and function of the normal capillary basement membrane

STRUCTURE

On light microscopy, the CBM is an amorphous sheath which encloses the capillary endothelial cells. Electron microscopy reveals a fibrillary structure, with inner and outer clear zones (*lamina lucida* or *rara interna*, and *externa*) and an intermediate *lamina densa* (Fig. 53.1). The thickness of the CBM correlates with the intracapillary pressure, the thickest membranes being found in the capillaries of the leg muscles.

Type IV collagen is the most abundant protein found in the CBM. Other constituents include the proteoglycans heparan, chondroitin and dermatan sulphates, and glycoproteins such as laminin, fibronectin and entactin [7, 8]. The sulphate groups carried by a number of these proteins confer a net anionic charge which is thought to contribute to the charge-dependent permselectivity of the vessels, especially in the glomerular capillaries (see Chapter 65). In the glomerular basement membrane, proteoglycans have a half-life of approximately 1 week; chemical modification resulting in altered charge-permselectivity characteristics can therefore induce functional changes relatively rapidly [9].

FUNCTION

The basement membrane acts as a structural support for the vessel wall, preventing overdistension under normal conditions, and forming a scaffolding during endothelial cell repair and regeneration. Although the charge characteristics and porosity of the CBM may partly determine the permeability of the capillary wall, the endothelial cells themselves provide the major barrier limiting permeation of macromolecules in most capillary beds. In the glomerular capillary', the epithelial foot processes also contain heparan sulphate proteoglycans which may contribute to charge-selective permeability.

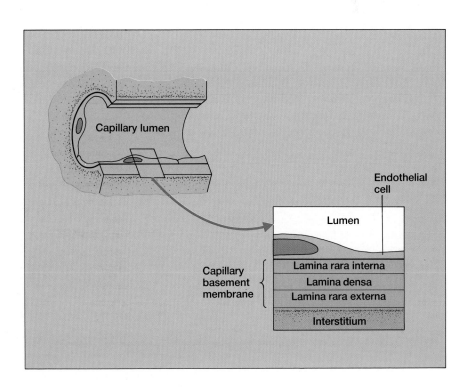

Fig. 53.1. Structure of the capillary basement membrane.

The capillary basement membrane in diabetes

Increased thickness of the CBM in diabetic patients has been demonstrated by morphometric techniques in the kidney, retina, skin, skeletal muscle, brain and heart [5, 6, 10−13]. Increased accumulation of basement membrane material in the kidney has also been confirmed by chemical analysis.

Several constituents of the CBM are chemically modified in diabetes (see Table 53.1) [8]. Immunofluorescent techniques have demonstrated increased amounts of a variety of plasma proteins including albumin, IgG, IgM and C3 in glomerular basement membranes and mesangium, renal tubular basement membranes, skeletal muscle sarcolemmal and capillary basement membranes of diabetic animals and humans [14, 15]. It is possible that non-enzymatic glycosylation of basement membrane constituents in diabetes may favour increased binding of plasma proteins (Chapter 54).

Pathogenesis of the capillary basement membrane changes in diabetes

Biochemical changes

The pathogenesis of diabetic microangiopathy is likely to be multifactorial. Detailed biochemical mechanisms are discussed in Chapter 54.

HYPERGLYCAEMIA AND PROTEIN KINASE C ACTIVITY

It is not clear whether hyperglycaemia *per se* or hyperglycaemia-induced functional vascular changes initiate or promote diabetic microangiopathy. The late complications of diabetes appear to affect cells and tissues which do not require insulin for glucose uptake. This suggests that hyperglycaemia has an important pathogenic role.

Recently, hyperglycaemia has been shown to cause an increase in cellular protein kinase C activity in cultured bovine retinal, renal and aortic endothelial cells, which results from enhanced *de novo* synthesis of diacylglycerol from glucose [16]. Protein kinase C is involved in a variety of important cellular functions, including signal transduction of responses to hormones, growth factors, neurotransmitters and drugs. In vascular smooth muscle cells, protein kinase C modulates growth rate, DNA synthesis and hormone receptor turnover, in addition to contraction. Protein kinase C may therefore be an intracellular mediator whose activity is stimulated by prolonged exposure to hyperglycaemia.

THE POLYOL PATHWAY

Enhanced polyol pathway activity, with increased metabolism of glucose to sorbitol catalyzed by the rate-limiting enzyme, aldose reductase, has been suggested as a possible mechanism of microvascular disease in diabetes. Inhibition of aldose reductase (Fig. 53.2) by various drugs reduces tissue levels of sorbitol and prevents the development of certain chronic diabetic complications such as cataracts and neuropathy in diabetic animals; aldose reductase inhibitors have also been shown to reduce levels of proteinuria in an animal model of diabetic nephropathy [17−19]. Studies in human diabetic patients are in progress and the results are awaited with interest, although preliminary data do not suggest an obvious beneficial effect (see Chapters 54 and 104).

NON-ENZYMATIC GLYCOSYLATION

Increased levels of glucose promote synthesis of proteins, including those of the basement mem-

Table 53.1. Some chemical changes in capillary basement membrane reported in diabetes (see [8]).

- Increased Type IV collagen and its glycosylation products
- Decreased heparan sulphate proteoglycan and a reduction in its degree of sulphation
- Decreased sialic acid
- Increased hydroxylysine/hydroxylysine-disaccharide units
- Decreased lysine
- Increased or decreased laminin and fibronectin
- Increased plasma protein binding (albumin, IgG, IgM, C3)

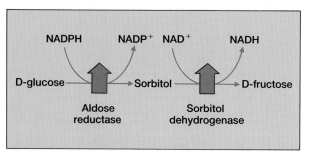

Fig. 53.2. The sorbitol (polyol) pathway.

brane, and continued hyperglycaemia leads to increased levels of non-enzymatic glycosylation products in a variety of vascular constituents [20–22].

As described in Chapter 54, cross-linked end-products of non-enzymatic glycosylation may accumulate in various cells and tissues. It has been shown that the administration of amino-guanidine to diabetic rats prevents increased cross-linking of aortic collagen [23, 24]. The effects of such compounds in other diabetic complications, or their possible use in man, are unknown.

Functional changes

INCREASED BLOOD FLOW

Increased capillary permeability and haemodynamic disturbances can be demonstrated in subjects with diabetes of short duration, long before any structural tissue or organ damage is evident. For example, the glomerular filtration rate (GFR) and the urinary excretion of plasma proteins are abnormally high in a proportion of short-term insulin-dependent patients, especially during periods of poor metabolic control [25–28] (see Chapter 65). Current evidence, based mainly on micropuncture studies in the rat, suggests that the raised GFR ('hyperfiltration') is related to an elevation of both renal plasma flow (RPF) and the transglomerular pressure gradient [29]. Strict metabolic control for 12 months has been shown to normalize glomerular hyperfiltration in IDDM patients, the GFR returning to the previously elevated level if glycaemic control is relaxed [30]. Experience is too limited at present to be able to define precisely the role of glomerular hyperfiltration in the pathophysiology of diabetic nephropathy: prospective and controlled studies of matched cohorts of diabetic patients with and without hyperfiltration have revealed that the GFR fell more quickly in the hyperfiltering group, although there was no evidence of accelerated progression to the later stage of clinical proteinuria in this group [31] (S.L. Jones et al., unpublished observations).

The resting forearm blood flow in newly diagnosed, untreated IDDM patients is almost twice that of non-diabetic controls and is normalized by 1–2 weeks of strict metabolic control [27]. As blood pressure is unchanged, elevated blood flow must indicate a reduction in vascular resistance (i.e. vasodilatation) in the forearm.

Retinal blood flow is increased, mean circulation time in the retina is reduced and retinal vessels are dilated in diabetic subjects [32–34] (see Chapter 57). The possibility that the elevated retinal blood flow and intravascular pressure may be important in the pathogenesis of diabetic retinopathy is supported by the finding of an association between the level of systolic blood pressure and the rate of development of diabetic retinopathy in Pima Indians [35]. Furthermore, patients with a unilateral reduction in retinal blood flow caused, for example, by raised intra-ocular pressure, show slower progression of diabetic retinopathy on the affected side [36].

VASCULAR PERMEABILITY

The role of increased glomerular permeability in the pathogenesis of diabetic nephropathy is more clearly established. In both IDDM and NIDDM patients, a subclinical elevation in the albumin excretion rate (AER) is predictive of later clinical proteinuria and organ damage [37–41] (see Chapters 64 and 65). Increased urinary losses of albumin and IgG are thought to originate from the glomerulus, as urinary excretion of β_2-microglobulin, an indicator of tubular function, is normal in diabetes. Recently, urinary transferrin levels have also been shown to be elevated in some diabetic patients and to be significantly correlated with urinary albumin excretion rates [42].

A strong correlation has been described between glycosylated haemoglobin levels and the urinary excretion rates of albumin and IgG [43]. Although associations do not necessarily imply cause (or effect), these findings suggest that the subclinical elevation of the glomerular filtration of these plasma proteins is, in fact, related to metabolic control. This concept has been further strengthened in recent years by the finding that prolonged correction of hyperglycaemia using various techniques can either lower AER or prevent it from increasing [44–46].

Elevations in AER not only predict renal disease but are also associated with proliferative retinopathy and increased cardiovascular mortality [47, 48]. Recently, it has been proposed that an increased AER reflects a more generalized vascular dysfunction which involves capillaries of the glomerulus and retina and the intima of large vessels [49]. In support of this hypothesis, the transcapillary escape rates of albumin and fibrinogen have been shown to be increased in patients with modest elevations of the urinary AER [50, 51]. A genetically-determined alteration of the composition of the extracellular matrix, resulting in loss of heparan sulphate proteoglycan, is proposed as an important mechanism in these processes; although plausible, this concept is supported at present by only a few data (Fig. 53.3).

Retinal capillaries display increased leakage of fluorescein early in the course of diabetes. Using the technique of vitreous fluorophotometry, accumulation of fluorescein in the vitreous after intravenous injection has been demonstrated in young diabetic patients who have either no retinopathy or only mild background changes [52, 53]. Fluorescein leakage is greater in patients with poor metabolic control and is reduced by improved control [54].

RHEOLOGICAL FACTORS

Abnormal blood viscosity and platelet function have also been proposed as possible causes or mediators of microangiopathy in diabetes. Plate-

lets from diabetic patients show an increased sensitivity to aggregation induced by ADP, adrenaline or collagen, and there is some evidence that this increased sensitivity correlates with certain diabetic complications [55]. Activation of the prostaglandin synthetase system resulting in either elevated levels of prostaglandins or decreased levels of prostacyclin could underlie altered platelet sensitivity [56, 57]. Furthermore, changes in other rheological properties of blood have been described, including increased plasma and whole blood viscosity and decreased red cell deformability. These defects would act to impede blood flow and hence increase intravascular hydrostatic pressure [58, 59], and could also predispose to sludging of blood in capillaries and therefore to hypoxia and poor nutrition of the tissues.

Endothelial cells produce prostaglandins and endothelial-derived relaxing factor (EDRF) which inhibit the adherence of platelets to the vascular wall as well as modulating vascular tone. Studies of human diabetes have produced conflicting evidence of altered levels of these endothelial

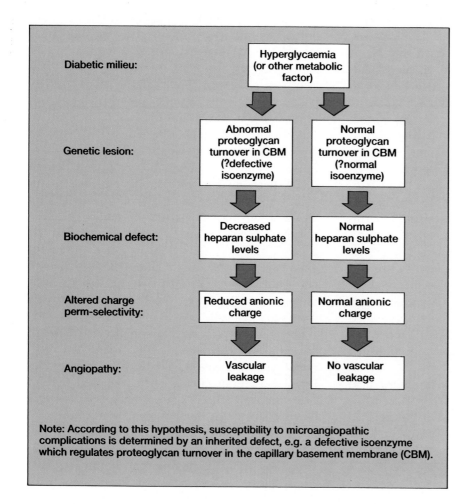

Fig. 53.3. Possible basis for susceptibility to microangiopathic complications of diabetes (redrawn from Deckert *et al.* [49]).

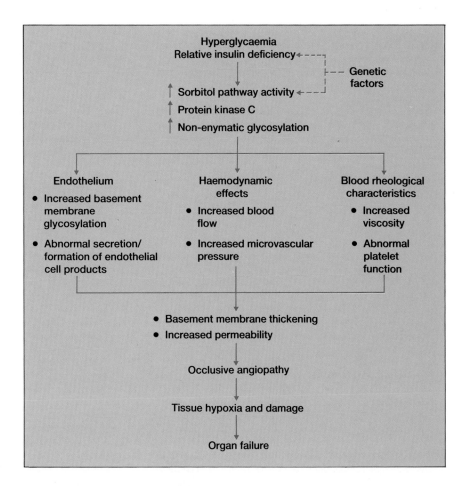

Fig. 53.4. A possible pathogenetic pathway of diabetic microangiopathy.

products, although some recent reports suggest a reduction in EDRF production (for a review of this area, see [60]).

Other endothelial products have been shown to be abnormal in diabetic subjects with evidence of diabetic microangiopathy. The tissue plasminogen activator response to exercise is impaired, whereas levels of von Willebrand factor, a glycoprotein synthesized by endothelial cells and responsible for platelet adhesion to the subendothelium, is increased in diabetic subjects with microalbuminuria or clinical nephropathy [61]. Together, these disturbances would favour an increased tendency to coagulation and a reduced ability to resolve microthrombi in diabetic subjects with an increased AER.

In view of the cross-sectional nature of these studies, it is not possible to determine whether these changes are of primary importance in the pathogenesis of diabetic microangiopathy or arise as a consequence of this.

Conclusions

Many metabolic and other factors may therefore contribute to the structural and functional abnormalities which characterize diabetes microangiopathy. Fig. 53.4 shows a possible pathway through which insulin deficiency and hyperglycaemia could lead to abnormalities in the basement membrane and endothelium, and disturbed haemodynamic and rheological properties in diabetes. The end points of this pathway are the tissue damage and organ failure caused by diabetic microangiopathy.

JAMES D. WALKER
GIAN CARLO VIBERTI

References

1 Ashton N. Vascular changes in diabetes with particular reference to retinal vessels. *Br J Ophthalmol* 1949; **33**: 407–20.
2 Friedenwald JS. A new approach to some old problems of retinal vascular disease. *Am J Ophthalmol* 1949; **32**: 487–98.
3 Friedenwald JS. Diabetic retinopathy. *Am J Ophthalmol* 1950; **33**: 1187–99.
4 Hidayat AA, Fine BS. Diabetic choroidopathy: light and electron microscopic observations of seven cases. *Ophthalmology* 1985; **92**: 512–22.

5 Johnson PC, Brendel K, Meezan E. Human diabetic perineurial cell basement membrane thickening. *Lab Invest* 1981; **44**: 265–70.

6 Johnson PC, Brendel K, Meezan E. Thickened cerebral cortical capillary basement membranes in diabetics. *Arch Pathol Lab Med* 1982; **60**: 214–17.

7 Scott PG. Macromolecular constituents of basement membranes: A review of current knowledge on their structure and function. *Can J Biochem Cell Biol* 1983; **61**: 942–8.

8 Williamson JR, Tilton RG, Chang K, Kilo C. Basement membrane abnormalities in diabetes mellitus: relationship to clinical microangiopathy. *Diabetes/Metabolism Reviews*; 1988; **4**: 339–70.

9 Cohen MP, Surma ML, Wu VY. *In vivo* biosynthesis and turnover of glomerular basement membrane in diabetic rats. *Am J Physiol* 1982; **242**: F385–9.

10 Østerby R, Hansen R. A quantitative estimate of the peripheral glomerular basement membrane in recent juvenile diabetes. *Diabetologia* 1965; **1**: 97–100.

11 Tilton RG, LaRose LS, Kilo C, Williamson JR. Absence of degenerative changes in retinal and uveal capillary pericytes in diabetic rats. *Invest Ophthalmol Vis Sci* 1986; **27**: 716–21.

12 Silver MD, Huckell VF, Lorber M. Basement membranes of small cardiac vessels in patients with diabetes and myxodema: Preliminary observations. *Pathology* 1977; **9**: 213–20.

13 Siperstein MD, Unger RG, Madison LL. Studies of muscle capillary basement membranes in normal subjects, diabetic, and prediabetic patients. *J Clin Invest* 1968; **47**: 1973–99.

14 Mauer SM, Michael AF, Fish AJ, Brown DM. Spontaneous immunoglobulin and complement deposition in glomeruli of diabetic rats. *Lab Invest* 1972; **27**: 488–94.

15 Chavers B, Etzwiler D, Michael AF. Albumin deposition in dermal capillary basement membrane in insulin-dependent diabetes mellitus. A preliminary report. *Diabetes* 1981; **30**: 275–8.

16 Lee T-S, Saltsman A, Ohashi H, King GL. Activation of protein kinase C by elevation of glucose concentration; proposal for a mechanism in the development of diabetic vascular complications. *Proc Natl Acad Sci* 1989; **86**: 5141–5.

17 Robison WG Jr, Kador PF, Akagi Y, Kinoshita JH, Gonzalez R, Dvornik D. Prevention of basement membrane thickening in retinal capillaries by a novel inhibitor of aldose reductase, tolrestat. *Diabetes* 1986; **35**: 295–9.

18 Beyer-Mears A, Cruz E, Edelist T, Varagiannis E. Diminished proteinuria in diabetes mellitus by sorbinil, an aldose reductase inhibitor. *Pharmacology* 1986; **32**: 52–60.

19 Chandler ML, Shannon WA, DeSantis L. Prevention of retinal capillary basement membrane thickening in diabetic rats by aldose reductase inhibitors. *Invest Ophthalmol Vis Sci* 1984; **25**: 159.

20 Li W, Shen S, Khatami M, Rockey JH. Stimulation of retinal capillary pericyte protein and collagen synthesis in culture by high-glucose concentration. *Diabetes* 1984; **33**: 785–9.

21 Li W, Khatami M, Rockey JH. The effects of glucose and an aldose reductase inhibitor on the sorbitol content and collagen synthesis of bovine retinal capillary pericytes in culture. *Exp Eye Res* 1985; **40**: 439–44.

22 Brownlee M, Cerami A, Vlassara H. Advanced glycosylation end products in tissue and the biochemical basis of diabetic complications. *N Engl J Med* 1988; **318**: 1315–21.

23 Brownlee M, Vlassara H, Cerami A. Nonenzymatic glycosylation and the pathogenesis of diabetic complications. *Ann Intern Med* 1984; **101**: 527–37.

24 Brownlee M, Vlassara H, Kooney A, Ulrich P, Cerami A.

Aminoguanidine prevents diabetes-induced arterial wall protein cross-linking. *Science* 1986; **232**: 1629–32.

25 Mogensen CE. Kidney function and glomerular permeability to macromolecules in juvenile diabetes. *Dan Med Bull* 1972; **19** (suppl 3): 1–40.

26 Ditzel J, Junker K. Abnormal glomerular filtration rate, renal plasma flow, and protein excretion in recent and short-term diabetics. *Br Med J* 1972; **2**: 13–19.

27 Parving H-H, Noer I, Deckert T et al. The effect of metabolic regulation on microvascular permeability to small and large molecules in short-term juvenile diabetics. *Diabetologia* 1976; **12**: 161–166.

28 Christiansen JS, Gammelgaard J, Tronier B et al. Kidney function and size in diabetics, before and during initial insulin treatment. *Kidney Int* 1982; **21**: 683–8.

29 Hostetter TH, Troy JL, Brenner BM. Glomerular hemodynamics in experimental diabetes. *Kidney Int* 1981; **19**: 410–15.

30 Wiseman MJ, Saunders AJ, Keen H, Viberti GC. Effect of blood glucose glomerular filtration rate and kidney size in insulin-dependent diabetics. *N Engl J Med* 1985, **312**: 617–21.

31 Lervang HH, Jensen S, Brochner Mortensen J, Ditzel J. Early glomerular hyperfiltration and the development of late nephropathy in Type 1 (insulin-dependent) diabetes mellitus. *Diabetologia* 1988; **31**: 723–9.

32 Kohner EM, Hamilton AM, Saunders SJ et al. The retinal blood flow in diabetes. *Diabetologia* 1975; **11**: 27–33.

33 Soeldner JS, Christacopoulos PD, Gleason RE. Mean retinal circulation time as determined by fluorescein angiography in normal, prediabetic and chemical diabetic subjects. *Diabetes* 1976; **25** (suppl 2): 903–8.

34 Skovborg F, Nielsen Aa V, Lauritzen E et al. Diameters of the retinal vessels in diabetic and normal subjects. *Diabetes* 1969; **18**: 292–8.

35 Knowler WC, Bennett PH, Ballintine EJ: Increased incidence of retinopathy in diabetics with elevated blood pressure. *N Engl J Med* 1980; **302**: 645–50.

36 Behrendt T, Duane TD. Unilateral complications in diabetic retinopathy. *Trans Am Acad Ophthalmol Otol* 1970; **74**: 28–32.

37 Viberti GC, Hill RD, Jarrett RD, Argyropoulos A, Mahmud U, Keen H. Microalbuminuria as a predictor of clinical nephropathy in insulin-dependent diabetes mellitus. *Lancet* 1982; i: 1430–2.

38 Mogensen CE, Christensen CK. Predicting diabetic nephropathy in insulin-dependent patients. *N Engl J Med* 1984; **311**: 89–93.

39 Jarrett RJ, Viberti GC, Argyropoulos A et al. Microalbuminuria predicts mortality in non-insulin dependent diabetics. *Diabetic Med* 1984; **1**: 17–19.

40 Mogenesen CE. Microalbuminuria predicts clinical proteinuria and early mortality in maturity-onset diabetes. *N Engl J Med* 1984; **310**: 356–60.

41 Mathiesen ER, Oxenbøll K, Johansen PAa, Svendsen PA, Deckert T. Incipient nephropathy in Type 1 (insulin-dependent) diabetes. *Diabetologia* 1984; **26**: 406–10.

42 O'Donnell MJ, Martin P, Florkowski CM, Toop MJ, Chapman C, Barnett AH. Transferrinuria and tubular proteinuria in Type 1 (insulin-dependent) diabetes mellitus. *Diabetic Med* 1988; **5**: 15A.

43 Viberti GC, Mackintosh D, Bilous RW, Pickup JC, Keen H. Proteinuria in diabetes mellitus: role of spontaneous and experimental variation of glycaemia. *Kidney Int* 1982; **21**: 714–20.

44 The Kroc Collaborative Study Group. Blood glucose control

and the evolution of diabetic retinopathy and albuminuria
N Engl J Med 1984; **311**: 365−72.

45 Feldt-Rasmussen B, Mathiesen E, Deckert T. Effect of two years of strict metabolic control on progression of incipient nephropathy in insulin-dependent diabetics. *Lancet* 1986; ii: 1300−4.

46 Dahl-Jørgensen K, Hanssen KF, Kierfulf P, Bjoro T, Sandvik L, Aageraes O. Reduction of urinary albumin excretion after 4 years of continuous subcutaneous insulin infusion in insulin-dependent diabetes mellitus; the Oslo study. *Acta Endocrinol* 1988; **117**: 19−25.

47 Kofoed-Envoldsen A, Jensen T, Borch-Johnsen K, Deckert T. Incidence of retinopathy in Type 1 (insulin-dependent) diabetes; associations with clinical nephropathy. *J Diab Complic* 1987; **3**: 96−9.

48 Borch-Johnsen K, Kreiner S. Proteinuria: a predictor of cardiovascular mortality in insulin-dependent diabetes-mellitus. *Br Med J* 1987; **294**: 1651−4.

49 Deckert T, Feldt-Rasmussen B, Borch-Johnsen K, Jensen T, Kokoed-Envoldsen A. Albuminuria reflects widespread vascular damage; the Steno hypothesis. *Diabetologia* 1989; **32**: 219−26.

50 Feldt-Rasmussen B. Increased transcapillary escape rate of albumin in Type 1 (insulin-dependent) diabetic patients with microalbuminuria. *Diabetologia* 1986; **29**: 282−6.

51 O'Hare JA, Twoney BM, Ferris JB *et al*. Metabolic control, hypertension and microvascular complications independently affect transcapillary escape of albumin in diabetes. *Diabetologia* 1982; **22**: 391−2.

52 Cunha-Vaz J, De Abreu F, Compos JR *et al*. Early breakdown of blood-retinal barrier in diabetics. *Br J Ophthalmol* 1975; **59**: 649−56.

53 Waltman SR, Oestrich C, Krupin T *et al*. Quantitative vitreous fluorophotometry: a sensitive technique for measuring early breakdown of blood-retinal barrier in young diabetic patients. *Diabetes* 1978; **27**: 85−7.

54 White NH, Waltman SR, Krupin T *et al*. Reversal of abnormalities in ocular fluorophotometry in insulin-dependent diabetes after five to nine months of improved metabolic control. *Diabetes* 1982; **31**: 80−5.

55 Mustard JF, Packham MA. Platelets and diabetes mellitus. *N Engl J Med* 1977; **297**: 1345−7.

56 Halushka PV, Lune D, Colwell JA. Increased synthesis of prostaglandin-E-like material by patients with diabetes mellitus. *N Engl J Med* 1977; **297**: 1306−10.

57 Silberbauer K, Schernthaner G, Sinzinger H, Piza-Katzer H, Winter M: Increased vascular prostacyclin in juvenile onset diabetes. *N Engl J Med* 1979; **300**: 367−8.

58 Barnes AJ, Locke P, Scudder PR *et al*. Is hyperviscosity a treatable component of diabetic microcirculatory disease? *Lancet* 1977; ii: 789−91.

59 McMillan DE, Utterback NG, La Puma J. Reduced erythrocyte deformability in diabetes. *Diabetes* 1978; **27**: 895−901.

60 Tooke JE. The microcirculation in diabetes. *Diabetic Med* 1987; **4**: 189−96.

61 Jensen T, Feldt-Rasmussen B, Bjerre-Knudsen J, Deckert T. Features of endothelial dysfunction in early diabetic nephropathy. *Lancet* 1989; i: 461−3.

54   Biochemical Basis of Microvascular Disease

Summary

● Prolonged exposure to elevated glucose concentrations damages tissues by causing either acute, reversible metabolic changes (mostly related to increased polyol pathway activity, decreased myoinositol and altered diacylglycerol levels, or glycosylation of proteins), or cumulative irreversible changes in long-lived molecules (formation of advanced glycosylation end-products on matrix proteins such as collagen and in nucleic acids and nucleoproteins).

● In insulin-independent tissues such as nerve, the renal glomerulus, lens and retina, hyperglycaemia causes elevated tissue glucose levels. The enzyme aldose reductase catalyses reduction of glucose to its polyol, sorbitol, which is subsequently converted to fructose.

● Sorbitol does not easily cross cell membranes and its accumulation may cause damage by osmotic effects (e.g. in the lens) and altered redox state of pyridine nucleotides.

● In addition, increased sorbitol production is partly responsible for tissue depletion of myoinositol, a molecule structurally related to glucose. Hyperglycaemia itself also inhibits myoinositol uptake into cells.

● Animal studies indicate that tissue myoinositol depletion may cause abnormalities in peripheral nerve function; myoinositol is a precursor of phosphatidylinositol, the turnover of which activates $Na^+-K^+-ATPase$ via diacylglycerol production and thus stimulation of protein kinase C.

● Lowered $Na^+-K^+-ATPase$ activity probably causes increased intracellular Na^+ concentrations and slows nerve conduction velocity.

● In other tissues such as endothelial cells and aortic smooth muscle cells in culture, protein kinase C is activated by high glucose levels, because of synthesis of diacylglycerol from glucose; these changes in protein kinase C may be involved in abnormal growth and synthesis in these tissues.

● Early glycosylation products form on proteins as glucose attaches to amino groups. These Schiff base adducts then undergo 'Amadori' rearrangement to form stable products analogous to glycosylated haemoglobin. Such glycosylation may affect the function of a number of proteins and be partly responsible for free radical-mediated damage in diabetes.

● Glycosylation may be limited by oxidative cleavage of Amadori products to peptide-bound carboxymethyllysine and erythronic acid.

● In long-lived molecules, early glycosylation products slowly and irreversibly form complex cross-linkings called advanced glycosylation end-products (AGE).

● One type of AGE is probably formed from the condensation of two Amadori products and is related to furoyl-furanyl-imidazole. Another type probably derives from reaction of Amadori products with the Amadori-derived 3-deoxyglucosone, to form several types of pyrrole-based cross-links.

● Pathological consequences of AGE cross-linking include covalent binding of proteins (e.g. LDL, albumin and IgG) to vessel walls; cross-linking of matrix components in vessel walls causing resistance to enzymatic degradation; and disturbed three-dimensional structure and altered binding of anionic proteoglycans which influence charge on the vessel wall and its interaction with bloodborne protein.

● Monocyte macrophages have a high-affinity

receptor for AGE and binding may release cytokines such as tumour necrosis factor (TNF) and interleukin-1 (IL-1).
• AGE also form on nucleic acids and histones and may cause mutations and altered gene expression.
• Pharmacological modulation of AGE formation may be possible using agents such as aminoguanidine which prevent cross-linking.

The pathogenesis of diabetic complications

Although the insulin deficiency of diabetes mellitus can be ameliorated by diet, oral hypoglycaemic agents or insulin administration, standard therapy has not been able to prevent the development of chronic complications affecting multiple organ systems. In the eye, retinal capillary damage leading to oedema, new vessel formation and haemorrhage results in visual impairment, and cataracts also develop at an accelerated rate. Chronic renal failure occurs because of capillary damage in the glomerulus associated with basement membrane and mesangial matrix accumulation. In the diabetic nerve, axonal dwindling and segmental demyelination associated with changes in the vasa nervorum produce motor, sensory and autonomic dysfunction. Large- and medium-sized vessel atheromatous disease are responsible for an increased incidence of coronary artery cerebrovascular and peripheral vascular disease.

These diverse clinical syndromes share a common pathophysiological feature: a progressive narrowing of vascular lumina in diabetes leading to inadequate perfusion of target organs. This narrowing appears to be the cumulative effect of three processes. First, an abnormal leakage of PAS-positive, carbohydrate-containing plasma proteins causes a progressive constriction of luminal area in both small and large vessels. Secondly, an increase in extracellullar matrix is seen in all types of diabetic vessels. The basement membrane is thickened in many tissues, including retinal capillaries and the vasa nervorum, mesangial matrix is expanded in the renal glomerulus, and collagen is increased in developing atherosclerotic plaques. Endothelial, mesangial and arterial smooth muscle cell hypertrophy and hyperplasia comprise the third pathological process [1–3].

What causes these pathological processes? Numerous investigations (see Chapter 52) have concluded that the primary causal factor responsible for the development of most diabetic complications is probably prolonged exposure to hyperglycaemia (Fig. 54.1). Marked differences in susceptibility to glucose-mediated tissue damage observed in different diabetic patients exposed to the same degree and duration of hyperglycaemia might be accounted for by genetic polymorphism, although the identity and function of these genes have yet to be determined. Hypertension is now recognized as the most significant independent accelerating factor for diabetic microvascular disease, while both hypertension and hyperlipidaemia accelerate the development of macrovascular disease [4].

Hyperglycaemia appears to damage tissues by causing both acute, reversible changes in cellular metabolism and cumulative, irreversible alterations in stable macromolecules (Fig. 54.1). Among the reversible abnormalities are abnormal polyol metabolism and the formation of early glycosylation products on matrix, cellular and plasma proteins (Table 54.1). The cumulative, irreversible changes caused by hyperglycaemia appear to affect long-lived molecules such as extracellular matrix components and nucleic acids. In model systems, these irreversible changes cause defective matrix binding of growth-inhibiting heparan

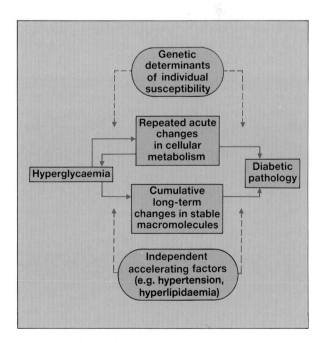

Fig. 54.1. Schematic representation of the mechanisms by which hyperglycaemia and independent risk factors interact to cause diabetic complications.

Table 54.1. Biochemical consequences of hyperglycaemia.

Acute reversible metabolic changes
Increased polyol pathway activity
Altered redox state of pyridine nucleotides
Decreased pools of myoinositol
Increased *de novo* synthesis of diacylglycerol
Increased activation of protein kinase C
Greater formation of early glycosylation products (EGP)
and EGP-derived free radicals.

Cumulative changes in stable macromolecules
Increased formation of advanced glycosylation end-
products (AGE) on extracellular matrix components
Increased formation of advanced glycosylation end-
products on nucleic acids and nucleoproteins
Disordered three-dimensional structure of basement
membrane and collagen
Impaired matrix associative/binding properties
Increased rate of genetic mutations (in prokaryotes)

sulphate proteoglycan [5], disordered three-dimensional structure of both basement membrane and collagen [6], and increased rates of genetic mutation [7]. Early in the course of diabetes, pathological changes are most likely due to the acute, reversible changes induced by hyperglycaemia. With increasing duration of diabetes, however, the cumulative, irreversible abnormalities play an increasingly prominent role.

Acute reversible metabolic changes

The acute reversible changes in metabolism that result from hyperglycaemia include increased polyol pathway activity [8], altered redox state of pyridine nucleotides [9], decreased myoinositol in selected subcellular pools [10], increased *de novo* synthesis of diacylglycerol [11], increased activation of protein kinase C [8, 11], and greater formation of early glycosylation products [12] (Table 54.1).

Polyol production

The polyol pathway includes a family of aldo-keto reductase enzymes which can utilize hexoses as a substrate for reduction by NADPH to their respective sugar alcohols (polyols), e.g. glucose to sorbitol, galactose to galactitol (Fig. 54.2). Because the Km of aldose reductase is high, elevated glucose levels are needed to produce high activity of the pathway.

In insulin-independent tissues where such enzymatic activity is present, hyperglycaemia increases the intracellular concentration of glucose, and thus the net flux through the polyol pathway. In many tissues, the sorbitol produced is subsequently oxidized to fructose by a specific dehydrogenase, using NAD as a cofactor (Fig. 54.2) [8]. Sorbitol does not easily diffuse across cell membranes and osmotic damage to cells may occur where accumulated sorbitol levels are high, such as in the lens during the development of diabetic cataracts. In other tissues, such as peripheral nerve, sorbitol levels are probably too low in diabetes to cause osmotic damage and here other consequences of increased polyol pathway flux might be important. One suggestion is that the altered redox state of pyridine nucleotides is critical, since pyruvate administration, which restores NAD$^+$ levels, can prevent endothelial cell dysfunction [9]. Another suggestion, based on animal data, is that increased polyol pathway activity results in a decrease in myoinositol, perhaps limited to a specific subcellular compartment involved in phosphoinositide metabolism [8, 10].

Polyols, myoinositol and protein kinase C

Myoinositol is structurally related to glucose (Fig. 54.3) and is present in most animal and plant

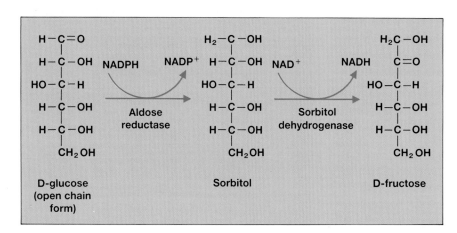

Fig. 54.2 The polyol pathway.

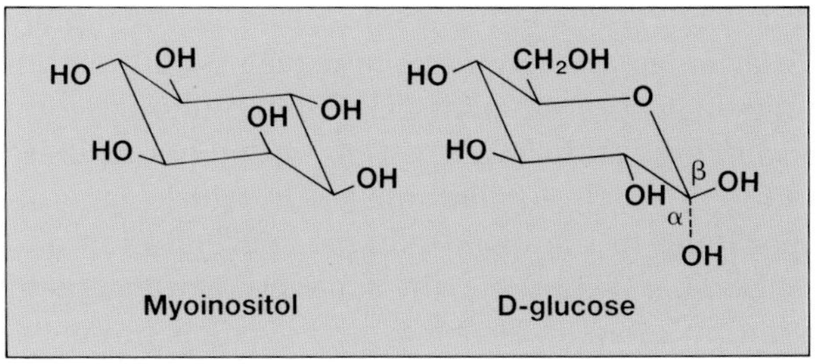

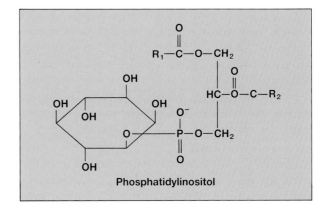

Fig. 54.3 The structures of myoinositol and glucose.

Fig. 54.4 The structure of phosphatidyl inositol. R_1 is usually stearate and R_2 arachidonate.

tissues, at higher intracellular than extracellular concentrations. It is mostly derived from the diet but is also synthesized in the cell from glucose-6-phosphate. It is actively transported inwards across cell membranes.

In rats made diabetic with streptozotocin, both motor nerve conduction velocity (NCV) and sciatic nerve myoinositol levels are decreased. Treatment with insulin to restore near-normoglycaemia increases both NCV and myoinositol content. Moreover, dietary supplements of myoinositol given to untreated diabetic rats also increase NCV and nerve myoinositol, even though nerve and blood glucose concentrations remain unaltered [8, 10].

One explanation for intracellular myoinositol depletion in diabetes is that glucose competes with myoinositol for uptake into cells. However, aldose reductase inhibitors have also been found to block the tissue depletion of myoinositol, suggesting a link between sorbitol accumulation and lowered myoinositol levels. Indeed, changes in myoinositol in diabetes are confined to those tissues susceptible to long-term complications and in which the polyol pathway is active (nerve, retina and glomerulus). The mechanism by which sorbitol affects myoinositol is unclear but may involve diminished myoinositol uptake into the cells.

Present evidence suggests that myoinositol depletion causes neuronal abnormalities by decreasing $Na^+-K^+-ATPase$ activity (see Chapter 61). Myoinositol is a precursor of phosphoinositides such as phosphatidylinositol (Fig. 54.4) which activate $Na^+-K^+-ATPase$ either directly or through the production of mediators (second messengers) such as inositol polyphosphates and diacylglycerol. The latter binds to and activates protein kinase C, a calcium-dependent activator of $Na^+-K^+-ATPase$. Inositol polyphosphates mobilize calcium and may thus

also modulate $Na^+-K^+-ATPase$ activity (see Fig. 54.5). Diminished $Na^+-K^+-ATPase$ is thought to impede Na^+ extrusion from the nerve cell, the resultant high intracellular Na^+ levels blocking nodal depolarization and slowing NCV. Altered Na^+ levels may also affect myoinositol uptake, which is Na^+-dependent.

Sorbitol−myoinositol derangement has also been implicated in glomerular hyperfiltration (an early renal abnormality in diabetes), increased permeability of the blood/retinal barrier and possibly the association of hypertension with

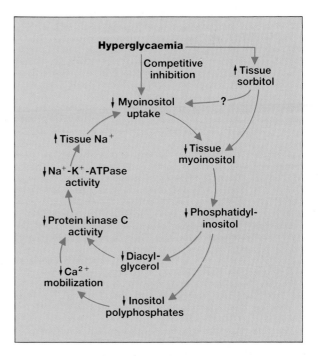

Fig. 54.5 A simplified scheme which shows some possible ways in which myoinositol depletion is involved in diabetic nerve damage. (Modified from Greene et al. 1987 [8] with permission from The New England Journal of Medicine.)

diabetes, as Na⁺−K⁺−ATPase in vascular smooth muscle may control the contractile response to hormones and neurotransmitters. In nerve, protein kinase C activity appears to be reduced and is associated with decreased Na⁺−K⁺−ATPase activity (see above), whereas in vascular tissues and in cell culture, hyperglycaemia is associated with an *increase* in diacylglycerol level and a corresponding increase in protein kinase C activation [8, 11]. This activation could be crucially involved in abnormal growth and synthesis in the diabetic vasculature. Increased *de novo* synthesis of diacylglycerol from glucose has been demonstrated directly in vascular tissue from diabetic animals.

Early glycosylation products

Another acute reversible change induced by hyperglycaemia is the excessive formation of early glycosylation products [12], which form continu-ously both outside and inside cells. Glucose rapidly attaches to amino groups of proteins via the non-enzymatic process of nucleophilic addition to form Schiff base adducts (Fig. 54.6). Within hours, these adducts reach equilibrium levels which are proportional to the blood glucose concentration and subsequently undergo the Amadori rearrangement to form more stable early glycosylation products, typified by glycosylated haemoglobin (see Chapter 34), which reach equilibrium levels over a period of weeks. Excessive formation of early glycosylation products may adversely affect a variety of functions relevant to diabetic complications, including the uptake of low-density lipoprotein [13] and the regulation of free radical-mediated vascular damage [14, 15]. Glycosylated proteins can undergo auto-oxidation, generating free radicals which may contribute to protein cross-linking and degradation and other forms of molecular damage in diabetes (see below).

The two major factors determining the extent of

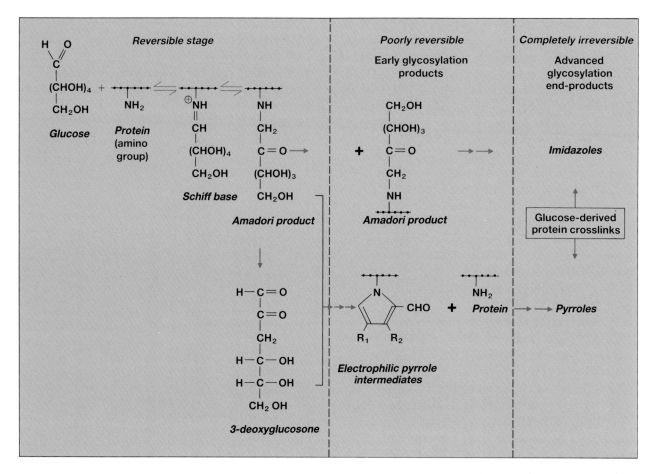

Fig. 54.6. Formation of reversible, early non-enzymatic glycosylation products, and of irreversible advanced glycosylation end-products (AGE). Through a complex series of chemical reactions, Amadori products can form families of imidazole-based and pyrrole-based glucose-derived cross-links.

early glycosylation product formation *in vivo* are the glucose concentration and duration of exposure to glucose. As glucose concentrations rise, the rate and equilibrium level of early glycosylation products increase proportionally through a mass action effect. One possible factor opposing this process may be a newly described pathway through which Amadori products are degraded by oxidative cleavage into peptide-bound carboxymethyllysine and erythronic acid [16]. Genetic variability in the regulation of this or analogous pathways might contribute to the wide differences in individual susceptibility to hyperglycaemia-mediated tissue damage.

Chronic irreversible changes in stable macromolecules

Some early glycosylation products dissociate or are degraded but those formed on collagen, DNA and other long-lived macromolecules slowly undergo further complex chemical rearrangements, which are irreversible, to form advanced glycosylation end-products (AGE) [17]. Unlike the short-lived and reversible products described above, AGE are stable and therefore accumulate throughout the lifetime of the tissue or vessel wall; their levels do not return to normal if hyperglycaemia is corrected.

Glucose-derived advanced glycosylation products apparently result from covalent cross-linking of protein molecules, which apparently follows one of two patterns (Fig. 54.6) [18, 19]. One type closely resembles the heterocyclic imidazole derivative, 2-furoyl-4(5)-(2-furanyl)1-*H*-imidazole (FFI) (Fig. 54.6). This yellow-brown compound has a fluorescence spectrum characteristic of AGE proteins. This type of AGE has been found in enzymatically hydrolyzed tissue [18] and appears to form from the condensation of two Amadori products. The other pattern of AGE cross-linking apparently results from the reaction of an Amadori product with the Amadori-derived compound 3-deoxyglucosone [19]. This highly reactive dicarbonyl compound cyclizes to form electrophilic pyrrole intermediates with reactive hydroxyl groups in benzylic positions which then react with amino groups to form pyrrole-based cross-links. Examples of this latter type of AGE include the 1-alkyl-2-formyl-3, 4-diglycosyl pyrroles (AFGP), an arginine-ribose-lysine cross-linked compound called 'pentosidine', a fluorescent HPLC peak designated 'peak L1', and the newly identified

Maillard Fluorescent Product 1 (MFP-1). Formation of other AGE apparently involves generation of glycolaldehyde from Schiff bases through a reversed aldol condensation reaction; the resulting product is an even more reactive cross-linking agent than 3-deoxyglucosone.

Pathological consequences of advanced glycosylation product formation

A number of these irreversible advanced glycosylation products are capable of forming covalent bonds with nearby amino groups on other proteins and nucleotides, resulting in glucose-derived cross-links. The formation of advanced glycosylation products could contribute to the development of diabetic tissue damage in several ways including effects on extracellular matrix proteins, specific cellular receptors, or nucleic acids and nucleoproteins.

CROSS-LINKING OF EXTRACELLULAR MATRIX PROTEINS (see Table 54.2)

Diabetic blood vessels characteristically show early and progressive accumulation of various plasma proteins. In the arterial subintima, extracellular accumulation of extravasated low-density lipoprotein (LDL) makes up the bulk of such material, whereas PAS-positive plasma glycoprotein deposits are most prominent in the media [20]. This accumulated lipoprotein can only be released from atherosclerotic plaques by treatment with proteolytic enzymes, suggesting that it is chemically attached to vessel wall matrix components [21].

In vitro, human LDL binds covalently to collagen modified by advanced glycosylation in direct proportion to the content of AGE, indicating that LDL binds specifically to AGE [22]. These findings suggest that excessive cross-linking by hyperglycaemia-induced AGE may accelerate atherosclerosis in diabetic patients, even at normal levels of plasma LDL.

Table 54.2. Pathological consequences of advanced glycosylation product accumulation: extracellular protein cross-linking.

Extracellular protein cross-linking:
• Irreversibly traps deposited plasma proteins
• Reduces susceptibility to enzymatic degradation
• Interferes with basement membrane self-assembly
• Decreases binding affinity for growth-modulating heparan sulphate proteoglycans

In the diabetic microcirculation, PAS-positive material is deposited in retinal, glomerular and endoneurial arterioles together with plasma proteins such as IgG, albumin and IgM which accumulate in the basement membrane [23, 24]. These proteins are tightly bound to matrix components and cannot be extracted even with high-salt buffers or thiocyanate treatment. Similarly, serum albumin or IgG added *in vitro* to non-enzymatically glycosylated collagen or basement membrane become covalently bound to matrix [25, 26]. Once normally short-lived plasma proteins such as LDL and IgG become covalently attached to vascular matrix AGE, further AGE form on these incorporated proteins and in turn serve as attachment sites for additional molecules of extravasated plasma proteins.

AGE on matrix proteins can also cross-link adjacent matrix components such as collagen, forming covalent and heat-stable bonds throughout the collagen molecule [27]; aortic collagen from diabetic rats is three times more cross-linked than that from non-diabetic animals [28].

Matrix components cross-linked by glucose probably accumulate in diabetic vessel walls because they are less susceptible to normal enzymatic degradation. *In vitro*, non-enzymatically glycosylated glomerular basement membrane is considerably more resistant to digestion by pepsin, papain, trypsin and endogenous glomerular proteases than is normal basement membrane [29]. Overall, accumulation within large- and small-vessel walls of cross-linked material involving matrix, plasma proteins, collagen and other proteins would directly cause progressive luminal narrowing. Further tissue injury could result from AGE-catalysed oxygen radical formation.

As well as impeding its enzymatic removal, cross-linking by AGE has detrimental effects on other matrix protein properties. For example, self-assembly of the basement membrane structure, which normally involves precise geometrical interactions between Type IV collagen, laminin, heparan sulphate proteoglycan and entactin, is disordered [5, 6]. There is an associated increase in the effective intermolecular pore size, which together with alterations in anionic proteoglycans of the vascular matrix, may damage the integrity of the charge-selective matrix filtration barrier which prevents circulating proteins from escaping into the vessel wall.

The anionic proteoglycans, such as heparan sulphate, also appear to inhibit the proliferation of adherent cells [30], either through direct transmembrane inhibition of cellular activity via specific glycosaminoglycan (GAG) receptors, or indirectly by down-regulating receptors for growth factors such as interleukin-1 (IL-1), insulin-like growth factor-1 (IGF-1) and platelet-derived growth factor (PDGF). In long-standing diabetes, the basement membrane content of anionic proteoglycan is markedly decreased in several tissues including the renal glomerulus [31, 32] (Chapter 65), and there is evidence that loss of this inhibitory matrix signal results in a compensatory increase in basement membrane production [33].

Accumulation of AGE on collagen and basement membrane contributes to this permanent loss of proteoglycan by reducing the ability of these long-lived matrix proteins to bind heparin.

These glycosylation-induced matrix defects would both increase leakage of plasma proteins and stimulate matrix overproduction. AGE-induced conformational changes in matrix components such as fibronectin, laminin, vitronectin and collagen are likely to cause further abnormalities in diabetic blood vessels by altering the interactions between the matrix and platelets and vessel-wall cells. These abnormalities, mediated by specific transmembrane signalling receptors called integrins [34], may result in microthrombus formation, hyper-responsiveness to growth factors, and enhanced secretion of vasoconstrictor molecules.

EFFECTS ON CELLULAR RECEPTORS (see Table 54.3)

Accumulation of vascular matrix in diabetes is due not only to reduced degradation but also to a significant increase in the synthesis of its components [35], which is frequently accompanied by proliferation of adjacent cells such as retinal endothelium, glomerular mesangial cells and arterial smooth muscle. These processes may be chronically stimulated by increased local production of growth-promoting factors such as IGF-1 [36], tumour necrosis factor (TNF), IL-1 and PDGF.

Both murine and human monocyte macrophages are now known to carry a high-affinity receptor for AGE proteins [37], which may also exist on endothelial cells [38]. As it does not recognize proteins with early glycosylation products alone, this receptor enables macrophages to identify and remove preferentially vascular matrix macromolecules which have been cross-linked through long-term exposure to glucose.

In non-diabetic individuals, AGE-protein binding to its cellular receptor appears to release TNF, IL-1 and possibly other monokines [39], which then initiate a cascade of homeostatic events within the vessel wall. The monokines act upon mesenchymal cells, which release extracellular hydrolases including collagenase [39] and a mesangial neutral protease [40], and upon endothelial cells to produce growth factors which enhance the growth-promoting effects of the monokines themselves [41, 42] (Fig. 54.7). Normally, these degradative and proliferative responses are balanced and the turnover of AGE-containing vascular elements is carefully regulated. The proliferative responses may, however, predispose to thrombus formation. The binding of TNF to its specific endothelial cell receptors induces a procoagulatory state, which in turn promotes the release of PDGF-like activity in response to stimulation of endothelial cells by thrombin and factor Xa [43]. In diabetic vessels, platelet aggregation and thrombosis might be induced by the rapid fall in thrombomodulin activity caused directly by binding of AGE proteins to endothelial cells [44]. The relative activity of the proliferative responses and therefore the tendency to thrombosis in response to glucose-derived AGE in vessel walls may be modulated by genetic

Table 54.3. Pathological consequences of advanced glycosylation product accumulation: interaction with cellular receptors.

Interaction with cellular receptors increases production of growth-promoting cytokines that:
• Augment matrix synthesis
• Stimulate hypertrophy/hyperplasia
• Induce procoagulatory changes in endothelial surface

factors, perhaps affecting the magnitude of the monokine response elicited by AGE-protein binding to macrophages, or the sensitivity of the endothelial and mesenchymal cells to the monokines. Such factors could account for some of the great individual variation in susceptibility to hyperglycaemia-mediated cell damage.

INTRACELLULAR NUCLEIC ACID
CROSS-LINKING (see Table 54.4)

The primary amino groups of nucleotides are chemically less reactive nucleophiles than the epsilon-amino groups of lysine. Nonetheless, reducing sugars found intracellularly can react *in vitro* with amino groups on DNA nucleotides in a manner analogous to the non-enzymatic glycosylation of protein amino groups [45], forming AGE whose spectral and fluorescent properties are similar to those of AGE on proteins. AGE also form readily on all classes of histones, suggesting that hyperglycaemia may also result in cross-linking of DNA with nucleoproteins [46].

In prokaryotic cells, formation of AGE on DNA is associated with mutations (either deletions or insertions) and altered gene expression [7]. Hyperglycaemia also affects DNA from eukaryotic cells [47]. Human endothelial cells cultured in 30 mmol/l glucose display an increase in single-strand DNA breaks and in DNA repair synthesis. Increased single-strand DNA breaks also occur in lymphocytes from chronically hyperglycaemic diabetic patients, but the extent of AGE formation in these human DNA preparations is not yet known. Accumulation of AGE on nucleic acids of diabetic vascular wall cells may eventually interfere with normal physiology, perhaps resulting in the early loss of pericytes from diabetic retinal capillaries (Chapter 58) and possibly explaining the expression of transforming genes by human coronary artery plaque cells [48].

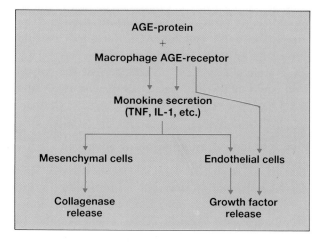

Fig. 54.7. Schematic representation of the proposed mechanism by which monokine production stimulated by AGE-protein binding to its macrophage receptor may regulate normal vessel wall homeostasis. (Redrawn with permission from Brownlee *et al*. 1988 [17].)

Table 54.4. Pathological consequences of advanced glycosylation product accumulation: intracellular nucleic acid cross-linking.

- Increases single-strand breaks in DNA
- Increases DNA excision/repair
- Increases mutation frequency
- Decreases transcriptional regulatory protein binding

Relationship of AGE formation to other pathogenic factors

Hypertension

In recent years, hypertension has been increasingly recognized as one of the most significant secondary risk factors for both microvascular and macrovascular diabetic complications (Chapter 52) [4, 49]. Effective anti-hypertensive treatment significantly reduces the rate of renal function decline in nephropathic patients (Chapter 65); a natural corollary is that unilateral ophthalmic or renal artery stenosis greatly reduces the severity of retinopathy or nephropathy on the affected side. Increased intravascular pressure probably accelerates the development of AGE-induced pathological changes by increasing the extravasation of plasma proteins. This would both accelerate the accumulation of AGE cross-linked protein deposits in the vascular matrix and increase the concentration of AGE proteins available to stimulate growth-factor production by cells carrying AGE receptors.

Aldose reductase inhibitors

Aldose reductase inhibitors (ARI) produce various biochemical effects which may retard the progression of diabetic complications [50]. For example, ARI can improve the 1.5-fold increase in vascular permeability associated with diabetes of short duration [51] and would thereby reduce the deposition of AGE proteins. Recent evidence indicates that ARI may also directly inhibit the excess formation of fructose-derived AGE in tissues with increased polyol pathway activity. Administration of ARI to rats induces both a decrease in collagen AGE content [52] and a reduction in collagen cross-linking [53]. However, such fructose-derived products appear to constitute only 10−20% of the total AGE in long-lived proteins [54].

Hypercoagulability and platelet aggregation

Diabetes is associated with several thrombogenic abnormalities, including a probable increase in coagulation cascade activity, hyperaggregable platelets, and decreased fibrinolysis [55]. Together, these processes are thought to accelerate the development of both microvascular and macrovascular disease. Excessive AGE formation is now known to promote thrombogenic changes at the endothelial cell surface by stimulating TNF and IL-1 secretion by macrophages. These monokines induce endothelial cells to produce a tissue-factor-like procoagulant (which suppresses the activity of the anticoagulant protein C pathway) and to synthesize an inhibitor of plasminogen activator [43]. These changes generate thrombin and activated factor Xa, which stimulate the release of PDGF which in turn accelerates both hyperplasia and hypertrophy in the diabetic vessel wall. Other thrombogenic effects include endothelial cell binding to AGE proteins causing a rapid reduction in thrombomodulin activity [44] and AGE-protein cross-linking which encourages platelet aggregation [56].

Dyslipoproteinaemia

Although diabetes is associated with greatly increased risks of developing coronary, cerebral and peripheral arteriosclerosis, plasma LDL levels are not consistently abnormal [57]. At any level of plasma LDL, however, accumulation of AGE on arterial wall collagen would enhance the extracellular deposition of lipoprotein [22], which would act as a nucleus for AGE formation and, by interaction with cellular AGE receptors, would stimulate growth-factor release (Fig. 54.7) [39]. AGE attached to LDL or collagen in the vessel wall could aggravate vascular injury by catalysing the formation of toxic free radicals [14, 15].

Pharmacological modulation of advanced glycosylation reactions

As AGE formation has been implicated in the pathogenesis of chronic diabetic complications, pharmacological agents have been sought to inhibit this process. Aminoguanidine HCl, a nucleophilic hydrazine derivative, selectively blocks reactive carbonyl groups on early glycosylation products and on their derivatives such as 3-deoxyglucosone and glycolaldehyde (see Fig.

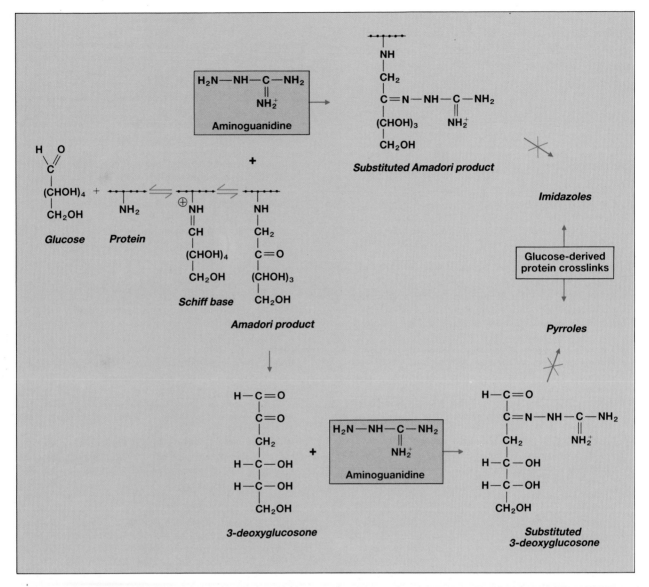

Fig. 54.8. Prevention of AGE-protein cross-link formation by aminoguanidine. Aminoguanidine binds preferentially to reactive AGE cross-link precursors, forming unreactive substituted products which can no longer participate in AGE cross-link formation.

54.8). Aminoguanidine is essentially non-toxic (LD_{50}=1800 mg/kg in rodents) and does not interfere with the formation of normal, enzymatically derived collagen cross-links, as determined both indirectly [28] and by direct quantitation of lysyl oxidase-dependent cross-link products.

In vitro, aminoguanidine effectively inhibits the formation of AGE, and blocks the AGE cross-linking of soluble proteins to matrix and of collagen. It also prevents defects due to cross-linking in the binding of heparin to collagen/fibronectin and of heparan sulphate proteoglycan to basement membrane [28, 58] (Brownlee M *et al*. unpublished data).

In vivo, the effect of aminoguanidine on diabetic early vascular lesions has been examined in diabetic rats. After 16 weeks of untreated diabetes, the matrix contents of AGE and of cross-linked plasma proteins in both aorta and kidney were four-fold higher than in non-diabetic controls [28, 59]. By contrast, these defects were nearly normalized in tissues from aminoguanidine-treated diabetic animals. Preliminary data from long-term studies suggest that aminoguanidine treatment also inhibits the development of experimental diabetic retinopathy (Hammes M-P *et al*. Unpublished observations).

The therapeutic potential of aminoguanidine

and its analogues is currently being further evaluated in several animal and cell culture model systems, while the pharmacokinetics and potential toxicity of this agent are being determined in human studies.

CATHLEEN J. MULLARKEY

MICHAEL BROWNLEE

References

1 Keen H, Jarrett J, eds. *Complications of Diabetes* 2nd ed. London: Edward Arnold, 1982: 1–331.

2 Bloodworth JMB Jr, Greider MH. The endocrine pancreas and diabetes mellitus. Bloodworth JMB Jr., ed. In: *Endocrine Pathology, General and Surgical*, 2nd ed. Baltimore: Williams and Wilkins, 1982: 556–721.

3 Dyck PJ. Hypoxic neuropathy: Does hypoxia play a role in diabetic neuropathy? *Neurology* 1989; **39**: 111–18.

4 Krolewski A, Canessa M, Warram JH et al. Predisposition to hypertension and susceptibility to renal disease in insulin-dependent diabetes mellitus. *N Engl J Med* 1988; **318**: 140–6.

5 Tarsio JF, Reger LA, Furcht LT. Decreased interaction of fibronectin, type IV collagen and heparin, due to non-enzymatic glycosylation. Implications for diabetes mellitus. *Biochemistry* 1987; **26**: 1014–20.

6 Tsilibary EC, Charonis AS, Reger LA, Wohlhueter RM, Furcht LT. The effect of non-enzymatic glucosylation on the binding of the main non-collagenous NC1 domain to type IV collagen. *J Biol Chem* 1988; **263** (suppl 9): 4302–8.

7 Lee AT, Cerami A. Elevated glucose 6-phosphate levels are associated with plasmid mutations *in vivo*. *Proc Natl Acad Sci USA* 1987; **84**: 8311–14.

8 Greene DA, Lattimer SA, Sima AAF. Sorbitol, phophoinositides, and sodium–potassium–ATPase in the pathogenesis of diabetic complications. *N Engl J Med* 1987; **316**: 599–606.

9 Williamson JR, Change K, Ostrow E, Allision W, Harlow J, Kilo C. Sorbitol-induced increases in vascular albumin clearance are prevented by pyruvate but not by myoinositol. *Diabetes* 1989; **38** (suppl 2): 94A.

10 Winegrad AI. Does a common mechanism induce the diverse complications of diabetes? *Diabetes* 1987; **36**: 396–406.

11 Lee TS, Saltsman KA, Ohashi H, King GL. Activation of protein kinase C by elevation of glucose concentration: Proposal for a mechanism in the development of diabetic vascular complications. *Proc Natl Acad Sci USA* 1989; **86**: 5141–5.

12 Brownlee M, Vlassara H, Cerami A. Non-enzymatic glycosylation and the pathogenesis of diabetic complications. *Ann Intern Med* 1984; **101**: 527–37.

13 Witztum JL, Mahoney EM, Branks MJ et al. Non-enzymatic glucosylation of low-density lipoprotein alters its biologic activity. *Diabetes* 1982; **3**: 283–91.

14 Gillery P, Monboisse JC, Maquart FX, Borel JP. Glycation of proteins as a source of superoxide. *Diabètes Métab* 1988; **14**: 25–30.

15 Hicks M, Delbridge L, Yue DK, Reeve TS. Catalysis of lipid peroxidation by glucose and glycosylated collagen. *Biochem Biophys Res Commun* 1988; **151**: 649–55.

16 Ahmed MU, Thorpe SR, Baynes JW. Identification of N-carboxymethyllysine as a degradation product of fructo-syllysine in glycated protein. *J Biol Chem* 1986; **261**: 4889–94.

17 Brownlee MB, Cerami A, Vlassara H. Advanced glycosylation end-products in tissue and the biochemical basis of diabetic complications. *N Engl J Med* 1988; **318**: 1315–21.

18 Chang JCF, Ulrich PC, Bucala R, Cerami A. Detection of an advanced glycosylation product bound to protein *in situ*. *J Biol Chem* 1985; **260**: 7970–4.

19 Baines JW, Monnier VM, eds. *The NIH Conference on the Maillard Reaction in Ageing, Diabetes and Nutrition*. New York: Alan R. Liss, 1989.

20 Dybdahl H, Ledet TS. Diabetic macroangiopathy: Quantitative histopathological studies of the extramural coronary arteries from Type 2 (non-insulin-dependent) diabetic patients. *Diabetologia* 1987; **30**: 882–6.

21 Smith EB, Massie IB, Alexander KM. The release of an immobilized lipoprotein fraction from atherosclerotic lesions by incubation with plasmin. *Atherosclerosis* 1976; **25**: 71–84.

22 Brownlee M, Vlassara H, Cerami A. Non-enzymatic glycosylation products on collagen covalently trap low-density lipoprotein. *Diabetes* 1985; **34**: 938–41.

23 Michael AF, Brown DM. Increased concentrations of albumin in kidney basement membranes in diabetes mellitus. *Diabetes* 1981; **30**: 843–6.

24 Graham AR, Johnson PC. Direct immunofluorescence findings in peripheral nerve from patients with diabetic neuropathy. *Ann Neurol* 1985; **17**: 450–4.

25 Brownlee M, Pongor S, Cerami A. Covalent attachment of soluble proteins by non-enzymatically glycosylated collagen: Role in the *in situ* formation of immune complexes. *J Exp Med* 1983; **158**: 1739–44.

26 Sensi M, Tanzi P, Bruno MR et al. Human glomerular basement membrane: altered binding characteristics following *in vitro* non-enzymatic glycosylation. *Ann NY Acad Sci* 1986; **488**: 549–52.

27 Kent MJC, Light ND, Bailey AJ. Evidence for glucose-mediated covalent cross-linking of collagen after glycosylation *in vitro*. *Biochem J* 1985; **225**: 745–52.

28 Brownlee M, Vlassara H, Kooney T, Ulrich P, Cerami A. Aminoguanidine prevents diabetes-induced arterial wall protein cross-linking. *Science* 1986; **232**: 1629–32.

29 Lubec G, Pollak A. Reduced susceptibility of non-enzymatically glucosylated glomerular basement membrane to proteases: is thickening of diabetic glomerular basement due to reduced proteolytic degradation? *Renal Physiol* 1980; **3**: 4–8.

30 Klahr S, Schreiner G, Ichikawa I. The progression of renal disease. *N Engl J Med* 1988; **318**: 1657–66.

31 Klein DJ, Brown DM, Oegema TR. Glomerular proteoglycans: partial structural characterization and metabolism of *de novo* synthesized heparan-$^{35}SO_4$ proteoglycan in streptozotocin-induced diabetic rats. *Diabetes* 1986; **35**: 1130–42.

32 Shimomura H, Spiro RG. Studies on macromolecular components of human glomerular basement membrane and alterations in diabetes: decreased levels of heparan sulfate proteoglycan and laminin. *Diabetes* 1987; **36**: 374–81.

33 Rohrbach DH, Hassel JR, Kleinman HK, Martin GR. Alterations in basement membrane (heparan sulfate) proteoglycan in diabetic mice. *Diabetes* 1982; **31**: 185–8.

34 Ruoslahti E, Pierschbacher MD. New perspectives in cell adhesion: RGD and integrins. *Science* 1987; **238**: 491–7.

35 Brownlee M, Spiro RG. Glomerular basement membrane metabolism in the diabetic rat. *In vivo* studies. *Diabetes* 1979; **28**: 121–5.

36 King GL, Goodman AD, Buzney S, Moses A, Kahn CR. Receptors and growth-promoting effects of insulin and insulin-like growth factors on cells from bovine retinal capillaries and aorta. *J Clin Invest* 1985; **75**: 1028−36.

37 Vlassara H, Brownlee M, Cerami A. High-affinity receptor-mediated uptake and degradation of glucose-modified proteins: A potential mechanism for the removal of senescent macromolecules. *Proc Natl Acad Sci USA* 1985; **82**: 5588−92.

38 Williams SK, Devenny JJ, Bitensky MW. Micropinocytic ingestion of glycosylated albumin by isolated microvessels: possible role in pathogenesis of diabetic microangiopathy. *Proc Natl Acad Sci USA* 1981; **78**: 2393−7.

39 Vlassara H, Brownlee M, Monogue K *et al*. Cachectin/TNF and IL-1 induced by glucose-modified proteins: role in normal tissue remodelling. *Science* 1988; **240**: 1546−8.

40 Lovett DH, Sterzel M, Kashgarian M, Ryan JL. Neutral proteinase activity produced *in vitro* by cells of the glomerular mesangium. *Kidney Int* 1983; **23**: 342−9.

41 Lovett DH, Ryan JL, Sterzel RB. Stimulation of rat mesangial cell proliferation by macrophage interleukin 1. *J Immunol* 1983; **136**: 3700−5.

42 Libby P, Warner SJC, Freidman GB. Interleukin 1: a mitogen for human vascular smooth muscle cells that induces the release of inhibitory prostanoids. *J Clin Invest* 1988; **81**: 487−98.

43 Bevilacqua MP, Pober JS, Majeau GR, Fiers W, Cotran RS, Giambrone MA. Recombinant tumor necrosis factor induces procoagulant activity in cultured human vascular endothelium: Characterization and comparison with the actions of interleukin 1. *Proc Natl Acad Sci USA* 1986; **83**: 4533−7.

44 Vlassara H, Esposito C, Gerlach H, Stern D. Receptor-mediated binding of glycosylated albumin to endothelium induces tissue necrosis factor and acts synergistically with TNF procoagulant activity. *Diabetes* 1989; **38** (suppl 2): 32A.

45 Bucala R, Model P, Cerami A. Modification of DNA by reducing sugars: a possible mechanism for nucleic acid aging and age-related dysfunction in gene expression. *Proc Natl Acad Sci USA* 1984; **81**: 105−9.

46 De Bellis D, Horowitz MI. *In vitro* studies of histone glycation. *Biochem Biophys Acta* 1987; **926**: 365−8.

47 Lornezi M, Montisano DF, Toledo S, Barrieux A. High glucose and DNA damage in endothelial cells. *J Clin Invest* 1986; **77**: 322−5.

48 Penn A, Garte SJ, Warren L, Nesta D, Mindich B. Transforming gene in human atherosclerotic plaque DNA. *Proc Natl Acad Sci USA* 1986; **83**: 7951−5.

49 *Diabetes in America: Diabetes Data Compiled 1984*. NIH Publication No. 85−1468, 1985.

50 Kador PF, Robison WG, Kinoshita JH. The pharmacology of aldose reductase inhibitors. *Ann Rev Pharmacol Tox* 1985; **25**: 691−714.

51 Williamson JR, Chang K, Tilton RC *et al*. Increased vascular permeability in spontaneously diabetic BB/W rats and in rats with mild versus severe streptozocin-induced diabetes: prevention by aldose reductase inhibitors and castration. *Diabetes* 1987; **36**: 813−21.

52 Suarez G, Rajaram R, Bhuyan KC, Oronsky AL, Goidl JA. Administration of an aldose reductase inhibitor induces a decrease of collagen fluorescence in diabetic rats. *J Clin Invest* 1988; **82**: 624−7.

53 Tamas C, Monnier VM. Aldose reductase inhibition partly prevents the browning and cross-linking of collagen in chronic experimental hyperglycemia. In: Baines JW, Monnier VM, eds. *Proceedings of the NIH Conference on the Maillard Reaction in Aging, Diabetes and Nutrition*, New York: Elsevier (in press).

54 McPherson JD, Shilton BH, Walton DJ. Role of fructose in glycation and cross-linking of proteins. *Biochemistry* 1988; **27**: 1901−7.

55 Brownlee M, Cerami A. The biochemistry of the complications of diabetes mellitus. *Annu Rev Biochem* 1981; **50**: 385−432.

56 Le Pape A, Gutman N, Guitton JD, Legrand Y, Muh JP. Non-enzymatic glycosylation increases platelet aggregating potency of collagen from placenta of diabetic human beings. *Biochem Biophys Res Commun* 1983; **111**: 602−10.

57 Briones ER, Mao SJT, Palumbo WM *et al*. Analysis of plasma lipids and apolipoproteins in insulin-dependent and non-insulin-dependent diabetes. *Metabolism* 1984; **33**: 42−9.

58 Brownlee M, Vlassara H, Cerami A. Aminoguanidine prevents hyperglycemia-induced defect in binding of heparin by matrix molecules. *Diabetes* 1987; **36**: 85A.

59 Nicholls K, Mandel TE. Advanced glycosylation end-products in experimental murine diabetic nephropathy: effect of islet isografting and aminoguanidine. *Lab Invest* 1989; **60**: 486−93.

55   The Regulation of Microvascular Function in Diabetes Mellitus

Summary

• Blood flow through the microcirculation is normally tightly regulated by central neural mechanisms, local reflexes, circulating mediators and locally produced vasoactive substances including nitric oxide (vasodilator) and endothelin (vasoconstrictor).

• Haemodynamic disturbances accompany and precede the natural history of diabetic microangiopathy and may contribute to its pathogenesis.

• Early haemodynamic abnormalities include increased basal blood flow in skin, retina and kidney, together with relatively impaired responses to various hyperaemic stimuli in skin. These abnormalities occur early in IDDM, before evidence of structural microvascular damage appears.

• Haemodynamic disturbances often worsen during puberty or pregnancy, paralleling the tendency of microvascular disease to deteriorate.

• Like microvascular disease, haemodynamic abnormalities are generally related to the duration of diabetes and the degree of hyperglycaemia. Early in the disease, haemodynamic changes may be reversible with tight glycaemic control but later become irreversible.

• Patients with uncomplicated diabetes of long duration often show preserved haemodynamic responses. Microvascular disease may therefore develop specifically in a susceptible subgroup of patients.

• Failure of autoregulation of capillary blood flow, together with a reduction in perfusion which tends to follow a fall in blood glucose levels, may compromise tissue nutrition when diabetic control is suddenly tightened. This may explain the acute deterioration in microvascular disease (the 'glycaemic re-entry' phenomenon) which sometimes occurs at this time.

• Haemodynamic changes, notably increased capillary pressure and flow, could stimulate capillary basement membrane thickening and cause arteriolar sclerosis. These changes could lead to failure of autoregulation, leakage of albumin and ultimately to impaired tissue nutrition.

It is generally accepted that damage to the smallest blood vessels underlies most of the late complications of diabetes but the nature of diabetic microangiopathy is far less certain. Clarification of the disease process depends upon understanding the normal physiology of the microvasculature, which in health is able to balance a series of conflicting demands. Flow must match local metabolic needs, yet pressure must be carefully regulated in order to prevent large shifts of fluid across the capillary endothelium. At the same time, general body functions which depend critically upon blood flow in various vascular beds — such as arterial blood pressure and core temperature — must be tightly controlled. These complicated specifications demand a sophisticated array of local and extrinsic mechanisms controlling flow through the microcirculation.

Microvascular control systems

Extrinsic control

Blood vessel diameter is regulated by both neural and humoral factors. The degree to which an organ is subject to central neural control is a function of both its metabolic needs and its capacity to withstand circulatory deprivation. Accordingly, the cerebral circulation is under little neurogenic control by comparison with the splanchnic bed. On the other hand, core temperature is largely regulated by the sympathetic nervous control of skin blood flow in the extremities, and arterial pressure by the sympathetic innervation supplying the various vascular beds which determine peripheral vascular resistance.

Receptors exist on the endothelium and vascular smooth muscle cells for a wide variety of peptide and non-peptide neurohumoral mediators, and the distribution of receptors may determine in part the reactivity of a particular vascular bed [1].

Intrinsic control mechanisms

Local systems which affect flow through capillaries by influencing pre- and postcapillary resistance could clearly be important in supplying the tissues' needs while maintaining tissue fluid economy, especially in the face of changing arterial blood pressure. There is considerable evidence that the local accumulation of metabolites may modify local vascular tone and hence blood flow. Furthermore, vascular smooth muscle responds directly to stretch and/or tension by contracting, thereby limiting any imposed increase in pressure or flow [2]. Recent work suggests that the sensor for this process may reside in the endothelial cell [3], although isolated vascular smooth muscle cells also possess this capacity, the so-called 'myogenic response' of Bayliss [4]. It is now firmly established that the vascular endothelium produces vasoactive mediators, notably the vasodilator, endothelium-derived relaxing factor (EDRF, recently identified as nitric oxide [5]) and endothelin, an extremely powerful vasoconstrictor peptide [6], as well as a variety of prostanoids. Endothelin receptors have also recently been identified on retinal capillary pericytes [7], supporting the possibility that these enigmatic cells are involved in vasoconstriction (see Chapter 57).

Local nervous mechanisms may also exist. Stimulation of pain fibres results in the axon reflex responsible for the flare component of Lewis's triple response in the skin [8] and a sympathetic axon reflex has been proposed to explain the precapillary vasoconstriction which accompanies a rise in venular pressure. The latter, the veno-arteriolar response, can be demonstrated in both skin [9] and subcutaneous tissue [10], and prob-

ably acts in health as a mechanism preventing oedema [11].

From the above, it is clear that microvascular control depends upon the integrity of the peripheral and central autonomic nervous systems, sensory nerves, vascular smooth muscle, pericytes and endothelium, all of which may be adversely affected by diabetes. The profound haemodynamic disturbances in the microcirculation of various tissues, particularly the kidney, retina and skin, are therefore to be anticipated. Indeed, haemodynamic abnormalities accompany and often precede the natural history of microangiopathy and, although other biochemical, rheological and cellular factors are also undoubtedly involved, haemodynamic factors fulfil several key criteria for a fundamental cause of microvascular disease. These observations are outlined in Table 55.1 and are discussed in more detail below.

Relationship of haemodynamic changes to microangiopathy

Early expression

To be considered a prime mover, a putative' aetiological factor must be present from the outset of diabetes. Early haemodynamic abnormalities have been demonstrated in IDDM patients, including increased basal blood flow in various organs, including the kidney [12], retina [13] and limbs [14]. In the skin, which is accessible to various measurement techniques, haemodynamic disturbances have been characterized in detail. Characteristically,

Table 55.1. Evidence suggesting that haemodynamic abnormalities may cause or contribute to diabetic microvascular disease.

Time-course of haemodynamic abnormalities:
- Present from early in untreated IDDM (i.e. precede microvascular disease)
- Accelerated progression during puberty (similar to microvascular complications)
- Related to duration of diabetes (similar to microvascular complications)

Relationship of haemodynamic abnormalities to glycaemic control:
- Reversible initially with improved metabolic control; poorly reversible in established disease (similar to microvascular disease)
- Consistent with 'glycaemic re-entry' phenomenon

Evidence for a susceptible subgroup
(as with microvascular disease)

resting flow is increased [15], particularly in areas with numerous arteriovenous shunts, and probably reflects the increased metabolic rate [16] and the need to dissipate heat in the newly diagnosed patient with uncontrolled IDDM. In addition to high resting values, impaired microvascular responses can be demonstrated within the first year of diabetic life [17]: the time taken to reach the peak of reactive hyperaemia (determined in single capillaries) is prolonged and the veno-arteriolar response is blunted. Even in children with IDDM, the maximum transcutaneous oxygen tension observed after release of ischaemia is reduced in the first few months of the disease [18].

In NIDDM, early expression of haemodynamic abnormalities is difficult to demonstrate because of the uncertain duration of the disease before presentation. NIDDM patients display a spectrum of microvascular haemodynamic defects which may represent the various stages of the evolution of microangiopathy.

Acceleration of abnormalities with passage through puberty

Clinically significant microangiopathic complications are rarely seen before puberty, but the rate of development of retinopathy is faster in the postpubertal years even when corrections are made for the overall duration of diabetes. In animal models, sex hormones and growth factors have been shown to influence the activity of the polyol pathway and the degree of collagen cross-linking [19], which may both be implicated in the development of microangiopathy (see Chapter 54).

Functional haemodynamic abnormalities also progress with passage through puberty, in parallel with the tendency of microvascular disease to deteriorate. Figure 55.1 shows maximum skin microvascular blood flow values in pre- and postpubertal children of similar disease duration. The significant reduction in the postpubertal group cannot be attributed to age differences alone.

Relationship to disease duration

The likelihood of developing microangiopathy rises with increasing disease duration, and abnormalities in microvascular reactivity demonstrate the same relationship. Maximum cutaneous microvascular blood flow falls with increasing disease duration in both children [20] and young adults [21]. Limitation of blood flow which is

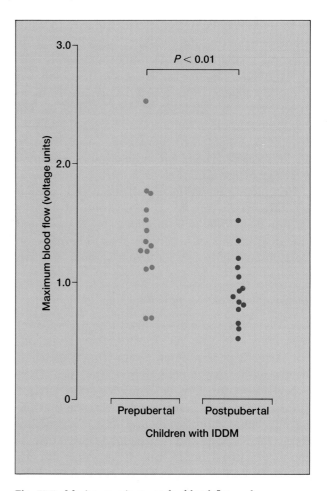

Fig. 55.1. Maximum microvascular blood flow values determined by laser Doppler flowmetry on the dorsum of the foot in pre- and postpubertal diabetic children matched for age and duration of IDDM.

related to the duration of diabetes may also be demonstrated in the renal [22] and retinal circulations using indirect techniques.

Relationship to glycaemic control

Although protracted hyperglycaemia is a prerequisite, the relationship between the development of microangiopathy and glycaemic control is not direct, and correcting hyperglycaemia does not necessarily reverse the damage. The pattern of microvascular functional impairment exhibits a similar relationship. Relatively early in diabetic life, effective control of diabetes will correct the impairment of maximum transcutaneous oxygen tension [18]. With increasing disease duration, however, the relationship to current diabetic control becomes more tenuous. After 10 years of diabetes, a protracted period (at least one year) of

REGULATION OF MICROVASCULAR FUNCTION/549

'good' control improves microvascular reactivity in some tissues but not others [17]. Short-term treatment (12 weeks) with an aldose reductase inhibitor in patients of short to moderate disease duration has conferred no apparent benefit on a variety of cutaneous microvascular responses (J. E. Tooke, M. Boolell: unpublished observations).

Is there a susceptible subgroup?

One possible explanation for the lack of a direct relationship between glycaemic control and the development of microangiopathy is that there may exist subsets of patients who are less vulnerable to the effects of sustained hyperglycaemia. Studies of patients who have survived IDDM for more than 40 years without developing nephropathy or significant retinopathy have revealed that microvascular responses which do not depend upon neural-integrity are normal in this group, although neurally-dependent mechanisms may be impaired [23]. Maximum cutaneous perfusion capacity is also relatively preserved in patients with uncomplicated disease of long duration [24].

Relationship to the 'glycaemic re-entry' phenomenon

Changes in microvascular reactivity may also provide an explanation for the acute deterioration in microvascular disease sometimes observed when glycaemic control is suddenly and markedly improved, the so-called 'glycaemic re-entry' phenomenon. A characteristic of the diabetic microcirculation after a moderate disease duration is impairment of autoregulation [25–27], i.e. the capacity to maintain constant flow in the face of a changing pressure head. A fall in blood glucose is accompanied by changes in plasma volume, sympathetic nervous activity and endothelial function, all of which may influence capillary pressure and flow if local control systems are impaired. Allied to this is the fact that improved diabetic control inevitably results in more episodes of hypoglycaemia, which not only influence the rheological properties of blood and encourage a prothrombotic tendency [28], but may also cause a transient increase in arterial blood pressure. In the presence of impaired autoregulation, increased systemic pressure may be transmitted to the microvascular bed and so cause tissue damage. Furthermore, in the retina (where nutrient supply is very closely matched to metabolic demand),

a sudden reduction in glucose availability may seriously compromise tissue nutrition until adaptive changes can occur.

Exacerbation during pregnancy

A transient but sometimes marked advancement of nephropathy [29] and retinopathy [30] may occur during pregnancy; the physiological changes in microvascular haemodynamics which accompany pregnancy may offer a ready explanation. In normal pregnancy, plasma volume is increased and vascular resistance in the periphery and kidney is reduced, overall causing a rise in peripheral capillary pressure [31]. Similar increases in capillary pressure are seen in women receiving the oral contraceptive pill [32], which may also be associated with an exacerbation of microangiopathy.

The haemodynamic hypothesis

These compelling data may suggest a primary role for microvascular haemodynamic changes in the pathogenesis of diabetic microangiopathy [33] (Table 55.2). According to this 'haemodynamic' hypothesis, capillary pressure and flow are increased in the relevant tissues, early in the disease. This acts as a stimulus to the basement membrane thickening and arteriolar sclerosis which are characteristic of long-standing diabetes and which, in turn, limit maximum perfusion and the capacity to autoregulate. Several studies have now demonstrated a link between microvascular histological changes and the later functional abnormalities [34, 35].

The central tenet of the hypothesis, that capillary pressure is pathologically raised, has until recently lacked direct experimental proof in humans, although direct micropuncture measurements in diabetic rats have demonstrated elevated glomerular capillary pressures [36]. Recent human studies have shown that nailfold capillary pressure

Table 55.2. The 'haemodynamic hypothesis' for the development of diabetic microangiopathy

Increased microvascular pressure and flow
→
Microvascular sclerosis
→
Limitation of maximum perfusion
→
Loss of autoregulation

is elevated in dependent feet [37] and that complication-prone patients may fail to prevent rises in arterial blood pressure from being transmitted to the capillary bed (Fig. 55.2). Not only is mean capillary pressure increased, but subtle changes in capillary pulse timing and wave-form are demonstrable which may have a bearing on endothelial cell function and transcapillary exchange.

The relationship between haemodynamic disturbances and other factors involved in the pathogenesis of diabetic microangiopathy

As discussed in Chapters 53 and 54, various biochemical, rheological and other factors are also

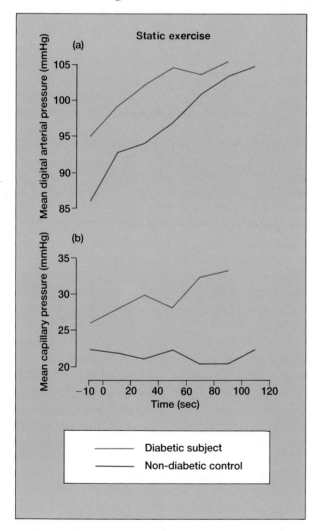

Fig. 55.2. Changes in digital arterial pressure (a) and capillary pressure (b) during isometric exercise in a diabetic subject and a matched control. Arterial blood pressure rises in both but only in the diabetic subject is a pressure increment transmitted to the capillary. This is evidence of loss of pressure autoregulation.

convincingly implicated in the development of diabetic microvascular disease. Fig. 55.3 represents a possible sequence of events in which microangiopathy results from interactions between these various factors and haemodynamic abnormalities. Initially, precapillary resistance is reduced, increasing flow through the capillary bed. Hyperaggregable red cells are forced to disaggregate as the vessel diameter narrows, resulting in greater tangential stress on the microvascular endothelium. In functional terms, this will result in greater filtration of fluid (for which there is experimental evidence) [38] as well as increased passage, mainly through solvent drag [39], of plasma albumin across the capillary wall. Alterations in endothelial charge characteristics will also facilitate the passage of albumin. Increased tangential stress also stimulates the endothelial cell to release vasodilator compounds such as nitric oxide and prostacyclin and to synthesize basement membrane components. As well as becoming thicker, the chemical composition of the capillary basement membrane will be chemically modified by the glycaemic and humoral environment (see Chapter 54).

In established disease (Fig. 55.4), sclerosis (thickening) of the capillary wall has supervened and effectively limits maximum vasodilation. The endothelium has been denuded, exposing the subintima and allowing the activation and aggregation of platelets. The break in the endothelial barrier further increases permeability, which is not offset by basement membrane thickening as the latter is architecturally distorted and has lost its chemical and electrostatic integrity. The autoregulation of pressure and flow becomes progressively impaired, exposing the microvascular bed to the vagaries of arterial blood pressure. The local 'fine tuning' of precapillary resistance which normally regulates vasomotion and ensures a uniform distribution of blood flow breaks down, causing heterogenous flow [40] and microvascular 'steal' which compromises the capillary supply to the tissues.

Implications for therapy

Consistent with the haemodynamic hypothesis is the fact that various agents which alter haemodynamic variables can also influence the course of microvascular disease in diabetes and certain other conditions. An important example is the lowering of arterial blood pressure, which has

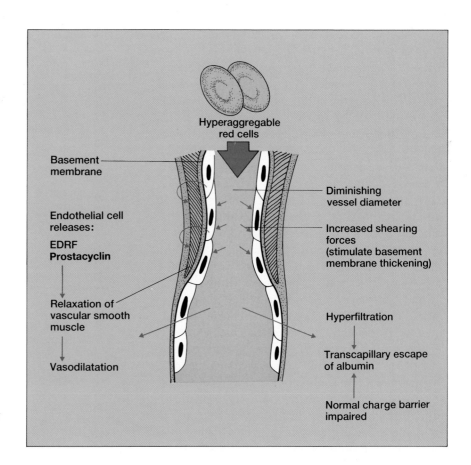

Fig. 55.3. Schematic diagram of pathogenic mechanisms which may operate early in diabetic microangiopathy.

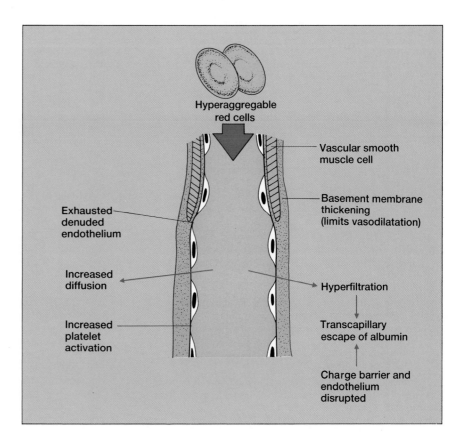

Fig. 55.4. Schematic diagram of possible pathogenic mechanisms operating in advanced microangiopathy.

been shown to decrease capillary pressure in patients with essential hypertension [41] and to reduce the abnormally enhanced passage of retinal fluorescein in diabetes [42]. Furthermore, blood pressure regulation is the only strategy that has been demonstrated to slow the progression of a clinical complication of diabetes, namely nephropathy [43] (see Chapters 65 and 67). Insulin may alter the distribution of peripheral blood flow in favour of the capillary bed [44]; theoretically, this may represent a disadvantage during evolving disease but may be a positive advantage in the foot threatened by ischaemia. It may ultimately be possible to manipulate capillary pressure separately from arterial blood pressure by using low doses of certain hypotensive drugs, but at present, the early control of blood glucose — before the development of irreversible impairment of microvascular control mechanisms — is of key importance. In the future, it may become possible to detect subtle microvascular functional changes before the appearance of clinical microangiopathy, or even of the early stage of microalbuminuria. This in turn may enable us to intervene in susceptible subjects at a stage when they may be more responsive to therapy.

JOHN E. TOOKE

ANGELA C. SHORE

References

1 Vanhoutte PM. Serotonin, adrenergic nerves, endothelial cells and vascular smooth muscle. *Prog Appl Microcirc* 1986; **10**: 1–11.

2 Johansson B. Myogenic tone and reactivity: definitions based on muscle physiology. *J Hypertens* 1989; **7** (suppl 4): 55–8.

3 Harder DR. Pressure-induced myogenic activation of cat cerebral arteries is dependent on intact endothelium. *Circ Res* 1987; **60**: 102–7.

4 Bayliss WM. On the local reactions of the arterial wall to changes of internal pressure. *J Physiol* (Lond) 1902; **28**: 230–41.

5 Furchgott RF. Role of the endothelium in responses of vascular smooth muscle. *Circ Res* 1983; **53**: 557–73.

6 Yanagisawa M, Kurihara H, Kimura S *et al*. A novel potent vasoconstrictor peptide produced by vascular endothelial cells. *Nature* 1988; **332**: 411–15.

7 Takahashi K, Brooks R, Kanse S *et al*. Production of endothelin 1 by cultured bovine retinal endothelial cells and presence of endothelin receptors on associated pericytes. *Diabetes* 1989; **38**: 1200–2.

8 Lewis T. *Blood Vessels of the Human Skin and their Responses*. London: Shaw and Sons, 1927.

9 Rayman G, Hassan AAK, Tooke JE. Blood flow in the skin of the foot related to posture in diabetes mellitus. *Br Med J* 1986; **292**: 87–90.

10 Henriksen O. Local nervous mechanism in regulation of blood flow in human subcutaneous tissue. *Acta Physiol Scand* 1976; **97**: 385–91.

11 Hassan AAK, Tooke JE. The relationship between foot swelling rate and postural vasoconstriction in man. *J Physiol* (Lond) 1987; **387**: 76P.

12 Christiansen JS, Gammelgaard J, Tronier B, Svendsen PAa, Parving H-H. Kidney function and size in diabetes, before and during initial insulin treatment. *Kidney Int* 1982; **21**: 683–8.

13 Kohner EM, Hamilton AM, Saunders SJ, Sutcliffe BA, Bulpitt CJ. The retinal blood flow in diabetes. *Diabetologia* 1975; **11**: 27–33.

14 Gundersen HJG. Peripheral blood flow and metabolic control in juvenile diabetes. *Diabetologia* 1974; **10**: 225–31.

15 Tymms DJ, Tooke JE. The effect of continuous subcutaneous insulin infusion (CSII) on microvascular blood flow in diabetes mellitus. *Int J Microcirc Clin Exp* 1988; **7**: 347–56.

16 Leslie P, Jung RT, Isles TE *et al*. Effect of optimal glycaemic control with subcutaneous insulin infusion on energy expenditure in type 1 diabetes mellitus. *Br Med J* 1986; **293**: 1121–6.

17 Tooke JE, Lins P-E, Østergren J, Fagrell B. Skin microvascular autoregulatory responses in Type I diabetes: the influence of duration and control. *Int J Microcirc Clin Exp* 1985; **4**: 249–56.

18 Kobbah AM, Ewald U, Tuvemo T. Impaired vascular reactivity during the first 2 years of diabetes mellitus after initial restoration. *Acta Universitatis Uppsaliensis*, Doctoral Thesis, 1988.

19 Williamson JR, Chang K, Tilton RG, Kilo C. Sex steroid modulation of vascular leakage and collagen metabolism in diabetic rats. *Pediatr Adolesc Endocr* 1988; **17**: 12–17.

20 Shore AC, Price KS, Tripp JH, Tooke JE. Impaired microvascular hyperaemia in children with diabetes mellitus (abstract). *Clin Sci* 1989; **76** (suppl 20): 15P.

21 Rayman G, Williams SA, Spencer PD *et al*. Impaired microvascular hyperaemic response to minor skin trauma in Type I diabetes. *Br Med J* 1986; **292**: 1295–8.

22 Mogenson CE, Christensen CK, Vittinghus E. The stages in diabetic renal disease. *Diabetes* 1983; **32** (suppl 2): 64–78.

23 Tooke JE, Østergren J, Lins P-E, Fagrell B. Skin microvascular blood flow control in long duration diabetics with and without complications. *Diabetes Res* 1987; **5**: 189–92.

24 Walmsley D, Wales JK, Wiles PG. Reduced hyperaemia following skin trauma: evidence for an impaired microvascular response to injury in the diabetic foot. *Diabetologia* 1989; **32**: 736–9.

25 Grunwald JE, Riva CE, Sinclair SH, Brucker AV. Altered retinal vascular response to 100% O_2 breathing in diabetes mellitus. *Microvasc Res* 1983; **25**; (abstract 35): 236.

26 Parving H-H, Kastrup H, Smidt UM, Andersen AR, Feldt-Rasmussen BF, Sandahl Christiansen J. Impaired autoregulation of glomerular filtration rate in Type I (insulin dependent) diabetic patients with nephropathy. *Diabetologia* 1984; **27**: 247–552.

27 Faris I, Vagn Nielsen H, Henriksen O, Parving H-H, Lassen NA. Impaired autoregulation of blood flow in skeletal muscle and subcutaneous tissue in long-term Type 1 (insulin-dependent) diabetic patients with microangiopathy. *Diabetologia* 1983; **25**: 486–8.

28 Frier BM, Hilsted J. Does hypoglycaemia aggravate the complications of diabetes? *Lancet* 1985; ii: 1174–6.

29 Zitzmiller JL, Brown ER, Phillipe M *et al*. Diabetic nephropathy and perinatal outcome. *Am J Obstet Gynecol* 1981; **141**: 741–6.

30 Phelps RL, Sakol P, Metzger BE *et al*. Changes in diabetic retinopathy during pregnancy: correlations with regulation of hyperglycaemia. *Arch Ophthalmol* 1986; **104**: 1806–10.

31 Tooke JE. The study of human capillary pressure. In: Tooke JE, Smaje LH, eds. *Clinical Investigation of the Microcirculation*. Massachusetts, USA: Martinus Nijhoff, 1987.

32 Tooke JE, Tindall H, McNicol GP. The influence of a combined oral contraceptive pill and menstrual cycle phase on digital microvascular haemodynamics. *Clin Sci* 1981; **61**: 91–5.

33 Henriksen O. Effect of chronic sympathetic denervation upon local regulation of blood flow in human subcutaneous tissue. *Acta Physiol Scand* 1976; **97**: 377–84.

34 Parving H-H, Viberti GC, Keen H, Christiansen JS, Lassen NA. Haemodynamics factors in the genesis of diabetic microangiopathy. *Metabolism* 1983; **32**: 943–9.

35 Rayman G, Malik RA, Metcalfe J *et al*. Relationship between impaired skin microvascular responses to injury and abnormal capillary morphology in the feet of Type I diabetics (abstract). *Diabetic Med* 1989; **6** (suppl 1): 7.

36 Zatz R, Dunn R, Meyer TW *et al*. Prevention of diabetic glomerulopathy by pharmacological amelioration of glomerular capillary hypertension. *J Clin Invest* 1986; **77**: 1925–30.

37 Rayman G, Williams SA, Hassan AAK, Gamble J, Tooke JE. Capillary hypertension and overperfusion in the feet of young diabetics (abstract). *Diabetic Med* 1985; **2**: A30.

38 Parving H-H, Noer I, Deckert T *et al*. The effect of metabolic regulation on microvascular permeability to small and large molecules in short-term juvenile diabetics. *Diabetologia* 1976; **12**: 161–6.

39 Renkin EM. Relation of capillary morphology to transport of fluid and large molecules: a review. *Acta Physiol Scand* 1979; **463**: 81–91.

40 Junger M, Frey-Schnewlin G, Bollinger A. Microvascular flow distribution and transcapillary diffusion at the forefoot in patients with peripheral ischaemia. *Int J Microcirc Clin Exp* 1989; **8**: 3–24.

41 Tooke JE. Microvascular dynamics in diabetes mellitus. *Diabète Métab* 1988; **14**: 530–4.

42 Parving H-H, Larsen M, Hommel E, Lund-Andersen H. Effect of antihypertensive treatment on blood–retinal barrier permeability to fluorescein in hypertensive Type I (insulin-dependent) diabetic patients with background retinopathy. *Diabetologia* 1989; **32**: 440–4.

43 Parving H-H, Andersen AR, Smidt UM, Svendsen PAa. Early aggressive antihypertensive treatment reduces rate of decline in kidney function in diabetic nephropathy. *Lancet* 1983; i: 1175–9.

44 Tooke JE, Lins P-E, Østergren J, Adamson U, Fagrell B. The effects of intravenous insulin infusion on skin microcirculatory flow in Type I diabetes. *Int J Microcirc Clin Exp* 1985; **4**: 69–83.

PART 13.2
DIABETIC EYE DISEASE

56   The Epidemiology of Diabetic Retinopathy

Summary

• The *prevalence* of retinopathy (of any degree) is highest in young-onset, insulin-treated diabetic patients and lowest in older-onset diabetic patients not taking insulin.

• The prevalence of retinopathy increases with duration of diabetes. In young-onset, insulin-treated diabetic patients, proliferative retinopathy is generally absent below 5 years' duration of diabetes and present in about 25% at 15 years and over 50% at 20 years of diabetes. In older-onset diabetic patients, retinopathy can be present in the first few years of diabetes (about 3–4% for proliferative retinopathy) but the prevalence is lower than in young-onset diabetic patients after 15 or more years (about 15–20%).

• Macular oedema is also associated with increasing duration of diabetes. It is commoner in older-onset diabetic patients, particularly in the first few years after diagnosis.

• The *incidence* of retinopathy is highest in younger-onset patients.

• In younger-onset patients, the incidence of proliferative retinopathy is close to zero with less than 5 years' duration of disease. The 4-year incidence of proliferative retinopathy rises to 28% after 13–14 years of diabetes and is stable at 14–16% after 15 years.

• In older-onset patients, the 4-year incidence of proliferative retinopathy is 2–3%, even in those with disease of short duration (2 years or less).

• These findings suggest that full ophthalmological examination should be carried out at the time of diagnosis and at least annually thereafter in patients diagnosed after 30 years of age. In those diagnosed diabetic before this age, examination should be performed at least annually after 5–9 years of diabetes.

Epidemiological data are essential for estimating the frequency, severity, development and progression of diabetic retinopathy in a given population. Such data are also needed in order to predict the demand for medical counselling and rehabilitative services, for developing screening programmes, for projecting costs, and for measuring temporal trends. Moreover, causal and risk factors may be identified, raising the possibility that such factors might be modified to ameliorate or prevent diabetic retinopathy.

Data on the frequency and incidence of diabetic retinopathy have come from specialized clinics for diabetes [1, 2] or eye disease [3], hospitals [4], and clinical trials [5]. Unfortunately, data from many of these studies cannot be extrapolated to a larger unselected population of diabetic patients. Other factors such as intervention, failure to use standardized protocols, inconsistent follow-up times and inadequate documentation of the retinopathy further limit the use of such data. For these reasons, the present description of prevalence and incidence of diabetic retinopathy is focused on a population-based study, the Wisconsin Epidemiologic Study of Diabetic Retinopathy (WESDR), which used grading of photographs to determine objectively the presence and severity of retinopathy [6–9].

Incidence and progression

Few population-based data exist which describe the prevalence and/or incidence of diabetic retinopathy [6–20]. Some recent and continuing studies

Table 56.1. Selected list of population-based studies describing the prevalence and/or incidence of diabetic retinopathy.

Author	Reference	Site	Type of diabetes	Duration of diabetes (y)	Retinopathy detection*	Crude prevalence	Crude incidence
Nilsson et al.	10	Kristianstad, Sweden	–	0–16+	O	35%	–
Dorf et al.	11	Pima Indians Arizona, USA	II	0–10+	O	18%	–
Leibowitz et al.	12	Framingham Massachusetts, USA	II	–	O	20%	–
West et al.	13	Oklahoma Indians, USA	II	–	O	–	–
Houston	14	Poole, England	I & II	0–30+	O, P	Not reported	–
King et al.	15	Nauru, Central Pacific	II	0–10+	O	24%	–
Dwyer et al.	16	Rochester, Minnesota USA	I	–	–	–	45.8/1000 person-y
			II	–	O	–	15.6/1000 person-y
Sjolie	17	County of Fynn, Denmark	I	0–30+	O	47.7%	?
Nielsen	18, 19	Falster, Denmark	I	0–58	P	66.3%	1 y = 3.7%
			II	0–42	P	40.9%	1 y = 3.7%
Teuscher et al.	20	Switzerland	I	0–30+	O	51%	8 y = 39%
			II			9%	8 y = 15%

*O = ophthalmoscopy; P = photography. I = IDDM; II = NIDDM.

Table 56.2. Prevalence and severity of retinopathy by sex (Wisconsin Epidemiologic Study of Diabetic Retinopathy).

Retinopathy status	Younger-onset taking insulin			Older-onset taking insulin			Older-onset not taking insulin		
	Male (%) (n=512)	Female (%) (n=484)	Total (%) (n=996)	Male (%) (n=321)	Female (%) (n=352)	Total (%) (n=673)	Male (%) (n=313)	Female (%) (n=379)	Total (%) (n=692)
None	31.1	27.5	29.3	26.8	32.7	29.9	64.5	58.6	61.3
Early non-proliferative	26.4	34.7	30.4	34.0	27.6	30.6	25.9	28.5	27.3
Moderate to severe non-proliferative	18.2	16.9	17.6	27.7	23.9	25.7	6.4	10.3	8.5
Proliferative – without DRS high-risk characteristics	12.3	14.0	13.2	8.1	9.9	9.1	1.9	1.1	1.4
Proliferative – with DRS high-risk characteristics or worse	12.1	6.8	9.5	3.4	6.0	4.8	1.3	1.6	1.4

DRS: Diabetic Retinopathy Study [23].

of retinopathy are listed in Table 56.1, together with their method of detecting retinopathy, and their reported crude rates of prevalence and incidence of diabetic retinopathy. Caution must be observed in attempting to compare studies, because of the differences in the populations and the methods used to detect retinopathy (for example, direct ophthalmoscopy versus grading of stereoscopic colour photographs of standard retinal fields).

In the WESDR, a large population of diabetic persons living and receiving their primary medical care in an 11-county area of south-western Wisconsin was identified in 1979−80. The population, consisting of all younger-onset, insulin-taking diabetic persons diagnosed before 30 years of age ($n=996$) and a probability sample of older-onset diabetic persons taking insulin ($n=673$) and not taking insulin ($n=692$), diagnosed at or after 30 years of age, was first examined in 1980−2 and again 4 years later. At both examinations, the presence and severity of diabetic retinopathy was identified by masked grading of stereoscopic colour fundus photographs using modifications of the Wisconsin '191' system and the Airlie House classification system [3].

Prevalence

Prevalence rates of retinopathy in different populations are shown in Table 56.1. In the WESDR baseline examination, the highest rates of prevalence of any degree or of severe retinopathy were found in the younger-onset, insulin-taking group; the lowest rates were found in the older-onset group not taking insulin (Table 56.2) [6, 7]. The

relationship of the prevalence of any or proliferative retinopathy to the duration of diabetes is shown in Figs 56.1 and 56.2.

For the younger-onset group, the prevalence of any retinopathy varied from 2% in persons with fewer than 2 years of diabetes to 98% in persons with 15 or more years of disease. The prevalence of proliferative retinopathy varied from 0% in persons with fewer than 5 years of disease to 26% in patients with 15−16 years, and to 56% in those with 20 or more years of disease. The lower prevalence of proliferative retinopathy after 35 years of diabetes (Fig. 56.1) was most likely due to the higher mortality in this group as well as to a decreased progression to proliferative retinopathy after 19 years of disease.

In the older-onset groups, the prevalence of diabetic retinopathy was also positively associated with duration of diabetes [7]. During the first 2 years of diabetes, higher rates of retinopathy (23% in those taking insulin and 20% in those not taking insulin) were found in the older-onset groups compared with the younger-onset group (2%). The higher rates in the older-onset group probably reflect the difficulty of accurately determining the actual onset of disease in these persons; they might also be due to increased sensitivity of retinal tissue to the diabetic process in older people. Four per cent of older-onset persons taking insulin and 3% of those not taking insulin, who had a history of diabetes of 4 years or less, had proliferative retinopathy. The prevalence of any retinopathy or of proliferative retinopathy was significantly lower in older-onset people compared with younger-onset patients with 15 or more years of diabetes (Figs 56.1 and 56.2).

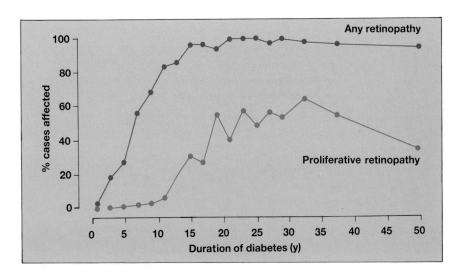

Fig. 56.1. Frequency of retinopathy (any degree) or proliferative retinopathy by duration of diabetes (in years) in persons taking insulin who were diagnosed as diabetic before 30 years of age and who participated in the Wisconsin Epidemiologic Study of Diabetic Retinopathy, 1980−2. (From Klein R *et al.* 1984 [6]. Reproduced by permission of the American Medical Association.)

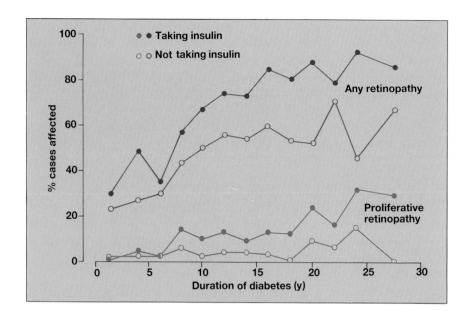

Fig. 56.2. Frequency of retinopathy (any degree) or proliferative retinopathy by duration of diabetes (in years) in persons receiving or not receiving insulin who were diagnosed to have diabetes at or after 30 years of age. (From Klein R *et al.* 1984 [7]. Reproduced by permission of the American Medical Association.)

Clinically significant macular oedema (defined as the presence of any one of the following: thickening of the retina located 500 μm or less from the centre of the macula; hard exudates with thickening of the adjacent retina, 500 μm or less from the centre of the macula; or a zone of retinal thickening one disc area or larger in size, located one disc diameter or less from the centre of the macula) [21] was also found to be significantly associated with increasing duration of diabetes in all three groups in the WESDR (Fig. 56.3). The prevalence of clinically significant macular oedema was consistently higher in older-onset patients taking insulin. In comparison with younger-onset diabetic patients, macular oedema was found to be present more frequently in older-onset people during the first few years after diagnosis of the disease. In addition, visual acuity was worse in older-onset persons as compared with younger-onset subjects when macular oedema was present [22].

Incidence and practical guidelines for ophthalmological care

The 4-year incidence rates and rates of progression of retinopathy for the three groups are reported in Table 56.3. Incidence rates were highest for the younger-onset group taking insulin (59%) and lowest for the older-onset group not taking insulin (34%). There was no significant difference between the males and females.

Information on the relationship of incidence to the duration of diabetes is of importance in determining guidelines for ophthalmological care. Because proliferative diabetic retinopathy is often asymptomatic and difficult to detect accu-

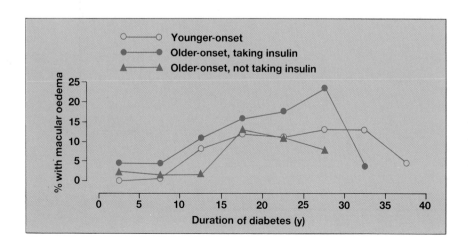

Fig. 56.3. Frequency of clinically significant macular oedema (CSME, as defined in the Early Treatment Diabetic Retinopathy Study) by duration of diabetes in younger-onset persons taking insulin (*n*=996) and older-onset persons taking insulin (*n*=674) or not taking insulin (*n*=696) who participated in the Wisconsin Epidemiologic Study of Diabetic Retinopathy (WESDR), 1980−2 [21].

Table 56.3. Four-year incidence of retinopathy or progression to proliferative retinopathy by sex (from the WESDR).

Diabetic group	No. at risk	Incidence (%)	No. at risk	Progression to proliferative retinopathy (%)
Younger-onset, taking insulin				
Male	143	56	354	11
Female	128	63	359	10
Total	271	59	713	11
Older-onset, taking insulin				
Male	62	47	193	7
Female	92	48	225	8
Total	154	47	418	7
Older-onset, not taking insulin				
Male	151	32	216	3
Female	169	36	270	2
Total	320	34	486	2

rately by non-specialists, and because pan-retinal photocoagulation treatment has been proven to be effective in preventing visual loss, it is important to be aware of the best time to refer diabetic patients to ophthalmologists [23]. The relationship of incidence of any retinopathy and progression to proliferative retinopathy to the duration of diabetes in the WESDR population is presented in Figs 56.4 and 56.5. None of the younger-onset, insulin-taking participants in the study who had less than 5 years duration at the baseline examination developed proliferative diabetic retinopathy over the 4-year follow-up period. Thereafter,

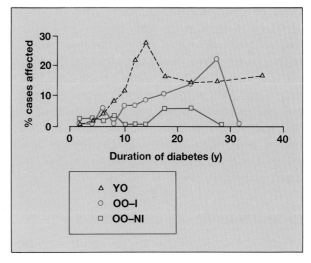

Fig. 56.5. Four-year incidence of proliferative retinopathy by duration of diabetes (in years) in younger-onset persons (YO, n=713), and older-onset persons taking insulin (OO−I, n=418) or not taking insulin (OO−NI, n=486) who participated in both baseline and follow-up examinations of the WESDR.

the incidence of proliferative retinopathy rose from 0.6% in younger-onset persons with 5−6 years of diabetes at the baseline examination to 27.9% in persons with 13−14 years of diabetes; after 15 or more years of diabetes, the incidence of proliferative retinopathy remained stable at 14−16%. For older-onset patients not taking insulin, some cases of proliferative retinopathy were found even in those with fewer than 2 years of diabetes at the baseline examination. Because of the possibility of developing proliferative retinopathy shortly after diagnosis of diabetes in this group,

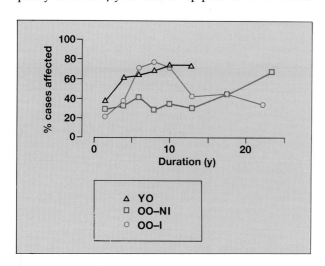

Fig. 56.4. Four-year incidence of any retinopathy by duration of diabetes in persons taking insulin who were diagnosed as diabetic before 30 years of age (YO, n=271) and older-onset persons taking insulin (OO−I, n=154) or not taking insulin (OO−NI, n=320) who participated in both baseline and follow-up examinations of the WESDR.

current guidelines for ophthalmological care for diabetic retinopathy should include careful ophthalmological examination at the time of diagnosis for *all* older-onset diabetic persons (i.e. those diagnosed after 30 years of age) followed by regular yearly (or more frequent) review, as determined by the findings on examination. The WESDR data suggest the need for careful ophthalmological examinations for younger-onset persons 5–9 years after the diagnosis of diabetes. After 10 years of diabetes, because of the increased incidence of proliferative diabetic retinopathy and clinically significant macular oedema, younger-onset patients should be examined on a yearly basis or more often, depending on the severity of the retinopathy present [24].

While incidence rates are significantly higher in the younger than the older-onset diabetic groups in the WESDR, the estimated number of incident cases of proliferative retinopathy (and of severe proliferative retinopathy with high risk for visual loss to 5/200 or worse) over a 4-year period is higher in the older compared with the younger-onset diabetic group (120 versus 83, estimated for a total population of persons living in the 11-county area of 839 000 in south-western Wisconsin). These data suggest that a greater burden will be imposed on the health care delivery system by the treatment of ocular complications developing in older-onset diabetic persons.

Ophthalmological care in the WESDR

The WESDR also provided an opportunity to evaluate ophthalmological care in the population [23]. In the WESDR, 22% of younger-onset diabetic people and 40% of older-onset diabetic patients had not seen an ophthalmologist. In addition, 11% of younger and 7% of older-onset people with high-risk characteristics for severe visual loss (as defined by the Diabetic Retinopathy Study) had never been seen by an ophthalmologist or were seen more than 2 years before the time of the study. These data suggest the need for further education of diabetic patients about the importance of periodic examinations by those experienced in evaluating the retina, and referral to retinal specialists or ophthalmologists interested in retinal disease, of all those individuals found to have either severe non-proliferative retinopathy, proliferative retinopathy and/or macular oedema, or decreased vision not correctable by refraction. This is important because patients with severe

retinopathy are often asymptomatic and timely treatment with pan-retinal photocoagulation and/or focal photocoagulation may prevent visual loss.

RONALD R. KLEIN

References

1 Pirart J. Diabetes mellitus and its degenerative complications: A prospective study of 4,400 patients observed between 1947 and 1973. *Diabetes Care* 1978; **1**: 168–88.
2 Krolewski AS, Warram JH, Rand LI *et al*. Risk of proliferative diabetic retinopathy in juvenile-onset Type I diabetes: A 40-year follow-up study. *Diabetes Care* 1986; **9**: 443–52.
3 Klein BEK, Davis MD, Segal P *et al*. Diabetic retinopathy: Assessment of severity and progression. *Ophthalmology* 1984; **91**: 10–17.
4 Miki E, Fukuda M, Kuzuya T *et al*. Relation of the course of retinopathy to control of diabetes, age, and therapeutic agents in diabetic Japanese patients. *Diabetes* 1969; **18**: 773–80.
5 University Group Diabetes Program. A study of the effects of hypoglycemic agents on vascular complications in patients with adult-onset diabetes. *Diabetes* 1982; **5** (suppl 31): 1–81.
6 Klein R, Klein BEK, Moss SE *et al*. The Wisconsin Epidemiologic Study of Diabetic Retinopathy: II. Prevalence and risk of diabetic retinopathy when age at diagnosis is less than 30 years. *Arch Ophthalmol* 1984; **102**: 520–6.
7 Klein R, Klein BEK, Moss SE *et al*. Wisconsin Epidemiologic Study of Diabetic Retinopathy: III. Prevalence and risk of diabetic retinopathy when age at diagnosis is 30 or more years. *Arch Ophthalmol* 1984; **102**: 527–32.
8 Klein R, Klein BEK, Moss SE *et al*. The Wisconsin Epidemiologic Study of Diabetic Retinopathy: IX. Four-year incidence and progression of diabetic retinopathy when age at diagnosis is less than 30 years. *Arch Ophthalmol* 1989; **107**: 237–43.
9 Klein R, Klein BEK *et al*. The Wisconsin Epidemiologic Study of Diabetic Retinopathy: X. Four-year incidence and progression of diabetic retinopathy when age at diagnosis is 30 or more years. *Arch Ophthalmol* 1989; **107**: 244–9.
10 Nilsson SE, Nilsson JE, Frostberg N *et al*. The Kristianstad Survey II. *Acta Med Scand* 1967; **469** (suppl): 1–42.
11 Dorf A, Ballintine EJ, Bennett PH *et al*. Retinopathy in Pima Indians. Relationships to glucose level, duration of diabetes, age at diagnosis of diabetes, and age at examination in a population with a high prevalence of diabetes mellitus. *Diabetes* 1976; **25**: 554–60.
12 Leibowitz HM, Krueger DE, Maunder LR *et al*. The Framingham Eye Study monograph. *Survey Ophthalmol* 1980; **24**: 335–610.
13 West KM, Erdreich LJ, Stober JA *et al*. A detailed study of risk factors for retinopathy and nephropathy in diabetes. *Diabetes* 1980; **19**: 501–8.
14 Houston A. Retinopathy in the Poole area: An epidemiological inquiry. In: Eschwege E, ed. *Advances in Diabetes Epidemiology*. INSERM Symposium No 22. Amsterdam: Elsevier Biomedical Press, 1982: 199–206.
15 King H, Balkau B, Zimmet P *et al*. Diabetic retinopathy in Nauruans. *Am J Epidemiol* 1983; **117**: 659–67.
16 Dwyer MS, Melton LJ, Ballard DJ *et al*. Incidence of diabetic

retinopathy and blindness: A population-based study in Rochester, Minnesota. *Diabetes Care* 1985; **8**: 316–22.

17 Sjolie AK. Ocular complications in insulin treated diabetes mellitus. An epidemiological study. *Acta Ophthalmol* 1985; **172** (suppl): 1–72.

18 Nielsen NV. Diabetic retinopathy. I. The course of retinopathy in insulin-treated diabetics. A one-year epidemiological cohort study of diabetes mellitus. The island of Falster, Denmark. *Acta Ophthalmol* 1984; **62**: 256–65.

19 Nielsen NV. Diabetic retinopathy. II. The course of retinopathy in diabetics treated with oral hypoglycaemic agents and diet regime alone. A one-year epidemiological cohort study of diabetes mellitus. The island of Falster, Denmark. *Acta Ophthalmol* 1984; **62**: 266–73.

20 Teuscher A, Schnell H, Wilson PWF *et al*. Incidence of diabetic retinopathy and relationship to baseline plasma glucose and blood pressure. *Diabetes Care* 1988; **11**: 246–51.

21 Early Treatment Diabetic Retinopathy Study Research Group. Photocoagulation of diabetic macular edema. *Arch Ophthalmol* 1985; **103**: 1796–1806.

22 Klein R, Klein BEK, Moss SE *et al*. The Wisconsin Epidemiologic Study of Diabetic Retinopathy. IV. Diabetic macular edema. *Ophthalmology* 1984; **91**: 1464–74.

23 Diabetic Retinopathy Study Group. Photocoagulation treatment of proliferative diabetic retinopathy: clinical application of Diabetic Retinopathy Study (DRS) findings (DRS Report No 8). *Ophthalmology* 1981; **88**: 583–600.

24 Klein R, Moss SE, Klein BEK. New management concepts for timely diagnosis of diabetic retinopathy treatable by photocoagulation. *Diabetes Care* 1987; **10**: 633–8.

25 Witkin SR, Klein R. Ophthalmologic care for persons with diabetes. *J Am Med Assoc* 1984; **251**: 2534–7.

57   The Pathogenesis of Diabetic Retinopathy and Cataract

Summary

• The earliest lesions of diabetic retinopathy, detectable histologically, are thickening of the capillary basement membrane and loss of pericytes which may have a contractile function.

• Capillary dilatation is the first abnormality recognizable on fluorescein angiography and is probably partly functional (secondary to increased retinal blood flow) and partly due to true anatomical widening of the vessel; dilatation is most marked in areas of pericyte fallout. Microaneurysms are localized capillary dilatations; they may give rise to haemorrhages or exudates.

• Capillary leakage of plasma lipids and proteins is probably due to a functional increase in permeability across the cells in early stages. Interruption of the tight junctions may occur later.

• Increased polyol pathway activity in pericytes (which contain aldose reductase, the pathway's rate-limiting enzyme) generates sorbitol under hyperglycaemic conditions. Accumulation of sorbitol, or of other polyols in galactosaemic animals, is associated with basement membrane thickening and pericyte loss; associated abnormalities such as myoinositol depletion and reduced Na^+-K^+ ATPase activity may also contribute.

• Aldose reductase inhibitors can prevent certain early features of galactosaemic retinopathy in animals but so far have no proven benefit in man, possibly because treatment is not started early enough in the course of retinopathy.

• Vascular occlusion, initially of capillaries and later of arteries and veins, leads to non-perfusion of areas of retina. Large ischaemic areas are the stimulus to new vessel formation.

Vascular occlusion may be due to microthrombi; the possible contributions of increased platelet aggregability, coagulation factor activity and endothelial damage are uncertain. Treatment with drugs which prevent platelet aggregation has only a small beneficial effect in reducing microaneurysm formation.

• Neovascularization begins with dissolution of extracellular matrix and proliferation of vascular cells into a solid cord which later canalizes. New vessel growth may be stimulated by factors such as retina-derived growth factor (fibroblast growth factor) which is produced locally, and insulin-like growth factor-1 (IGF-1) which is produced in the liver under the influence of growth hormone. Various factors which inhibit neovascularization are also released by the retina.

• Retinal blood flow is increased in untreated or poorly controlled diabetes and may damage endothelial cells. Retinal blood flow is reduced by correcting hyperglycaemia; an acute and profound glycaemic fall may cause retinal ischaemia and a deterioration in retinopathy.

• The presence of diabetes accelerates the development of senile cataracts, by two- to three-fold in patients in their 50s and 60s. 'Juvenile' cataracts with a snowflake appearance may be precipitated acutely by a period of poor metabolic control.

• The maintenance of lens shape and transparency depends on active metabolism by the lens epithelium, which contains aldose reductase and therefore accumulates sorbitol under high glucose concentrations. Sorbitol accumulation, myoinositol depletion or other associated factors may contribute to cataract formation.

• Non-enzymatic glycation of the lens protein,

crystallin, could also interfere with light transmission by forming disulphide-linked aggregates.

Diabetic retinopathy is a long-term sequel or complication of diabetes. While the exact cause of the abnormalities seen is not known, in recent years a considerable amount of work has been done to unravel the sequence of events which finally lead to sight-threatening forms of the disease. The three principal abnormalities are capillary occlusion, leakage (usually associated with vascular dilatation), and finally new vessel formation. This last event only occurs when, in addition to the capillaries, larger vessels, both arteries and veins, are also occluded. When considering pathogenic mechanisms in the evolution of diabetic retinopathy, these three steps, which are not independent from one another, have to be explained.

Structure of the capillary wall

Throughout the vascular network, the capillaries have two types of cells in their wall, endothelial cells and pericytes. In most tissues the number of endothelial cells is far larger than that of the pericytes, and only in the retina is there a one-to-one relationship between the two. This is important because it has been shown that, the higher the number of pericytes in relation to the number of endothelial cells, the slower is the turnover of the cells under normal conditions [1]. The endothelial cells in the retina are also different from other vascular cells in the body (with the exception of the brain endothelial cells) in that they have tight junctions between adjacent cells, zonae occludentes, which under normal circumstances prevent leakage of certain substances such as sodium fluorescein and horseradish peroxidase from the intravascular to the extravascular space.

The endothelial cells have many functions, and these have recently been surveyed by Petty and Pearson [2]. They include both thrombotic and anticoagulant, fibrinolytic, antiplatelet and immunological properties, secretion of basement membrane, production of growth factors and vasoactive properties. In addition, the cells, together with the basement membrane, are responsible for the permeability of the capillaries.

The function of the pericytes is less clear. In the 1960s, Cogan and Kuwabara developed the technique of the retinal digest preparation [3]. This enabled the study of the vasculature of the retina without interference from neuronal elements. These authors noted the selective loss of pericytes in the diabetic retina [4], and observed a number of other changes, such as dilatation of some capillaries, while others lost their endothelial cells and became simple basement membrane tubes. Earlier work by Ashton [5] using Indian ink injection, showed that there were large areas of nonperfused retina in diabetes, these areas being the acellular capillaries demonstrated by Cogan and Kuwabara. Because of the changes noted, in particular the dilatation of some capillaries without pericytes in their wall, Cogan and Kuwabara suggested that the pericytes may have a muscle cell-like action on the capillaries, controlling their diameter. They also suggested that some capillaries may become occluded because these dilated vessels act as shunt vessels, diverting blood away from the capillaries. Kohner et al. [6] demonstrated that only rarely did dilated vessels act as true shunts, in the sense of high-flow, low-resistance channels. However, recent work supports the muscle cell-like activity of pericytes. In most vascular systems, smooth muscles control vascular tone. In the retinal vessels, there are relatively few muscle cells. Endothelin, a recently isolated vasoactive peptide [7], is secreted by endothelial cells and acts on smooth muscle cells causing vascular constriction. Though initially thought to be absent in brain, and by inference in retinal vessels [8], this has not subsequently proved to be the case. The Hammersmith Hospital group found that bovine retinal endothelial cells, but not pericytes, secreted endothelin in vitro and that the receptors normally found on smooth muscle cells were on pericytes [9]. Thus, pericytes may well control small vessel tone in the retina.

The controlling role of the pericytes on endothelial cells was demonstrated in elegant co-culture studies by Orlidge and D'Amore [10]. These workers were able to demonstrate that pericytes and smooth muscle cells grown in co-cultures allowing cell-to-cell contact with endothelial cells inhibited endothelial cell growth and multiplication. In the absence of contact, but with free access of diffusible factors, this inhibition was absent. Other cells such as epithelial cells, fibroblasts and 3T3 cells did not have this effect. Further work by the same group identified the inhibiting factor as activated transforming growth factor β (TGF-β). Purified antibodies to TGF-β added to the co-culture abolished the inhibitory effect on cell growth [11]. We still do not know whether the TGF-β is produced by the endothelial cells and then activated by the pericytes, or whether pericytes produce TGF-β.

This recent work indicates why the capillaries could become abnormal when pericytes are lost. The exact cause of the pericyte damage, and indeed of the damage to endothelial cells, has not been fully established.

Metabolic causes of damage to endothelial cells and pericytes

Since pericyte loss is the earliest abnormality seen in histological preparations of the diabetic retina (with perhaps the exception of basement membrane thickening), it is important to explain this abnormality. Until recently, there were no good explanations, but in 1977 Buzney et al. demonstrated in cell culture work the presence of the polyol pathway in pericytes [12]. In 1984, Engerman and Kern [13] reported that dogs fed a high galactose diet developed a diabetic-like retinopathy, consisting of pericyte loss, micro-aneurysms and acellular capillaries. In galactosaemia, the galactose is converted by aldose reductase to dulcitol. This substance then accumulates in cells which contain aldose reductase. This finding led to a large amount of work by many investigators, mainly those of the National Eye Institute, and the St. Louis group. Williamson's group, in elegant studies, showed that thickening of basement membrane in both BB and streptozotocin-induced diabetic rats could be inhibited by aldose reductase inhibitors [14]. Increased basement membrane production is probably more related to an endothelial cell abnormality than abnormal pericyte function, but Li et al. [15] showed in cell culture work of bovine retinal pericytes, that in high glucose medium more basement membrane collagen was produced. Williamson's group [16] also showed decreased degradation of type IV collagen in basement membrane in renal glomeruli of diabetic rats. The fact that rats fed a galactose-rich diet develop increased basement membrane thickening and that this can be prevented by aldose reductase inhibitors has been shown by various observers [17−19]. It again suggests that the basement membrane excess comes from pericytes rather than endothelial cells, as there is no evidence that the polyol pathway plays an important role in the

endothelial cells. Although most workers have not found aldose reductase in endothelial cells of the retina, a notable exception is the work of Chakrabati et al. [20] who found aldose reductase in the retinal endothelial cells of BB rats.

Kinoshita's group has shown recently that there is not only basement membrane thickening in galactosaemic rats, but also formation of micro-aneurysms, and this too is prevented by aldose reductase inhibitors [21]. Kador et al. have performed most interesting experiments; they used galactosaemic dogs, and randomly allocated them to galactose only or to galactose and an aldose reductase inhibitor. They found that micro-aneurysms were seen after 3 to 6 months in those on the high galactose diet, but this was prevented by aldose reductase inhibitors. In particular, they noted that pericyte loss did not occur in the first several months in animals fed with the inhibitors as well as the high galactose. However, at 32 months high galactose feeding resulted in at least some microaneurysms, even in those on aldose reductase inhibitors [22]. Unfortunately, the experiments were not continued after 36 months, and therefore the long-term effect of aldose reductase inhibitors cannot be certain, even in the galactosaemic animals. Engerman, whose experiments were of longer duration, and who also studied diabetic animals receiving aldose reductase inhibitors, did not find the dramatic effects seen by Kador [23]. It appears that most of the lesions only appear after about 42 months. In addition, human studies with the aldose reductase inhibitor sorbinils in some 600 diabetic patients with minimal or no retinopathy have not yet produced any striking results. The work of Kador suggests that studies in humans with diabetes of some years duration may be non-productive because by then many of the pericytes are lost, and thus the disease is probably self-perpetuating. Indeed, a study to show the effectiveness of aldose reductase inhibitors would have to start when diabetes was diagnosed.

How the polyol pathway is involved in pericyte damage is not completely clear. It is unlikely to be the accumulation of sorbitol itself (although in galactosaemic animals dulcitol accumulation may be harmful); it could be a consequence of the associated reduction in myoinositol or the reduced Na^+-K^+ ATP-ase activity which damages cells [24, 25].

Retinal endothelial cells are probably not directly affected by the polyol pathway, as aldose reductase has not been found in these cells by most observers. Endothelial cells of larger vessels may contain this enzyme, as the Newcastle group [26] found it in umbilical vein endothelial cells. Even in the absence of aldose reductase, high glucose concentrations may nevertheless affect endothelial cell function, as suggested by the work of Lorenzi et al. [27], who found reduced cell replication and increased cell death of cultured umbilical vein endothelial cells in a high glucose medium. Prolonged exposure of these cultured cells also resulted in changes in the DNA which manifested an accelerated rate of unwinding in alkali, suggestive of an increased number of single-strand breaks [28]. Such changes have not yet been demonstrated in retinal endothelial cells. Damage may also occur if there is interference with the controlling influence of pericytes. This could of course occur simply by increased basement membrane thickening, which interrupts cell-to-cell interaction between endothelial cells and pericytes.

Although these metabolic abnormalities can explain many of the features of endothelial cell damage in diabetes, changes in blood flow may also be involved.

Haemodynamic changes in diabetic retinopathy

In early and uncontrolled diabetes, blood flow in the retina is probably increased [27–29]. Experimental work by Atherton et al. [30] suggested that high blood glucose levels (approximately 26 mmol/l), achieved by bolus injection in experimental animals, increased blood flow significantly. Recent studies by Sullivan et al. (unpublished observations), using laser Doppler velocimetry (LDV) for blood flow measurement in miniature swine, demonstrated that a gradual rise in blood glucose concentrations caused an even bigger rise in blood flow already noticeable at 17 mmol/l. Reducing the glucose to hypoglycaemic levels also caused an increase in blood flow [31]. This latter finding was somewhat unexpected. Though, on the one hand nerve tissue needs glucose for metabolism (and if this is reduced, autoregulation would be expected to cause a compensatory increase in blood flow) on the other hand Grunwald and co-workers [32] noted that in NIDDM patients with poor control normalization of glucose over a 2 hour period reduced blood flow, and at the same time improved vessel reactivity to oxygen. Using the blue light entoptic technique, Fallon et al. found that in diabetic

patients with early retinopathy blood flow was increased compared with normal controls [33], and this has recently been confirmed by work from the Joslin Clinic [34]. Thus, increases in blood flow occur in diabetes at high and at very low glucose levels, and at these levels the flow may be associated with reduced vascular reactivity. The blood flow changes noted by Kohner et al. [29], and those seen in experimental animals are of sufficient magnitude to damage the vascular endothelium [35]. It is not only the increased blood flow, but also the frequent changes in flow which may cause much of the damage. Once retinopathy is present, flow in the peripheral retina is probably reduced [35] as a result of the reduced capillary bed, and this serves to maintain blood flow in the functionally more important central, perifoveal retina. Only when there are large areas of capillary non-perfusion, as seen in preproliferative and proliferative diabetic retinopathy, is there significant reduction in the perifoveal blood flow [33]. Diabetic control is often improved in patients when they become aware of the presence of retinopathy, and in studies with continuous subcutaneous insulin infusion (CSII) this was also achieved [36–38]. By this time there is already significant vascular damage, and reduction of blood flow may actually worsen retinopathy, as was seen in these studies. The lesions noted to deteriorate were microaneurysms, haemorrhages and cotton wool spots, all indicative of increasing ischaemia. Indeed, the work of Sleightholm et al. (unpublished observations), also using the blue light entoptic technique, showed that retinopathy did not deteriorate in those patients in whom blood flow increased during the first week following CSII.

Thus, endothelial cells could be damaged by the increased blood flow through them, which could be due to abnormal glucose levels initially, but also to reduced peripheral resistance in dilated capillaries when pericytes are lost. Damage to the endothelial cells is always present when there is capillary occlusion.

Capillary dilatation and leakage

Capillary dilatation is an early manifestation of diabetic retinopathy. Vink found this to be the earliest feature recognizable on fluorescein angiograms [39]. Work by Sosula in diabetic rats [40] confirmed that dilatation did indeed occur early, that the endothelial cells were not flattened, while the vessel diameter was increased, suggesting true dilatation with anatomical changes. Even before there are anatomical alterations, the increased blood flow associated with high glucose could cause capillary dilatation of a functional nature in patients. As noted by Kuwabara and Cogan [3, 4], capillary dilatation occurs when there is loss of pericytes, but it could occur before if the pericyte control over the endothelial cells is lost. Thickening of the basement membrane, another early manifestation of retinopathy, could interfere with cell-to-cell contact between pericytes and endothelial cells, and thus endothelial cells may lose the controlling influence of the pericytes. Transient leakage can occasionally be seen at this early stage in diabetic patients investigated with fluorescein angiograms. This leakage is probably also functional, and indicates transfer of fluorescein through endothelial cells into the extracellular space.

That leakage is initially functional is suggested by the work of Parving et al. [41], who showed that in diabetic patients with mild hypertension, the normal or only slightly increased leakage, as measured by vitreous fluorophotometry, could be reduced by an angiotensin-converting enzyme (ACE) inhibitor. Parving proposed that this was due to the reduced intravascular pressure, but it could also be due to an effect of the drug on the endothelial cells, since these produce angiotensin converting enzyme. A direct effect on the endothelial cells is suggested by the fact that ACE inhibitors are therapeutically useful in idiopathic peripheral oedema.

Later, after long-standing disease, there is damage to the tight junctions between endothelial cells, at least in diabetic dogs [42], and this will allow free escape of fluorescein. New vessels invariably leak fluorescein, and this may indicate that tight junctions are missing at the time of active growth of vessels, though fenestrated junctions were only rarely seen in new vessels of fibrovascular membranes removed at vitrectomy [43].

The leakage seen in diabetic maculopathy is almost invariably associated with dilated vessels, and this dilatation is also associated with loss of some capillaries. It has not been established whether the leakage is across the cells or between them.

Vascular occlusion

The causes of capillary occlusion have not yet been established. The most plausible explanation remains the more active haemostasis and platelet coagulation of the blood of patients with retinopathy. The formation of microthrombi could be facilitated by the reduced fibrinolytic and antithrombin activities of the vessel wall, a direct result of the endothelial cell damage, consequent on increased blood flow and altered physical properties of the blood, such as increased viscosity and reduced red cell deformability.

Recent work, however, has questioned whether platelets are hyperactive in patients with diabetic complications. Alessandrini et al. [44] measured the levels of urinary 2,3-dinor metabolites of thromboxane A2, the major promoter, and prostacyclin, the major inhibitor, of platelet aggregation. No differences were found between normal controls and diabetic patients with or without retinopathy. Other widely used in vitro and in vivo indicators of platelet function also failed to discriminate between these groups. The measurement of 2,3-dinor metabolites appears to be more reliable than previous methods, overcoming the problems of cross-reactivity with other prostaglandins present in higher quantities in the plasma. By suggesting that the thromboxane/prostacyclin balance is not altered in diabetic retinopathy, these results fail to support the hypothesis that platelets are involved in capillary plugging in the retina, or elsewhere. Further negative evidence derives from the observed normal survival of ^{111}In-labelled platelets in patients with retinopathy [45], confirming earlier reports from the Hammersmith Hospital [46].

There is no uniform agreement about the role of platelets in diabetic retinopathy, but there are several reports of abnormal in vitro behaviour of platelets. In trying to identify the abnormality Watanabe et al. [47] reported that LDL isolated from patients with IDDM significantly potentiates platelet aggregation induced by thrombin, and that this activity correlates directly with the degree of LDL glycosylation in vivo. LDL glycosylated in vitro enhances thrombin-, collagen- and ADP-induced platelet aggregation. Platelets exhibit higher uptake for glycosylated rather than native LDL and this may lead to alteration of their membrane lipid composition in poorly controlled diabetes. Insulin, on the other hand, may modify platelet membranes so as to decrease aggregability, as observed in the course of clamp studies at steady-state levels as low as 40 mU/l [48]. Other mechanisms suggested to account for *in vitro* platelet hyperactivity include an increased content of histamine [49], increased Ca^{++} influx [50], potentiation by catecholamines released during hypoglycaemia [51], and reduced vitamin E content. This last observation was originally reported by Karpen *et al.* [52], and led to trials of vitamin E supplements. Normalization of thromboxane A2 production by platelets in response to ADP and collagen *in vitro* was reported by Gisinger *et al.* [53], after 4 weeks of treatment with 400 mg/day tocopherol acetate and by Colette *et al.* [54] after 5 weeks on the rather large dose of 1 g daily.

Thus, platelet abnormalities in diabetic retinopathy are more evident *in vitro* than *in vivo*. One way of ascertaining whether such changes are indeed relevant to the pathogenesis of diabetic retinopathy is by randomized controlled clinical trials where antiaggregating agents and placebo are administered and the effects on disease progression studied. The result of one major trial of aspirin alone, aspirin together with dipyridamole and placebo was reported recently by the DAMAD study group [55]. This study showed that aspirin alone or in conjunction with dipyridamole significantly (though marginally) reduced the formation of new microaneurysms in early background retinopathy.

The main problem remains the relevance of phenomena observed *in vitro* to the situation in life. Most tests look at platelet function either indirectly or under highly artificial experimental conditions, such as during anti-coagulation and after separation of platelets from red and white cells. This alone makes it difficult to translate observations into general pathogenic terms. In addition, patient selection and laboratory techniques are not standardized, contributing to the heterogeneity of reports in the literature. Major doubts still remain as to whether platelets play a significant role in the vascular occlusion of diabetic retinopathy.

New vessel formation

New vessel formation is not unique to diabetic retinopathy; it occurs in several conditions where there is widespread vascular occlusion which is not sufficient to cause total death of the retina. Thus, it is seen in sickle cell disease, retinal vas-

culitis and retinal vein occlusion. In all these conditions, as in diabetes, occlusion of arterioles and venules, as well as capillaries, occurs before the new vessels develop.

The steps in the development of new vessels are: first, dissolution of extracellular matrix, followed by cellular migration and proliferation, and finally the formation of a vascular lumen. Proteoglycans secreted by endothelial cells cause dissolution of the basement membrane, which allows migration of endothelial cells. The first suggestion that a retina-derived angiogenic factor was produced to initiate and promote these changes came from Michaelson [56] as long ago as 1948. But only in the last few years have real advances been made in the isolation of several growth-promoting and -inhibiting substances. Retina-derived angiogenic factor [57] and retina-derived growth factor [58] have been found to be homologous to fibroblast growth factor (FGF), which exists in two closely related forms, acidic and basic FGF [59]. Basic FGF (bFGF) is widely distributed and endothelial cells from brain and adrenal cortex have been shown to express the bFGF gene. bFGF is produced by the endothelial cells and is stored in the extracellular matrix, from where it is released at the time of cell death [59].

Herman and D'Amore have shown that retina-derived growth factor, by implication FGF, has the ability of transforming endothelial cells from a stationary to a motile spindle shape [60]. FGF also stimulates cell proliferation [61]. There are other angiogenic substances, insulin-like growth factor-1 (IGF-1) being a prime candidate, especially, as this substance has been found in the vitreous of patients with proliferative retinopathy [62]. The pigment epithelium also induces growth promotion under certain circumstances [63]. In health, there is a balance between the growth-promoting and growth-inhibiting substances produced by endothelial cells and pigment epithelium [62, 63], and it is this balance which is upset at the time of new vessel growth.

Among the many regulatory peptides, growth hormone (GH) is the one which has been most implicated in retinal neovascularization. Following a case report by Poulsen in 1953 [64] reporting regression of retinopathy following postpartum pituitary haemorrhage, hypophysectomy came to be used for the treatment of proliferative diabetic retinopathy. Long-term follow-up of patients treated with yttrium-90 implantation was reported by Sharp *et al.* [65]. This showed a dramatic regression and cessation of new vessel growth of the optic disc, and by 10 years there was no disc neovascularization in any eye. Since the benefits of pituitary destruction were related to the degree of GH deficiency [66, 67] it was reasonable to suggest that GH had some influence on the neo-vascular process. As GH acts through IGF-1 this latter peptide has become of paramount interest. It was, therefore, suprising that patients with dia-betes had no higher IGF-1 levels than normals, and even patients with proliferative retinopathy had levels in the normal range [68]. This could be due in part to the fact that lower levels of IGF-1 are produced in poorly controlled diabetic children in response to a standard dose of GH than in those with better control [69]. Since insulin regulates the expression of hepatic GH receptors in more severe diabetes, there may be reduction in these receptors [70]. That IGF-1 could be of importance, at least in the proliferative stage of diabetic retinopathy, has been suggested by Merimee et al. [71], who found increased levels of IGF-1 in those patients with rapidly advancing 'florid' retinopathy. Recently, Hyer et al. [72] reported on a longitudinal study of patients with preproliferative diabetic retinopathy, and found that these patients had IGF-1 levels in the normal range. During the period of follow-up, eight of the patients developed active vascular prolifer-ation. At the time of active neovascularization, IGF-1 levels rose in these patients, though they still remained in the normal range. The elevation of IGF-1 was restricted to these eight patients, and it returned to normal soon after effective photocoagulation. This fact, together with the finding that following photocoagulation patients with retinopathy have lower than normal IGF-1 levels [72], suggests the possibility that IGF-1 is produced in the retina. Indeed, IGF-1 receptors have been found by King et al. [73] in both cultured retinal endothelial cells and pericytes.

In summary, it appears that the neovascular process starts with loss of the pericyte–endothelial cell interaction, allowing proliferation of the endothelial cells. This leads to vascular dilatation and increased retinal blood flow which is also stimulated by the high glucose levels. Metabolic changes and sheer stress damage endothelial cells, and endothelial–platelet interaction, together with decreased fibrinolytic activity, leads to vascular occlusion. Cell death releases FGF and imbalance between inhibitory and stimulatory factors results in neovascularization.

Although many details in the neovascular process are still not known, and the interrelation-ships between the factors produced by retinal endothelial and other cells are uncertain, the picture is gradually becoming clearer, and it is hoped that a full understanding of all the pro-cesses is not too far away.

Pathogenesis of cataract in diabetes

Diabetes is undoubtedly a significant risk factor for the development of cataracts [74–78]. In the Framingham Eye Study [74–76], senile lens change was consistently commoner in diabetic than in non-diabetic subjects up to the age of 69 years and other reports have shown an increased fre-quency of senile cataract in diabetic patients in their 40s and a two- to three-fold increase in patients in their 50s and 60s. Beyond the age of 69 years, however, there is little increased risk [74–78]. Overall, the available epidemiological data strongly suggest that the presence of diabetes ac-celerates the development of senile cataracts in man.

In addition, typical diabetic cataracts with a characteristic 'snowflake' appearance have long been recognized, particularly in adolescents with poor diabetic control. They are rarely seen today.

Lens metabolism

The lens retains its shape and transparency by virtue of active metabolic processes. Nutrients and oxygen required for metabolism are taken up from the aqueous humour across a single-cell layer of cuboidal epithelial cells which maintain the ionic equilibrium within the lens [79]. These cells derive energy from glucose metabolism, mainly through anaerobic glycolysis. Control of lens glycolysis, which must be precisely regulated to avoid excess-ive lactate production, apparently depends on two enzymes, phosphofructokinase and hexokinase. Phosphofructokinase activity is regulated by ATP availability and hexokinase by the level of its product, glucose-6-phosphate [80]. At physiologi-cal glucose levels, both enzymes are saturated. Raising the glucose concentration in blood or aqueous humour does not, therefore, lead to in-creased glycolytic activity [81] and intracellular glucose levels will tend to rise. Excess glucose within the lens is metabolized by the hexose monophosphate shunt or, more importantly, by the polyol pathway which is made possible by the presence of aldose reductase in the lens epithelium. The low activities of glycolytic enzymes and polyol (sorbitol) dehydrogenase in lens epithelium also favour sorbitol accumulation during exposure to high glucose levels [82] (see Chapter 54).

THE POLYOL PATHWAY AND CATARACT FORMATION IN EXPERIMENTAL DIABETES

Polyol pathway activity has been implicated in cataract formation in animals. Those species with high lenticular aldose reductase activity (such as the Mongolian gerbil, the degu and the rat) develop cataracts when diabetes is induced using streptozotocin or alloxan; the cataracts develop faster if the hyperglycaemia is more severe and the animals are young [83–85]. Sorbitol accumulation in the lens can be demonstrated in these models [86]. Similar cataracts can also be induced in these species by feeding diets with high contents (35%) of galactose or xylose which are converted by aldose reductase into their respective polyols, dulcitol and xylitol [86]. This suggests a common mechanism, namely accumulation of polyol within the lens. By contrast, in animals with absent or very low aldose reductase activity in the lens (e.g. CFW, db/db and ob/ob mice), cataract formation cannot be induced by either prolonged hyperglycaemia for up to six months or diets containing as much as 50% galactose [87, 88]. Polyol levels remain very low in the lenses of these animals.

Cell membranes are relatively impermeable to polyols and, once formed, these substances will accumulate, creating a hypertonic environment within the lens epithelium and lens fibres, which will attract water by osmosis. Opacification of the lens and cataract formation could result from secondary changes, such as loss of amino acids, myoinositol, and potassium ions due, in turn, to membrane damage associated with cellular swelling. Kinoshita's postulate that aldose reductase is pivotal in the pathogenesis of 'sugar cataract' [89] stimulated a search for inhibitors of the enzyme which might prevent this complication. Aldose reductase inhibitors have been reported to delay or prevent the onset of cataracts in diabetic and galactosaemic rats [90]. The effectiveness of these agents is critically dependent on the timing of their administration relative to the onset of galactose-feeding or induction of diabetes,

suggesting an effect on an early, reversible phase before membrane damage has occurred [91].

THE POLYOL PATHWAY AND THE HUMAN DIABETIC LENS

A direct correlation between plasma glucose concentration and the levels of sorbitol and fructose in the lenses of diabetic patients has been reported [92]. A further study has demonstrated a strong correlation between sorbitol levels in human cataracts and both fasting blood glucose and HbA_1 levels [93]. The reduction in phosphofructokinase activity which occurs in the human diabetic cataract [94] will result in less efficient clearing of accumulated sorbitol. As in animals, sorbitol accumulation is therefore apparently related to cataract formation, but its pathogenic role is uncertain. It also remains to be shown whether aldose reductase inhibitors will delay or prevent cataract formation in human diabetes. It is possible that such agents will need to be administered soon after the diagnosis of diabetes if they are to be effective, a stratagem which is difficult to justify in current clinical trials.

Non-enzymatic glycation of lens proteins

The soluble protein of the lens, crystallin, contained within the fibre cells, has a much slower turnover than other proteins in the body. As it ages, human lens crystallin undergoes various post-translational modifications including non-enzymatic glycation [95] (see Chapter 54). The extent of crystallin glycation in human diabetic lenses is reported to be 2–3%, about twice as high as in non-diabetic lenses [95]. In another study [96] glycation of lens cortical proteins but not of nuclear proteins was significantly higher in diabetic patients than in control subjects with senile cataracts. This implies that the lens nucleus is exposed to less metabolic variation than the lens cortex. Glycation has also been demonstrated in the human lens capsule and again was significantly greater in diabetic patients [97].

Glycation offers another possible mechanism for cataract formation. Changes in the tertiary structure of crystallin after glycation expose sulphydryl groups to oxidation, thus favouring the formation of disulphide-linked aggregates within the lens [98]. Such cross-linkages could form the basis of lens opacities and eventually cataract, although the available evidence is not sufficient to establish a definite link between the extent of lens protein glycation and the initiation of cataract formation. There is no evidence that non-enzymatic glycation is involved in the development of cataract in experimental animals fed on a high galactose diet [99].

Conclusions

These two postulated biochemical mechanisms of cataract formation — polyol pathway activity and non-enzymatic glycation of lens proteins — are not mutually exclusive. Prevention of this complication will probably require therapeutic intervention early in the natural history of the disease before irreversible damage has taken place.

EVA M. KOHNER
MASSIMO PORTA
STEPHEN L. HYER

References

1 Tilton RG, Miller EJ, Kilo C, Williamson JK. Pericyte form and distribution in rat retinal and uveal capillaries. *Invest Ophthalmol Vis Sci* 1985; **26**: 60–73.
2 Petty RG, Pearson JD. Endothelium — the axis of vascular health and disease. *J Roy Coll Physicians London* 1989; **23**: 92–102.
3 Cogan DG, Toussaint D, Kuwabara T. Retinal vascular patterns IV: diabetic retinopathy *Arch Ophthalmol* 1961; **60**: 100–12.
4 Kuwabara T, Cogan DG. Retinal vascular patterns VI. Mural cells of the retinal capillaries. *Arch Ophthalmol* 1963; **69**: 492–502a.
5 Ashton N. Injection of the retinal vascular system in enucleated eyes in diabetic retinopathy. *Br J Ophthalmol* 1950; **54**: 38–44.
6 Kohner EM, Dollery CT, Patterson JW, Oakley WN. Arterial fluorescein studies in diabetic retinopathy. *Diabetes* 1967; **16**: 1–10.
7 Yanagisawa M, Kurihara H, Kimura S et al. A novel potent vasoconstrictor peptide produced by vascular endothelial cells. *Nature* 1988; **332**: 411–15.
8 Yanagisawa M, Inoue A, Ishikawa T et al. Primary structure synthesis and biological activity of rat endothelin as endothelium derived vasoconstrictor peptide. *Proc Natl Acad Sci USA* 1988; **85**: 6964–7.
9 Takahashi K, Brooks RA, Kanse SM, Ghatei MA, Kohner EM, Bloom SR. Endothelin I is produced by cultured bovine retinal endothelial cells and endothelin receptors are present on the associated pericytes. *Diabetes* 1989; **38**: 1200–2.
10 Orlidge A, D'Amore PA. Inhibition of capillary endothelial cell growth by pericytes and smooth muscle cells. *J Cell Biol* 1987; **105**: 1455–62.
11 Antonelli-Orlidge A, Saunders KB, Smith SR, D'Amore P. An activated form of transforming growth factor β is produced by cocultures of endothelial cells and pericytes. *Proc Natl Acad Sci USA* 1989; **86**: 4544–8.
12 Buzney SM, Frank RN, Varma SD. Aldose reductase in retinal mural cells. *Invest Ophthalmol* 1977; **16**: 392–6.
13 Engerman RL, Kern TS. Experimental galactosemia produces a diabetic like retinopathy. *Diabetes* 1984; **33**: 97–100.
14 Williamson JR, Chang K, Tilton RG et al. Increased vascular permeability in spontaneously diabetic BB/W rats with mild versus severe streptozotocin induced diabetes: prevention by aldose reductase inhibitors and castration. *Diabetes* 1987; **36**: 813–21.
15 Li W, Shen S, Khatami M, Rochley JH. Stimulation of retinal capillary pericyte protein and collagen synthesis in culture by high glucose concentration. *Diabetes* 1984; **33**: 785–9.
16 Williamson JR, Kilo C. Extracellular matrix changes in diabetes mellitus. In: Scarpelli DG, Migaki G, eds., *Comparative Pathobiology of Major Age-related Disease.* New York: Alan R. Liss Inc., 1984, 269.
17 Robinson WG Jr, Kador PF, Kinoshita JH. Retinal capillaries: Basement membrane thickening by galactosemia prevented with aldose reductase inhibitors. *Science* 1983; **221**: 1177–9.
18 Lightman S, Rechthand E, Teruyabshi H, Palestine A, Rapaport S. Permeability changes in blood retinal barrier of galactosemic rats are prevented by aldose reductase inhibitors. *Diabetes* 1986; **36**: 1271–5.
19 Akagi Y, Yajima Y, Kador PF, Kuwabara T, Kinoshita JH. Localisation of aldose reductase in the human eye. *Diabetes* 1984; **33**: 562–6.
20 Chakrabati S, Sima AAF, Nakajima T, Yagihashi S, Green DA. Aldose reductase in the BB rat — isolation, immunological identification and localisation in the retina and peripheral nerve. *Diabetologia* 1987; **30**: 244–57.
21 Kador PF, Akagi Y, Terubayashi H, Nyman M, Kinoshita JH. Prevention of pericyte ghost formation in retinal capillaries of galactose fed dogs by aldose reductase inhibitors. *Invest Ophthalmol Vis Sci* 1988; **29** (suppl 1): 180.
22 Kador PF, Akagi Y, Ikebe H, Takahasi Y, Ymar M, Kinoshita SH. Prevention of retinal vessel changes associated with diabetic retinopathy in galactose fed dogs by aldose reductase inhibitor. *Invest Ophthalmol Vis Sci* 1989; **30** (suppl 1): 139.
23 Engerman RL, Kern TS. Retinal vasculature in sorbinil treated galactosaemic dogs. *Invest Ophthalmol Vis Sci* 1989; **30** (suppl 1): 139.
24 Greene DA, Lattimer SA, Sima AAF. Sorbitol, phosphoinositides, and sodium-potassium ATP-ase in the pathogenesis of diabetic complications. *N Engl J Med* 1987; **316**: 559–606.
25 MacGregor LC, Matschinsky FM. Treatment with aldose reductase inhibitor of myoinositol arrests deterioration of the electroretinogram of diabetic rats. *J Clin Invest* 1985; **24**: 1250–8.
26 Hawthorne GC, Bartlett K, Hetherington CS, Alberti KGMM. The effect of high glucose on polyol pathway activity and myoinositol mechanism in cultured human endothelial cells. *Diabetologia* 1989; **32**: 163–6.
27 Lorenzi M, Cagliero E, Toledo S. Glucose toxicity for human endothelial cells in culture. *Diabetes* 1985; **34**: 621–3.
28 Lorenzi M, Montisano DF, Toledo S, Barrieux A. High glucose induces DNA damage in cultured human endothelial cells. *J Clin Invest* 1986; **77**: 322–5.
29 Kohner EM. The problems of retinal blood flow in diabetes. *Diabetes* 1976; **25** (suppl 2): 839–44.
30 Atherton A, Hill DW, Keen H, Young S, Edwards EJ. The effect of acute hyperglycaemia on the retinal circulation of the normal cat. *Diabetologia* 1980; **18**: 233–7.

31 Caldwell G, Davies EG, Sullivan P, Morris A, Kohner EM. The effect of hypoglycaemia on retinal blood flow measured by the laser doppler velocimeter. (Submitted for publication).

32 Grunwald JE, Riva CE, Martin DB, Quint AR, Epstein PA. Effect of an insulin induced decrease in blood glucose on the human diabetic retinal circulation. *Ophthalmology* 1987; **94**: 1614–20.

33 Fallon TJ, Chowiencyzk P, Kohner EM. Measurement of retinal blood flow in diabetes by the blue light entoptic phenomenon. *Br J Ophthalmol* 1986; **70**: 43–6.

34 McMillan DE. Rheological and related factors in diabetic retinopathy. In: Kohner EM, ed., *International Ophthalmology Clinics*. Boston: Little, Brown and Co, 1978, 35.

35 Grunwald JE, Riva CE, Sinclair SH, Bruckner SJ, Petrig BL. Laser doppler velocimetry study of retinal circulation in diabetes mellitus. *Arch Ophthalmol* 1986; **104**: 991–6.

36 Lauritzen T, Frost Larson K, Larson HW, Deckert T, the Steno Study Group. Effect of 1 year of near normal blood glucose levels on retinopathy in insulin dependent diabetics. *Lancet* 1983; i: 200–4.

37 The KROC Collaborative Study Group. Blood glucose control and the evolution of diabetic retinopathy and albuminuria. *N Engl J Med* 1984; **311**: 365–72.

38 Ballegooie van E, Hooymans J, Timmerman Z, Reitsma W, Sluiter WJ, Schweitzer NMJ, Doorenbas H. Rapid deterioration of diabetic retinopathy during treatment with continuous subcutaneous insulin infusion. *Diabetes Care* 1984, **7**: 236–43.

39 Oosterhuis JA, Vink R. Fluorescein photography in diabetic retinopathy. *Perspectives in Ophthalmol Excerpta Medica Fed.* 1967; **186**: 115–32.

40 Sosula L, Beaumont P, Hollows FC, Jonson KM. Dilatation and endothelial proliferation of retinal capillaries in streptozotocin-diabetic rats: quantitative electron microscopy. *Invest Ophthalmol* 1972; **11**: 926–35.

41 Parving HH, Larson M, Hommel E, Lund-Anderson H. Effect of antihypertensive treatment on blood retinal permeability to fluorescein in hypertensive type I diabetic patients with background retinopathy (in press).

42 Wallow IHL, Engerman RL. Permeability and patency of retinal blood vessels in experimental diabetes. *Invest Ophthalmol Vis Sci* 1977; **16**: 447–54.

43 Williams JM, de Juan E, Machemer R. Intrastructural characteristics of new vessels in proliferative diabetic retinopathy. *Am J Ophthalmol* 1988; **105**: 491–9.

44 Alessandrini P, McRae J, Feman S, Fitzgerald GA. Thromboxane biosynthesis and platelet function in diabetes mellitus. *N Engl J Med* 1988; **319**: 208–12.

45 Luikens B, Forstrom LA, Johnson T, Johnson G. Indium-111 platelet kinetics in patients with diabetes mellitus. *Nucl Med Comm* 1988; **9**: 223–34.

46 Porta M, Peters AM, Cousins SA, Cagliero E, Fitzpatrick ML, Kohner EM. A study of platelet-relevant parameters in patients with diabetic microangiopathy. *Diabetologia* 1983; **25**: 21–5.

47 Watanabe J, Wohltmann HJ, Klein RL, Colwell JA, Lopes-Virella MF. Enhancement of platelet aggregation by low density lipoprotein from IDDM patients. *Diabetes* 1988; **37**: 1652–7.

48 Trovati M, Anfossi G, Cavalot F, Massucco P, Mularoni E, Emanuelli G. Insulin directly reduces platelet sensitivity to aggregating agents. Studies *in vitro* and *in vivo*. *Diabetes* 1988; **89**: 780–6.

49 Gill DR, Barradas MA, Fonseca VA, Gracey L, Dandona P. Increased histamine content in leukocytes and platelets of patients with peripheral vascular disease. *Am J Clin Pathol* 1988; **89**: 622–6.

50 Bergh CH, Hjalmoarson A, Holm G, Angwald E, Jacobsson B. Studies on calcium exchange in platelets in human diabetes. *Eur J Clin Invest* 1988; **18**: 92–7.

51 Trovati M, Anfossi G, Cavelot F *et al*. Studies on mechanisms involved in hypoglycemia induced platelet activation. *Diabetes* 1986; **35**: 818–25.

52 Karpen CW, Pritchard KA, Arnold JH, Cornwell DG, Panganamala RV. Restoration of prostacyclin/thromboxane A₂ balance in the diabetic rat: influence of dietary vitamin E. *Diabetes* 1982; **31**: 947–51.

53 Gisinger C, Jeremy J, Speiser P, Mikhailidis D, Dandona P, Schernthaner G. Effect of vitamin E supplementation on platelet thromboxane A₂ production in type I diabetic patients. Double-blind cross-over trial. *Diabetes* 1988; **37**: 1260–4.

54 Colette C, Pares-Herbute N, Monnier LH, Cartry E. Platelet function in type 1 diabetes: effect of supplementation with large doses of vitamin E. *Am J Clin Nutr* 1988; **47**: 256–61.

55 DAMAD Study Group. Effect of aspirin alone and aspirin plus dipyridamole in early diabetic retinopathy. A multicentre randomised controlled clinical trial. *Diabetes* 1989; **38**: 491–8.

56 Michaelson IC. The mode of development of the vascular system of the retina. *Trans Ophthalmol Soc UK* 1948; **68**: 137–80.

57 D'Amore PA, Klagsbrun M. Endothelial cell mitogens derived from retina and hypothalamus, biochemical and biological stimulants. *J Cell Biol* 1984; **99**: 545–9.

58 Baird A, Esch F, Gospodarowicz D, Guillemin R. Retina and eye derived endothelial cell growth factors: partial molecular characterisation and identity with acidic and basic fibroblast growth factor. *Biochemistry* 1985; **24**: 7855–60.

59 Gospodarowicz D, Massoglia S, Cheng J, Fuji DK. Effect of retina-derived basic and acidic fibroblast growth factor and lipoproteins on the proliferation of retina-derived capillary endothelial cells. *Exp Eye Res* 1986; **43**: 459–76.

60 Herman IM, D'Amore PA. Capillary endothelial cell migration: loss of fibres in response to retina derived growth factor. *J Muscle Res Cell Motil* 1989; **5**: 697–709.

61 Schweigerer I, Neufeld G, Friedman J, Abraham JA, Fiddes JC, Gospodarowicz D. Capillary endothelial cells express basic fibroblast growth factor, a mitogen that promotes their growth. *Nature* 1987; **325**: 257–9.

62 Grant M, Russel B, Fitzgerald C, Merimee TJ. Insulin-like growth factors in vitreous. *Diabetes* 1986; **35**: 416–20.

63 Glaser BM, Campochiaro PA, Davis JL, Sato M. Retinal pigment epithelial cells release an inhibitor of neovascularization. *Arch Ophthalmol* 1985; **103**: 1870–5.

64 Poulsen JE. Recovery from retinopathy in the case of diabetes with Simmonds' disease. *Diabetes* 1953; **2**: 7–12.

65 Sharp PS, Fallon TJ, Brazier OJ, Sandler L, Joplin GF, Kohner EM. Long term follow up of patients who underwent yttrium-90 pituitary implantation for treatment of proliferative retinopathy. *Diabetologia* 1987; **33**: 199–207.

66 Wright AD, Kohner EM, Oakley NW, Hartog M, Joplin GF, Fraser TR. Serum growth hormone levels and the response of diabetic retinopathy to pituitary ablation. *Br Med J* 1969; **2**: 364–8.

67 Adams DA, Rand RW, Roth NH, Dashe AM, Gipstein RM, Heuser G. Hypophysectomy in diabetic retinopathy — the relationship between the degree of pituitary ablation and ocular response. *Diabetes* 1974; **23**: 698–707.

68 Hyer SL, Sharp PS, Brooks RA, Burrin JM, Kohner EM. Serum IGF-I concentration in diabetic retinopathy. *Diabetic Med* 1988; **5**: 356–60.
69 Lanes R, Recher B, Fort B, Liftschitz F. Impaired somatomedin generation test in children with insulin dependent diabetes mellitus. *Diabetes* 1985; **34**: 156–60.
70 Baxter RC, Brown AJ, Turtle JR. Association between serum insulin, serum somatomedin and liver receptors for human growth hormone in streptozotocin diabetes. *Horm Metab Res* 1980; **12**: 371–81.
71 Merimee TJ, Zapf F, Froesch ER. Insulin like growth factors: studies in diabetics with and without retinopathy. *N Engl J Med* 1983; **309**: 527–30.
72 Hyer SL, Sharp PS, Brooks RA, Burrin JM, Kohner EM. A two year follow up study of serum insulin like growth factors in diabetics with retinopathy. *Metabolism* 1989; **38**: 586–9.
73 King GL, Goldman AD, Buzney S, Moses A, Kahn CR. Receptors and growth promoting effects of insulin and insulin like growth factors on cells from bovine retinal capillaries and aorta. *J Clin Invest* 1985; **75**: 108–1036.
74 Kahn HA, Leibowitz HM, Ganley JP *et al*. The Framingham Eye Study I. Outline and major prevalence findings. *Am J Epidemiol* 1977; **106**: 17–32.
75 Kahn HA, Leibowitz HM, Ganley JP *et al*. The Framingham Eye Study II. Association of ophthalmic pathology with single variables previously measured in the Framingham Heart Study. *Am J Epidemiol* 1977; **106**: 33–41.
76 Leibowitz HM, Krueger DE, Maunder LR *et al*. The Framingham Eye Study monograph. *Surv Ophthalmol* 1980; **24** (suppl): 335–610.
77 Hiller R, Kahn HA. Senile cataract extraction and diabetes. *Br J Ophthalmol* 1976; **60**: 283–6.
78 Ederer F, Hiller R, Taylor HR. Senile lens changes and diabetes: two population studies. *Am J Ophthalmol* 1981; **91**: 381–95.
79 Cheng HM, Chylack LT Jr. Lens metabolism. In: Maisel H, ed. *The Ocular Lens*. New York: M. Dekker Inc, 1985, 223–64.
80 Lou MF, Kinoshita JH. Control of lens glycolysis. *Biochem Biophys Acta* 1967; **141**: 545–59.
81 Levari R, Wertheimer E, Kornblueth W. Interrelation between the various pathways of glucose metabolism in the rat lens. *Exp Eye Res* 1964; **3**: 99–104.
82 Ahmad SS, Tsou KC, Ahmad SI *et al*. Studies on cataractogenesis in humans and rats with alloxan-induced diabetes. II. Histochemical evaluation of lenticular enzymes. *Ophthalmic Res* 1985; **17**: 12–20.
83 Patterson JW. Cataractogenic sugars. *Arch Biochem Biophys* 1955; **58**: 24–30.
84 Varma SD, Mizuno A, Kinoshita JH. Diabetic cataracts and flavonoids. *Science* 1977; **195**: 205–6.
85 El-Aguizy HK, Richards RD, Varma SD. Sugar cataracts in Mongolian gerbils. *Exp Eye Res* 1983; **36**: 839–44.
86 Van Heyningen R. Formation of polyols by the lens of the rat with sugar cataract. *Nature* 1959; **184**: 194–5.
87 Kuck JFR. Response of the mouse lens to high concentrations of glucose or galactose. *Ophthalmol Res* 1970; **1**: 166–74.
88 Varma SD, Kinoshita JH. The absence of cataracts in mice with congenital hyperglycaemia. *Exp Eye Res* 1974; **19**: 577–82.
89 Kinoshita JH. Mechanisms initiating cataract formation. *Invest Ophthalmol* 1974; **13**: 713–24.
90 Kador PF, Kinoshita JH. Diabetic galactosaemic cataracts. *Human Cataract Formation* (Ciba Foundation Symposium 106). London: Pitman, 1984; 110–31.
91 Simard-Duquesne N, Greselin E, Dubuc J *et al*. The effect of a new aldose reductase inhibitor (Tolrestat) in galactosemic and diabetic rats. *Metabolism* 1985; **34**: 885–92.
92 Varma SD, Schocket SS, Richards RD. Implications of aldose reductase in cataracts in human diabetes. *Invest Ophthalmol Vis Sci* 1979; **18**: 237–41.
93 Lerner BC, Varma SD, Richards RD. Polyol pathway metabolites in human cataracts. Correlation of circulating glycosylated hemoglobin content and fasting blood glucose levels. *Arch Ophthalmol* 1984; **102**: 917–20.
94 Jedziniak J, Arredondo LM, Meys M. Polyol dehydrogenase in the human lens. *Invest Ophthalmol Vis Sci* 1986; **27** (suppl 1): 137.
95 Garlick RL, Mazer JS, Chylack LT Jr *et al*. Non-enzymatic glycation of human lens crystallin. *J Clin Invest* 1984; **74**: 1742–9.
96 Liang JN, Hershorin LL, Chylack LT Jr. Nonenzymatic glycosylation in human diabetic lens crystallins. *Diabetologia* 1986; **29**: 225–8.
97 Mandel SS, Shiu DH, Newman BL *et al*. Glycosylation *in vivo* of human lens capsule (basement membrane) and diabetes mellitus. *Biochem Biophys Res Comm* 1983; **117**: 51–6.
98 Liang JN, Chylack LT Jr. Change in the protein tertiary structure with nonenzymatic glycosylation of calf crystallin. *Biochem Biophys Res Comm* 1984; **123**: 899–906.
99 Chou S, Chylack LT Jr, Bunn HF *et al*. Role of nonenzymatic glycosylation in experimental cataract formation. *Biochem Biophys Res Comm* 1980; **95**: 894–901.

58 The Lesions and Natural History of Diabetic Retinopathy

Summary

• The lesions of diabetic retinopathy can be grouped into those associated with background, preproliferative and proliferative retinopathy.

• Background retinopathy is characterized by: capillary dilatation (later with leakage), capillary occlusion, microaneurysms, 'blot' haemorrhages and lipid-rich hard exudates (commonly in the macular area and associated with oedema).

• In preproliferative retinopathy, there are cotton-wool spots (interruption of axoplasmic transport indicating retinal ischaemia), venous abnormalities (loops, beading and reduplication), arterial abnormalities (variation of calibre, narrowing of segments and occlusion) and intraretinal microvascular abnormalities (IRMA — clusters of dilated abnormal capillaries lying within the retina).

• In proliferative retinopathy, new vessels arise in the periphery and/or on the optic disc, eventually with a fibrous tissue covering. The visual complications are caused by vitreous retraction which leads to haemorrhage and to traction and detachment of the retina.

• New vessels on the optic disc are a 'high-risk' feature as they are particularly prone to cause complications of haemorrhage and retinal detachment.

• Uncomplicated background retinopathy is common and in most patients remains mild for many years. Turnover of microaneurysms, haemorrhages and hard exudates is relatively rapid.

• Maculopathy is heralded by rings of hard exudates approaching the fovea.

• Maculopathy occurs mostly in NIDDM and can cause severe visual loss which is often central, with preserved peripheral navigational vision. It can be exudative, oedematous (at times cystoid) or ischaemic.

• Proliferative retinopathy is the commonest sight-threatening lesion in IDDM. Advanced diabetic eye disease is its end stage, defined by long-standing vitreous haemorrhage, macular traction or detachment, or thrombotic glaucoma.

• Thrombotic glaucoma is due to new vessels and fibrous tissue proliferating in the angle of the anterior chamber, preventing drainage of the aqueous. It is associated with rubeosis iridis (neovascularization of the iris) and causes severe pain and irreversible blindness.

There are few conditions which have been studied as intensely as diabetic retinopathy. There is hardly a week in which there are not several papers on the subject in the medical literature. The tremendous effort expended on this subject has not been in vain. During the last 20 years the lesions of diabetic retinopathy have been well recognized, and the natural history described in detail. Though the condition still surprises us from time to time in its manifestations or progression, by and large there is little that we do not know about the clinical features. In addition, the last 15 years have seen the development of treatment, in the form of photocoagulation, for the sight-threatening forms of diabetic retinopathy. Microsurgery, in particular vitrectomy and membrane stripping, has also allowed eyes that are already blind to regain some vision. In spite of these advances, there is still very little that we know about the pathogenic mechanisms leading to the lesions, particularly the sight-threatening ones, and we have as yet no ideas about how to avoid the development of these events.

In this chapter, the lesions themselves and their natural history will be described. Their treatment is discussed in Chapter 59.

The lesions of diabetic retinopathy

The lesions of diabetic retinopathy can be divided into two major groups: those associated with background or non-proliferative retinopathy, and those with proliferative retinopathy (see Table 58.1). *Background* changes include capillary dilatation, capillary occlusion, microaneurysms, haemorrhages, hard exudates and retinal (especially macular) oedema. *Proliferative* retinopathy includes the formation of new vessels, arising from the disc or the retinal periphery, and fibrous tissue which accompanies and eventually replaces the new vessels. There is an additional sub-group of lesions which although considered as background changes indicate that proliferative retinopathy is likely to develop within the next 6–12 months. These *preproliferative* changes include cotton-wool spots, intraretinal microvascular abnormalities (IRMA), and venous and arterial abnormalities.

Non-proliferative lesions

CAPILLARY DILATATION

Capillary dilatation is probably the earliest manifestation of diabetic retinopathy. True dilatation of the capillaries is suggested by the findings in diabetic rats that the number of cells forming the capillary wall was increased, and that the wall was thinned, compared with non-diabetic controls [1]. Fluorescein angiograms in diabetic patients demonstrate retinal capillaries more clearly than in non-diabetic subjects, suggesting either true dilatation or leakage of fluorescein into the capillary wall [2].

The significance of capillary dilatation early in diabetes, before any other signs of retinopathy, is not clear. It may reflect increased retinal blood flow, which has been observed by some workers [3] but not by others [4]. Other causes of the dilatation could include metabolic factors such as increased lactic acid production or reduced oxygen utilization.

At this early stage, when dilatation is uniform, it carries no prognostic significance. Later, how-

ever, when dilatation of some capillaries is secondary to occlusion of others, the dilated capillaries become leaky and are responsible for retinal and macular oedema and the formation of lipid-rich 'hard' exudates.

Capillary dilatation is not visible on fundoscopy and must be demonstrated by fluorescein angiography. Dilatation of the retinal *veins* is an early fundoscopic feature of diabetic retinopathy.

CAPILLARY OCCLUSION

Capillary occlusion is probably the most important of the early and even the late lesions. It precedes the development of microaneurysms, and when the area occluded is large enough, the non-perfused area is responsible for the development of new vessels. In the early stages, however, capillary non-perfusion can only be detected on high-quality fluorescein angiograms (Fig. 58.1). When extensive, especially in the retinal periphery, the featureless appearance of the retina, bereft of the normal striations, can be recognized easily on retinal photographs, and with experience on fundoscopic examination.

MICROANEURYSMS

Microaneurysms, the hallmark of diabetic retinopathy [5] (Fig. 58.2), are localized dilatations of the capillaries which were first described in detail in 1948 by Ballantyne and Lowenstein [6]. It is important to realize that, although the appearance of the first microaneurysm indicates the appearance of diabetic retinopathy, microaneurysms are not themselves of sinister prognostic importance: as long as there are only microaneurysms, with some capillary closure and dilatation, there is no danger of loss of sight.

More severe retinopathy follows as the number of microaneurysms increases. Large numbers almost never occur as the only manifestation of diabetic retinopathy. Later, when there are increasing areas of capillary non-perfusion, the number of microaneurysms may actually fall, but this is a relatively late, preproliferative stage of diabetic retinopathy.

The pathogenesis of microaneurysms is not clearly established. The most plausible current theory is that microaneurysms only arise when pericytes are lost from the capillary wall. Normal retinal capillaries have two different cell types in their walls, endothelial cells and pericytes. In dia-

Table 58.1. Appearances of diabetic retinopathy on fundoscopy and corresponding features on fluorescein angiography.

Stage	Features on fundoscopy	Angiographic appearances

Non-proliferative (background)	Featureless retina	Capillary dilatation
		Capillary occlusion
		   (with areas of
		   non-perfusion)

	Venous dilatation (generalized)	Confirmed

	Microaneurysms	Greater number
		   visualized than by
		   fundoscopy

	Haemorrhages*:
	• flame (superficial)
	• blot (deep in retina)
		Haemorrhages appear
		   as dark areas (fluorescence
		   absorbed by haemorrhage)

	Exudates ('hard')	

Preproliferative	Cotton-wool spots**	Non-perfused areas,
		   usually larger than
		   cotton-wool spots and
		   surrounded by dilated, leaky
		   vessels

	Specific venous abnormalities: • loops • beading • reduplication	Appearances confirmed
	Arterial abnormalities: • segmental narrowing • 'sheathing' • occlusion	Reduced luminal size, irregularity
Proliferative	New vessels (neovascularization): • on disc • elsewhere	Abnormal configuration of leaky vessels
	Fibrous tissue	
	Advanced complications: Haemorrhage • preretinal • vitreous	
	Retinal detachment	Diffuse leakage

Notes
* A single retinal haemorrhage, in the absence of other features, is not diagnostic of diabetic retinopathy.
** A single cotton-wool spot, in the absence of other features, is not diagnostic of preproliferative retinopathy.

betes, there appears to be an early loss of pericytes, at a time when endothelial cell numbers are normal. The role of the pericytes is not clearly established, but recent work suggests they have a controlling influence over endothelial cell growth. In elegant co-culture studies, Orlidge and D'Amore [7] demonstrated that when pericytes and endothelial cells were in direct contact, endothelial cell proliferation was inhibited. When the cells were separated, even though diffusion of materials was still possible, the inhibition was lost. Inhibition of cell proliferation was specific

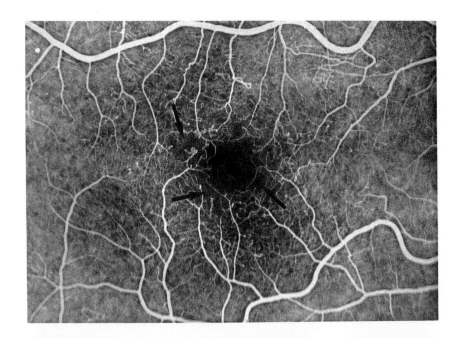

Fig. 58.1. Fluorescein angiogram of the perifoveal area of a patient with early diabetic retinopathy, showing small areas of non-perfusion (arrows).

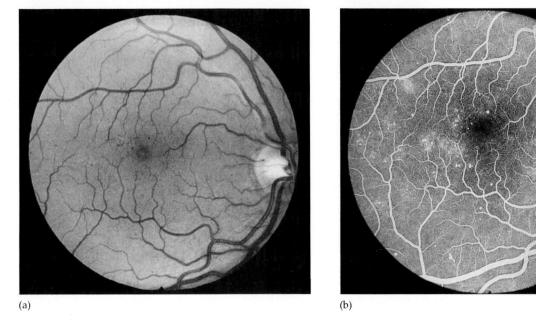

(a)   (b)

Fig. 58.2. (a) From a colour photograph of the right macular area of a diabetic patient with mild retinopathy, showing only a few microaneurysms and early hard exudates. (b) Fluorescein photograph of area shown in (a). Note many more microaneurysms showing up as white dots.

to smooth muscle cells and pericytes; loss of pericytes, for whatever reason, may therefore be responsible for the formation of microaneurysms.

HAEMORRHAGES

Haemorrhages in diabetic retinopathy occur early. A single haemorrhage in the deep or superficial retinal layer, in the absence of microaneurysms, can occur in the absence of diabetes, and accordingly is given a score on the Wisconsin grading system which is lower than that of the earliest retinopathy [8]. Once microaneurysms are present, multiple haemorrhages indicate increasing severity of diabetic retinopathy. Superficial flame-shaped haemorrhages were previously thought to indicate hypertension, but this is not necessarily the case. Deep, blot-shaped haemorrhages are more common in diabetes, and almost invariably indicate retinal ischaemia. In the early phases they are usually most numerous lateral to the macula but later are present throughout the posterior pole, very often lying on the demarcation line between perfused and non-perfused areas (Fig. 58.3). In NIDDM, multiple blot-shaped haemorrhages are common early in the disease, when they usually carry a poor prognosis. In general, haemorrhages have a short life, usually resolving within 6–8 weeks, but large blot haemorrhages at the margin of the perfused area may persist for much longer, especially in elderly patients.

Preretinal haemorrhages may be associated with hypertension and arise from small vessels. More commonly, they are associated with new vessels, and result from the retracting vitreous pulling on the vessels, which grow on the posterior vitreous surface. The haemorrhages may be quite large, obscuring the vessels from which they arise; they may track down to the lower half of the retina, but usually remain attached to the vessels from which they arise. If the new vessels are treated by photocoagulation, they clear up rapidly. Occasionally, the preretinal haemorrhage is partially encapsulated in fibrous tissue, in which case it may persist for a long time. Preretinal haemorrhages are only associated with visual loss if the haemorrhage covers the foveal area. Haemorrhages arising from new vessels, if large enough may fill the entire retrovitreal space or may break into the vitreous. Such haemorrhages are usually associated with severe visual loss.

HARD EXUDATES

Hard exudates are also early lesions in diabetic retinopathy and are true exudates due to leakage from abnormal vessels. Such leakage is clearly demonstrated by fluorescein angiography but the hard exudates themselves are not visualized (Fig. 58.4). In the earliest cases, hard exudates are small and scattered, but soon tend to coalesce and form plaques and ring patterns. Hard exudates can develop in any part of the retina but are most common in the macular area between the superior and inferior temporal vessels. They usually appear some distance from the fovea and gradually advance towards it, the vessels behind being leaky. Because hard exudates are true exudates, they are always associated with leakage of plasma constituents and therefore with some degree of retinal oedema, which may be focal or in later cases, more generalized and usually affects the macular area. On stereo retinal photographs, these areas appear as retinal thickening. Indeed, the Early Treatment of Diabetic Retinopathy Study defined macular oedema as macular thickening and advised focal treatment if any part of the macula was so affected [9].

The lesions described so far are all lesions of non-proliferative diabetic retinopathy. With the exception of extensive hard exudates, they do not

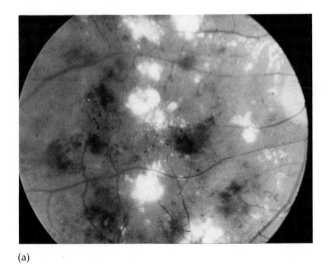

(a)

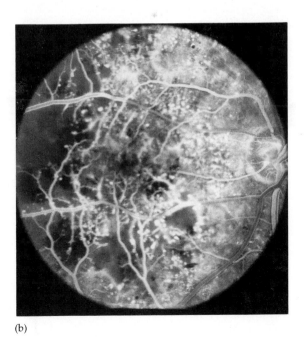

(b)

Fig. 58.3. (a) Right macular area of a patient with large blot haemorrhages and hard exudates. (b) Fluorescein angiogram of area shown in (a). Note large areas of non-perfusion and the darker areas indicating ischaemic haemorrhages between perfused and non-perfused retina.

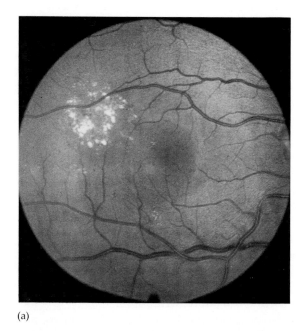

(a)

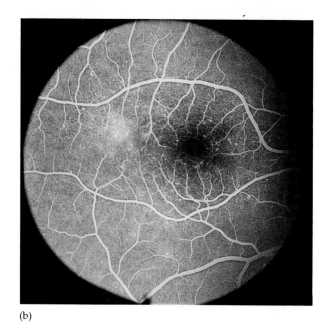

(b)

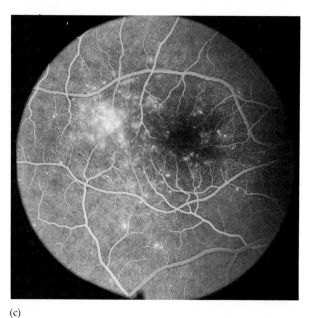

(c)

Fig. 58.4. (a) Vascular tree lateral to right macular area, showing an isolated hard exudate ring. (b) Fluorescein angiogram of a similarly affected area in a different patient. The capillary phase shows focal capillary dilatation, leakage and loss associated with the hard exudate rings. (c) Later phase of angiogram from same area as in (b) showing focal leakage.

cause visual loss unless they involve the fovea, which is rare. The remaining lesions are associated with impending or actual proliferative retinopathy (see Table 58.2).

Preproliferative lesions

These lesions warn of, and may already be accompanied by, new vessel formation. They only rarely cause visual loss themselves but indicate the urgent need for treatment to prevent the development of proliferative changes (see Table 58.2).

Preproliferative lesions are listed in Table 58.1 and illustrated in Fig. 58.5.

COTTON-WOOL SPOTS

Cotton-wool spots represent areas of interrupted axoplasmic transport, in which material from both orthograde and retrograde transport accumulates within an area of retinal ischaemia [10]. They are not unique to diabetes, occurring in many other conditions such as embolism, hypertension, collagen−vascular diseases and retinal vein occlusion. A single cotton-wool spot in a diabetic

Table 58.2. Warning signs in diabetic retinopathy.

Maculopathy
- Hard exudates in rings approaching fovea
- Retinal thickening at macula
- Falling visual acuity without other obvious cause

Imminent new vessel formation
- Five or more cotton-wool spots
- Multiple IRMA
- Venous reduplication and beading

eye in the absence of microaneurysms or any other lesions is not of prognostic importance and does not necessarily herald impending diabetic retinopathy; as with a single haemorrhage, an isolated cotton-wool spot therefore has a low score according to the Wisconsin grading system. On the other hand, multiple cotton-wool spots (more than 5) in an eye indicate rapidly advancing retinopathy. In a prospective study at the Hammersmith Hospital, visual prognosis at 5 years was worse in those with five or more cotton-wool spots in an eye than in those with fewer. Because of the small number of patients with over ten cotton-wool spots, it was not possible to determine whether prognosis worsened with increasing numbers of cotton-wool spots.

When fully developed, cotton-wool spots appear as shiny white areas with ragged edges, some-

times with a greyish area between the white edges where axoplasmic transport is disrupted. On fluorescein angiography cotton-wool spots always appear as non-perfused areas (Fig. 58.5), which may be considerably larger than the visible white spots. Long-standing cotton-wool spots are surrounded by microaneurysms which, on late-phase angiograms, are seen to leak fluorescein into the non-perfused area.

Cotton-wool spots persist for longer in diabetes than in hypertension and other diseases, but eventually disappear as the accumulated axoplasmic debris is cleared by macrophages. In diabetes, the circulation in areas of cotton-wool spots is often markedly reduced; this probably accounts for their prolonged half-life, which may be as much as 15 months in young IDDM patients and over 40 months in older patients [11].

Multiple cotton-wool spots in an eye are of prognostic importance (see Table 58.2). However, it should be emphasized that, in the absence of venous abnormalities or IRMA (see below), the prognosis is not uniformly serious and new vessels may take over a year to appear.

VENOUS ABNORMALITIES

Dilated veins, like capillaries, appear early in diabetes, before there is any other evidence of retino-

(a)
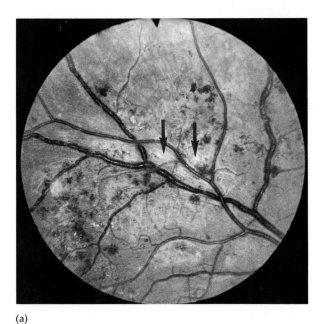

(b)
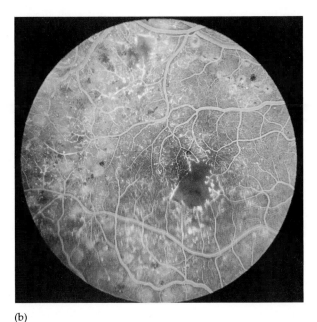

Fig. 58.5. (a) Right superior temporal area of patient with marked preproliferative changes, showing venous beading, haemorrhages, IRMA and a few early cotton-wool spots. The peripheral retina also appears atrophic. (b) Late phase of fluorescein angiogram of a macular area. Note blind ends of occluded small vessels, IRMA leakage and large areas of non-perfusion, some corresponding to cotton-wool spots.

pathy. Whether this indicates increased blood flow, increased viscosity, or perhaps an autoregulatory adaptation to hyperglycaemia, has not been established. Simple dilatation of retinal veins does not carry any prognostic significance in the evolution of diabetic retinopathy.

In contrast to simple venous dilatation, more severe lesions include venous loops, reduplication and beading (Fig. 58.5). These lesions are invariably associated with more severe forms of retinopathy and are always associated with occlusion of some of the veins, often only in the periphery. Of these lesions, reduplication is the least common and the most important prognostically, while loops alone are of less importance. Reduplication suggests that new vessels are not long delayed. The significance of venous beading falls between the two. It is an important preproliferative lesion and, together with clusters of blot haemorrhages and cotton-wool spots, heralds the imminent development of proliferative lesions.

ARTERIAL ABNORMALITIES

Arterial abnormalities usually start in the retinal periphery and extend gradually towards the posterior pole. The first notable change is marked calibre variation of the arteries, with increasing numbers of narrowed segments. Side-branches become narrowed at their origin, a feature which pre-dates eventual occlusion of the vessel. Before they become occluded, vessels are often 'sheathed' as well as irregular. The sheathing indicates that the blood flow in the vessel is reduced and there is a relative thickening of the vessel wall in comparison to the blood column. It does not necessarily mean true thickening.

Eventually, the vessels become occluded. When there is arterial occlusion, capillary perfusion in that area ceases. When the occlusion is rapid there are usually cotton-wool spots. Sudden occlusion leads to retinal infarction, and no cotton-wool spots develop. If occlusion is gradual or occurs in the retinal periphery where the retinal nerve fibre layer is thin, the disappearance of the normal striated appearance of the retina is the most marked feature, the retina looking featureless and dull. A paucity of vessels may be noted, and haemorrhages tend to occur at the junction of the perfused and non-perfused areas (Fig. 58.3).

The crucial importance of arterial occlusion is that new vessels will not form in its absence.

INTRARETINAL MICROVASCULAR ABNORMALITIES (IRMA)

These are perhaps the most sinister of the preproliferative lesions. They occur in areas of widespread capillary occlusion, often associated with occlusion of larger vessels, and consist of dilated, abnormal capillaries which are often leaky and lie in the plane of the retina.

When widespread, their prognosis is similar to that of new vessels. Indeed, widespread IRMA are usually associated with cotton-wool spots and venous beading, often with extensive blot haemorrhages, when the prognosis is very severe indeed (Fig. 58.5). This condition is known as 'florid' diabetic retinopathy, and usually affects young patients with poorly controlled diabetes. Untreated, it leads to blindness in some 90% of cases within 1 year, and if treated with photocoagulation, requires very heavy burns and extensive treatment. This fact was not initially appreciated at the introduction of photocoagulation and explains why pituitary ablation was for a long time considered the treatment of choice for this condition [12].

Proliferative lesions

NEW VESSELS AND FIBROUS RETINITIS PROLIFERANS

New vessels appear in the retinal periphery (Fig. 58.6) or on the optic disc (Fig. 58.7). Their origin is usually a major vein but occasionally they arise from arteries and those on the disc may grow from the choroidal circulation. Proliferative retinopathy is the commonest sight-threatening complication of retinopathy in IDDM. In the Wisconsin epidemiological study, up to 60% of patients diagnosed before the age of 30 years developed such lesions after about 20 years of diabetes [13]. The prevalence decreased after 30 years, probably because the patients with the worst lesions also had severe nephropathy or other fatal complications (see Chapter 56). Proliferative changes are less common in NIDDM, affecting about 40% of those treated with insulin and less than 20% of those treated by diet with or without oral agents [14].

When peripheral new vessels first form, they lie in the plane of the retina but, with accompanying mesenchyme, soon pierce the internal limiting membrane to lie in front of the retina and become

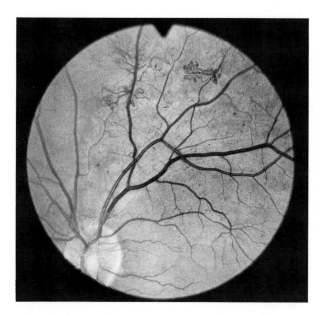

Fig. 58.6. New vessels arising from superior temporal vein.

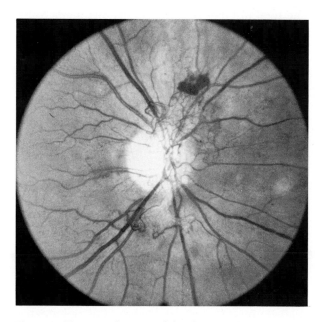

Fig. 58.7. New vessels arising from the optic disc.

attached to the posterior face of the vitreous. They may then enter the cortex of the vitreous, forming firm adhesions. The outcome of new-vessel growth depends on what happens to the vitreous. While the vitreous remains attached to the retina, the vessels are asymptomatic. Usually, however, the presence of the vessels leads to retraction of the vitreous, pulling the vascular mesenchyme forward from the site of its firm fibrovascular

adhesion to the retina, forming epiretinal membranes. This event leads to the complications of new vessels which cause visual symptoms. In their early stages, vessels may break as the vitreous retracts, producing preretinal or vitreous (intragel) haemorrhage. The vessels and their fibrous tissue covering may be pulled forward, causing traction on the internal limiting membrane and retina and resulting in distortion of vision. Fibroglial tissue proliferates on the posterior vitreous face and tends to contract, applying antero-posterior traction to its attachment to vascularized fronds at the base of the vitreous. If severe, traction may result in retinal detachment, which always causes some degree of visual loss and is profound if the macula is involved. Disc vessels undergo the same process, but much faster. One reason for this may be that the vitreous is attached to the disc margin but not the surface of the disc, perhaps allowing the new vessels to grow forward at an early stage. New vessels on the disc (unless of minimal severity) are the most important 'high-risk characteristic' identified by the Diabetic Retinopathy Study [15], as they rapidly lead to visual loss if untreated. If haemorrhage is associated with new vessels, visual loss is imminent even if the initial bleed is small and retained within the new vessel fibrovascular tissue.

Clinically, new vessels are recognized by their haphazard configuration, often with microaneurysm-like dilatations at their growing ends. Later, when well established, they may form branching arborizing patterns. It must be remembered that new vessels *never* arise in an otherwise healthy retina; there are always other lesions, such as microaneurysms, haemorrhages and signs of retinal ischaemia, such as an atrophic-looking peripheral retina, cotton-wool spots, occluded arteries and veins (showing up as white lines), other venous abnormalities, and IRMA. While untreated, new vessels carry a poor prognosis for vision, but they are also the lesions most responsive to photocoagulation, when this is carried out early and adequately.

Fibrous tissue is easily recognized by its white colour. It tends to be vascular in its early stages and dry and featureless after the vessels have closed. Attached fibrous tissue puckers the retina, and traction lines can be followed to a fibrous tissue base (Fig. 58.8).

Once fibrous tissue is extensive, photocoagulation is potentially dangerous as it may cause further traction and retinal detachment. Fibrous

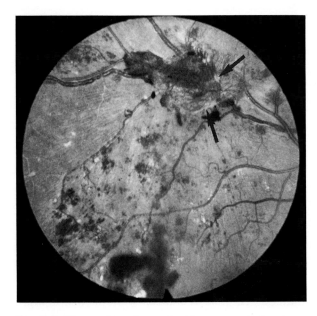

Fig. 58.8. Fibrous tissue (arrows) with new vessels forming the origin of traction lines distorting the internal limiting membrane.

tissue and the accompanying traction can be removed by vitrectomy, membrane splitting and peeling (see Chapter 59).

The natural history of diabetic retinopathy

The lesions of diabetic retinopathy as indicated above can be broadly grouped into background and proliferative lesions. On a clinical basis, it is useful to subdivide retinopathy into uncomplicated background retinopathy, background retinopathy with macular oedema, proliferative retinopathy and advanced diabetic eye disease. These subdivisions also help to illustrate the natural history of the condition.

Uncomplicated background retinopathy

This is the commonest form of retinopathy. It is present in up to 97% of young-onset patients after about 20 years of diabetes [13] and has been found within the first years of the disease in those diagnosed at over 30 years of age [14]. In the ongoing United Kingdom Prospective Diabetes Study, up to 30% of newly diagnosed NIDDM patients had some degree of retinopathy. Some reports suggest genetic predisposition to retinopathy, but it is difficult to believe that a condition which occurs in up to 97% of patients and is similar in appearance in IDDM, NIDDM

and secondary diabetes has a genetic rather than a metabolic pathogenesis.

Although retinopathy is common, its development in patients not previously affected is more difficult to characterize and to date, has been addressed by only two good prospective studies. In Denmark, Sjolle [16], using stepwise logistic analysis, concluded that the probability of developing retinopathy depended on the duration of diabetes and insulin dosage and was greater in smokers. In a Swiss population of patients without retinopathy at an initial examination, Teuscher *et al.* [17] reported that, after 8 years of follow-up, background retinopathy had developed in 39% of 53 IDDM patients, 40% of late-onset patients treated with insulin and in only 15% of subjects treated by diet with or without oral agents.

In most patients, background retinopathy remains mild for many years. The turnover of all background lesions — microaneurysms, haemorrhages and hard exudates — is relatively high. The total number of microaneurysms tends to increase, although there is great variation between patients. Haemorrhages have a much shorter half-life, as mentioned above. Hard exudates develop gradually and tend to extend towards the fovea. It is often difficult to predict who will deteriorate within a short period of time. In general, maculopathy is imminent when hard exudates start to form rings and approach the fovea. Increasing numbers of haemorrhages suggest increasing ischaemia. In IDDM patients, preproliferative or at least more active retinopathy is heralded by increasing numbers of haemorrhages and new microaneurysms and the first appearance of IRMAs.

Diabetic maculopathy

Diabetic maculopathy is background retinopathy with macular oedema. Mild degrees of macular oedema are not uncommon in IDDM, but the great majority of patients suffering from visual loss from this condition are those with NIDDM. The British Multicentre Study on Photocoagulation [18] illustrated this clearly, in that 56 of the 99 patients with maculopathy were aged 30–59 years and only nine patients were under the age of 30 years when diabetes was diagnosed.

Visual loss with maculopathy can be severe, and legal blindness is not uncommon. In the British study [18], even of those with initially good vision, 50% became blind within 5 years. The Early Treatment of Diabetic Retinopathy Study found that over 20% of patients lost two or more lines of visual acuity in eyes in which treatment was deferred [9]. It should, however, be remembered that the blindness of macular oedema is not total, as, for example, with a large vitreous haemorrhage, but is confined to central visual loss, with preservation of peripheral, navigational vision. Many of these patients can therefore be greatly helped by low-vision aids and remain able to cope with much of their everyday life (see Chapter 60).

Diabetic maculopathy can be subdivided into three groups. The commonest, and the most amenable to treatment, is *exudative maculopathy* (Fig. 58.9), in which hard exudate rings form usually lateral to the foveal area and gradually approach it. In the centre of the rings are leaky microvascular lesions which are responsible for the deposition of the exudates. The centres of the rings, and often their advancing edge are oedematous and therefore seen as retinal thickening on stereo photographs or biomicroscopy. The lesions usually progress gradually but, unless treated, will eventually affect the fovea either by forming a hard exudate plaque in its centre, or through leakage from microvascular lesions at its edge. The natural history of these rings, with new exudates forming while others disappear, was first described by Dobree [19]. Once the fovea has been

involved, treatment becomes more difficult and is often impossible. Hard exudate plaques, even when in the centre of the fovea, eventually disappear but any resulting visual loss will remain. Similarly, long-standing oedema usually causes permanent visual loss, often with pigment epithelial changes.

Oedematous maculopathy, consisting of widespread and often cystoid oedema, is the other common form of maculopathy. Little is known about the natural history of this condition. In young patients, cystoid oedema can coexist with reasonable vision for long periods of time, before vision is eventually lost. In older patients, however, visual loss is more rapid and profound. In many instances of oedematous maculopathy, there is a decrease of capillaries in the perifoveal area and the remaining capillaries become dilated and leaky (Fig. 58.10).

Ischaemic maculopathy carries the worse prognosis for vision (Fig. 58.11). In this condition, perifoveal capillaries are destroyed, so that the non-perfused area at the fovea is enlarged. This is compatible with normal or near-normal vision in young patients but in older patients, visual loss occurs after a relatively short period of time. In ischaemic maculopathy, peripheral as well as perifoveal capillaries are often lost. Such eyes are in danger of developing new vessels, and present a particularly difficult treatment problem, since the

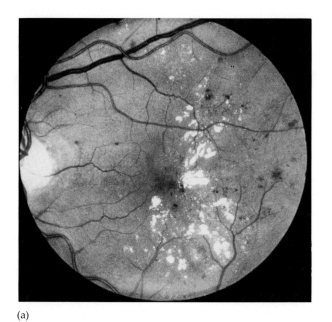

(a)

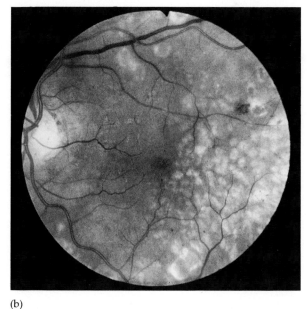

(b)

Fig. 58.9. (a) Hard exudate ring near the left macula, before treatment. Visual acuity 6/18. (b) Hard exudate ring has disappeared after treatment by pan-retinal photocoagulation. Visual acuity 6/9.

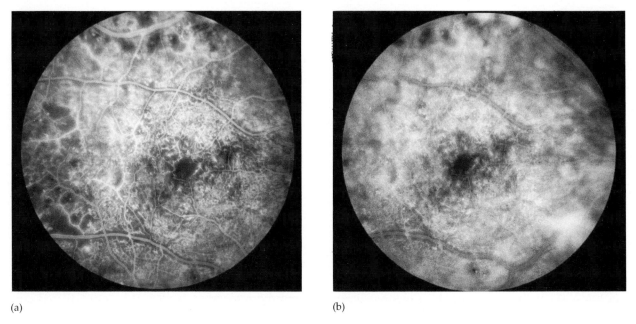

Fig. 58.10. (a) Fluorescein angiogram from a patient with oedematous maculopathy, showing dilated leaky capillaries. (b) Late phase of fluorescein angiogram shown in (a) with widespread leakage in perifoveal area.

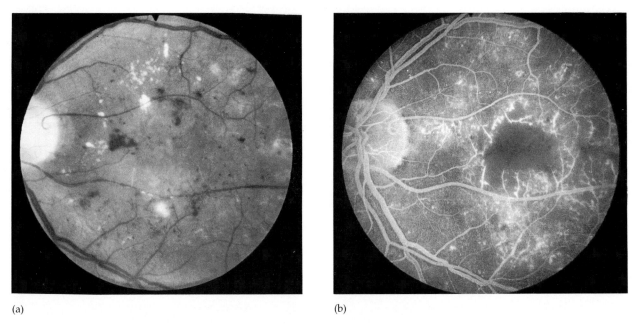

Fig. 58.11. (a) Right macular region of patient with ischaemic maculopathy. Note large blot haemorrhages suggesting ischaemia. (b) Fluorescein angiogram of area shown in (a). Note large perifoveal and peripheral ischaemic areas.

use of pan-retinal photocoagulation will cause loss of peripheral vision. Ischaemia is almost invariably progressive, which explains the poor prognosis.

The probability of developing maculopathy when there is no retinopathy or only mild background retinopathy has not been established,

largely because the importance of maculopathy as a cause of visual loss has only recently been recognized and long-term follow-up has not been reported. Moreover, many affected patients are treated, because several studies indicate that photocoagulation is better than no treatment.

Proliferative diabetic retinopathy

Proliferative diabetic retinopathy, as indicated above, is the commonest sight-threatening lesion in IDDM. The chances of developing new vessels in patients not previously affected was 3% per year in the Joslin clinic study of IDDM patients [20]. In the 8-year follow-up study by Teuscher et al. [17], 9% of IDDM patients initially without retinopathy developed new vessels, which also appeared in 8% of insulin-treated NIDDM and 3% of non-insulin treated NIDDM patients. For those patients with background retinopathy at the initial examination, the chances of developing proliferative retinopathy increased to 25% of IDDM, 22% of insulin-treated NIDDM and 13% of non-insulin-treated NIDDM patients.

Proliferative retinopathy carries a poor prognosis for vision, especially if the new vessels arise from the disc. Thus, in the British Multicentre Study, no eyes with disc vessels showed improved vision during follow-up and 33 out of 38 eyes deteriorated, 20 of these becoming blind when untreated [21]. In a study performed at the Hammersmith Hospital before photocoagulation became available, less than one-third of eyes became blind over 5 years when new vessels arose from the retinal periphery only, and most maintained normal vision. When new vessels arose from the disc, however, 13 out of 21 eyes became blind over this period of time. The Diabetic Retinopathy Study [15] of over 1700 patients associated the worst prognosis with 'high-risk' characteristics, including more than minimal disc vessels, disc vessels with present or previous vitreous haemorrhage, and peripheral new vessels with haemorrhage.

In the natural history of new vessels, vitreous haemorrhage is usually the first complication to cause visual loss. Caird et al. [22] found that within 1 year of the first vitreous haemorrhage, one-third of the affected eyes were blind and that within 3 years, one-third of the patients were blind in both eyes. The large follow-up study reported by Beetham in 1963 [23] found that 10% of patients with proliferative retinopathy maintained useful vision after over 10 years of follow-up.

The most important feature to note in the management of proliferative retinopathy is that new vessels by themselves do not cause significant visual loss, although leakage from them may cause macular oedema with reduction of vision. In most cases, however, vision remains normal until haemorrhage or tractional complications supervene. By then, treatment may be difficult and sometimes ineffective. Regular screening of patients at risk is therefore crucial.

Advanced diabetic eye disease

Advanced diabetic eye disease is the end stage of proliferative retinopathy. Until recently, it was invariably associated with profound visual loss, leading to complete irreversible blindness. In recent years, the development of improved intra-ocular microsurgical techniques such as vitrectomy and membranectomy have made it possible to improve vision in most patients, as long as the diagnosis is made and treatment undertaken early. The complications of proliferative retinopathy which constitute this group of complications are long-standing vitreous haemorrhage, traction on the macula and retinal detachment, especially that involving the macula (see Chapter 59).

The other form of advanced diabetic eye disease which leads to blindness is thrombotic (neovascular) glaucoma. This condition tends to occur in the most profoundly ischaemic eyes, and is associated with rubeosis iridis (new vessel growth in the iris). New vessels and contracting fibrous tissue proliferate in the angle of the anterior chamber and interfere with normal drainage of aqueous from the anterior chamber. The raised intra-ocular pressure causes pain, often intractable, and blindness, which is permanent.

The natural history of diabetic retinopathy is therefore unfavourable. Fortunately, however, many patients now maintain their vision due to photocoagulation. Nonetheless, as the pathogenic mechanisms are not fully known, prevention of the usual progression of retinopathy is not yet possible.

EVA M. KOHNER

References

1 Sosula L. Capillary radius and wall thickness in normal and diabetic rat retinae. Microvasc Res 1974; 7: 274–7.
2 Oosterhuis JA, Lammens AJJ. Fluorescein photography of the ocular fundus. Ophthalmologica 1965; 179: 210–18.
3 Kohner EM, Hamilton AM, Saunders SJ, Sutcliffe BA, Bulpitt CJ. The retinal blood flow in diabetes. Diabetologia 1975; 11: 27–33.
4 Grunwald JE, Riva CE, Sinclair SH, Bruckner SJ, Petrig BL. Laser doppler velocimetry study of retinal circulation in diabetes mellitus. Arch Ophthalmol 1986; 104: 991–6.

5 Bowman W. Capillary microaneurysms in diabetic retinopathy. *Trans Ophthalmol Soc UK* 1965; **85**: 199–205.

6 Ballantyne AJ, Lowenstein A. The pathology of diabetic retinopathy. *Trans Ophthalmol Soc UK* 1943; **63**: 95–115.

7 Orlidge A, D'Amore PA. Inhibition of capillary endothelial cell growth by pericytes and smooth muscle cells. *J Cell Biol* 1987; **105**: 1455–62.

8 Early Treatment of Diabetic Retinopathy Study, *Manual of Operations*, Virginia, USA: Department of Commerce National Technical Information Service, 1985.

9 Early Treatment of Diabetic Retinopathy Study Research Group. Photocoagulation for diabetic macular edema. *Arch Ophthalmol* 1985; **103**: 1796–1806.

10 McLeod D. Clinical signs of obstructed axoplasmic transport. *Lancet* 1975; ii: 954–6.

11 Kohner EM, Dollery CT, Bulpitt CJ. Cotton wool spots in diabetic retinopathy. *Diabetes* 1969; **18**: 691–704.

12 Kohner EM, Hamilton AM, Joplin GF, Fraser TR. Florid diabetic retinopathy and its response to treatment by photocoagulation or pituitary ablation. *Diabetes* 1976; **25**: 104–10.

13 Klein R, Klein BEK, Moss SE, Davies MD, deMets DL. The Wisconsin Epidemiologic Study of Diabetic Retinopathy. II. Prevalence and risk of diabetic retinopathy when age of diagnosis is less than 30 years. *Arch Ophthalmol* 1984; **102**: 520–6.

14 Klein R, Klein BEK, Moss SE, Davis MD, deMets DL. The Wisconsin Epidemiologic Study of Diabetic Retinopathy. III. Prevalence and risk of diabetic retinopathy when age of diagnosis is 30 or more years. *Arch Ophthalmol* 1984; **102**: 527–32.

15 The Diabetic Retinopathy Study Group. Preliminary report on effects of photocoagulation therapy. *Am J Ophthalmol* 1976; **81**: 383–97.

16 Sjolle AK. Ocular complications in insulin-treated diabetes mellitus. *Acta Ophthalmol* 1985; **172**: (suppl) 1–77.

17 Teuscher A, Schnelle H, Wilson PWT. Incidence of diabetic retinopathy and relationship to baseline plasma glucose and blood pressure. *Diabetes Care* 1988; **11**: 246–51.

18 British Multicentre Study Group. Photocoagulation for diabetic maculopathy: A randomised controlled clinical trial using the xenon arc. *Diabetes* 1983; **32**: 1010–16.

19 Dobree JH. Simple diabetic retinopathy — evolution of lesions and therapeutic considerations. *Br J Ophthalmol* 1970; **54**: 1–10.

20 Rand LI, Krolewski AS, Aiello LM, Warram JH, Baker RS, Maki T. Multiple factors in the prediction of risk of proliferative retinopathy. *N Engl J Med* 1985; **313**: 1433–8.

21 British Multicentre Study Group. Photocoagulation for proliferative diabetic retinopathy: a randomised controlled clinical trial using the xenon arc. *Diabetologia* 1984; **26**: 109–15.

22 Caird FI, Burditt AF, Draper GJ. Diabetic retinopathy: a further study of prognosis of vision. *Diabetes* 1968; **17**: 121–3.

23 Beetham WP. Visual prognosis of proliferating diabetic retinopathy *Br J Ophthalmol* 1963; **47**: 611–19.

59 The Surgical Management of Diabetic Eye Disease

Summary

• It is now possible to treat the major sight-threatening complications of diabetic retinopathy (proliferative changes and macular oedema) using laser photocoagulation.

• Photocoagulation employs either the xenon arc lamp, which produces a relatively large, painful retinal burn, or the argon laser, which has a smaller spot size.

• Photocoagulation can be used either to destroy specific targets (e.g. new vessels) or to treat the whole retina except for the central macula and the papillo-macular bundle essential for central vision; this 'pan-retinal' photocoagulation reduces overall retinal ischaemia and thus the stimulus to new vessel formation.

• Pan-retinal photocoagulation reduces by over 50% the likelihood of severe visual loss (acuity 1/60 or worse) developing in eyes with high-risk proliferative retinopathy. The place of photocoagulation in *pre*proliferative changes is not yet established.

• Photocoagulation to the peripheral macula can also seal points of capillary leakage and so reduce macular oedema; photocoagulation treatment of clinically significant macular oedema (i.e. involving or threatening the fovea) reduces the risk of visual loss by over 50%.

• 'Closed' vitreo-retinal surgery is performed using instruments and a light source inserted into the vitreous cavity through the pars plana to avoid damaging the lens or retina. The eye is kept distended by a saline infusion. Fibrous membranes, haemorrhages and vitreous can be removed and detached areas of retina can be re-attached.

• Detached retina only remains viable for some weeks; detachment must therefore be diagnosed immediately if surgical re-attachment is to restore vision. B-scan ultrasonography can identify retinal detachments behind dense vitreous haemorrhages.

• Vitreo-retinal surgery can restore and maintain useful vision in up to 70% of eyes with advanced diabetic disease.

• Diabetic patients' eyes must be examined at least annually, with formal measurements of distant and near acuity; checking for an afferent pupillary defect (a sign of serious retinal or optic nerve disease); and inspection of the lens, vitreous and retina through fully dilated pupils.

• Ophthalmological referral is indicated soon for preproliferative changes; urgently for maculopathy, new vessel formation or retinal detachment; and immediately for vitreous haemorrhage or neovascular glaucoma.

'Next to life itself, the loss of sight is most harrowing' (Von Helmholtz)

The principal objectives in the surgical management of diabetic eye disease are: the preservation of vision in eyes threatened by proliferative retinopathy or macular oedema; the lasting restoration of sight to eyes blinded by vitreous haemorrhage or retinal detachment; and the prevention of the ultimate horror of an eye not only blind but painful from the ravages of neovascular glaucoma. The advent and development of laser photocoagulation and closed intra-ocular microsurgery, particularly within the last decade, have made it possible to achieve these objectives in many cases.

The purpose of this chapter is to put laser treatment and vitreous surgery into clinical perspective for the physician and to discuss the nature, timing and outcome of these treatments against the background of the natural history of diabetic retinopathy. Above all, it is hoped to enable the clinician to identify the imminence of visual loss and the indications for referring specific patients for surgical management.

Clinical classification of diabetic retinopathy

The classification of diabetic retinopathy outlined in Chapter 58 can be modified (Table 59.1) to provide a rational basis for determining treatment and for interpreting the results of recent treatment trials.

Background diabetic retinopathy without macular oedema

This is simply the presence of scattered microaneurysms and intra-retinal haemorrhages ('dots and blots') with hard exudates which do not involve the macula (Fig. 59.1). Attempts to distinguish microaneurysms from small haemorrhages are unnecessary and unrewarding. At this stage, there is no threat to vision *per se* and monitoring is required solely to detect the possible complications of macular oedema or preproliferative changes.

Diabetic macular oedema

This is defined as the presence of retinal thickening and/or hard exudate within one disc diameter (approximately 1500 μm) of the centre of the macula [1]. Macular oedema may be classified as *focal* (Fig. 59.2), where the leaking capillaries

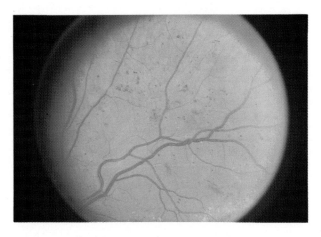

Fig. 59.1. Background diabetic retinopathy, showing scattered red 'dots and blots' (microaneurysms and haemorrhages) and exudates.

and microaneurysms are relatively discrete; *diffuse* (Fig. 59.3) where the leakage is extensive, ill-defined and accompanied by cystoid change; and *ischaemic*, in which oedema is associated with extensive areas of capillary non-perfusion, best identified by fluorescein angiography (Fig. 59.4).

This definition is independent of visual acuity, although this is generally predictable within each subgroup [2]. Visual acuity tends to be good (6/6 to 6/12) if the leakage is focal and the hard exudate is not deposited in the fovea. Acuity is moderately reduced (6/12 to 6/24) if the leakage is diffuse and the fovea oedematous, and poor (6/24 to 6/60) if the macula is ischaemic with enlargement of the normal avascular zone at the fovea (Fig. 59.4).

Clinically significant macular oedema

Clinically significant macular oedema is that which

Table 59.1. Clinical classification of diabetic retinopathy.

Background retinopathy without macular oedema

Macular oedema — focal, diffuse, ischaemic

Clinically significant macular oedema

Proliferative retinopathy

Preproliferative retinopathy

Advanced diabetic eye disease:
  Vitreous haemorrhage
  Macular distortion
  Tractional retinal detachment
  Combined rhegmatogenous/tractional retinal detachment
  Neovascular glaucoma

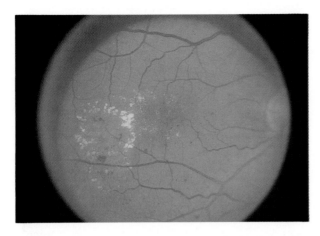

Fig. 59.2. Focal macular oedema, showing thickening and a greyish appearance of the retina (more easily appreciated by binocular indirect fundoscopy) restricted to the macular area adjacent to a ring of hard exudates.

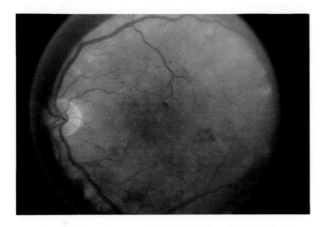

Fig. 59.3. Diffuse macular oedema, with widespread changes surrounding the macula. Scars from previous photocoagulation are visible peripherally.

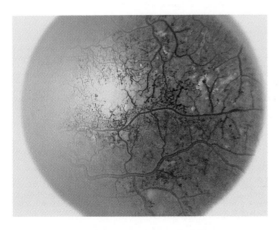

Fig. 59.4. Ischaemic macular oedema. The fluorescein angiogram demonstrates capillary non-perfusion and enlargement of the foveal avascular zone.

threatens the fovea and central vision [3, 4] and is precisely (but lengthily) defined [3] as any one of the following:

1 Thickening of the retina at or within 500 μm of the centre of the macula (Fig. 59.5).

2 Hard exudate at or within 500 μm of the centre of the macula, only if associated with thickening of adjacent retina (Fig. 59.6). This excludes any hard exudate remaining after retinal thickening has disappeared (Fig. 59.7).

3 A zone or zones of retinal thickening one disc area or larger in size, any part of which falls within one disc diameter of the centre of the macula (Figs 59.8 and 59.9).

Again, this definition is purely anatomical and takes no account of visual acuity, which in patients entering the Early Treatment Diabetic Retinopathy Study (ETDRS), ranged from 6/4 to 6/60; the severity of macular oedema also varied considerably [3, 5]. The concept of *clinically significant macular oedema* is crucial to the understanding and application of the ETDRS results (see below) [3, 5–7].

Proliferative diabetic retinopathy

This stage is defined as the presence of new blood vessels within the eye, which may form on the optic disc ('NVD'; Fig. 59.10), elsewhere on the retina ('NVE'; Fig. 59.11) or on the iris and drainage angle (rubeosis iridis; Fig. 59.12).

Preproliferative diabetic retinopathy

Preproliferative changes comprise one or more of the following, in the absence of new vessels (Figs 59.13 and 59.14):

• Deep round haemorrhages.

• Cotton-wool spots (two or more).

• Intra-retinal microvascular abnormalities (IRMA).

• Changes in the calibre of the major vessels: venous beading, reduplication or looping and attenuation or obliteration of the smaller branch arterioles, which then appear as white lines (see Fig. 59.11).

• 'Empty' retina: the featureless appearance of ischaemic retina, devoid of its normal striations, adjacent to the above lesions.

The concept of preproliferative retinopathy is important in designing and interpreting trials of treatment to prevent or delay the onset of proliferative changes [1, 6].

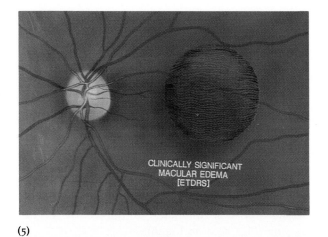

(5)

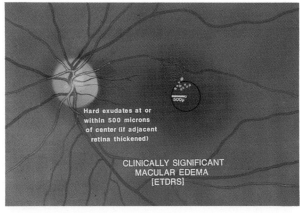

(6)

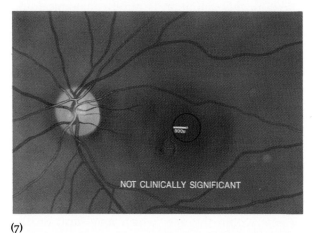

(7)

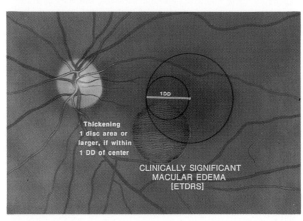

(8)

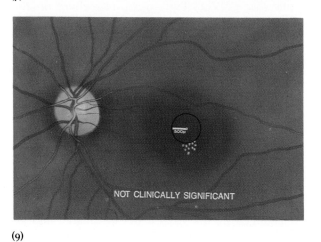

(9)

Fig. 59.5–9. Clinically significant macular oedema, showing the variety of lesions which may threaten central vision. Retinal thickening (oedema) is shown in grey. See text for explanations. (Courtesy of Dr R. Murphy, Wilmer Institute, Baltimore, Maryland, USA.)

Advanced diabetic eye disease

This is end-stage disease, defined by the presence of any of the potentially blinding complications of proliferative diabetic retinopathy:

- Severe vitreous haemorrhage (Fig. 59.15).
- Macular distortion (Fig. 59.16), due to traction by contracting fibrous tissue, which may progress to macular detachment.

- Tractional retinal detachment (TRD). This may be extramacular (Fig. 59.17), which is compatible with good vision, or involve the macula (Fig. 59.18), when vision is severely impaired.
- Combined rhegmatogenous and tractional retinal detachment. The formation of a tear or hole (Greek, *rhegma*, meaning a rent) in the retina (Fig. 59.19) permits the rapid exchange of fluid between the vitreous cavity and the subretinal

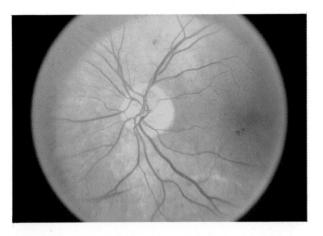

Fig. 59.10. Diabetic Retinopathy Study (DRS) standard photograph indicating new vessels on the disc, and showing a preretinal haemorrhage (at 7 o'clock).

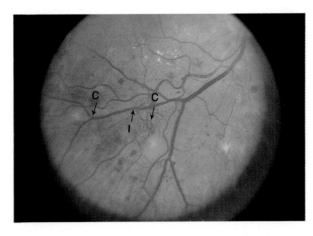

Fig. 59.13. Shows cotton-wool spots (C), IRMA (I), deep round haemorrhages and the 'empty retina' of preproliferative retinopathy.

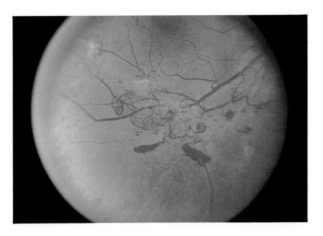

Fig. 59.11. New vessels elsewhere in the retina (NVE), in this case inferior to the macula. The picture also shows arteriolar obliteration and retinal ischaemia; the columns of blood are attenuated and some occluded arterioles are reduced to whitish lines (e.g. between the two haemorrhages lying below the new vessels).

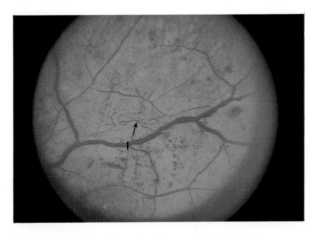

Fig. 59.14. Shows venous beading and IRMA (I) of preproliferative retinopathy.

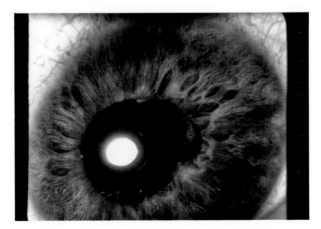

Fig. 59.12. Rubeosis iridis, most easily seen at 6 o'clock on the pupil margin. There is also circumcorneal injection of the sclera.

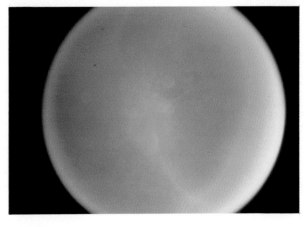

Fig. 59.15. Shows severe vitreous haemorrhage. The fundus is virtually invisible.

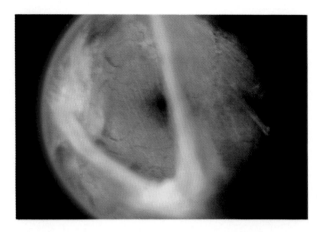

Fig. 59.16. Tractional macular distortion. Traction lines running obliquely are clearly visible in the retina lateral to the disc.

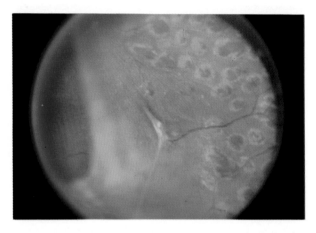

Fig. 59.17. Focal vitreo-retinal adhesion, with a small area of localized extramacular tractional retinal detachment, lateral to the macula. Photocoagulation scars are clearly visible.

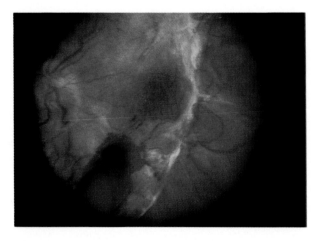

Fig. 59.18. Confluent epiretinal membrane with several foci of vitreo-retinal adhesion and tractional detachment involving the macula.

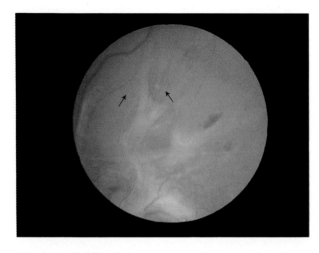

Fig. 59.19. Combined rhegmatogenous/tractional detachment with horseshoe-shaped retinal tear (indicated by arrowheads).

space, causing sudden and extensive retinal detachment accompanied by catastrophic visual loss.

● Neovascular glaucoma. This results from obstruction of the drainage angle by new vessels and accompanying fibrous tissue (Fig. 59.20). It is the final common result of untreated retinal ischaemia, progressive retinal detachment, rubeosis iridis or failed surgery and ultimately results in an eye which is often both irretrievably blind and intractably painful.

Clinical examination

Visual symptoms

Visual symptoms are extremely variable and must be elicited by careful questioning. The osmotic

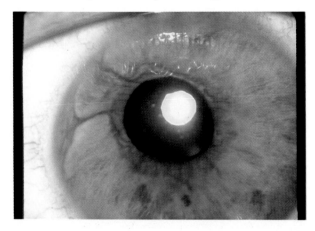

Fig. 59.20. Neovascular glaucoma, showing growth of new vessels and associated fibrous tissue into the drainage angle (best seen on the left of the picture). The pupil is oval and the cornea slightly hazy, suggesting corneal oedema.

effects of hyperglycaemia cause transient blurring of vision, often with hyperopia ('I cannot see the television without my *reading* glasses'). This is a common presenting symptom of diabetes but will improve with stabilization of treatment and has no long-term ill-effects.

A gradual decline in central vision ('I cannot read at all now; my new glasses are not strong enough') is often due to associated presenile cataract but demands the exclusion of diabetic macular oedema. Mild macular oedema often has no symptoms.

Sudden loss of vision — usually terrifying, especially in previously asymptomatic patients — generally denotes an extensive vitreous haemorrhage or retinal detachment; when the retina detaches behind a vitreous haemorrhage (which happens quite frequently), the patient may report a sensation 'like the light going out behind the thundercloud'. This is a crucial symptom which must not be neglected, as the duration of retinal detachment directly determines the viability of the photoreceptors and therefore the likelihood of eventual surgery failing to restore vision; long-standing, unsuspected retinal detachment is one of the greatest disappointments to the vitreo-retinal surgeon and his patient.

Symptoms may be entirely absent even in patients with extensive proliferative changes, until haemorrhage or detachment occur. A lack of symptoms is therefore not necessarily reassuring and the possibility of occult retinopathy with the potential for acute severe visual loss emphasizes the importance of routine screening.

Physical signs

The purpose of clinical examination (Table 59.2) is to allocate each eye to one of the above classes of retinopathy and to detect risk factors for visual loss before complications occur. It is imperative, for example, to seek retinal detachment behind a vitreous haemorrhage, proliferative changes before vitreous haemorrhage occurs, preproliferative features before neovascularization supervenes, and macular oedema before visual acuity declines.

Measurement of visual acuity is mandatory, as it is not only the end-point of clinical trials [3, 7–20] but also the property of vision most important to the patient. Acuity for distance is measured with a Snellen chart and for near vision with a standard reading chart. Distance acuity should be checked with the patient wearing his spectacles for distant vision, or with a pinhole to counteract any reduction in acuity due to purely refractive problems. Poor acuity which is not improved in this way is likely to be due to serious retinal or macular disease or to dense opacities in the lens or vitreous.

Having measured the visual acuity, the presence of a relative afferent pupillary defect should be sought. If present, this sign indicates severe underlying retinal or optic nerve damage, such as retinal detachment. This applies even in the presence of vitreous haemorrhage, as opacities in the media (such as cataract or vitreous haemorrhage) do not produce such a defect.

Formal measurement of the intra-ocular pressure

Table 59.2. Examination of the eyes in diabetic patients.

When to examine:
- On diagnosis
- Annually after 3 years of diabetes
- Annually if background retinopathy alone is present
- Three- to 6-monthly if retinopathy is more severe than background
- Immediately if any change in vision or visual symptoms occur

Examination should include:
- Visual acuity — distant vision (Snellen chart + spectacles or pinhole)
  — near vision (reading chart)
- Afferent pupillary defect
- Ophthalmoscopy through dilated pupils (1% tropicamide), unless glaucoma or previous eye surgery are present: examine lens, vitreous and retina

Specialized ophthalmological examination will also include slit-lamp microscopic examination of the iris, anterior chamber and retina, indirect binocular fundoscopy and measurement of intra-ocular pressure.

is the next step. Elevated intra-ocular pressure may be caused by vitreous haemorrhage or neovascular glaucoma. A slit lamp is then used to detect rubeosis iridis and, if present, a contact lens is used to examine the drainage angle for possible occlusion by new vessels or fibrous tissue. Both pupils are then dilated with 1% tropicamide eye drops (with or without 10% phenylephrine). Patients should be warned to return should they develop symptoms of acute glaucoma; the chances of this happening are generally remote, but mydriatics should only be used by experts in patients with a known history of glaucoma or of eye surgery. Following full pupillary dilatation, the binocular indirect ophthalmoscope is used to scan the retina for the presence of background retinopathy. This is also the best instrument to detect vitreous haemorrhage or retinal detachment and, with practice, can even visualize the retina through relatively dense cataract or vitreous haemorrhage.

The traditional hand-held monocular direct ophthalmoscope can identify cataract and vitreous opacities and is particularly useful for identifying small clusters of new vessels, which are best seen by focusing slightly anterior of the retina. NVD are sought by carefully examining the disc, and NVE by following the retinal veins and their major branches out from the optic disc in each quadrant; NVE invariably arise from retinal veins, most commonly at their bifurcations (Fig. 59.11).

Detailed stereoscopic biomicroscopy of the posterior pole of the eye is performed with the slit-lamp microscope and a corneal contact lens or a 90-dioptre hand-held lens. The detection of hard exudate at the macula is easy (Fig. 59.2) but identification of retinal oedema (seen as retinal thickening) *without* hard exudate is more difficult (Fig. 59.8).

Clinical testing of colour vision and visual fields is unnecessary in routine practice, although colour vision is subtly impaired in diabetic retinopathy and could theoretically interfere with the ability to read blood glucose testing strips.

The important physical signs are illustrated in Figs 59.1–20.

Ancillary investigations

If the retina cannot be seen through vitreous haemorrhage or dense cataract, B-scan ultrasonography can be used to determine the presence or absence of underlying retinal detachment. This technique is of great value but is expensive and requires an experienced examiner.

Fundus photography, especially stereoscopic photography, of standard retinal fields is also expensive but provides clear and permanent records and permits more detailed study of the retina than clinical examination [1]. 'Non-mydriatic' cameras can photograph the central and part of the peripheral retina through undilated pupils. The quality is not as high as with formal photography through fully dilated pupils and the photographs require skilled interpretation. However, the examination is quick and easy to perform and non-mydriatic cameras are currently being evaluated in screening for diabetic retinopathy.

Adjunctive fluorescein angiography confirms early proliferative disease and helps to confirm and classify macular oedema. The angiogram is a useful guide to the treatment of macular oedema (Figs 59.22, 59.24 and 59.25) and is essential for follow-up treatment (see below).

Electrophysiological tests such as the electroretinogram and visual evoked responses are essentially research tools and contribute little to routine clinical evaluation.

Treatment of diabetic retinopathy

Laser photocoagulation

The rationale for using photocoagulation in proliferative retinopathy is that it destroys ischaemic areas of retina which are thought to produce vasoproliferative factors which act locally to stimulate new vessel growth [21–25]. A high-energy light beam is focused through a corneal contact lens on to the target area of retina. The first device to be used was the xenon arc lamp, which produces a relatively large (1000 μm diameter) burn suitable for ablating large areas but too imprecise for small targets. Xenon arc photocoagulation is also painful and usually needs retrobulbar (or general) anaesthesia. The instrument in widest current use is the argon laser, which produces very short flashes (20 ms) of monochromatic blue-green light with a spot size of one-third of a disc diameter which allows very precise targeting. The colour is complementary to that of haemoglobin, so that vascular structures (e.g. new vessels or normal retina) will maximally absorb the radiation.

Laser photocoagulation can be used to destroy specific targets (e.g. clusters of new vessels at risk of haemorrhage) but is now generally used to perform *pan-retinal photocoagulation*, in which the entire retina is treated, with the exception of the macula and papillo-macular bundle which are essential to central vision (Figs 59.21 and 59.26). Pan-retinal photocoagulation may require 1500–2000 burns and is divided into several treatment sessions to minimize possible adverse effects [20]. By partly destroying the retina, the remaining retina can survive and function on its limited blood supply; the stimulus to neovascularization is removed, existing new blood vessels regress and further neovascularization is aborted. As the new vessels shrink or disappear, the incidence and severity of vitreous haemorrhage are reduced. The benefits of this treatment are evident from the results discussed below.

Apart from pain with the xenon arc, the most disturbing adverse effect of photocoagulation is exacerbation of pre-existing macular oedema, leading to a fall in central visual acuity [26]. This can destroy the patient's faith in photocoagulation, especially when he has asymptomatic new vessels, but can largely be avoided by careful staging of treatment. There must also be detailed discussion with the patient about the natural history of the condition and the potential benefits and limitations of photocoagulation. Patients generally welcome laser photocoagulation after their first vitreous haemorrhage, when it is often too little and too late; asymptomatic subjects must be treated carefully and considerately, or many will be lost to follow-up.

As well as its use in proliferative retinopathy, photocoagulation has also been found to improve macular oedema. Leaking capillaries and micro-aneurysms are directly treated and sealed. Indirect effects on the retinal pigment epithelial pump and secondary alterations in capillary integrity result in the clearing of macular oedema and hard exudate [21, 22]. Again, technical skill is crucial, particularly in patients with normal or nearly normal vision.

Recent trials of photocoagulation have suggested guidelines for the routine clinical management of these two indications.

Photocoagulation treatment of proliferative retinopathy

Several studies have now demonstrated beyond all doubt that laser photocoagulation improves the outcome of proliferative diabetic retinopathy. The Diabetic Retinopathy Study (DRS), which withstands any criticism [27], showed that pan-retinal photocoagulation reduces by more than 50% the risk of severe visual loss in proliferative retinopathy, as compared with untreated control eyes [8, 9].

The DRS identified three high-risk characteristics for severe visual loss (Table 59.3) [8, 9], defined as a visual acuity of 1/60 at two consecutive visits 4 months apart. The high-risk characteristics, which serve as indications for photocoagulation to be performed soon, are:

1 New vessels on the optic disc (NVD) which are more extensive than in a standard photograph (Fig. 59.10).
2 NVD less extensive than this standard, but accompanied by *any* vitreous or preretinal haemorrhage (Fig. 59.10).
3 New vessels elsewhere (NVE), more than two disc areas in size, together with *any* vitreous or preretinal haemorrhage.

The incidence of severe visual loss with high-risk characteristics and the benefits of treatment are shown in Table 59.4.

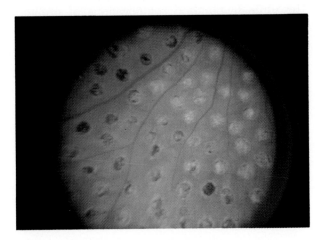

Fig. 59.21. Standard pan-retinal photocoagulation. The papillo-macular bundle is not treated, in order to preserve central vision (see Fig. 59.26).

Table 59.3. High-risk characteristics identified by the Diabetic Retinopathy Study [8, 9].

NVD	≥	DRS standard photo 10 A (Fig. 59.10)
NVD	<	Standard photo 10 A (Fig. 59.10) but with *any* vitreous/preretinal haemorrhage.
NVE	≥	2 disc areas with any vitreous/preretinal haemorrhage.

Key: NVD = optic disc new vessels; NVE = new vessels elsewhere.

Table 59.4. Outcome of patients with high-risk characteristics (from the Diabetic Retinopathy Study [8, 9]).

	Percentage with severe visual loss
Without treatment	25% at 2 years 50% at 5 years
With treatment	11% at 2 years 26% at 5 years

Table 59.5. Proliferative and preproliferative diabetic retinopathy. Indications for laser photocoagulation.

Condition	Recommended action
NVD*	Pan-retinal photocoagulation before vitreous haemorrhage occurs
NVE*	Pan-retinal photocoagulation before retinal detachment occurs
Rubeosis*	Pan-retinal photocoagulation before neovascular glaucoma develops
Preproliferative	Pan-retinal photocoagulation, of first eye
Peroperative*	Pan-retinal endolaser photo-coagulation of all attached retina

Key: NVD: optic disc new vessels; NVE: new vessels elsewhere; *: benefit proven by Diabetic Retinopathy Study [8, 9].

Photocoagulation treatment of preproliferative retinopathy

It is not known whether photocoagulation should be given early, at the preproliferative stage, of deferred until high-risk characteristics develop. This question was not considered by the DRS but is currently being addressed by the ETDRS [1].

There are, however, theoretical advantages in treating preproliferative retinopathy. Treatment can be staged rather than rushed for fear of imminent vitreous haemorrhage, and pretreatment of existing macular oedema reduces the risk of its later exacerbation by pan-retinal photocoagulation. Moreover, there are indications that treating preproliferative retinopathy may often be curative, whereas treating established proliferative disease is frequently only palliative.

While awaiting the outcome of the ETDRS, it is the author's personal practice to treat the first eye of a patient with preproliferative retinopathy with pan-retinal photocoagulation [7, 20]. Any existing macular oedema is treated first (see below). If treatment is effective and there are no adverse effects, the other eye is then treated similarly.

Indications for laser photocoagulation of proliferative and preproliferative diabetic retinopathy are suggested in Table 59.5.

Photocoagulation treatment of macular oedema

The ETDRS finished recruiting 3928 patients in 1985 [3]. Although the study was primarily designed to determine the appropriate timing and type of pan-retinal photocoagulation, its results to date have been confined to the photocoagulation of macular oedema [3, 6, 7]. Patients with macular oedema were either not treated or given photocoagulation on diagnosis, with focal treatment for discrete lesions and diffuse 'grid' treatment for widespread capillary leakage and non-perfusion. Any residual leakage was re-treated every 4 months; follow-up treatment was commonly needed during the ETRDS study [4]. Case examples of focal treatment are illustrated in Figs 59.22−24, and of 'grid' photocoagulation in Fig. 59.26.

The outcome of photocoagulation treatment of clinically significant macular oedema in the ETDRS study is summarized in Table 59.6. Overall, the risk of severe visual loss in treated eyes was less than one-half of that in control eyes [3].

Vitreo-retinal surgery

The ultimate blinding complications of proliferative diabetic retinopathy are severe vitreous haemorrhage and secondary retinal detachment. The latter is determined by certain important anatomical considerations [28]. In the normal eye, the vitreous is loosely applied to the entire retina, with firm bonds only at the optic disc, adjoining major retinal vessels and at the peripheral vitreous base (Fig. 59.27a). Neovascular tissue invading from the optic disc and elsewhere through the retina produces a fibro-vascular carpet spreading to line the vitreo-retinal interface. This carpet is 'nailed down' to the underlying retina by the original fibro-vascular ingrowths and is fused to the overlying cortical vitreous. Detachment of the posterior surface of the vitreous from the retina (Fig. 59.27b), which occurs normally in the elderly,

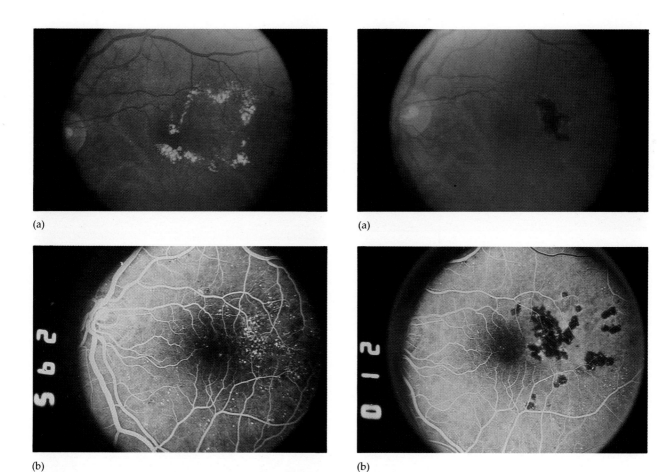

(a)

(b)

Fig. 59.22. Focal treatment of macular oedema. Pretreatment photograph (a) and matching angiogram (b) showing features of localized macular oedema.

(a)

(b)

Fig. 59.24. (a, b) One year posttreatment photograph (a) of the same area with matching angiogram (b), showing improvement in features of macular oedema. Visual acuity improved from 6/12 to 6/6.

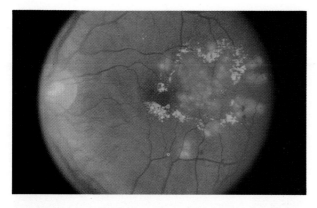

Fig. 59.23. Immediate posttreatment photograph of area shown in Fig. 59.22a.

Table 59.6. Clinically significant macular oedema. Outcome of treatment at diagnosis compared with deferral of treatment on visual loss*. (Adapted from ETDRS — see text.)

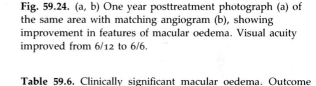

	Treated group	Untreated group
1 year	5%	10%
2 years	8%	21%
3 years	13%	30%

* Visual loss was defined as doubling of the initial visual angle, e.g. from 6/6 to 6/12, 6/36 to 6/60.

will result in tractional forces being applied to the neovascular membrane. These tractional forces, combined with intrinsic contraction of the membrane itself, may result in vitreous haemorrhage from shearing of the fragile new vessels, tractional retinal detachment and, if sufficient to tear a hole in the retina, in a combined rhegmatogenous and tractional retinal detachment (Figs 59.15–19). The role of the vitreous in the pathogenesis of these tractional complications is shown in Fig. 59.28.

Although vitrectomy can be performed electively for severe vitreous haemorrhage alone [11], urgent surgery is required for operable retinal detachment [12, 13, 17–19]. As mentioned above, the

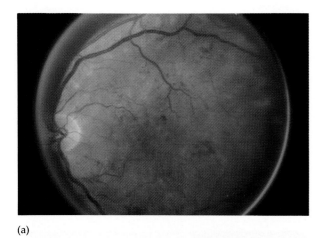

(a)

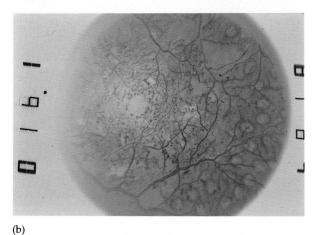

(b)

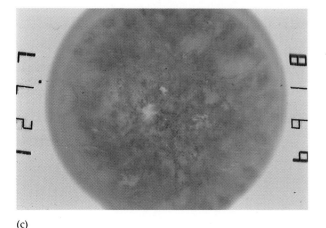

(c)

Fig. 59.25. (a) Pretreatment photograph of diffuse macular oedema. (b) Early-phase fluorescein angiogram of area in (a) showing extensive capillary non-perfusion. (c) Late-phase angiogram showing diffuse capillary leakage.

viability of the retina declines with increasing duration of detachment and in general, re-attaching the macula after 3 months will not use-fully improve central vision.

All the techniques used in vitreo-retinal micro-surgery require a closed intra-ocular approach [28].

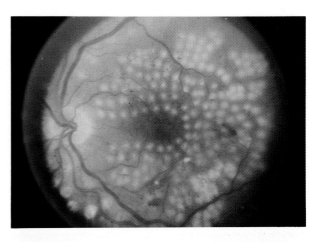

Fig. 59.26. Grid treatment of diffuse/ischaemic macular oedema, sparing the central macula and papillo-macular bundle.

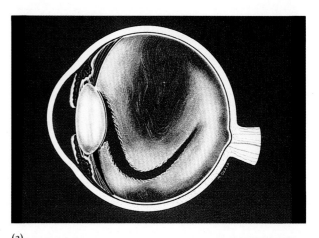

(a)

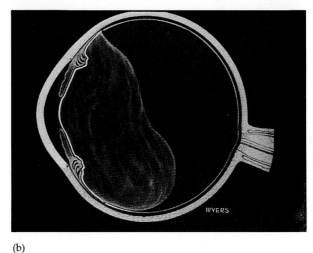

(b)

Fig. 59.27. (a) The normal vitreo-retinal relationships in a young person. The posterior surface of the vitreous is in total contact with the retina. (b) Complete posterior vitreous detachment from the retina occurs normally in the elderly.

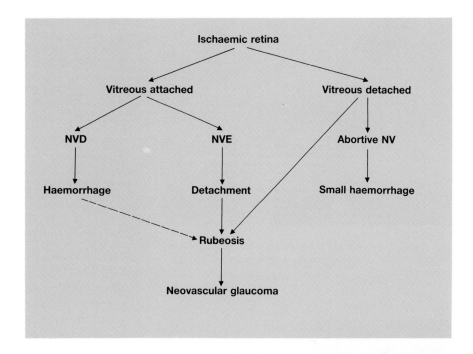

Fig. 59.28. The pathogenesis of diabetic blindness. NV = new vessels; NVD = on disc; NVE = elsewhere on retina.

The vitreous cavity can be entered safely through the *pars plana*, a 2-mm zone centred 4.5 mm lateral to the corneo-scleral junction which is sufficiently posterior to avoid damaging the crystalline lens and yet clear of the anterior edge of the retina (Fig. 59.29). Isotonic saline is infused into the ocular cavity through a cannula pushed through the pars plana, in order to maintain and control intra-ocular pressure. Operative instruments (cutters and aspirators) and a light source are introduced through two further sclerotomies; all instruments are common-gauge so that the sclerotomies are watertight. Using a corneal contact lens, the retina may be clearly seen and an operating microscope allows precise intra-ocular manipulation (Figs 59.30 and 59.31.) The vitreous and its contained haemorrhage are first removed, either with mechanical cutters or an yttrium−aluminium garnet (YAG) laser, and then replaced with infused saline. The retina can be physically re-attached to the choroid and is then treated peroperatively with endolaser photocoagulation to prevent both further detachment and subsequent neovascularization. Operative techniques are discussed in detail elsewhere [28−33].

Visual recovery can be both dramatic and sustained [11, 12, 17−19, 29], the pooled success rate for anatomical and functional success being around 65−70%. However, the principal complications of retinal detachment (either persistent or iatrogenic) and resultant neovascular glaucoma can result in an eye that is blind and painful;

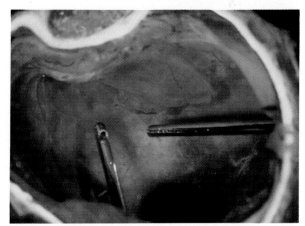

Fig. 59.29. Principles of vitreo-retinal surgery, illustrated by common-gauge instruments inserted through the pars plana of a transected cadaver eye.

surgery is therefore not undertaken lightly.

The major indications for vitrectomy are shown in Table 59.7. Recent results from the Diabetic Retinopathy Vitrectomy Study [DRVS] indicate that early vitrectomy should be considered in eyes retaining useful vision but with advanced active proliferative retinopathy [12, 13]. In the author's experience, the most important factors in deciding whether to subject an eye to vitrectomy are the duration of macular detachment and the likelihood of achieving the surgical goals; failed surgery makes re-operation considerably more difficult.

The normal successful postoperative appear-

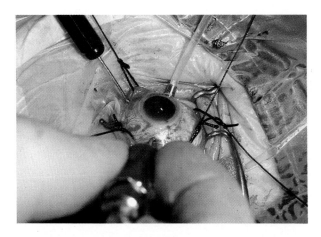

Fig. 59.30. Trans-pars plana vitrectomy with common-gauge instrumentation and infusion of saline to maintain intra-ocular pressure.

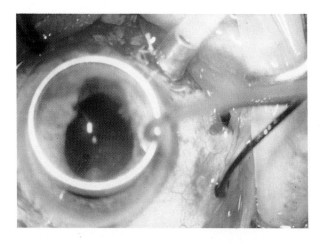

Fig. 59.31. Trans-pars plana vitrectomy. Peroperative view of retina through contact lens placed on cornea.

Table 59.7. Surgical indications for diabetic vitrectomy.

Long-standing severe vitreous haemorrhage (visual acuity worse than 6/60 for 6 months)

Recent tractional macular detachment

Combined rhegmatogenous/tractional detachment

Possibly in severe active proliferative retinopathy with good vision

Likelihood of achieving surgical goals.

ances are shown in Fig. 59.32. Most of the epi-retinal membrane has been removed, leaving only minor residual islands of tissue, and the retina has remained re-attached for two years. Note the extensive laser scars and profound retinal ischaemia with avascular arterioles.

Indications for ophthalmological referral

The need for vitrectomy in diabetic patients would largely disappear if adequate laser photocoagulation were applied promptly at an early stage. This can only be achieved if diabetic patients are regularly and effectively screened for ocular complications. The timing of eye examinations is outlined in Table 59.2, together with a schedule which is appropriate to a busy diabetic clinic. The indications for referral to an ophthalmologist are listed in Table 59.8, which also indicates the necessary urgency for each problem.

Table 59.8. Indications for referring a diabetic patient to an ophthalmologist.

Condition	Urgency
Cataract	Routine (few months)
Hard exudates: close to macula or numbers increasing Retinal haemorrhages: numbers increasing Preproliferative changes	Soon (few weeks)
Fall in visual acuity (two lines or more) Visible maculopathy (oedema, exudates) New vessels Rubeosis iridis Advanced diabetic eye disease, especially retinal detachment	Urgent (1 week)
Vitreous haemorrhage Neovascular glaucoma	Immediate (same or next day)

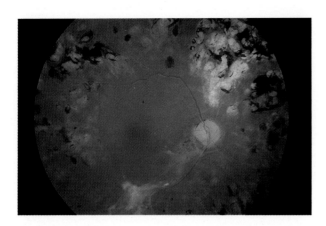

Fig. 59.32. Successful outcome of vitreo-retinal surgery, showing residual islands of epiretinal membrane (temporal to macula, nasal to disc, and on upper vascular arcade), retinal re-attachment and laser photocoagulation scars. There is still profound retinal ischaemia. Visual acuity has been restored to 6/12 from 1/60 preoperatively.

Conclusions

Photocoagulation is now of indisputable value in treating two major threats to the vision of diabetic patients, namely proliferative retinopathy and macular oedema. Moreover, intra-ocular microsurgery can restore vision to some eyes with blindness which, only a few years ago, would have been untreatable. It is obvious that photocoagulation and microsurgery services must be made available to all diabetic patients, but the immense importance of early detection of diabetic eye disease and its correct monitoring cannot be overemphasized. It is to be hoped that measures such as these will go a long way towards eliminating and preventing blindness in diabetes.

PETER J. BARRY

References

1 Early Treatment Diabetic Retinopathy Study (ETDRS). *Manual of Operations.* Baltimore: ETDRS Coordinating Center, Department of Epidemiology and Preventive Medicine, University of Maryland, 1985.
2 Whitelocke RAF, Kearns M, Blach RK, Hamilton AM. The diabetic maculopathies. *Trans Ophthalmol Soc UK* 1979; **99**: 314–20.
3 Early Treatment Diabetic Retinopathy Study Research Group. Photocoagulation for diabetic macular edema. ETDRS Report No 1. *Arch Ophthalmol* 1985; **103**: 1796–1806.
4 Murphy RP, Ferris FL. The current status of the Early Treatment Diabetic Retinopathy Study. *Ophthalmic Forum* 1984; **2**: 149–52.
5 Early Treatment Diabetic Retinopathy Study Research Group. Treatment techniques and clinical guidelines for photocoagulation of diabetic macular oedema: ETDRS Report No 2. *Ophthalmology* 1987; **94**: 761–74.
6 Early Treatment Diabetic Retinopathy Study Research Group. Techniques for scatter and local photocoagulation treatment of diabetic retinopathy: ETDRS Report No 3. *Int Ophthalmol Clin* 1987; **27** (No **4**): 254–64.
7 Early Treatment Diabetic Retinopathy Study Research Group. Photocoagulation for diabetic macular edema: ETDRS Report No 4. *Int Ophthalmol Clin* 1987; **27** (No **4**): 265–333.
8 The Diabetic Retinopathy Study Research Group. Design, methods and baseline results. Report No 6. *Invest Ophthalmol Vis Sci* 1981; **21** (suppl 1) (part 2): 1–209.
9 The Diabetic Retinopathy Study Research Group. Photocoagulation treatment of proliferative diabetic retinopathy. Clinical application of DRS findings. Report No 8. *Ophthalmology* 1981; **88**: 583–600.
10 Diabetic Retinopathy Vitrectomy Study Research Group. Two year course of visual acuity in severe proliferative diabetic retinopathy with conservative management. Diabetic Retinopathy Vitrectomy Study (DRVS) Report No 1. *Ophthalmology* 1985; **92**: 492–502.
11 Diabetic Retinopathy Vitrectomy Study Research Group. Early vitrectomy for severe vitreous haemorrhage in diabetic retinopathy. Two-year results of randomized trial. DRVS Report No 2. *Arch Ophthalmol* 1985; **103**: 1644–52.
12 Diabetic Retinopathy Vitrectomy Study Research Group. Early vitrectomy for severe proliferative diabetic retinopathy in eyes with useful vision: Results of a randomized trial. DRVS Research Report No 3. *Ophthalmology* 1988; **95**: 1307–20.
13 Diabetic Retinopathy Vitrectomy Study Research Group. Early vitrectomy for severe proliferative diabetic retinopathy in eyes with useful vision: Clinical application of results of a randomized trial. DRVS Report No 4. *Ophthalmology* 1988; **95**: 1321–34.
14 British Multicentre Study Group. Photocoagulation for proliferative diabetic retinopathy: a randomized control clinical trial using the xenon arc. *Diabetologia* 1984; **26**: 109–15.
15 British Multicentre Study Group. Photocoagulation in the treatment of diabetic retinopathy. *Lancet* 1975; ii: 1110–13.
16 British Multicentre Study Group. Photocoagulation for diabetic maculopathy. *Diabetes* 1983; **32**: 1010–16.
17 Michels R. Vitrectomy for complications of diabetic retinopathy. *Arch Ophthalmol* 1978; **96**: 237–46.
18 Blankenship G, Machemer R. Pars plana vitrectomy for management of severe diabetic retinopathy. *Am J Ophthalmol* 1978; **85**: 553–62.
19 Mandelcorn MS, Blankenship G, Machemer R. Pars plana vitrectomy for the management of severe diabetic retinopathy. *Am J Ophthalmol* 1976; **81**: 561–70.
20 The Diabetic Retinopathy Study Research Group. Indications for photocoagulation treatment of diabetic retinopathy: Report No 14. *Int Ophthalmol Clin* 1987; **27** (suppl 4): 239–53.
21 Marshall J, Glover G, Rothery S. Some new findings on retinal irradiation by krypton and argon lasers. *Doc Ophthalmol* 1984; **36**: 21–37.
22 Weiter JJ, Zuckerman R. The influence of the photoreceptors—RPE complex on the inner retina; an explanation for the beneficial effects of photocoagulation. *Ophthalmology* 1980; **87**: 1133–9.
23 Glaser BM, Hayashi H, Krause WG. A protease inhibitor accumulates within the vitreous following panretinal photocoagulation (PRP) in primates: possible mechanisms for

the effect of PRP on retinal neovascularization. *Invest Ophthalmol Vis Sci* 1988; **29** (suppl): 1180.

24 Glaser BM, D'Amore PA, Michels RG, Patz A, Fenselau A. Demonstration of vasoproliferative activity from mammalian retina. *J Cell Biol* 1980; **84**: 298–30.

25 Glaser BM, Campochiaro PA, Davis JL, Jerdan JA. Retinal pigment epithelial cells release inhibitors of neovascularization. *Ophthalmology* 1987; **94**: 780–4.

26 McDonald HR, Schatz E. Macular oedema following panretinal photocoagulation. *Retina* 1985; **5**: 5–10.

27 Edererer F, Hiller R. Clinical trials, diabetic retinopathy and photocoagulation. A reanalysis of 5 studies. *Survey Ophthalmol* 1975; **19**: 267–86.

28 Charles S. *Vitreous Microsurgery*, 2nd edn. Baltimore: Williams & Wilkins, 1987.

29 DeBustros S, Thompson JJ, Michels RG, Rice TA. Vitrectomy for progressive proliferative diabetic retinopathy. *Arch Ophthalmol* 1987; **105**: 196–9.

30 McLeod D, James CRH. Viscodelamination at the vitreoretinal juncture in severe diabetic eye disease. *Br J Ophthalmol* 1988; **72**: 413–19.

31 Barry PJ, Hiscott PS, Grierson I, Marshall J, McLeod D. Reparative epiretinal fibrosis after diabetic vitrectomy. *Trans Ophthalmol Soc UK* 1985; **104**: 285–96.

32 Acheson RW, Capon M, Cooling RJ, Leaver PK, Marshall J, McLeod D. Intraocular argon laser photocoagulation. *Eye* 1987; **1**: 97–105.

33 McLeod D. Silicone oil injection during closed microsurgery for diabetic retinal detachment. *Graefes Arch Klin Exp Ophthalmol* 1986; **224**: 55–9.

60 Psychological, Social and Practical Aspects of Visual Handicap for the Diabetic Patient

Summary

• Diabetes is the commonest cause of visual loss in the British working population.

• 'Blindness' is defined as the inability to perform any task for which eyesight is essential, and 'partial sighted' as substantial and permanent visual loss.

• Loss of vision is psychologically devastating, often causing prolonged shock, denial, anxiety, anger and depression.

• Many blind people use 'mental mapping', a combination of tactile input and visual imagery, to find their way around and perform daily activities. This encourages mobility, independence and self-assurance.

• Many aids are available to help blind and partially sighted patients to draw up insulin accurately and measure their blood glucose concentration.

• It is essential to register blind or partially sighted patients immediately to activate the many social services and facilities available to them.

Loss of vision — which often implies loss of status, independence, self-confidence and income — is a devastating experience for anyone. As shown in Table 60.1, diabetes is the commonest cause of blindness in people of working age in the UK. For diabetic patients, who have to relearn how to manage their diabetes as well as a new way of life, loss of vision presents added difficulties. However, much can be done for the diabetic person under these circumstances and, indeed, helping the patient to overcome the practical difficulties of diabetic management can often accelerate his or her progress towards independence and greater self-esteem.

This section will first describe the psychological and social aspects of losing vision, including the process of 'mental mapping' by which many blind people find their way around. Finally, the practical management of the partially sighted or blind diabetic patient will be discussed, with emphasis on the services, benefits and aids available.

Psychological and social aspects

As with all grieving processes, the psychological trauma associated with visual loss may comprise shock, denial, anxiety, anger and depression [1] (see Chapter 77). This is the usual response to loss of sight, and a process that all go through (to a variable extent) before they come to terms with their disability; there is a 'need to mourn the loss of vision before being able to accept the reality of blindness' [2]. The immediate shock following visual loss can last weeks or months and is followed by denial that this could happen and anxiety about how to cope with life and the future. Some may feel guilty and blame themselves for blindness, which is sometimes regarded as a punishment for past sins. Depression can last for a long time, even years. Some people lean heavily on their relatives, who may be overprotective, whereas others are determined to lead a normal life and soon become quite independent [2, 3; Conyers, unpublished]. The grieving process is influenced by personality, age, rapidity of visual loss and the quality of help available to the newly blind. Rapid visual loss in the young produces greater psychological trauma than gradually declining vision in the elderly, who have more

Table 60.1. Current UK statistics concerning loss of vision and diabetes. (Sources: Office of Population Censuses and Surveys, 1989, and *Health Bulletin* **41** [6]).

In the UK population as a whole:
- 1.75 million people suffer from significant visual loss
- 78% of visual handicap registrations are in people over 65 years of age

The role of diabetes:
- The overall prevalence of retinopathy in the diabetic population is 26–35%, and of severe (proliferative or advanced) retinopathy is 9–11%
- Diabetic retinopathy is the major cause of blindness in people under 65 years of age (about 300 visual handicap registrations per year)
- In visually handicapped diabetic patients, diabetic eye disease is responsible in 44% of younger-onset patients, 22% of older-onset patients treated with insulin and 11% of older-onset patients not receiving insulin

time to adjust to what is happening and possibly fewer expectations of life [2, 3].

It is essential to be honest with people who are losing their vision: to hold out false hopes only encourages the health workers, not the patient [2; Conyers, unpublished]. People able to accept blindness have much better psychological and social function [1, 2]. Allowing people to express their feelings of sadness, anger and fear may hasten the passing of depression [4, 5]. Another common problem, due partly to depression and partly to the loss of the close relationship between vision and sexual arousal, is decreased sexual activity and castration fears [2, 4]. Indirectly, visual loss can profoundly affect other family members, changing previous relationships and often imposing great strain on those who now have to care for the blind person. Nonetheless, rehabilitation is more difficult for those living alone than for those living within a family [2].

Rehabilitation, although essential, tends to segregate the disabled from normal society [6]. Many people feel anxious and uncomfortable when close to disability and need to recognize their prejudices, preconceptions and emotional reactions when dealing with blindness; 'the problem of the blind individual in dealing with the sighted may be greater than the problem of dealing with the blindness itself' [2]. It is easy to focus on the deficit of blindness, but vital not to overlook the person's other attributes which remain and may grow as he adjusts to his changed life.

Mental imagery

Loss of vision promotes the use and heightens the sensitivity of the other senses, possibly because these are now essential for navigation and spatial awareness. Congenitally blind people employ 'haptic' navigation (i.e. using touch), whereas those who have lost sight retain visual imagery, which greatly improves their orientation and spatial skills [7–9]. These forms of imagery represent alternative forms of coding information; a distinction has been made between 'videation' (an image created using information from senses other than sight, including other people's observations) and a recreated visual image, generated by memory alone [10, 11].

Visual images draw attention to particular cues in the environment and their spatial relationships, and together with information gathered from experiences in navigation and problem solving, are used as a basis for mental mapping [12]. People who lose their vision relearn how to find their way around their home, to the local shops, and around the workplace and the houses of friends and relatives. Learning to make mental maps helps the individual to become mobile again, encouraging independence and self-assurance.

Practical management of diabetes for the partially sighted and blind

Enabling the newly visually handicapped patient to take charge of his diabetic management again is often a significant first step in helping him to become generally independent.

Drawing up insulin

For the partially sighted, a 1-ml plastic syringe graduated in black is the easiest to read, especially against a pale background in a good light. Several syringe magnifiers, designed to be fitted on to a plastic syringe barrel, are available. The Magniguide (Becton–Dickinson) is useful as it magnifies the whole length of the barrel (Fig. 60.1a); Monoject and Hypoguard produce smaller magnifiers. Another aid to drawing up the correct dose is the syringe guide (Terumo), consisting of a strip of plastic with a hole to take one of the wings of the syringe barrel (Fig. 60.1b). The strip is marked along its length in units corresponding to the syringe and is cut to the length corresponding to the dose by a sighted person. Insulin is then drawn up level to the end of the plastic strip. It is possible to have a different strip for each insulin dosage, which can be written in large black numbers on the back. 'Count a Dose' is a gadget which enables blind people to draw up a combination of insulins in a plastic syringe.

Blind diabetic patients can use two special types of glass syringe, which require no vision. The *click-count* syringe (Hypoguard) is a conventional glass syringe whose plunger is scored at unit intervals and clicks against a ratchet incorporated into the base of the syringe as the plunger is withdrawn (Fig. 60.1c). The dosage of insulin, including different preparations, can be drawn up simply by counting the clicks. Insulin must be drawn up slowly in order to count the clicks, so there is less chance of drawing up air. The *preset syringe* (Rand Rocket) is a glass syringe with a threaded plunger carrying two screws (Fig. 60.1d). A sighted person sets the screws at the correct dose and insulin is then drawn up until the screws prevent any further movement. It is more likely that air will be drawn up using this syringe, as people tend to pull the plunger down more rapidly. Many blind people prefer to use plastic syringes because of their finer needles and disposability; the Terumo syringe guide can be used with a plastic syringe by the blind if the dosage is marked in braille or with Hymark on the back of the guide.

Different types of insulin can be distinguished by placing sticky tape or rubber bands around the neck of long-acting insulin vials. The NovoPen (I or II) is a great help for the partially sighted or blind patient. This can be carried around very easily, and the dosage easily counted either by depressing the cap (= 2 units on NovoPen I) or 'dialing' the number of units (NovoPen II). The 'neutral' and 'primed' positions on the NovoPen II are also identified by palpable marks on the barrel. With the pen devices, it is possible to test if there is any insulin left by ejecting one unit over the palm of the hand or wrist.

Oral medication

Taking oral hypoglycaemic agents and other

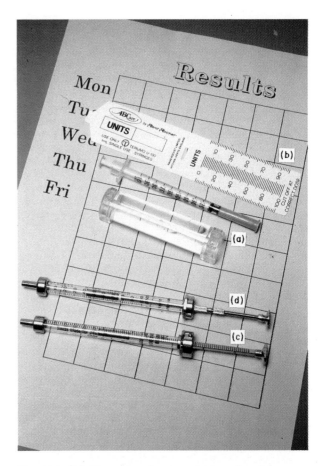

Fig. 60.1. This illustration shows a selection of useful gadgets: a large-print result sheet, magnifier and syringe guide. At the bottom is a click count and preset syringe.

tablets obviously presents fewer problems than injecting insulin, but may still be difficult. Various containers are available which are prefilled by a sighted person and distribute one batch of tablets at a time (Fig. 60.2). These devices, as well as large-print and braille labels, are available from the Royal National Institute for the Blind (see Table 60.4).

Home blood glucose monitoring

Partially sighted and blind diabetic patients can be taught to measure their own blood glucose levels [13]. For the partially sighted, the standard Hypocount meter (BCL) with its large red LED display is very useful. Blind patients can use various specially adapted blood glucose meters which buzz, beep or speak the result. The buzzing Hypocount meter (BCL) gives the result as a series of buzzes (e.g. one buzz represents 0−3 mmol/l, two buzzes 4−7 mmol/l, and so on). The Glucochek

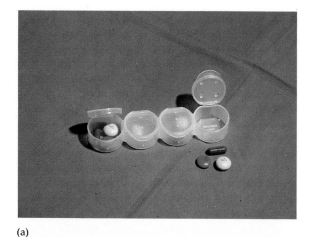

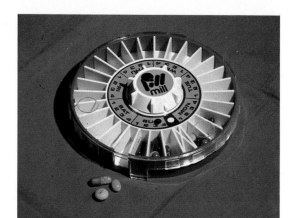

(a)

(b)

Fig. 60.2. (a) Daily pillminder, holding a day's supply of tablets. Compartments are differentiated by raised dots (not braille). (b) The Pillmill, a circular container with 28 compartments, holding one week's supply. The clear plastic top is turned to access successive doses. (Reproduced with permission from Mrs J. Williams, Fazakerley Hospital, Liverpool, and the Editors of *Practical Diabetes*.)

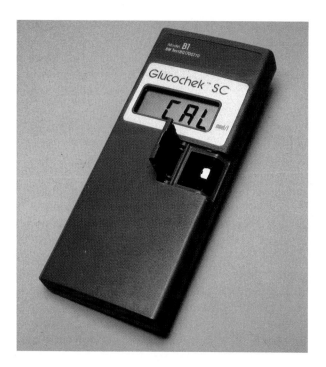

Fig. 60.3. The musical Glucochek machine uses a series of different codes of blips and buzzes to denote blood glucose values of between 2–22 mmol, and ascending and descending musical scales for values outside this range.

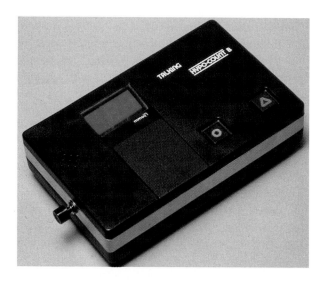

Fig. 60.4. The talking Hypocount meter. The large button on the left can be pressed at any time during the machine's sequence for the user to be told what is happening as well as speaking the result.

SC (Ames) (Fig. 60.3) conveys more detailed information with a combination of different musical tones, whereas the 'talking' Hypocount meter (Fig. 60.4) uses an electronically generated voice to give both instructions and the result. All of these machines are useful and patients enjoy using them.

There remains the problem of teaching someone with little or no vision to prick their finger and place a small drop of blood accurately on a reagent strip. Mental mapping can be exploited to produce an image of the finger, which has to be kept level to avoid losing the drop of blood. Orientating on the painful part of the finger which has been pricked, the reagent pad on the stick (identified with a fingernail) is then pressed against the finger so it can be felt just underneath the finger-prick site; the finger is then rolled on to the pad. Blank readings, where the drop of blood misses the stick completely, are quite common at first but with encouragement and perseverance, most people (except for those with severe sensory neuropathy, who cannot feel the needle) can learn this manoeuvre.

Results can be recorded by partially sighted patients on large-print, black-inked results sheets or on a tape recorder by the blind. The elderly are more difficult to teach than the young, chiefly because they have less confidence in their ability to learn new skills, and much patience and perseverence may be needed on the part of both the diabetic care team and the patient.

Blind registration and social services

The definitions of 'partial sight' and 'blindness' for the purposes of registration are purely economic. Blindness is defined as the inability to perform any work for which eyesight is essential, and partial sight as substantial and permanent visual handicap. In the UK, the blind registration form (BD8) is completed by a consultant ophthalmologist and forwarded to the patient's local Social Services department, where it is passed to the social worker responsible for the handicapped. Different areas show considerable variation in the services available and the personnel who actually provide them. The social worker dealing with a disability is the 'gatekeeper' for both the official local services and for information concerning voluntary and other organizations specializing in support for that disability. The social worker who visits the visually handicapped offers emotional support, encouragement and practical help, as well as organizing local services. The various allowances and benefits for which blind diabetic patients may be eligible in the UK are shown in Table 60.2. Some local authorities also have technical officers who teach the blind person everyday tasks such as cooking, advise on special pieces of equipment and teach braille and typing. Mobility officers teach the newly blind long-cane training and help them to plan the layout of their surroundings. In many areas, these three disciplines are undertaken by one social worker. Other useful services are listed in Table 60.3, and a list of relevant addresses is provided in Table 60.4.

Table 60.2. Allowances and benefits available.*

Benefit	Amount (£/week)
Unemployment Benefit	41.15
Statutory Sick Pay:	
lower rate	34.25
standard rate	49.20
Sickness Benefit	31.30
Mobility Allowance	23.05
Invalidity Benefit	41.15
Invalidity Allowance:	
higher rate	8.65
middle rate	5.50
lower rate	2.75
Invalid Care Allowance	24.75
Attendance Allowance:	
higher rate	32.95
lower rate	22.00

Blind people are also eligible for a British Rail Disabled Person's Railcard, a reduced-price TV licence and Disabled Person's car stickers, and may vote by post.

* 1989 UK figures.

Table 60.3. Useful services and facilities in the UK for partially sighted and blind patients (addresses are given in Table 60.4).

Talking books. Giant cassette tapes and the machines for playing them are available from RNIB, British Talking Book Service for the Blind, Royal National Library for the Blind and Calibre Library

Talking newspapers. Some Sunday papers and monthly magazines are available on standard cassettes from the Talking Newspaper Association. Some local authorities provide local papers on cassette

Library services. Most libraries have large-print books and some have a service for housebound readers

Residential establishments, courses, holiday homes and caravans for the blind are organized by the RNIB

Information and a wide range of aids to daily life are available from the RNIB and the Partially Sighted Society

Table 60.4. Useful addresses for visually handicapped patients in the UK.

Royal National Institute for the Blind (RNIB), 224 Great Portland Street, London W1N 6AA, UK
Partially Sighted Society, Queens Road, Doncaster DN1 2NX, UK
London Association for the Blind, 14–16 Vernay Street, London SE16, UK
Guide Dogs Association, Alexandra House, 9–11 Park Street, Windsor, Berkshire, UK
Talking Newspaper Association for the UK, 224 Mount Pleasant, Wembley, Middlesex, UK

The Guide Dogs for the Blind Association arrange trials to assess an individual's suitability for a guide dog, which can give a greater degree of independence as well as a valuable companion. The RNIB residential centre at Torquay offers retraining for people wishing to return to work and a general, intensive rehabilitation course, with the aim of encouraging as much independence and self-confidence as possible. Most Job Centres have a Disability Resettlement Officer, to help and advise on retraining and employment.

JACQUELINE N. JONES

References

1 Keegan DL, Ash D, Greenough T. Adjustment to blindness. *Canad J Ophthalmol* 1976; **11** (suppl 2): 22–9.
2 Diffenburg RS. The psychology of blindness. *Geriatrics* 1967; **22**: 127–33.
3 Clark-Carter D. Psycho-social aspects of mobility training. *New Beacon* 1987; **71**: 217–19.
4 Fitzgerald RG. The newly blind, mental distress, somatic illness, disability and management. *EENT Monthly* 1973; **52**: 99–102.
5 Jones JN, Uccellari H. Coping with visual loss. British Diabetic Association, London, 1989.
6 Goffman E. *Stigma*. Englewood Cliffs, New Jersey: Spectrum Books, 1963: Chapter 3.
7 Herman JE. Cognitive mapping in blind people, acquisition of spatial relationships in a large scale environment. *J Vis Impair Blind* 1983; **77**: 161–6.
8 Sylvester RH. The mental imagery of the blind: discussion. *Psychol Bull* 1983; **10**: 210–11.
9 Finke RA. Mental imagery and the visual system. *Sci Am* 1986; **254**: 88–95.
10 Miller S. In: Gelder BD, ed. *The Problem of Imagery and Spatial Development. Knowledge and Representation*. London: Routledge and Keegan Paul, 1982.
11 Ryerson N. Using and creating visual images, a new task for rehabilitation. *J Vis Impair Blind* 1982; **76**: 421–3.
12 Dodds AG, Carter DDC. Memory of movement in blind children: the role of previous visual experience. *J Motor Behav* 1983; **15**: 343–52.
13 Prior JC, Alojado NC, Hunt JA, Begg IS. Use of tactile techniques for self-monitoring of blood glucose in visually impaired patients with diabetes mellitus. *Diabetes Care* 1984; 7: 313–17.

PART 13.3
DIABETIC NEUROPATHY

61   Diabetic Neuropathy: Epidemiology and Pathogenesis

Summary

• Diabetic neuropathy can be classified as either reversible (e.g. reduced nerve conduction velocity) or established (focal, multifocal, symmetric and mixed neuropathies).

• The epidemiology of diabetic neuropathy is unclear because of inconsistent definitions of what constitutes neuropathy — frequencies of 10–100% of patients affected have been reported.

• Nerve biopsies show axonal degeneration and regeneration, demyelination and remyelination and abnormalities of the vasa nervorum; capillary closure is correlated with the severity of neuropathy.

• Neurophysiological studies show reduced motor and sensory nerve conduction velocities and resistance to ischaemic conduction failure.

• The pathogenesis is still uncertain: metabolic factors may predominate in early disease and vascular factors at a later stage and in focal neuropathies.

• In experimental diabetic neuropathy, a possible metabolic mechanism involves hyperglycaemia-induced sorbitol accumulation, myoinositol depletion, reduced Na^+-K^+- ATPase activity and an increase in intracellular Na^+ levels.

• The importance of non-enzymatic glycosylation of axonal proteins and changes in axoplasmic transport is uncertain.

A wide variety of disturbances of peripheral nerve function occur in relation to diabetes mellitus. Their precise classification is still not agreed, mainly because of persisting uncertainty as to their causation. In general, they can be divided into two categories (see Table 61.1). The first comprises rapidly reversible phenomena including distal paraesthesiae in the limbs and reduced nerve conduction velocity in newly diagnosed or poorly controlled diabetic subjects [1], and increased resistance to ischaemic conduction failure [2, 3]. The second category consists of more persistent phenomena ('established' neuropathy). These can be broadly subdivided into focal and multifocal neuropathies on one hand, and symmetric polyneuropathies on the other. Mixed syndromes are common.

This section considers the epidemiology, pathology, electrophysiology, pathogenesis and natural history of diabetic neuropathy.

Epidemiology

Satisfactory information is not so far available for the incidence and prevalence of diabetic neuropathy, largely because of inconsistency in defining

Table 61.1. A classification of diabetic neuropathy.

Rapidly reversible phenomena:
   Distal sensory symptoms
   Reduced nerve conduction velocity
   Resistance to ischaemic conduction failure

'Established' neuropathy:
   Focal and multifocal neuropathies
   • cranial mononeuropathies
   • thoracoabdominal neuropathy
   • focal limb neuropathies
   • asymmetric proximal lower limb motor neuropathy (diabetic amyotrophy)

   Symmetric neuropathies
   • sensory/autonomic polyneuropathy
   • proximal lower limb motor neuropathy

   Mixed syndromes

neuropathy. Ascertainment bias has also played a part. Currently available estimates of the frequency of diabetic neuropathy range between 10 and 100% [4], depending upon the criteria adopted. Those series reporting a prevalence of 100% have been based on the results of nerve conduction studies. Other series have given widely differing prevalences depending upon whether symptoms in the absence of signs, signs in the absence of symptoms, or the requirement that both should be present, have been taken as indicative of the presence of neuropathy. In a large prospective study of diabetic out-patients [5], the prevalence rose from 7.5% at the time of diagnosis of diabetes to 50% after 25 years. The prevalence after 20 years was over 40%. Yet in the prospective, community-based survey of Palumbo *et al.* [6], it was only half this value; this latter study, however, was a cohort analysis confined to NIDDM patients without neuropathy at entry. Attempts have recently been made [7] to define minimal criteria for the diagnosis of diabetic neuropathy and for staging the evolution of

neuropathy. Future prospective studies employing such criteria are likely to yield more consistent information.

Neuropathy is uncommon in children with diabetes, the prevalence rate being in the region of 2% [8]. Its prevalence increases progressively with age. The prospective study of Pirart [5] indicated that the risk of developing neuropathy is directly related to the duration of the diabetes so that the slopes for the increase in prevalence and annual incidence were approximately uniform (Fig. 61.1). The median time from the diagnosis of NIDDM to the development of neuropathy was found to be 9 years in one study [6].

There is no clear indication for any difference in liability to diabetic polyneuropathy between the sexes. Some series [5] have found a higher prevalence of males, but this was thought possibly to be related to confusion with other causes of neuropathy such as alcoholism. However, acute painful diabetic neuropathy and diabetic amyotrophy may be commoner in males. Little information is available for the relative prevalence

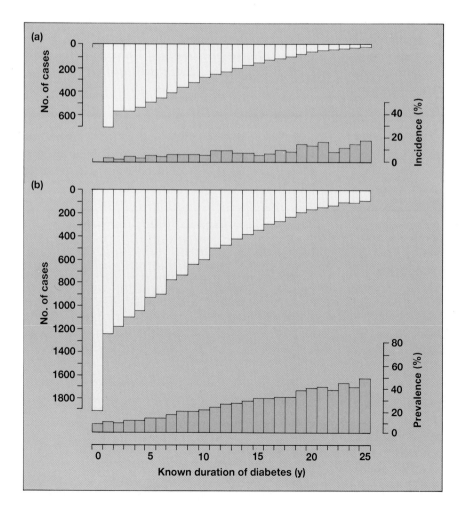

Fig. 61.1. Increase in the annual incidence and prevalence of diabetic neuropathy obtained from a prospective survey of 2795 cases observed from the time of diagnosis of diabetes. The suspended columns show the decrease in the number of subjects over time. (a) Incidence of neuropathy; (b) prevalence of neuropathy. (Redrawn with permission from Pirart 1978 [5].)

in different racial groups or geographical areas. Most studies have been conducted in Europe, Scandinavia or North America; Osuntokun [9] reported a prevalence of 40% in Nigeria.

The possible contribution of genetic factors in susceptibility to neuropathy requires further investigation, and may help to explain why some individuals with poorly controlled diabetes never develop significant neuropathy whereas others with mild or well-controlled disease develop troublesome neuropathy. The possibility of genetic linkage to acetylator status has not been confirmed [10].

Neuropathy occurs both in IDDM and NIDDM. It has been noted that the prevalence of neuropathy is less in the former than the latter at the time of diagnosis, presumably because of the shorter duration of antecedent undiscovered diabetes. Thus Mincu [11] found a prevalence of neuropathy of 1.4% in newly diagnosed cases of IDDM and 14.1% for NIDDM.

There is general agreement that the commonest type of diabetic neuropathy in both IDDM and NIDDM is a symmetric sensory and autonomic polyneuropathy. Some series [12] have reported a high prevalence of asymmetric motor syndromes, probably because of selection bias. Focal neuropathies are accepted as being more common in patients with diabetes, although this has never been established by a community-based epidemiological study.

Pathological changes

Most information on the pathology of diabetic neuropathy has been derived from investigations on nerve biopsies, which sample a relatively small portion of the peripheral nervous system (PNS). Full autopsy studies to assess the distribution of the changes throughout the PNS are few in number. Patients with diabetic polyneuropathy show axonal loss which increases in severity distally, accompanied by moderate demyelination. In one biopsy study of untreated diabetic subjects [13], the predominant changes in patients without symptoms of neuropathy were segmental demyelination and remyelination; patients with symptomatic neuropathy showed the combination of demyelination and remyelination together with axonal degeneration. Finally, in treated cases, often with long-standing diabetes, axonal degeneration was the commonest abnormality. In painful diabetic neuropathy, predominant loss of small myelinated fibres and evidence of degeneration and regeneration of unmyelinated axons has been described [14]. Such examples of diabetic 'small fibre neuropathy' probably do not represent a separate group, but rather one end of a spectrum in which fibres of all sizes may be lost [15]. Prominent axonal regeneration (Fig. 61.2) is a conspicuous feature of diabetic neuropathy, except in advanced cases, where few axons may remain in distal sensory nerves. Some loss of dorsal root

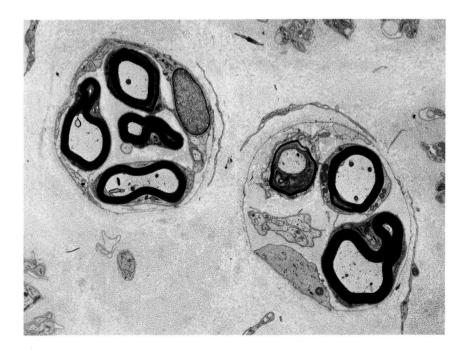

Fig. 61.2. Electron micrograph of transverse section of sural nerve biopsy from a patient with diabetic polyneuropathy, showing two regenerative clusters composed of groups of myelinated axons and associated Schwann cells.

and autonomic ganglion cells and of anterior horn cells occurs, but this is relatively modest. Degeneration of fibres is also detectable in the posterior columns of the spinal cord.

Fewer observations are available for patients with focal nerve lesions. In patients with third cranial nerve palsies, focal demyelination has been demonstrated in the nerve [16].

Attention to abnormalities of the vasa nervorum was drawn by Fagerberg [17] who found the walls of the endoneurial capillaries to be thickened by PAS-positive material. Electron microscopy showed this to be due to reduplication of the basal lamina (Fig. 61.3). Proliferation of endothelial cells, leading to narrowing of the vascular lumen has also been described, as have intraluminal deposits of fibrin. Dyck *et al.* [18] found that the numbers of closed capillaries in sural nerve biopsies were significantly greater than in age-matched control nerves and were positively correlated with the severity of the neuropathy (Fig. 61.4). More recently, however, Bradley *et al.* [19a] have failed to confirm capillary closure in a series of younger patients with diabetic polyneuropathy.

Neurophysiological changes

In asymptomatic diabetic patients, nerve conduction velocity, both motor and sensory, is frequently slightly reduced and sensory nerve action potentials are often of diminished amplitude, indicating subclinical neuropathy. Abnormalities may be detectable at common sites of compression or entrapment, reflecting an increased vulnerability of diabetic nerve to pressure damage [20]. The slight reduction of nerve conduction velocity which is present in newly diagnosed diabetic patients and which is rapidly reversed by institution of satisfactory glycaemic control [1] is of uncertain significance. It may reflect abnormalities of axolemmal function rather than indicating the presence of structural changes.

Diabetic nerves are abnormally resistant to the conduction failure normally caused by ischaemia, as can be demonstrated by electrophysiological means. Both evoked sensory nerve action potentials and conduction in motor fibres persist longer during ischaemia of a limb, produced by inflation of a pressure cuff above arterial pressure, than in normal subjects [3, 21].

In established diabetic polyneuropathy, the abnormalities are greater in sensory than motor fibres and are more prominent in the lower than in the upper limbs. The reduction in motor conduction velocity is mild or moderate, and severe slowing should raise the suspicion that the neuropathy has some other cause. Chronic inflammatory demyelinating polyneuropathy, hereditary motor and sensory neuropathy, and paraproteinaemic neuropathy are the three most important possibilities. Short-latency somatosen-

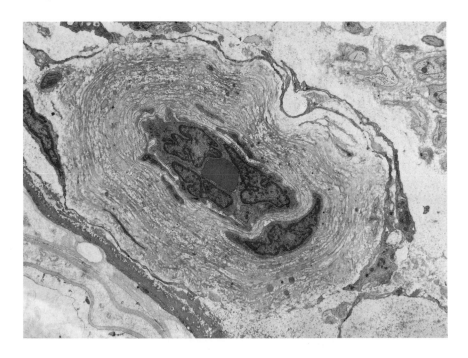

Fig. 61.3. Electron micrograph of endoneurial capillary from sural nerve biopsy from a patient with diabetic polyneuropathy, showing thickened surrounding zone composed of reduplicated basal lamina.

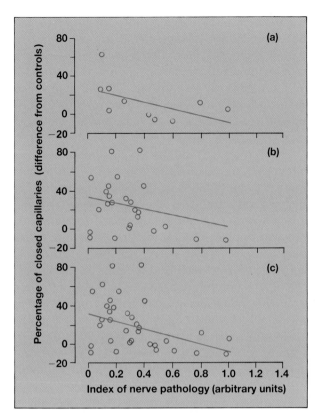

Fig. 61.4. Relationship between numbers of closed capillaries and the index of nerve pathology (IP) for sural nerve biopsies of patients with IDDM (a), NIDDM (b) and both combined (c). The number of closed capillaries is expressed as a percentage difference from controls. The IP combines the severity of loss of myelinated nerve fibres with abnormalities in surviving fibres. A higher IP value indicates less severe pathology. For all three groups, there is a significant negative slope, indicating a positive correlation between the numbers of closed capillaries and the severity of neuropathy. (Redrawn with permission from Dyck *et al.* 1985 [18] and the publisher.)

sory evoked responses may be delayed [22], indicating pathology in the spinal roots, dorsal columns, or both.

In patients with focal nerve lesions such as the carpal tunnel syndrome or ulnar neuropathy, localized abnormalities of nerve conduction are demonstrable. Similarly, conduction time may be prolonged in the femoral nerve in proximal lower limb motor neuropathy (diabetic amyotrophy).

Electromyography demonstrates denervation in affected muscles in patients with focal limb nerve lesions or proximal lower limb motor neuropathy. In the latter syndrome, denervation may be detectable in paraspinal muscles, suggesting involvement of spinal nerves as well as the lumbo-

sacral plexus and femoral nerves. Some denervation may be present in distal muscles (sometimes only in the small foot muscles) in diabetic sensory/autonomic polyneuropathy, even in the absence of clinically demonstrable weakness.

Pathogenesis

The causation of diabetic neuropathy is still not understood. Part of the difficulty stems from the fact that multiple abnormalities can be demonstrated in the PNS of human subjects with diabetes and in animals with experimentally induced or genetic diabetes. Identification of the causal chain of events leading to peripheral nerve damage is correspondingly difficult. Moreover, correlation does not imply causation. The major discussion concerns the relative contributions of metabolic and vascular factors.

Glycaemic control

The question as to whether improved control of glycaemia can prevent or ameliorate diabetic neuropathy has recently been reviewed [23]. The balance of evidence favoured the conclusion that hyperglycaemia is an important determinant of neuropathy and that improved glycaemic control benefits nerve function. This was based on four lines of evidence. The first derives from several retrospective studies (which are defective in various respects) which concluded overall that neuropathy was commoner in poorly controlled individuals. Further evidence comes from assessments of neuropathy before and after starting diabetic treatment. Minor improvements in nerve conduction velocity and reversal of resistance to ischaemic conduction failure are well documented, but neither of these phenomena is known to be related to the later development of established neuropathy. Acute painful diabetic neuropathy has been reported to improve after the institution of tight glycaemic control [24] and painful neuropathy has also been found to be benefited by continuous subcutaneous insulin therapy (CSII) [25]. Thirdly, untreated NIDDM patients show close correlations of nerve conduction velocity with plasma glucose and glycosylated haemoglobin levels [26]. Again, it is not yet clear whether such changes in nerve conduction velocity are a predictor for the later development of neuropathy. Finally, in a prospective randomized trial comparing standard and intensive diabetic (CSII) therapy [27], nerve conduction velocity and vibration sense threshold were found to improve after 8 months of CSII.

Polyol and myoinositol metabolism

Brain, peripheral nerve and other tissues which do not depend upon insulin for the entry of glucose into their cells, have cytoplasmic glucose concentrations which reflect the degree of glycaemia. Aldose reductase, the rate-limiting enzyme of the polyol pathway (see Fig. 54.2), is present in peripheral nerve. Aldose reductase has a low affinity for its hexose sugar substrates, including glucose. At low glucose concentrations (during normoglycaemia), concentrations within nerves of its reaction product, the polyol sorbitol, are low. Sorbitol is converted to fructose by the enzyme sorbitol dehydrogenase. Hyperglycaemia results in greatly increased concentrations of glucose in peripheral nerve and, consequently, through increased activity of aldose reductase, leads to elevated concentrations of sorbitol and fructose. The original suggestion was that sorbitol accumulation itself could cause osmotic damage, but there is no histological evidence of this, either from animal or human nerves.

In the peripheral nerves of diabetic animals, the elevations of sorbitol and fructose are accompanied by a decrease in the concentration of another polyol, myoinositol [28]. Myoinositol concentrations are normally substantially greater in peripheral nerve than in plasma, as it is taken up by a sodium-dependent, energy-consuming active transport mechanism. Nerve conduction velocity can be improved by the ad-ministration of aldose reductase inhibitors to diabetic animals and also by dietary supplementation with myoinositol. From this it has been concluded that myoinositol depletion, rather than sorbitol accumulation, is responsible for the changes in nerve conduction velocity. These various experimental studies have been reviewed by Gillon *et al.* [29].

The activity of sodium−potassium-dependent adenosine triphosphatase ($Na^+−K^+−ATPase$) is known to be reduced in the peripheral nerves of diabetic rats and this can be corrected by the administration of aldose reductase inhibitors or dietary supplementation with myo-inositol. It has been proposed that nerve $Na^+−K^+−ATPase$ is controlled by membrane phosphoinositides, possibly via protein kinase C. The following chain of pathogenetic events has been proposed (Fig. 61.5) [30]. Reduced nerve myo-inositol concentrations result in abnormal phosphoinositides, leading to reduced membrane $Na^+−K^+−ATPase$ activity. Since myo-inositol transport is dependent on this enzyme, a self-reinforcing cycle of reduced myo-inositol uptake and $Na^+−K^+−ATPase$ activity results, leading to increased intra-axonal Na^+ accumulation. This could affect nerve impulse generation, sodium-dependent amino acid uptake and other phenomena. It has been claimed [31] that intra-axonal accumulation of sodium in the paranodal region leads to axonal swelling and 'axoglial dysjunction', namely the separation of the terminations of the myelin lamellae from the axon, and further structural changes [31].

Although providing an attractive explanation for many of the phenomena observed in per-

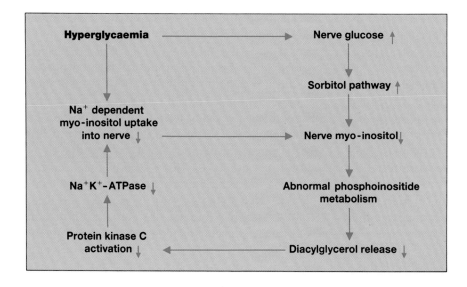

Fig. 61.5. Scheme summarizing proposed relationships between hyperglycaemia, sorbitol and myo-inositol metabolism in peripheral nerve.

ipheral nerves in diabetic animals, it is difficult to transfer this hypothesis to the pathogenesis of human diabetic neuropathy. First, although sorbitol accumulates in peripheral nerves in human diabetes, reductions in nerve myo-inositol concentrations have not been convincingly demonstrated [29, 32, 33]. Secondly, the morphological changes which characterize human diabetic neuropathy do not develop in the animal models so far studied. It has therefore not been possible to show that correction of nerve sorbitol, myo-inositol and $Na^+-K^+-ATPase$ activity in animals will prevent these changes. In man, aldose reductase inhibitors have so far been shown to improve nerve conduction velocity but produce no other convincing benefits. No definite benefit has been obtained by dietary myo-inositol supplementation (see Gillon et al. [29]). Finally, the results of recent observations on experimental galactose-induced neuropathy are important. Galactose is metabolized to galactitol by aldose reductase and accumulates in nerve. In this experimental model, in which nerve myoinositol is also reduced, $Na^+-Ka^+-ATPase$ activity has been found to be *increased* rather than reduced [34]. There is thus no simple relationship between myoinositol metabolism and $Na^+-K^+-ATPase$ activity.

Axonal transport

Protein synthesis in neurons is effectively confined to the cell body. Materials such as enzymes, neurotransmitters and structural proteins must then be translocated down the axons in the fast and slow anterograde transport systems, following which degenerate material, together with substances such as growth factors taken up by nerve terminals, are taken back to the cell body in the retrograde transport system.

Fast anterograde transport in peripheral nerves remains normal in experimental diabetes, but there is a slight impairment of slow component 'a' (SCa), which can be correlated with the reduced axonal calibre found in this model. The SCa defect is not corrected either by myoinositol supplementation or by aldose reductase inhibitors, whereas impaired transport of the enzyme choline acetyl transferase, which is carried in SCb, is corrected by treatment with either agent. Retrograde axonal transport is also impaired in streptozotocin-induced diabetes in rats.

The relevance of these observations to human diabetic neuropathy is again uncertain. Acetyl cholinesterase and dopamine β-hydroxylase, both of which are fast-transported enzymes, have been reported to be reduced in human diabetic neuropathy whereas their transport is normal in the animal models.

The abnormalities of axonal transport in human and experimental diabetes have recently been reviewed by Sidenius and Jakobsen [35].

Non-enzymatic glycosylation of nerve proteins

Abnormal glycosylation of axonal proteins has been demonstrated in experimental diabetes in animals [36]. The relevance of this to peripheral nerve function is so far uncertain. Non-enzymatic glycosylation of walls of the vasa nervorum and of the endoneurial connective tissue matrix [37] could also be important. Chronic changes in these tissues could eventually lead to ischaemic changes.

Ischaemia

Clinical considerations suggest a vascular basis for diabetic mononeuropathies of acute onset, such as lesions of the third cranial nerve. There is some pathological support for this concept, although, as discussed earlier, further evidence is desirable.

One of the main points of current controversy regarding the pathogenesis of diabetic neuropathy is the possible role of vascular factors in the production of the diabetic polyneuropathies. Thus, multifocal lesions in proximal nerves have been found at autopsy [38−40] which may have summated to produce a symmetric distal polyneuropathy. The pathological changes also suggested the presence of diffuse fibre loss and, as these studies were performed on elderly patients, the superimposition of vascular lesions on a diffuse neuropathy of metabolic origin cannot be excluded. In another study, patchy fibre loss was found in sural nerve biopsies from a series of patients with diabetic neuropathy [41]. However, such patchy fibre loss is also a feature of neuropathies in which a vascular basis can be discounted [42]. Perhaps the most cogent morphological evidence so far is the correlation between the severity of the neuropathy and the number of 'closed' capillaries in sural nerve biopsies, to which reference has already been made [18], although this may only apply to older individuals. Intraneural recordings have also demonstrated reduced oxygen tension [43]. There is some supportive evidence from animal studies in that nerve blood flow has been shown to be reduced in streptozotocin-diabetic rats, in which intraneural oxygen tension is also reduced [44] (Fig. 61.6).

The weight of the current evidence favours a combination of metabolic factors, probably more important at the earlier stages in younger diabetic subjects, and vascular factors which become increasingly important with duration of diabetes and advancing age. It would appear difficult to attempt to explain the totality of diabetic neuropathy on a vascular basis. The features of diabetic polyneuropathy, with a predominance of sensory and autonomic features over motor involvement, differ in pattern from those observed in other neuropathies of ischaemic origin.

Natural history

Few longitudinal surveys have been undertaken to follow the natural history of diabetic neuropathy. The more effective methods now available to quantify sensory, motor and autonomic deficits, together with nerve conduction studies, should make possible definitive observations on the evolution of the manifestations of the different types of peripheral nerve changes that occur. In general, these studies necessarily have to be of a long-term nature. Although some instances of diabetic sensory polyneuropathy have a relatively abrupt start, most have a slow and insidious onset. Acute painful diabetic neuropathy is an exception. This syndrome may be associated with precipitous weight loss. Following institution of glycaemic control and weight gain, the neuropathy resolves over some months [24] (Fig. 61.7). The same is true for the acute painful neuropathy which may follow the introduction of diabetic treatment or the establishment of euglycaemia in a previously poorly controlled patient [43]. It is general clinical experience that diabetic sensory polyneuropathy, once established, does not improve substantially, even with satisfactory glycaemic control. The Mayo Clinic CSII trial [27] documented only an improvement in nerve conduction velocity and vibration sensation without any change in symptoms over an 8-month period. Jakobsen *et al.* [46] have

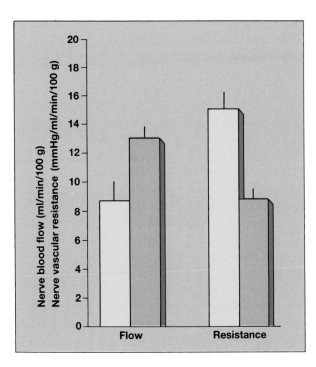

Fig. 61.6. Mean sciatic nerve blood flow and vascular resistance from seven streptozotocin-diabetic rats (yellow columns) and eight control rats (orange columns) showing reduced flow and increased vascular resistance in the diabetic animals. (Redrawn with permission from Tuck *et al.* 1984 [42] and from the Editor of *Brain*.)

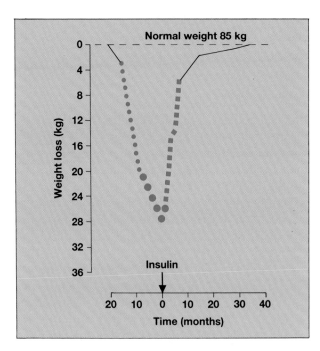

Fig. 61.7. Changes in body weight in a case of acute painful diabetic neuropathy. Initiation of treatment with insulin is indicated by the arrow, treatment before then having been with an oral hypoglycaemic agent. A precipitate loss of over 27 kg in weight is accompanied by the development of a mild (●) and then a severe (●) painful neuropathy. Restoration of body weight is associated with improvement (■) and then disappearance (———) of the neuropathy.

recently shown from studies employing quantitative sensory testing and assessment of autonomic function that over a 2-year period, in patients treated by CSII, neuropathy remained stable whereas in those receiving conventional insulin treatment it deteriorated.

Evidence of autonomic neuropathy may be present at the time of diagnosis of diabetes [47] or may appear within 1–2 years of diagnosis [48], but the precise relationship of autonomic dysfunction to duration of diabetes has not been established. Once symptomatic autonomic neuropathy is present, the prognosis for survival is substantially diminished. For a group of 73 patients followed prospectively for up to 5 years, mortality rates of 44% after 2½ years and 56% after 5 years were found (see Fig. 63.3). Half of the deaths were from renal failure and the other half from causes which could be related to autonomic neuropathy [49].

For focal and multifocal neuropathies, the diabetic third cranial nerve lesions of acute onset characteristically recover satisfactorily. Proximal lower limb motor neuropathy (amyotrophy), particularly if of acute onset, may also recover in some cases. In one series of 12 cases [50], three recovered fully, four showed a good functional result and five continued with residual disability. In the experience of the writer, symptoms of the carpal tunnel syndrome tend not to respond as satisfactorily to surgical decompression in diabetic as in non-diabetic subjects.

P.K. THOMAS

References

1 Ward JD, Barnes CG, Fisher DJ, Jessop JD, Baker RWR. Improvement in nerve conduction following treatment in newly diagnosed diabetics. *Lancet* 1971; i: 428–30.

2 Steiness IB. Vibratory perception in diabetics during arrested blood flow to the limb. *Acta Med Scand* 1959; **163**: 195–205.

3 Seneviratne KN, Peiris OA. The effect of ischaemia on the excitability of sensory nerves in diabetes mellitus. *J Neurol Neurosurg Psychiatr* 1968; **31**: 348–53.

4 Melton LJ, Dyck PJ. Epidemiology. In: Dyck PJ, Thomas PK, Asbury AK, Winegrad AI, Porte Jr D, eds. *Diabetic Neuropathy*. Philadelphia: W.B. Saunders, 1987: 27–35.

5 Pirart J. Diabetes mellitus and its degenerative complications: a prospective study of 4,400 patients observed. *Diabetes Care* 1978; **1**: 168–88, 252–63.

6 Palumbo PJ, Elveback LR, Whisnant JP. Neurologic complications of diabetes mellitus: transient ischemic attack, stroke, and peripheral neuropathy. In: Schoenberg BS, ed. *Neurological Epidemiology: Principles and Clinical Applications*. New York: Raven Press, 1978: 593–601.

7 Dyck PJ, Karnes JL, Daube J, O'Brien P, Service FJ. Clinical and neuropathological criteria for the diagnosis and staging of diabetic polyneuropathy. *Brain* 1985; **108**: 861–80.

8 Hoffman J. Peripheral neuropathy in children with diabetes mellitus. *Acta Neurol Scand* 1964; **40** (suppl 8): 1–23.

9 Osuntokun BO. *The Neurology of Diabetes Mellitus in Nigerians*. MD Thesis. University of London, 1971.

10 Boulton AJM, Hardisty CA, Worth RC, Drury J, Wolfe E, Cudworth AG, Ward JD. Metabolic and genetic factors in diabetic neuropathy. *Diabetologia* 1984; **26**: 15–19.

11 Mincu I. Micro- and macroangiopathies and other chronic degenerative complications in newly detected diabetes mellitus. *Rev Rom Med Int* 1980; **18**: 155–64.

12 Sullivan JF. The neuropathies of diabetes. *Neurology (Minneap)* 1958; **8**: 243–9.

13 Dyck PJ, Sherman WR, Hallcher LM, Service FJ, O'Brien PC, Grina LA, Palumbo PJ, Swanson CJ. Human diabetic endoneurial sorbitol, fructose, and *myo*-inositol related to sural nerve morphometry. *Ann Neurol* 1980; **8**: 590–6.

14 Brown MJ, Martin JR, Asbury AK. Painful diabetic neuropathy: a morphometric study. *Arch Neurol* 1976; **33**: 164–71.

15 Dyck PJ, Lais A, Karnes JL, O'Brien P, Rizza R. Fiber loss is primary and multifocal in sural nerves in diabetic polyneuropathy. *Ann Neurol* 1986; **19**: 425–39.

16 Asbury AK, Aldridge H, Hershberg R, Fisher CM. Oculomotor palsy in diabetes mellitus: a clinico-pathological study. *Brain* 1970; **93**: 555–66.

17 Fagerberg SE. Diabetic neuropathy: a clinical and histological study on the significance of vascular affections. *Acta Med Scand* 1959; **164** (suppl 345): 1–80.

18 Dyck PJ, Hansen S, Karnes J, O'Brien P, Yasuda H, Windebank A, Zimmerman B. Capillary number and percentage closed in human diabetic sural nerve. *Proc Natl Acad Sci USA* 1985; **52**: 2513–17.

19 Bradley JL, King RHM, Llewelyn JG, Thomas PK. Is diabetic polyneuropathy a vascular disease? *J Neurol Neurosurg Psychiatr* (in press).

20 Mulder DW, Lambert EH, Bastron VA, Sprague RG. The neuropathies associated with diabetes mellitus: a clinical and electromyographic study of 103 unselected diabetic patients. *Neurology (Minneap)* 1961; **11**: 275–84.

21 Gregersen G. Diabetic neuropathy: influence of age, sex, metabolic control, and duration of diabetes on motor conduction velocity. *Neurology (Minneap)* 1967; **17**: 972–80.

22 Kuribayashi T, Kurihara T, Tanaka M, Tsuruta K, Araki S. Diabetic neuropathy and electrophysiological studies: evoked potentials, nerve conduction, and short latency SEP. In: Goto Y, Horiuchi A, Kogure K, eds. *Diabetic Neuropathy*. Amersterdam: Excerpta Medica, 1982: 120–4.

23 Committee of Health Care Issues, American Neurological Association. Does improved control of glycemia prevent or ameliorate diabetic polyneuropathy? *Ann Neurol* 1986; **19**: 288–90.

24 Archer AG, Watkins PJ, Thomas PK, Sharma AK, Payan J. The natural history of acute painful diabetic neuropathy. *J Neurol Neurosurg Psychiatr* 1983; **46**: 491–9.

25 Boulton AJM, Drury J, Clarke B, Ward JD. Continuous subcutaneous insulin infusion in the management of painful diabetic neuropathy. *Diabetes Care* 1982; **5**: 386–91.

26 Porte D, Graf RJ, Halter JB, Pfeifer MA, Halar E. Diabetic neuropathy and plasma glucose control. *Am J Med* 1981; **70**: 195–200.

27 Service FJ, Rizza RA, Daube JR, O'Brien PC, Dyck PJ. Near normoglycaemia improves nerve conduction and vibration sensation in diabetic neuropathy. *Diabetologia* 1985; **28**: 722–7.

28 Greene DA, De Jesus PV Jr, Winegrad AI. Effects of insulin and dietary *myo*-inositol on impaired peripheral motor nerve conduction velocity in acute streptozotocin diabetes. *J Clin Invest* 1975; **55**: 1326–36.

29 Gillon KRW, King RHM, Thomas PK. The pathology of diabetic neuropathy and the effects of aldose reductase inhibitors. In: Watkins PJ, ed. *Long Term Complications of Diabetes. Clinics in Endocrinology and Metabolism.* Vol 15(4). London: W.B. Saunders, 1986: 837–54.

30 Greene DA, Lattimer SA, Sima AAF. Sorbitol, phospho-inositides, and sodium–potassium ATPase in the pathogenesis of diabetic complications. *N Engl J Med* 1987; **316**: 599–606.

31 Sima AAF, Nathaniel V, Bril V, McEwen TAJ, Greene DA. Histopathological heterogeneity of neuropathy in insulin-dependent and non-insulin-dependent diabetics and demonstration of axoglial dysjunction in human diabetic neuropathy. *J Clin Invest* 1988; **81**: 349–64.

32 Hale PJ, Nattrass M, Silverman SH, Sennit C, Perkins CM, Uden A, Sundkvist G. Peripheral nerve concentrations of glucose, fructose, sorbitol and myoinositol in diabetic and non-diabetic patients. *Diabetologia* 1987; **30**: 464–7.

33 Dyck PJ, Zimmerman BR, Vilen TH, Minnerath SR, Karnes JL, Yao JK, Poduslo JF. Nerve glucose, fructose, sorbitol, myo-inositol, and fiber degeneration and regeneration in diabetic neuropathy. *N Engl Med* 1988; **319**: 542–8.

34 Lambourne JE, Tomlinson DR, Brown AM, Willars GB. Opposite effects of diabetes and galactosaemia on adenosine triphosphatase activity in rat nervous tissue. *Diabetologia* 1987; **30**: 360–2.

35 Sidenius P, Jakobsen J. Axonal transport in human and experimental diabetes. In: Dyck PJ, Thomas PK, Asbury AK, Winegrad AI, Porte D Jr, eds. *Diabetic Neuropathy.* Philadelphia: W.B. Saunders, 1987: 260–5.

36 Williams SK, Howarth NL, Devenny JJ, Bitensky MW. Structural and functional consequences of increased tubulin glycosylation in diabetes mellitus. *Proc Natl Acad Sci USA* 1982; **79**: 6546–50.

37 Brownlee M, Cerami M, Vlassara H. Advanced glycosylation end products in tissue and the biochemical basis of diabetic complications. *N Engl J Med* 1988; **318**: 1315–21.

38 Sugimura K, Dyck PJ. Multifocal fiber loss in proximal sciatic nerve in symmetric distal diabetic neuropathy. *J Neurol Sci* 1982; **53**: 501–9.

39 Dyck PJ, Karnes JL, O'Brien P, Okazaki H, Lais A, Engelstad J. The spatial distribution of fiber loss in diabetic poly-neuropathy suggest ischemia. *Ann Neurol* 1986; **19**: 440–9.

40 Johnson PC, Doll SC, Cromer DW. Pathogenesis of diabetic neuropathy. *Ann Neurol* 1986; **19**: 450–7.

41 Dyck PJ, Lais A, Karnes JL, O'Brien P, Rizza R. Fiber loss is primary and multifocal in sural nerves in diabetic poly-neuropathy. *Ann Neurol* 1986; **19**: 425–39.

42 Llewelyn JG, Thomas PK, Gilbey SG, Watkins PJ, Muddle JR. Pattern of myelinated fibre loss in the sural nerve in neuropathy related to Type 1 (insulin-dependent) diabetes. *Diabetologia* 1988; **31**: 162–7.

43 Newrick PG, Wilson AJ, Jakubowski J, Boulton AJM, Ward JD. Sural nerve oxygen tension in diabetes. *Br J Med* 1986; **293**: 1053–4.

44 Tuck RR, Schmelzer JD, Low PA. Endoneurial blood flow and oxygen tension in the sciatic nerves of rats with experimental diabetic neuropathy. *Brain* 1984; **107**: 935–50.

45 Llewelyn JG, Thomas PK, Fonseca V, King RHM, Dandona P. Acute painful diabetic neuropathy precipitated by strict glycaemic control. *Acta Neuropathol (Berl)* 1986; **72**: 157–63.

46 Jakobsen J, Christiansen JS, Kristoffersen I, Christensen CK, Hermansen K, Schmitz A, Mogensen CE. Autonomic and somatosensory nerve function after 2 years of continuous subcutaneous insulin infusion in Type I diabetes. *Diabetes* 1988; **37**: 452–5.

47 Fraser DM, Campbell IW, Ewing DJ, Murray J, Neilson JMM, Clarke BF. Peripheral and autonomic nerve function in newly diagnosed diabetes. *Diabetes* 1977; **26**: 546–50.

48 Pfeifer MA, Cook D, Brodsky J, Tice D, Reenan A, Swedine S, Halter JB, Porte D Jr. Quantitative evaluation of cardiac parasympathetic activity in normal and diabetic man. *Diabetes* 1982; **31**: 339–45.

49 Ewing DJ, Campbell IW, Clarke BF. The natural history of diabetic autonomic neuropathy. *Q J Med* 1980; **193**: 95–108.

50 Casey EB, Harrison MJG. Diabetic amyotrophy: a follow-up study. *Br J Med* 1972; **1**: 656–9.

62 Clinical Aspects of Diabetic Somatic Neuropathy

Summary

- Diabetic peripheral neuropathy may present as several syndromes which often overlap.
- *Chronic insidious sensory neuropathy* causes progressive development of unpleasant sensations, often with pain, in the legs and feet. Muscle wasting and autonomic dysfunction are commonly associated. This form is common and usually unrelated to glycaemic control.
- *Acute painful neuropathy* and *diabetic amyotrophy* both cause sudden-onset pain in thighs and/or legs, usually unilateral in amyotrophy, associated with severe muscle wasting and occasionally profound weight loss; there is little objective sensory loss. These often begin during a period of hyperglycaemia and may improve with strict control.
- *Diffuse motor neuropathy* presents as severe, generalized muscle wasting and weakness, usually without pain or sensory loss. It commonly affects older NIDDM patients; recovery is usually poor.
- *Focal neuropathies* are probably due to *pressure damage* (especially the carpal tunnel syndrome, which usually responds poorly to surgical decompression) or *vascular damage* (e.g. third nerve palsy, which is often painful, sometimes associated with hyperglycaemia and may recover with improved control).
- Other coexistent and potentially treatable causes of peripheral neuropathy must always be excluded.
- Peripheral nerve function can be assessed adequately by routine physical examination. Specialized tests for diagnostic difficulties and research applications include electrophysiological measurements of sensory and motor nerve conduction, determinations of vibration and thermal discrimination thresholds, and sural nerve biopsy.
- Painful symptoms in diabetic neuropathy may respond to improved glycaemic control, simple analgesia and tricyclic drugs; other agents (e.g phenytoin, carbamazepine, mexiletine) are sometimes effective.

Clinical experience suggests that about 10% of insulin-treated diabetic patients have symptoms of peripheral neuropathy and that a further 10% also show obviously abnormal physical signs [1]. As well as being common, peripheral nerve damage is important because of its major contribution to the problems of the diabetic foot (see Chapter 70) and male impotence (Chapter 76).

Clinical presentations of diabetic neuropathy

Diabetic peripheral neuropathy has been subdivided on simple topographical grounds [2] into *symmetrical polyneuropathy* (comprising sensory, motor or combined forms) and *focal and multifocal neuropathies* (including damage to cranial, limb or trunk nerves, and proximal motor neuropathy) (see Chapter 61). In clinical terms, however, it is useful to describe the various ways in which neuropathic syndromes may present. Most patients with neuropathy have the symmetrical sensori-motor form with autonomic features, but several other syndromes and mixed patterns occur, firmly indicating that many aetiological factors must contribute to human diabetic neuropathy. Despite their classification as predominantly 'sensory' or 'motor' neuropathies, it will be appreciated from the descriptions below that many

623

patients show evidence of sensory, motor and autonomic involvement. The major clinical presentations, summarized in Fig. 62.1, are:

1 Chronic insidious sensory neuropathy.
2 Acute painful neuropathy.
3 Proximal motor neuropathy.
4 Diffuse motor neuropathy.
5 Pressure neuropathies.
6 Focal vascular neuropathies.

Chronic insidious sensory neuropathy

This is the commonest syndrome. The patient describes a slow, progressive build-up of unpleasant sensations consisting of tingling, burning, cramps and frank pain, often dramatically described as 'shooting', 'tearing' or 'excruciating'. Hyperaesthesia is common, and contact with clothing or bedclothes may cause great discomfort. The legs and feet are mainly affected; intriguingly, similar symptoms are very unusual in the arms and hands. For unknown reasons, all symptoms are much worse at night and often prevent sleep. This form of neuropathy usually develops gradually, with no clear-cut association with hyperglycaemia, and symptoms often persist after glycaemic control has been improved. Most sufferers report no improvement in symptoms 5 years after onset [3]. Understandably, depression often aggravates the situation.

Clinical examination reveals patchy sensory loss, predominantly distal ('stocking' and sometimes also 'glove' distribution), and affecting all modalities. Vibration sensation is usually markedly reduced, and proprioception may be so impaired as to cause Romberg's sign. Ankle and knee tendon reflexes are usually reduced or absent. Many patients show significant generalized muscular wasting, particularly of the small muscles of the hand, with variable degrees of weakness. Cardiovascular and other autonomic function tests (see Chapter 63) are frequently abnormal in these patients, and many males will also be impotent. Other features, attributable largely to sensory loss with or without associated autonomic damage, include neuropathic ulceration of the feet and Charcot arthropathy (Chapter 70).

Acute painful neuropathy

This is a relatively uncommon presentation which is probably a variant of proximal motor neuro-

pathy (see below). Severe pain appears suddenly, usually in the thighs, legs and feet, and has a particularly excruciating and distressing quality. Marked muscle wasting and weakness develop rapidly, often accompanied by weight loss ('neuropathic cachexia') and depression. Surprisingly, knee and ankle tendon reflexes may be preserved in some patients and there is often only little objective sensory deficit to be demonstrated. Certain subjects have very warm legs (with skin temperature sometimes approaching core temperature (Fig. 62.3)) and distended veins (Fig. 62.2), suggesting arterio-venous shunting of blood as has been described in the numb neuropathic foot ([5]; see Chapter 70).

This acute syndrome usually occurs in association with hyperglycaemia and improved control will result in symptomatic recovery in many cases, generally within a year or so. Rapidly developing pain is more likely to resolve than that which develops progressively over several months [6]. Acute painful neuropathy, with or without sensory loss, may also occasionally be precipitated by a sudden improvement in glycaemic control, which is usually the result of starting insulin treatment. It may last for some weeks or months and in most cases resolves spontaneously.

Proximal motor myopathy (amyotrophy)

Garland [7] described *diabetic amyotrophy* as the sudden onset of severe pain in one thigh, accompanied by profound wasting of the quadriceps muscles, usually during a period of marked hyperglycaemia. Other leg muscles, especially the anterior tibial and peroneal muscles, may be involved, and the condition may be bilateral (Fig. 62.4). The tendon reflexes of affected muscles are reduced. An unexplained feature is the extensor plantar reflexes displayed by a few patients. Despite the prominence of pain, objective evidence of sensory loss is only rarely found.

The cause of proximal motor myopathy is unknown. The condition was previously regarded as a femoral neuropathy or radiculopathy, which is suggested by the focal, unilateral onset in many patients. However, the bilateral involvement in some cases argues against this, and many subjects show significant features of widespread neuropathy. The combination of focal features superimposed on a diffuse neuropathy may suggest a vascular event complicating generalized biochemical nerve damage.

Syndrome	Chronic insidious sensory neuropathy	Acute painful neuropathy	Proximal motor myopathy	Diffuse motor neuropathy	Focal nerve palsies — Pressure (Median, Ulnar, Common peroneal)	Focal nerve palsies — 'Vascular' (III, IV, VI; VII; Phrenic; Thoracic)
Pattern	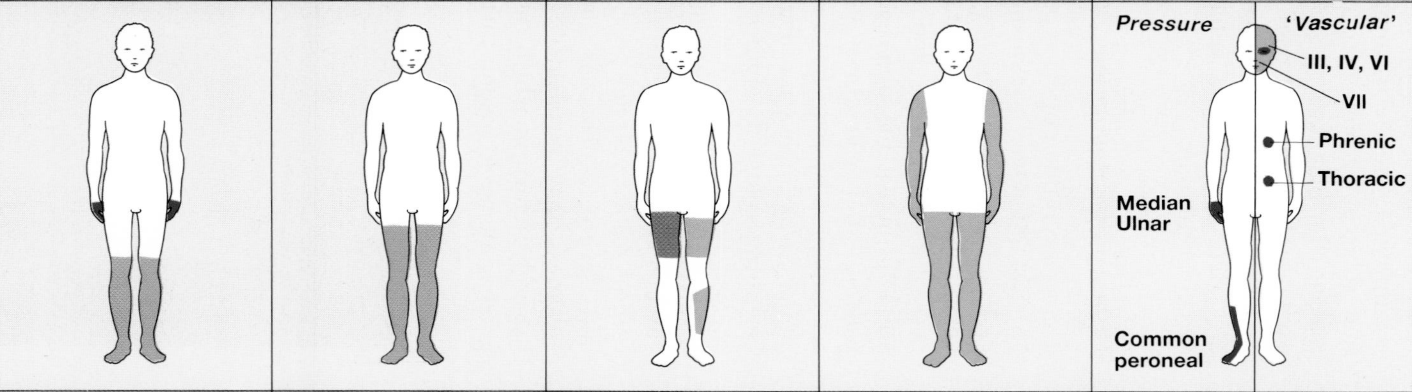 *(body diagram)*	*(body diagram)*	*(body diagram)*	*(body diagram)*	*(body diagram)*	
Sensory loss	+ → ++	+	O	O → +	++	++
Pain	O → +++	+++	+ → +++	O	++	O → ++
Tendon reflexes	→	→	→	→	+	+
Muscle wasting and weakness	O → ++	+ → ++	+++	++ → +++	+ → ++	O → ++
Autonomic features	+ → ++	May be present	May be present	May be present	May be present	May be present
Prevalence and relationship to glycaemia	Common; usually unrelated to glycaemia	Relatively rare; onset often during hyperglycaemia	Relatively rare; onset often during hyperglycaemia	Relatively rare; generally unrelated to hyperglycaemia	Relatively rare; usually unrelated to hyperglycaemia	Relatively rare; sometimes related to hyperglycaemia

Fig. 62.1. Clinical patterns of diabetic peripheral neuropathy.

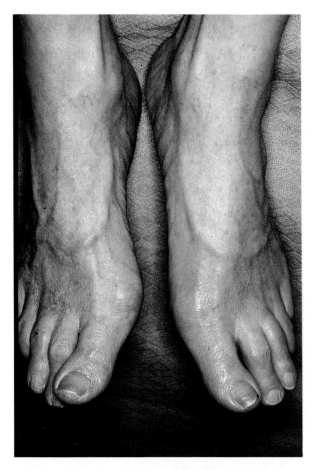

Fig. 62.2. Distended veins on the dorsum of the foot of a diabetic patient with painful peripheral neuropathy. (Reproduced by kind permission of Dr Geoff Gill, Arrowe Park Hospital, Wirral.)

Many patients, but by no means all, recover spontaneously, especially after glycaemic control is improved; muscle wasting may persist and a few subjects become permanently disabled. In making the diagnosis, it is vitally important to exclude other causes of pain and muscle wasting in the legs — especially when the plantar responses are extensor — such as anterior disc protrusions or spinal tumours.

Diffuse motor neuropathy

This is a condition of older patients, usually with NIDDM [8]. Over a 3–6 month period, severe generalized muscle wasting and weakness develop, often to an incapacitating degree, in the face of blood glucose and HbA_1 levels which are little above the non-diabetic range. Muscle wasting, often severe in the hands (Fig. 62.5), is accompanied by reduction or absence of reflexes and there is often some degree of sensory loss. Electrophysiological studies in these patients suggest diffuse nerve damage with significant focal involvement, perhaps indicating widespread vascular disease. Even with tightened glycaemic control, recovery is often poor. Rapidly progressing and severe generalized muscle wasting and weakness may occasionally be associated with hyperglycaemia, in which case there is usually a good response to insulin therapy.

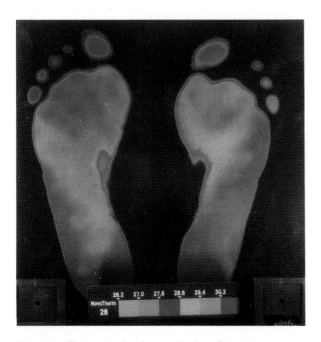
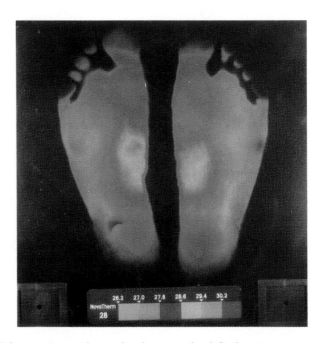

Fig. 62.3. Thermographs showing higher skin temperature in a diabetic patient with peripheral neuropathy (left) than in a non-diabetic subject (right). (Reproduced by kind permission of Dr Ah Wah Chan, Royal Liverpool Hospital.)

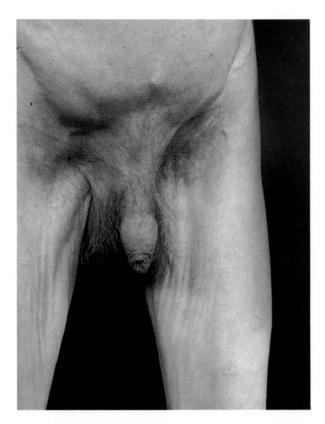

Fig. 62.4. Diabetic amyotrophy, showing marked wasting of both thighs.

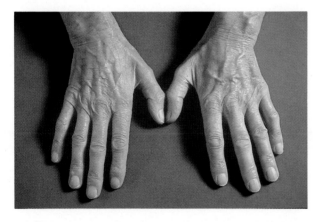

Fig. 62.5. Generalized wasting of small muscles of the hands due to diffuse motor neuropathy.

Pressure neuropathies

Diabetic nerves are particularly vulnerable to pressure damage. The commonest pressure palsy in diabetes involves the median nerve, producing a typical carpal tunnel syndrome. Characteristic symptoms include pain in the hands, which is worse at night and often radiates up the forearm. The hand may take up a stiffened posture, perhaps

aggravated by the cheiroarthropathy of diabetes (Chapter 73), which can be mistakenly attributed to rheumatological disease. Surgical decompression is often performed to relieve the symptoms, but pain seems more likely to return in the diabetic patient than in the non-diabetic [9]. Other peripheral nerve palsies commonly seen in diabetic patients affect the ulnar and common peroneal nerves.

Focal vascular neuropathies

It is assumed that other focal lesions, where there is no reason to suspect pressure damage, are due to occlusion of intraneural vessels; indeed, one autopsy case supports this view [10]. Third cranial nerve palsy (Fig. 62.6) is by far the commonest and is usually accompanied by pain in the orbit, when other causes of painful third nerve palsies (aneurysm, tumour) must be considered in the differential diagnosis. However, the pupillary innervation is frequently unaffected in third nerve palsies due to diabetes, unlike those due to compression or invasion. This pupillary sparing may suggest that nerve damage is due to intraneural vascular occlusion [2]. Fourth, sixth and seventh cranial nerve palsies are well described in diabetic subjects and there are reports of intercostal and phrenic nerve lesions. These are all presumably of a similar aetiology, although pressure damage cannot be excluded.

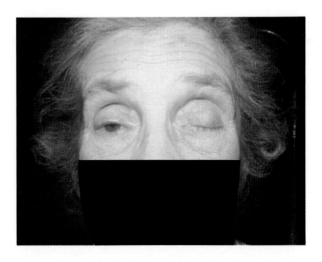

Fig. 62.6. Sudden onset of left ptosis (with diplopia) in a diabetic patient, due to third cranial nerve palsy. The patient complained of pain in the left orbit, and the left pupillary reactions were intact; pain and pupillary sparing are typical features of a third nerve palsy in diabetes.

Assessment of nerve function

Clinical examination alone is usually adequate to assess a diabetic patient suspected of having neuropathy. An outline of the relevant tests is shown in Table 62.1. Certain specialized tests of nerve function may help to resolve difficult diagnostic problems, but it must be remembered that asymptomatic patients may have considerable functional impairment, and that results in an individual patient may be misleading. Quantitative tests of nerve function, which are essential in research applications, include electrophysiological measurements, determinations of vibration perception threshold and thermal discrimination threshold, and sural nerve biopsy.

Electrophysiological measurements

These investigations should preferably be performed by a specialist neurophysiologist. Measurement of motor and sensory conduction velocity are the most commonly used but only assess myelinated fibres which constitute about 25% of peripheral fibres. Conduction velocity is related to the ambient blood glucose at the time of testing, tending to improve as glycaemia improves [11, 12], and shows various abnormalities even in people without a distinct clinical problem. However, the tests do correlate in groups of patients with the presence of clinical neuropathy [13]. More sophisticated measurements include evoked sensory action potentials (which provide a measure of fibre number), and the Hoffman reflex and F-wave responses to assess the total sensori-motor arc [14]. The real significance of impaired conduction velocity is not yet known; for example, a similar improvement (3 m/s) in conduction velocity following improved glycaemic control has been observed in newly diagnosed patients *without* neuropathy as in a group of patients with chronic, unremitting, painful neuropathy treated with continuous subcutaneous insulin infusion (CSII) [15]. It is possible that part of the alteration in conduction velocity relates simply to the fluid and electrolyte content of the nerve at the time of measurement.

Vibration perception threshold (VPT)

This is a quantitative measure of large-fibre function using an electromechanical device which causes a tactor to vibrate at fixed frequency but variable amplitude [16]. A Biothesiometer or Somedic Vibrameter may be used, the latter standardizing the pressure with which the tactor is applied to the test site [17]. These devices are obviously superior to the traditional tuning-fork and results are reasonably reproducible, although there may be considerable and unpredictable variation between different sites, and between different times at a given site, in the same individual [18, 19]. Measurements are usually made on the tip of the big toe, the medial malleolus and on one finger, and values must be related to both site and the patient's age, as VPT increases significantly with age [16, 18, 20]. This very simple test is probably of use in epidemiological studies or large clinical studies but it remains to be seen whether it is sensitive enough for long-term prospective studies.

Since it has been demonstrated that significant impairment of VPT correlates with points of high pressure in the diabetic foot, which itself predisposes to ulcer formation, it has been suggested that VPT could be used to screen for subjects vulnerable to foot ulceration [21]. The measurement of VPT requires the shoes and socks to be removed, which in itself may be the most important act in screening for those at risk from foot ulcers.

Temperature discrimination threshold (TDT)

This index of small-fibre function can be measured by several different instruments, based on the Peltier thermocouple whose temperature rises or falls depending on the direction of the electrical current flowing through it [22]. Using a forced-choice technique, the patient responds to a rise or fall in the temperature of the thermocouple plate, which is altered in a random manner. This is more time-consuming than assessment of vibration sensitivity, but also seems to be a more sensitive measure as it is abnormal in many patients with normal VPT who may be at an earlier stage in the natural history of neuropathy [23].

Sural nerve biopsy

This is the ultimate test to assess changes in structure and composition of nerves. Histological examination can document features such as axonal loss, demyelination and the state of the microvasculature, and biochemical analyses can be performed [24, 25]. However, it rarely has a place in

Table 62.1. Assessment of peripheral nerve function.

Pathway	Modality	Clinical screen	Specialized tests	Comments
Sensory — Dorsal columns	Vibration	Tuning fork	VPT (Biothesiometer)	Tuning fork unreliable; VPT varies with age and site and may be poorly reproducible
	Proprioception	Joint position, Romberg test	—	—
Spinothalamic	Light touch	Cotton wool	von Frey hairs	von Frey hairs still a research procedure and not widely available
	Temperature	—	TDT (Marstock thermode)	May be more sensitive than VPT; time-consuming
Single nerves	Pain	Pin-prick, deep pressure	Spring-loaded calipers to pinch skin; thermal pain threshold	Pain thresholds difficult to quantitate and poorly reproducible
		—	Electrophysiological measurements of sensory conduction velocity and action potential	Abnormalities early and common; include reduced conduction velocity and reduced amplitude with spreading of sensory action potential
Tendon reflexes		Ankles, knees (± reinforcement)	—	Ankle jerks often lost, but may be reduced or absent in elderly
		Bulk, tone, power of limb muscles	—	Wasting of small hand muscles common in neuropathy, often with minimal weakness
Motor		—	Electrophysiological measurements of motor conduction velocity	Motor nerve conduction velocity markedly reduced in clinical neuropathy, especially mixed forms

Notes: VPT, vibration perception threshold; TDT, thermal discrimination threshold.

clinical management and should be reserved for carefully planned research projects.

Staging of diabetic neuropathy

In routine clinical practice, it is quite sufficient to diagnose diabetic neuropathy and specify which neuropathic syndrome is present. However, if prospective studies of natural history or therapeutic intervention are to be carried out, it is essential to have some agreement as to the grade of neuropathy at the time of study. Most studies have wisely focused on the commonest neuropathy (chronic sensori-motor), and have avoided the acute syndromes which have a great potential for spontaneous fluctuation and recovery. It is now known that there is very reasonable correlation between symptoms and signs and functional neurophysiological investigations, although no single symptom or test is indicative of neuropathy in one individual. In a research setting, therefore, it is essential to perform electrophysiological tests on at least two nerves, as well as measurements of VPT and TDT. Assessment should also include a range of autonomic function tests (Chapter 63) and a very detailed quantitative assessment of symptoms and physical signs. Using this approach, P.J. Dyck [26] has proposed the following staging system:

0 — No neuropathy: No symptoms and fewer than two abnormalities of testing (including autonomic tests).
1 — Asymptomatic neuropathy: No symptoms but two or more abnormalities of functional testing.
2 — Symptomatic neuropathy: Symptoms of a lesser degree with two or more functional abnormalities.
3 — Disabling neuropathy: Disabling symptoms and two or more functional abnormalities.

Attempts such as this to standardize scores of both symptoms and neurophysiological measures should make it possible in the future to compare results between various studies.

A diagnostic approach to the diabetic leg

Pain, discomfort or weakness in the legs of the diabetic patient are not necessarily due to peripheral diabetic neuropathy. Other forms of neuropathy should be considered, e.g. uraemia, nutritional deficiency, carcinoma, collagen—vascular diseases, amyloidosis and hereditary (see Fig. 62.7) and toxic neuropathies. Special consideration should be given to the role of alcohol,

which despite conflicting evidence as to whether it is more commonly used by patients with diabetic neuropathy, probably plays a significant part in some clinical syndromes.

Intrinsic or extrinsic spinal cord disease (e.g. cauda equina tumour, spinal stenosis, anterior lumbar disc lesions) will occasionally present with pain and wasting in proximal leg muscles and may be confused particularly with diabetic amyotrophy.

The major diagnostic difficulty, however, is to evaluate the importance of peripheral vascular disease, which is commonly present in older patients. Clinical assessment of pulses in the legs and feet may be supplemented by the use of the Doppler ultrasound stethoscope to calculate the ankle pressure index (see Chapter 70) [27]. There is some evidence that the arterio-venous shunting

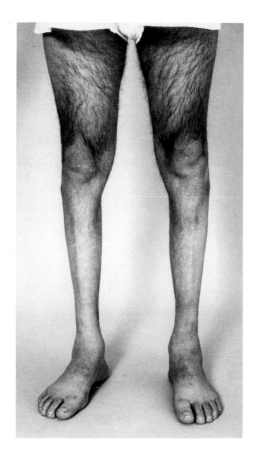

Fig. 62.7. Extreme muscular weakness with wasting in a 38-year-old man with diabetes for 11 years. Sensory loss was minimal and pain was absent. The 'inverted champagne bottle' pattern of wasting suggested the diagnosis of hereditary motor and sensory neuropathy Type 1 (Charcot–Marie–Tooth disease), which was confirmed by electrophysiological measurements.

seen in diabetic neuropathy may also cause discomfort, as the increased skin temperature and blood flow can be reversed by arterial occlusion, which surprisingly sometimes also relieves pain [5].

A good history may be diagnostic, especially if coupled with the characteristic physical signs described above. A totally anaesthetic foot may not cause complaint, but will show typical signs on examination. It is of interest that the totally numb neuropathic foot may also be the source of unpleasant tingling and burning sensations — the so-called 'painful–painless' foot.

Management of diabetic neuropathy

The main indication for intervention in neuropathy is pain and other troublesome sensory symptoms. A suggested management scheme is outlined in Fig. 62.8.

As mentioned above, it is first essential to exclude other coexistent conditions which are potentially treatable. The next step is to try to achieve the best glycaemic control possible. Many neuropathic syndromes are related to hyperglycaemia and will improve, often rapidly, following tightened glycaemic control. There has

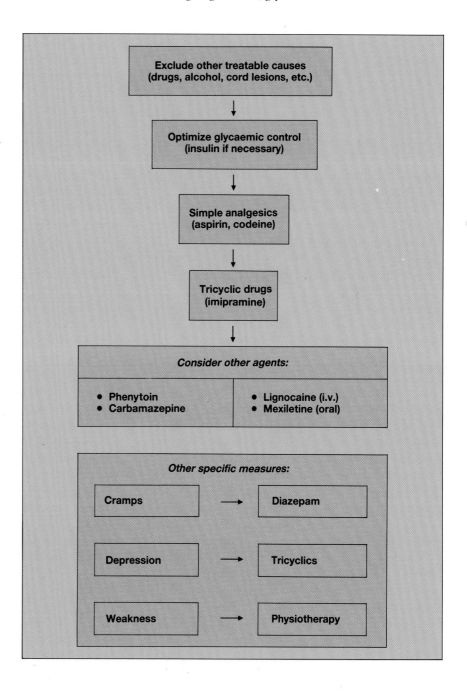

Fig. 62.8. Management of painful diabetic neuropathy.

been controversy regarding the possible effects of the blood glucose concentration on pain perception: an initial report that the pain threshold was lower in non-diabetic subjects during glucose infusion [28] has been contradicted by a recent study [29].

Specific drug treatment should begin with simple analgesics (e.g. aspirin, codeine phosphate), with diazepam or quinine sulphate for troublesome muscle cramps. If there is no improvement after a few weeks of these general measures, a tricyclic drug such as imipramine should be used. These drugs do not apparently act centrally in this situation but probably are effective by modulating the activity of nociceptive C fibres and their receptors. Nonetheless, depression accompanies any chronic painful condition, and their antidepressant effects may also contribute. The dosage range of 50–125 mg daily may induce drowsiness and in controlled trials, the addition of fluphenazine has been helpful [30–33]. Improvement, if it occurs, is usually seen within the first week or so. Sympathetic support of such patients is an important part of their management.

The use of local anaesthetic agents seems a logical way to approach discomfort due to peripheral nerve disease. Intravenous infusion of lignocaine is very effective in providing relief of symptoms which often persist for a period after withdrawal of the infusion [34]. Oral administration of a lignocaine analogue, mexiletine (200 mg thrice daily) has also been shown to be effective in double-blind clinical trials [35].

Other sedative agents have been variously reported to be of benefit and should be considered if improved blood glucose control, simple analgesics, tricyclics or mexiletine fail. Those with the best record of success (albeit with many failures) include phenytoin (200–300 mg daily) and carbamazepine (200 mg thrice daily). Motor symptoms are generally less troublesome in diabetic neuropathy, but physiotherapy and specific mechanical aids (such as ankle calipers or a toe spring for foot-drop) may be helpful in individual cases.

A number of other approaches may hold some hope for future therapy (see Chapter 104). Gangliosides — a complex of sialoglycolipids, found in high concentration in nervous tissue — are initiators of dendritogenesis and may stimulate nerve regeneration when administered after nerve damage. A few clinical trials have reported improvement in electrophysiological parameters and some symptomatic relief [36].

Aldose reductase inhibitors (ARI) are also currently under study. By preventing the vicious circle of sorbitol accumulation, myoinositol depletion and depression of $Na^+-K^+-ATPase$ (see Chapter 61), these agents have immense theoretical potential, and in animal models, their use has been associated with improvements in both biochemical abnormalities and in structural and electrophysiological indices of nerve damage [37–39]. However, final proof of their possible efficacy in clinically significant diabetic neuropathy in man is not yet available. Of the several trials carried out in diabetic patients with symptomatic neuropathy [40–42], only one uncontrolled study [40] claimed to find any useful symptomatic improvement. There has been no consistent effect on various objective measurements of peripheral nerve function, in either symptomatic [40–42] or asymptomatic [43] patients, although improvements in certain electrophysiological indices and morphometric features in sural nerve biopsies have recently been reported following 12 months' treatment with sorbinil [44]. Supplementation of myoinositol is also ineffective [45]. The stage at which these agents (or others aiming to influence structure or function) are administered may be crucial. In symptomatic neuropathy, axon fall-out, demyelination and hypoxia of the nerve are already considerable (Chapter 61) and it may be too late to use agents which modify fundamental biochemical processes. The potential usefulness of these drugs may be to prevent nerve damage, and they will probably have most benefit when given at a much earlier stage in the natural history of nerve disease. Unfortunately, the 7–10 year prospective studies which will be necessary to prove efficacy pose obvious economic and organizational problems.

Supplementation of the diet of diabetic subjects with γ-linolenic acid has been shown to improve nerve conduction, perhaps by normalizing the metabolism of the long-chain essential fatty acids derived from linoleic acid [46]. However, no extensive clinical studies have yet been carried out with regard to symptoms.

Prevention of diabetic neuropathy

The role of blood glucose control in preventing neuropathy must be stressed, although in many instances there is no clear-cut relationship between neuropathic manifestations and the degree of hyperglycaemia at the time of onset. Numerous studies have shown amelioration of various electrophysiological measures following improvement in glycaemia. In the Oslo study, the use of CSII to optimize blood glucose control resulted in better conduction velocities over a 3-year period [47], and a recent preliminary report found VPT to be lower in well-controlled than in poorly controlled young diabetic subjects [48]. In another group of adolescent diabetic subjects, impairment of motor conduction velocity at entry to the study was shown to predict the development of neuropathic symptoms 5 years later and that these subjects had higher glycosylated haemoglobin levels [49]. All this evidence, as with other complications of diabetes, obliges clinicians to help their patients to achieve the best possible blood glucose control at all times.

JOHN D. WARD

References

1 Boulton AJM, Knight J, Drury J, Ward JD. The prevalence of symptomatic diabetic neuropathy in an insulin-treated population. *Diabetes Care* 1985; **8**: 125−8.

2 Thomas PK, Ward JD, Watkins PJ. Diabetic neuropathy. In: Keen H, Jarrett J, eds. *Complications of Diabetes*, 2nd edn. London: Edward Arnold, 1982: 109−36.

3 Boulton AJM, Armstrong WD, Scarpello JHB, Ward JD. The natural history of painful diabetic neuropathy − a 4-year study. *Postgrad Med J* 1983; **59**: 556−9.

4 Archer AG, Watkins PJ, Thomas PK, Sharma AK, Payan J. The natural history of acute painful neuropathy in diabetes mellitus. *J Neurol Neurosurg Psychiatr* 1983; **46**: 491−6.

5 Archer AG, Roberts VC, Watkins PJ. Blood flow patterns in painful diabetic neuropathy. *Diabetologia* 1984; **27**: 563−7.

6 Young RJ, Ewing DJ, Clarke BF. Chronic remitting painful diabetic polyneuropathy. *Diabetes Care* 1988; **11**: 34−40.

7 Garland H. Diabetic amyotrophy. *Br Med J* 1955; **2**: 1287−90.

8 Timperley WR, Boulton AJM, Davies-Jones GAB, Jarratt JA, Ward JD. Small vessel disease in progressive diabetic neuropathy associated with good metabolic control. *J Clin Pathol* 1985; **38**: 1030−8.

9 Clayburgh RH, Beckenbaugh RD, Dobyns JH. Carpal tunnel release in patients with diffuse peripheral neuropathy. *J Hand Surg* 1987; **12**A: 380−3.

10 Asbury AK, Aldredge H, Herschberg R, Fisher CM. Oculomotor palsy in diabetes mellitus: a clinico-pathological study. *Brain* 1970; **93**: 555−7.

11 Gregerson G. Diabetic neuropathy: Influence of age, sex, metabolic control and duration of diabetes on motor conduction velocity. *Neurology* 1967; **17**: 972−6.

12 Service FJ, Rizza RA, Daube JR, O'Brien PC, Dyck PJ. Near normoglycaemia improved nerve conduction and vibration sensation in diabetic neuropathy. *Diabetologia* 1985; **28**: 722−7.

13 Dyck PJ, Karnes J, O'Brien PC. Diagnosis, staging and classification of diabetic neuropathy and associations with other complications. In: Dyck PJ, Thomas PK, Asbury AK, Winegrad AA, Porte D Jr, eds. *Diabetic Neuropathy*. Philadelphia: WB Saunders Co., 1987: 37−44.

14 Jarratt JA. The electrophysiological diagnosis of peripheral neuropathy. A brief review. *Bull Eur Physiopathol Res* 1987; **23** (Suppl 11): 195−8.

15 Boulton AJM, Drury J, Clarke B, Ward JD. Continuous subcutaneous insulin infusion in the management of painful diabetic neuropathy. *Diabetes Care* 1982; **5**: 386−90.

16 Steiness IB. Vibratory perception in normal subjects. A biothesiometric study. *Acta Med Scand* 1957; **158**: 315−25.

17 Lowenthal LM, Hockaday TDR. Vibration sensory thresholds depend on pressure of applied stimulus. *Diabetes Care* 1987; **10**: 100−4.

18 Bertelsmann FW, Heimans JJ, van Rooy JC, Heine RJ, van der Veen EA. Reproducibility of vibratory perception thresholds in patients with diabetic neuropathy. *Diabetes Res* 1986; **3**: 463−6.

19 Fagius J, Wahren LK. Variability of sensory threshold determination in clinical use. *J Neurol Sci* 1981; **51**: 11−27.

20 Bloom S, Till S, Sönksen PH, Smith S. Use of a biothesiometer to measure individual vibration thresholds and their variation in 519 non-diabetic subjects. *Br Med J* 1984; **288**: 1793−5.

21 Boulton AJM, Hardisty CA, Betts RP, Franks CI, Worth RC, Ward JD, Duckworth T. Dynamic foot pressure and other studies as diagnostic and management aids in diabetic neuropathy. *Diabetes Care* 1983; **6**: 26−32.

22 Fowler CF, Carroll MB, Burns D, Howe N, Robinson K. A portable system for measuring cutaneous thresholds for warming and cooling. *J Neurol Neurosurg Psychiatr* 1987; **50**: 1211−15.

23 Guy RJC, Clark CA, Malcolm PN, Watkins PJ. Evaluation of thermal and vibration sensation in diabetic neuropathy. *Diabetologia* 1985; **28**: 131−7.

24 Dyck PJ, Sherman WR, Hallcher LM. Human diabetic endoneurial sorbitol, fructose and *myo*-inositol related to sural nerve morphometry. *Ann Neurol* 1980; **8**: 590−4.

25 Dyck PJ, Zimmerman BR, Vilen TH *et al*. Nerve glucose, fructose, sorbitol, *myo*-inositol, and fiber degeneration and regeneration in diabetic neuropathy. *N Engl J Med* 1988; **319**: 542−8.

26 Dyck PJ. Detection, characterization, and staging of polyneuropathy: Assessed in diabetics. *Muscle Nerve* 1988; **11**: 21−31.

27 Yao JST, Hobbs JT, Irvine WT. Ankle systolic pressure measurement in arterial disease affecting the lower extremities. *Br J Surg* 1969; **56**: 676−8.

28 Morley GK, Mooradian MD, Levine AL, Morley JE. Mechanisms of pain in diabetic peripheral neuropathy: effect of glucose on pain perception in humans. *Am J Med* 1984; **77**: 79−82.

29 Chan AW, MacFarlane IA, Bowsher DR *et al*. Does acute hyperglycaemia influence heat pain thresholds? *J Neurol Neurosurg Psychiatr* 1988; **51**: 688−90.

30 Kvinesdal BB, Molin J, Frøland A, Gram LF. Imipramine treatment of painful diabetic neuropathy. *JAMA* 1984; **251**: 1727−30.

31 Davis JL, Lewis SB, Gerich JE, Kaplan AR, Schultz TA, Wallin JD. Peripheral diabetic neuropathy treated with amitriptyline and fluphenazine. *JAMA* 1977; **238**: 2291−2.

32 Young RJ, Clarke BF. Pain relief in diabetic neuropathy: the effectiveness of imipramine and related drugs. *Diabetic Med* 1985; **2**: 363−6.

33 Gomez-Perez FJ, Rull JA, Dies H *et al*. Nortriptyline and

fluphenazine in the symptomatic treatment of diabetic neuropathy. A double-blind cross-over study. *Pain* 1985; **23**: 395–400.

34 Kastrup J, Peterson P, Dejgård J, Hilsted J, Angelo HR. Treatment of chronic painful diabetic neuropathy with intravenous lidocaine infusion. *Br Med J* 1986; **292**: 173–6.

35 Dejgård J, Peterson P, Kastrup J. Mexiletine for treatment of painful diabetic neuropathy. *Lancet* 1987; i: 9–11.

36 Crepaldi G, Fedele D, Tiengo A *et al*. Ganglioside treatment in diabetic peripheral neuropathy. *Acta Diabetol Lat* 1983; **20**: 265–76.

37 Mayer JH, Tomlinson DR. Prevention of defects of axonal transport and nerve conduction velocity by oral administration of *myo*-inositol or an aldose reductase inhibitor in streptozotocin-diabetic rats. *Diabetologia* 1983; **25**: 433–8.

38 Greene DA, Lattimer SA. Action of sorbinil in diabetic peripheral nerve. Relationship of polyol (sorbitol) pathway inhibition to a *myo*-inositol-mediated defect in sodium–potassium ATPase activity. *Diabetes* 1984; **33**: 712–16.

39 Tomlinson DR, Townsend J, Fretten P. Prevention of defective axonal transport in streptozocin-diabetic rats by treatment with 'Statil' (ICI 128436), an aldose reductase inhibitor. *Diabetes* 1985; **34**: 970–2.

40 Jaspan J, Maselli R, Herold K, Bartkus C. Treatment of severely painful diabetic neuropathy with an aldose reductase inhibitor: relief of pain and improved somatic and autonomic nerve function. *Lancet* 1983; ii: 758–62.

41 Young RJ, Ewing DJ, Clarke BF. A controlled trial of sorbinil, an aldose reductase inhibitor, in chronic painful diabetic neuropathy. *Diabetes* 1983; **32**: 938–42.

42 Pitts NE, Vreeland F, Shaw GL *et al*. Clinical experience with sorbinil — an aldose reductase inhibitor. *Metabolism*

35 (suppl 1): 96–100.

43 Martyn CN, Reid W, Young RJ, Ewing DJ, Clarke BF. Six-month treatment with sorbinil in asymptomatic diabetic neuropathy. Failure to improve abnormal nerve function. *Diabetes* 1987; **36**: 987–90.

44 Sima AAF, Bril V, Nathaniel V, McEwen TAJ, Brown MB, Lattimer SA, Greene DA. Regeneration and repair of myelinated fibers in sural-nerve biopsy specimens from patients with diabetic neuropathy treated with sorbinil. *N Engl J Med* 1988; **319**: 548–55.

45 Gregerson G, Bertelsen B, Harbo H *et al*. Oral supplementation of myoinositol: effects on peripheral nerve function in human diabetics and on the concentration in plasma, erythrocytes, urine and muscle tissue in human diabetics and normals. *Acta Neurol Scand* 1983; **67**: 164–72.

46 Jamal GA, Carmichael H. The effect of gamma-linolenic acid on human diabetic peripheral neuropathy: a double-blind placebo-controlled. *Diabetic Med* 1990; **7**: 319–23.

47 Dahl-Jørgensen K, Bringhmann I, Hansen O, Hanssen KF, Ganes T, Kierul FP, Smeland E, Sandvik L. Effect of near normoglycaemia for two years on progression of early diabetic retinopathy, nephropathy and neuropathy: The Oslo Study. *Br Med J* 1986; **293**: 1195–9.

48 Frighi V, Loughnane JW, Pozzilli P, Tarn AC, Thomas JM, Taylor JE, Andreani D, Gale EAM. Early signs of neuropathy and microangiopathy in young Type 1 (insulin-dependent) diabetic patients: correlation with long-term metabolic control. *Diabetologia* 1987; **30** (abstract): 521A.

49 Young RJ, MacIntyre CCA, Ewing DJ, Prescott RJ. Prediction of neuropathy over 5 years in young insulin-dependent diabetic patients. *Diabetic Med* 1988 (abstract); 5A.

63   Autonomic Neuropathy

Summary

• Up to 40% of diabetic patients show some evidence of autonomic dysfunction, but only a few have symptoms of autonomic neuropathy.

• Autonomic neuropathy may evolve through defects in thermoregulation and sweating in the legs, followed by impotence and bladder dysfunction, to cardiovascular reflex abnormalities. Late manifestations include generalized sweating disorders, postural hypotension, gastrointestinal problems and reduced awareness of hypoglycaemia.

• Symptomatic autonomic neuropathy carries a poor prognosis; death is usually due to associated diabetic complications (especially nephropathy) but is occasionally sudden and unexplained.

• Autonomic dysfunction is best diagnosed by evaluating the cardiovascular reflex responses to various stimuli: changes in heart rate to the Valsalva manoeuvre, deep breathing and standing up, and blood pressure changes following standing and sustained handgrip. These tests are simple, non-invasive and can be performed in the clinic within 30 min. Computer programs are available to analyse the results.

• Other tests include measurements of pupillary function and sweating.

• The most prominent symptom is postural hypotension, which is due to loss of mainly sympathetic reflexes. It is aggravated by antihypertensive agents, antidepressants and insulin and may respond to fludrocortisone treatment.

• Bladder dysfunction usually causes asymptomatic enlargement but may cause overflow incontinence and recurrent urinary tract infections.

• Erectile failure is common in diabetic men, but is not always due to autonomic neuropathy.

Diabetes mellitus commonly affects the autonomic nervous system, with up to 40% of diabetic patients demonstrating some autonomic abnormality [1]. Historically, autonomic nerve damage in diabetes has been classified as an aspect of peripheral neuropathy but it is now apparent that it affects far more patients than those showing the well-known 'glove and stocking' symmetrical polyneuropathy. In recent years, the original concept of dual parasympathetic and sympathetic systems has been replaced by one in which the autonomic nervous system exercises a key integrating role [2]. It is not surprising, therefore, that when autonomic damage occurs its effects can be detected all over the body. Some effects are readily apparent clinically, but others can only be identified by using sensitive tests (Fig. 63.1).

Terminology may cause some confusion. Autonomic damage is sometimes classified by systems, as cardiovascular neuropathy, genitourinary neuropathy, gastrointestinal neuropathy and so on. This approach neglects the widespread nature of autonomic nerve damage in diabetes, and the global terms 'autonomic neuropathy' and 'autonomic dysfunction' are preferable. For the purposes of this chapter, 'autonomic neuropathy' refers to suggestive clinical features of autonomic involvement combined with objective evidence of abnormal autonomic function which is usually based on cardiovascular tests (see below). The term 'autonomic dysfunction' describes abnormal tests in the absence of clinical symptoms.

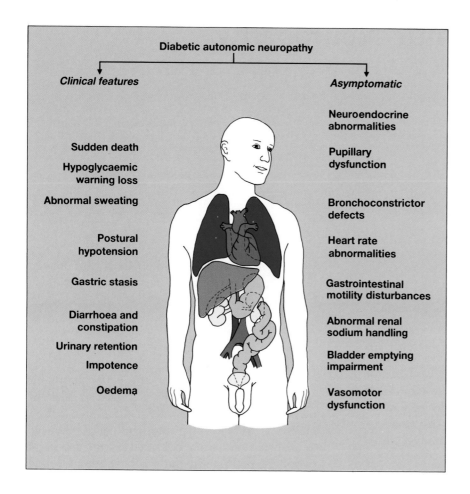

Fig. 63.1. Clinical features and asymptomatic effects of diabetic autonomic neuropathy.

Epidemiology of autonomic neuropathy

The prevalence of autonomic damage in diabetes is not clear. Autonomic dysfunction has been demonstrated in 20% or more of diabetic patients, the exact percentages depending on the tests used and the population selected. In a recent series of 500 IDDM patients, abnormal cardiovascular reflexes were found in 17% overall, with more abnormalities in those aged 40–49 years and those with diabetes for more than 20 years [3]. Another study of 700 patients reported an overall prevalence of postural hypotension of 12%, predominantly in older patients and in those young subjects with a longer duration of diabetes [4]. There have been no satisfactory studies of the prevalence of autonomic symptoms. Widely variable figures have been reported in different series, possibly because of the often vague and non-specific nature of such symptoms. Impotence is relatively common in diabetic men (Chapter 76) and almost invariably accompanies other clinical features of autonomic neuropathy, but the relative contributions of autonomic neuropathy and of

other causes are not known. Autonomic symptoms are uncommon in young diabetic patients, although there have been occasional case reports of severe symptomatic autonomic neuropathy [1].

Aetiology of autonomic neuropathy

The prevalence of autonomic abnormalities is similar in IDDM and NIDDM, suggesting that the metabolic consequences of hyperglycaemia rather than the type of diabetes lead to autonomic nerve damage [5, 6]. The importance of hyperglycaemia was underlined by a recent prospective study of young IDDM patients, which demonstrated a clear relationship between deteriorating cardiovascular reflex tests and poor glycaemic control [7]. Moreover, patients whose metabolic control was improved for 2 years by continuous subcutaneous insulin infusion (CSII) have shown small but significant improvements in autonomic function [8]. There appears, therefore, to be a definite link between deteriorating autonomic function and hyperglycaemia, which may be partly reversed by improved metabolic control. The possible biochemical and pathophysiological basis of nerve damage in diabetes is discussed in Chapter 61.

No genetic factor has yet been implicated in the development of autonomic neuropathy. It has, however, been suggested that diabetic autonomic neuropathy is associated with iritis and that both might be caused by immunological damage [9], but this has been disputed [10].

Relationship of autonomic neuropathy to other complications

Inevitably, as peripheral nerves contain both somatic and autonomic fibres, associations between somatic and autonomic neuropathy have been found [1]. Recently, this relationship was re-examined in diabetic subjects with various clinical manifestations of neuropathy [11] and in untreated NIDDM patients [12]. Both studies suggested that diffuse, symmetrical involvement of peripheral nerves occurred; selective damage to the various fibre types may account for the different clinical presentations.

It has traditionally been taught that diabetic nephropathy, retinopathy and neuropathy develop in parallel and that any patient with long-standing diabetes will have evidence of all three. However, the relationship between autonomic nerve damage and other diabetic complications is currently being reconsidered. Recent studies [13, 14] have suggested that autonomic damage itself may promote the development and progression of nephropathy and retinopathy, possibly through a direct effect of nerve damage on the microcirculation within these organs (Fig. 63.2).

Natural history

The natural history of autonomic involvement in diabetes is slowly being elucidated. Early autonomic dysfunction may in some cases progress to overt autonomic neuropathy. In one large series of patients assessed by cardiovascular reflex tests, approximately three-quarters had not deteriorated a few months to some years later, while the remaining quarter had developed new or additional autonomic symptoms and worsening autonomic function tests. Indices of autonomic function improved in only a very few [15]. In a 5-year prospective study of diabetic patients with abnormal cardiovascular reflexes and symptoms suggestive of autonomic neuropathy, the mortality rate was

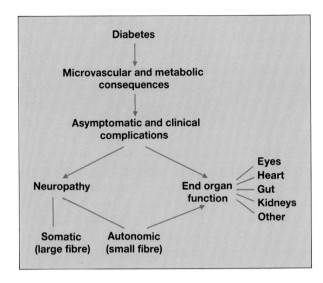

Fig. 63.2. Possible influence of autonomic nerve damage on other diabetic complications.

found to be 50% within 3 years (Fig. 63.3) [16]. Several other studies have now confirmed the poor prognosis of symptomatic autonomic neuropathy [17−19]. Many deaths are due to associated

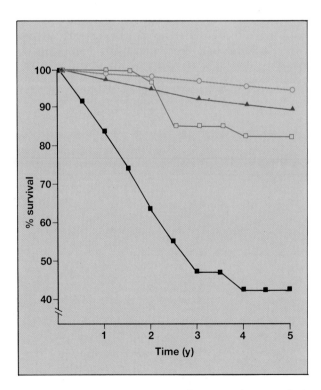

Fig. 63.3. Five-year survival curves for age- and sex-matched general population (○), age- and sex-matched diabetic population (▲), 33 diabetic patients with normal (□) and 40 diabetic patients with abnormal (■) autonomic function tests. (Redrawn with permission from Ewing *et al.* 1980 [16].)

renal failure but some, as discussed below, are sudden and unexpected.

A possible sequence of events is that thermoregulatory function and sweating in the feet may be impaired first, followed by impotence and bladder problems. Cardiovascular reflex abnormalities then appear, and finally the late severe symptomatic manifestations of upper body sweating disturbance, reduced awareness of hypoglycaemia, postural hypotension and gastrointestinal problems (Fig. 63.4). It is not yet clear whether all diabetic patients inevitably progress through all these various stages, or whether some develop only a few early features and do not deteriorate further. Possible factors affecting autonomic nerves, and their consequences, are illustrated in Fig. 63.5.

Clinical features of autonomic neuropathy

Autonomic symptoms are often vague, remain unrecognized for some time and are of limited diagnostic value. However, severe autonomic neuropathy can present with a variable combination of postural hypotension, nocturnal diarrhoea, gastric problems, bladder symptoms, abnormal sweating, impotence in males, and a failure to recognize hypoglycaemia (Fig. 63.1). Most diabetic patients with severe symptomatic features also have advanced nephropathy, retinopathy and somatic neuropathy. Elsewhere in this

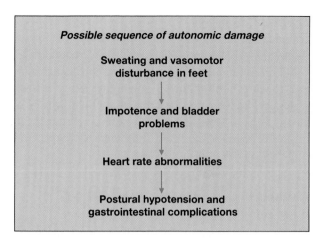

Fig. 63.4. Possible temporal sequence of the clinical progression of autonomic neuropathy in diabetes.

book, gastrointestinal symptoms (Chapter 71), impotence (Chapter 76) and problems associated with the diabetic foot (Chapter 70) are covered in detail. Other clinical features are discussed below.

Postural hypotension

Dizziness associated with a fall in blood pressure on standing up is the most obvious symptom of autonomic neuropathy, and is due to loss of predominantly sympathetically mediated reflexes. The patient may complain of postural weakness,

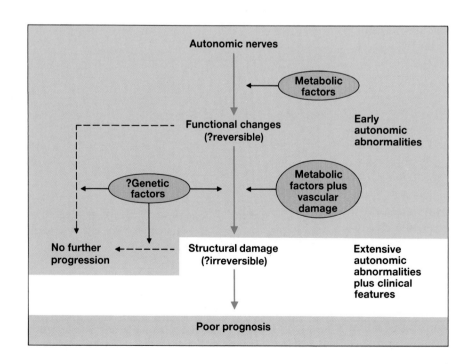

Fig. 63.5. Potential influences on autonomic nerves and their relation to the clinical progression of autonomic neuropathy in diabetes.

faintness, visual impairment or even loss of consciousness, symptoms which are sometimes wrongly attributed to hypoglycaemia. Many drugs, including antihypertensive agents, diuretics, tricyclic antidepressants, phenothiazines, vasodilators and nitrates worsen postural hypotension. Insulin treatment can also aggravate postural hypotension, possibly through a direct vasodilator action on peripheral blood vessels [20, 21]. Conversely, fluid retention, for example in cardiac failure or the nephrotic syndrome, may mask postural hypotension.

Sweating disturbances

Diminished or absent sweating in the feet, extending in more severe cases to the whole leg and lower trunk, is a well-recognized clinical feature of diabetic autonomic neuropathy. Increased sweating over the upper part of the body is also common. Drenching sweats, sometimes mistaken for hypoglycaemic attacks, may affect the head and upper body, particularly in warm weather, during exercise or in bed. Gustatory sweating, starting within minutes of eating and provoked by certain foods, may also occur. It usually affects the forehead first and then spreads to the face, scalp and neck, and is often profuse [22].

Vasomotor problems, oedema and Charcot joints

Autonomic damage impairs local microvascular reflexes which are mediated by vasoconstrictor and vasodilator fibres. Denervation and opening of arterio-venous anastomoses may cause shunting of blood into the skin, which could partly explain the high resting blood flow and skin temperature and dilated foot veins of some neuropathic patients [1, 23]. Paradoxically, they usually complain of cold feet. Peripheral oedema in patients with diabetic neuropathy is not uncommon and may also be related to increased arterio-venous shunting [1, 24]. Altered peripheral blood flow may also be a factor in the development of Charcot arthropathy (see Chapter 70).

Loss of hypoglycaemic warning symptoms

So-called 'hypoglycaemic unawareness' has traditionally been associated with autonomic neuropathy. It is now clear, however, that diabetic patients without other evidence of autonomic involvement may also be affected, possibly because of failure of hypothalamic control mechanisms (see Chapter 23). Normally, hypoglycaemia first causes an asymptomatic parasympathetic response with bradycardia and mild hypotension, followed by sympathetic activation which usually produces easily recognizable symptoms. If these warning signs are absent, the first manifestation of hypoglycaemia may be neuroglycopenic symptoms with a rapid progression to unconsciousness. In clinical practice, less stringent glycaemic control may have to be accepted to avoid this problem.

Sudden unexpected death

Some diabetic patients with autonomic neuropathy have died suddenly and unexpectedly. The reasons for this are unknown, but three possible explanations, none entirely convincing, have been suggested. Episodes of cardiorespiratory arrest have been observed in young diabetic patients with severe autonomic neuropathy [25], and it has been suggested that such subjects may not respond normally to hypoxia. However, laboratory studies of ventilatory control in diabetic patients have so far produced conflicting results [1]. Cardiac arrhythmias are a second possible explanation, but 24-h electrocardiogram monitoring has failed to demonstrate more frequent arrhythmias in diabetic patients than in normal subjects [26]. A third possibility is sleep apnoea, although patients with autonomic neuropathy do not appear to have abnormal breathing patterns during sleep [1, 27]. Failure of an as yet unidentified reflex mechanism under certain conditions may be responsible for unexpected deaths.

Any diabetic patient with autonomic neuropathy is a potential anaesthetic risk, and particular care needs to be taken during and after surgery to provide adequate oxygenation and appropriate monitoring. The same cautions apply to severe respiratory infections.

Bladder and erectile dysfunction

Bladder dysfunction is a well-recognized feature of autonomic neuropathy, but usually remains asymptomatic until the late stages. Characteristically, there is an enlarged bladder and increased residual urine volume after micturition. As autonomic neuropathy progresses, there are lengthened intervals between micturition, an increase in the overnight urine volume, and a weakened or prolonged urinary stream with postmicturition dribbling. In advanced autonomic neuropathy, the bladder may become palpable, with overflow incontinence and rarely, acute retention of urine. Bladder stasis predisposes to urinary tract infection, which may in turn accelerate renal damage.

Impotence is invariably found in men with other features of autonomic neuropathy (see Chapter 76).

Asymptomatic abnormalities

Diabetic patients have a higher resting heart rate than normal subjects (Figs 63.6 and 63.7), possibly due to autonomic damage [28]. A 'fixed' heart rate has also been described, although 24-h electrocardiographic monitoring has shown that very few diabetic patients have this abnormality and that most, including those with autonomic damage, have quite obvious diurnal heart rate variation [26].

Other asymptomatic abnormalities include

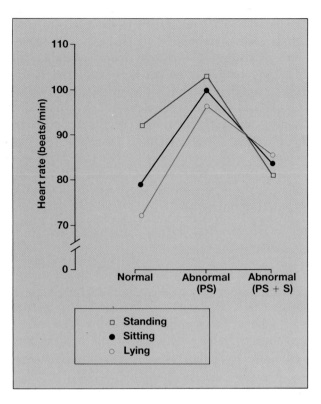

Fig. 63.7. Mean resting heart rates in three diabetic patients whose autonomic function changed with time from normal to definite (PS) and then severe (PS+S) damage. (Redrawn with permission from Ewing *et al.* 1981 [28].)

defective pupillary responses and impaired bronchomotor function. The pupil shows a reduction in resting diameter [29] and loss of spontaneous oscillations ('hippus') [30, 31], and commonly fails to dilate quickly in the dark [30, 31]. Diminished bronchoconstriction in response to provocation tests such as breathing cold air has also been found [32, 33], but no specific clinical respiratory abnormality has yet been identified.

Neuroendocrine changes

Disturbances in the secretion of pancreatic polypeptide and other gastrointestinal hormones are increasingly being recognized in diabetic subjects with autonomic neuropathy. Abnormalities in the release of catecholamines and vasopressin and in the regulation of the renin–angiotensin system have also been described [1, 34]. The clinical consequences of these and other neuroendocrine changes are not yet clear, although certain gastrointestinal symptoms associated with autonomic damage could, in part, be caused by abnormalities of gut regulatory peptides which have been demonstrated in experimental animals [35].

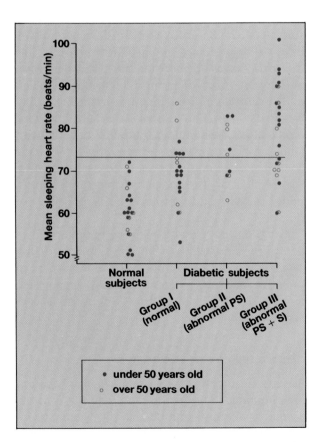

Fig. 63.6. Individual mean sleeping heart rates in normal subjects, diabetic patients with normal cardiovascular reflexes, with definite abnormalities (PS), and with severely abnormal cardiovascular reflexes (PS+S). The solid line represents two SDs above the group mean normal value. (Redrawn with permission from Ewing *et al.* 1983 [26].)

Central neuropathic damage

The question of whether there is involvement of central neuronal pathways is a vexed one. The term 'diabetic encephalopathy' was coined in the 1950s [36] and certain degenerative pathological changes have subsequently been observed in the brains and spinal cords of young diabetic patients [37]. At a clinical level, there have been suggestions of subtle and selective defects of cognitive function in diabetic patients [38]. Profound and prolonged hypoglycaemia can severely damage the central nervous system (see Chapter 50) but whether minor hypoglycaemia causes lesser effects is uncertain. The possible role of prolonged hyperglycaemia in central neuropathic damage is unknown.

The integrity of various central sensory pathways can be investigated using evoked potential techniques. Visual evoked potentials measure the latency and character of the electrical response of the visual cortex (recorded by electroencephalogram) to retinal stimulation using a checkerboard reversal pattern. The auditory pathways can similarly be investigated by the brain-stem auditory evoked potentials and conduction from the periphery to the sensory cortex by somatosensory evoked potentials. Results obtained in diabetic subjects have been conflicting [39, 40]. Some studies have suggested that central damage occurs early in the course of diabetes, while others have found no evidence at all of central involvement, even in patients with widespread complications.

Diagnosis of autonomic neuropathy

The diagnosis of diabetic autonomic neuropathy was first based on symptoms but now depends on various objective reflex tests. There has been considerable debate as to what constitutes the 'best' diagnostic test or set of tests. Some, while useful for physiological studies, are impracticable for use in a diabetic clinic and others are too complex, 'invasive', inherently risky or poorly reproducible [41]. Cardiovascular tests have been best characterized and now allow objective assessment of autonomic function through a series of well-validated, non-invasive and relatively simple manoeuvres. Implicit in their use, however, is the assumption that cardiovascular reflex abnormalities reflect damage throughout the autonomic nervous system. Although this appears largely

correct, early manifestations elsewhere may antedate certain cardiovascular reflex changes.

A consensus statement has recently been published to provide guidelines for the diagnosis and classification of diabetic neuropathy [42]. Recommendations relevant to the autonomic nervous system were that:

1 Symptoms, possibly reflecting autonomic neuropathy should not, by themselves, be considered markers for its presence.
2 Non-invasive validated measures of autonomic neural reflexes should be used as specific markers of autonomic neuropathy if end-organ failure is carefully ruled out and other important factors, such as concomitant illness, drug use, and age, are taken into account. An abnormality of more than one test on more than one occasion is desirable to establish the presence of autonomic dysfunction.
3 Independent tests of both parasympathetic and sympathetic function should be performed.
4 A battery of quantitative measures of autonomic reflexes should be used to monitor improvement or deterioration of autonomic nerve function, although their utility for monitoring patients over time has not clearly been established [42].

Cardiovascular tests

Five simple, non-invasive tests using cardiovascular reflexes are now widely accepted for both diagnostic and research assessment of autonomic neuropathy [15]. These tests examine the responses to various stimuli of either heart rate (the Valsalva manoeuvre, deep breathing and standing up) or blood pressure (standing up and sustained handgrip). These tests are described below, and the range of normal, borderline and abnormal values are shown in Table 63.1.

Other cardiovascular tests sometimes used are based on the baroreflex responses, the heart rate responses to atropine and propanolol or the cold pressor test. None of these appear to be as reliable or as easily performed as the five described here. Two new tests, the heart rate responses to coughing and lying down, have not yet been fully evaluated.

HEART RATE RESPONSE TO THE VALSALVA MANOEUVRE

The Valsalva manoeuvre — forced expiration against resistance — causes complex reflex circulatory changes mediated by both parasympathetic

Table 63.1. Normal, borderline and abnormal values for cardiovascular autonomic function tests [15].

	Normal	Borderline	Abnormal
Heart rate tests			
Heart rate response to Valsalva manoeuvre (Valsalva ratio)	≥1.21	—	≤1.20
Heart rate response to standing up (30:15 ratio)	≥1.04	1.01−1.03	≤1.00
Heart rate response to deep breathing (maximum minus minimum heart rate)	≥15 beats/min	11−14 beats/min	≤10 beats/min
Blood pressure tests			
Blood pressure response to standing up (fall in systolic BP)	≤10 mmHg	11−29 mmHg	≥30 mmHg
Blood pressure response to sustained handgrip (increase in diastolic BP)	≥16 mmHg	11−15 mmHg	≤10 mmHg

and sympathetic pathways. While straining, the blood pressure normally falls and the heart rate rises. After release of the strain, the blood pressure promptly rises and overshoots its resting value while the heart rate slows. With autonomic damage, the blood pressure falls during strain but only slowly returns to normal after release, with no overshoot; there is no change in heart rate. Heart rate is easily measured during and after the Valsalva manoeuvre, and gives a reliable guide to the overall integrity of the complex reflex pathways involved.

The test is performed by asking the subject to sit quietly and then to blow into a mouthpiece attached to an aneroid pressure gauge at a pressure of 40 mmHg for 15 s. Heart rate is recorded continuously using a standard electrocardiogram machine during and after the manoeuvre. The 'Valsalva ratio' is the ratio of the longest R−R interval found after (within about 20 beats of the end of the manoeuvre) to the shortest R−R interval during the manoeuvre. The result is taken as the mean ratio for three successive Valsalva manoeuvres. It is probably wise to avoid this test in diabetic patients with proliferative retinopathy because of the theoretical risk of provoking a retinal or vitreous haemorrhage. Subjects with cardiac failure may fail to show significant heart rate changes during the Valsalva manoeuvre.

HEART RATE RESPONSE TO STANDING UP

Standing up from lying normally causes reflex alterations in heart rate which are mainly under parasympathetic control, with a small sympathetic component. Normally, there is an immediate increase in heart rate, maximal at about the 15th beat after standing, followed by relative bradycardia which is maximal around the 30th beat. Subjects with autonomic neuropathy show only a gradual increase, or no change in heart rate on standing.

For this test, the subject lies quietly on a couch and then stands up unaided. The electrocardiogram is recorded continuously. The heart rate response is best expressed as the '30:15 ratio', i.e. the ratio of the longest R−R interval (around the 30th beat after starting to stand up) to the shortest R−R interval (around the 15th beat). It is important to begin counting beats (by marking the ECG chart) when the subject *starts* to stand up, and not several seconds later when the postural change has been completed.

HEART RATE RESPONSE TO DEEP BREATHING

In normal subjects, the heart rate continually varies, mostly in association with breathing. Heart rate increases during inspiration and decreases during expiration, with maximal variation at a respiratory rate of around six breaths/min. This so-called 'respiratory sinus arrhythmia' is under cardiac parasympathetic control. Autonomic neuropathy considerably reduces and may even abolish heart rate variation during breathing.

The test is conveniently performed by asking the patient to sit quietly and then breathe deeply and evenly at six breaths/min (i.e. 5 s in and 5 s out). The maximum and minimum heart rates during each 10-s breathing cycle are calculated from R−R intervals recorded by electrocardiogram. The mean of the differences during three successive breathing cycles gives the 'maximum−minimum heart rate'. An alternative way to express these changes is as a ratio of the heart rate at its slowest during expiration to that at its fastest during inspiration (the 'E:I ratio').

BLOOD PRESSURE RESPONSE TO STANDING UP

On standing, blood pools in the legs and causes a fall in blood pressure which is normally rapidly corrected by a reflex combination of tachycardia and peripheral and splanchnic vasoconstriction. The cardiovascular reflexes concerned with postural homeostasis are complex and involve both sympathetic and parasympathetic pathways. Defective sympathetic reflexes impair splanchnic vasoconstriction, leading to postural hypotension.

Blood pressure is simply measured while the subject is lying down and again 1 min after standing up, and the difference in systolic blood pressure noted.

BLOOD PRESSURE RESPONSE TO SUSTAINED HANDGRIP

During sustained handgrip, a sharp rise in blood pressure normally occurs due to a heart rate-dependent increase in cardiac output with unchanged peripheral vascular resistance. If the reflex pathways controlling this response are damaged, as in severe diabetic autonomic neuropathy, the blood pressure rise is attenuated.

The test is performed by asking the subject to squeeze a handgrip dynamometer as hard as possible for a few seconds and then to maintain steady pressure at 30% of that maximum for as long as possible, which is usually between 3−4 min. Blood pressure is measured each minute, and the difference between the diastolic blood pressure before starting and just before releasing handgrip is taken as the measure of response.

PRACTICAL ASSESSMENT OF CARDIOVASCULAR AUTONOMIC FUNCTION

This battery of tests can be performed easily in the clinic. All that is needed are a sphygmomanometer, electrocardiogram machine, aneroid pressure gauge attached to a mouthpiece by a rigid or flexible tube, and a handgrip dynamometer (available from Tephcotronics Ltd, 5 Hillview Drive, Edinburgh, EH12 8QW, UK). In practice, all the tests can be performed in a simple planned sequence within 15−20 min (Table 63.2). Data can be handled in two ways. Before the advent of the microcomputer, a ruler and electrocardiogram strip were adequate and are still sufficient where tests are only occasionally performed. However, a number of computer programs are now available which measure R−R intervals automatically, calculate the required ratios, and group the results.

Table 63.2. Flow-plan for performing cardiovascular autonomic function tests.

Tests (performed in this order)	Position of subject	Approximate time of test (min)	Apparatus required
Heart rate response to Valsalva manoeuvre	Sitting	5	Aneroid manometer, electrocardiograph
Heart rate response to deep breathing	Sitting	2	Electrocardiograph
Blood pressure response to sustained handgrip	Sitting	5	Handgrip dynamometer, sphygmomanometer
Heart rate response to standing up Blood pressure response to standing up	Lying, then standing	3	Electrocardiograph Sphygmomanometer

One package specifically designed for the five tests outlined above is the 'Autocaft' system (UnivEd Technologies Ltd, 16 Buccleuch Place, Edinburgh, EH8 9LN, UK), which operates with BBC- or IBM PC-compatible microcomputers. It has the advantages of allowing blood pressure measurements to be entered and of automatically classifying the results as normal, borderline or abnormal.

The results from these five tests enable the severity of autonomic damage (Fig. 63.8) to be categorized according to a system derived from observations on large numbers of subjects over a number of years [15]. The categories are:
1 Normal: all five tests normal, or one borderline.
2 Early involvement: one of the three heart-rate tests abnormal or two borderline.
3 Definite involvement: two or more of the heart-rate tests abnormal.
4 Severe involvement: two or more of the heart-rate tests abnormal, plus one or both of the blood pressure tests abnormal, or both borderline.
5 Atypical pattern: any other combination of abnormal tests (only about 6% of diabetic subjects are 'atypical').

An alternative to this classification is to give each individual test a score of 0, 1 or 2 depending on whether it is normal, borderline or abnormal. An overall 'autonomic score' of 0–10 can then be obtained. Increasing scores from 0 to 10 correlate

closely with the grades of severity given above [15]. Scoring of the tests in this way allows an 'atypical' pattern to be given a numerical value.

The classification proposed here avoids labelling the tests as specifically 'parasympathetic' or 'sympathetic', as the reflex pathways involved are extremely complex. The use of a single cardiovascular reflex test to assess autonomic function is misleading and should be avoided as it neglects the possible range of autonomic nerve damage.

Tests in other systems

While cardiovascular reflex tests are generally accepted as the 'gold standard' for the assessment of autonomic dysfunction in diabetes, tests in other systems can sometimes be of value [1, 41]. However, most are more complex and are mentioned here only in outline.

GASTROINTESTINAL TESTS

Oesophageal function can be assessed by cineradiography after swallowing barium, by manometry, or by scintiscanning using solid and liquid meals labelled with gamma-emitting isotopes (see Chapter 71). Abnormal motility and transit patterns have been found in diabetic autonomic neuropathy. Emptying of the stomach is a coordinated process involving both parasympathetic and sympathetic nerves. Gastric abnormalities in diabetic patients have been assessed by barium meal studies, by scintigraphic techniques, and by monitoring changes in gastric volume using electrical impedance measurements or ultrasonography [43, 44]. Within the small and large bowel there are no simple, reliable methods available to assess transit time or motor function, although certain marker techniques and breath hydrogen measurements have been used. Detailed studies of colonic motility have been reported, but such techniques are still research procedures.

BLADDER FUNCTION TESTS

Bladder function can be assessed using specialized cystometric and urodynamic methods, but these require expert interpretation. Three simpler tests are ultrasound imaging of the bladder to measure the approximate volume of residual urine, mictiography to quantitate urine flow time and volume, and intravenous pyelography. Their exact place

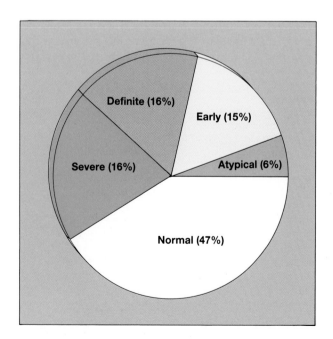

Fig. 63.8. Results of cardiovascular autonomic function tests in 1469 diabetic subjects, grouped according to the severity of autonomic damage.

Sweating can be assessed roughly (and messily) by applying powders which change colour on contact with moisture. Two quantifiable tests have recently been described. The first uses a special 'cell' which stimulates local sweating by iontophoresis of acetylcholine — the so-called 'quantitative sudomotor axon reflex test' (or Q-SART) [45]. A second approach is to count the number of imprints made by sweat drops in a soft Silastic film applied to the skin, after stimulating sweating with pilocarpine [46].

PUPILLARY TESTS

Abnormalities of pupillary diameter are described above. Sophisticated pupillary analysis requires a costly infrared pupillometer, but two simple methods are available. The diameter of the dark-adapted pupil can be measured from a polaroid photograph of the eye, which provides a quantitative estimate of sympathetic pupillary innervation [47]. Pupil cycle time can also be measured. Regular oscillations of the pupil can normally be induced with a slit-lamp beam and are a sensitive indicator of parasympathetic function. In diabetic autonomic neuropathy, pupil cycle time is considerably prolonged [48].

NEUROENDOCRINE TESTS

These tests measure the stimulated levels of hormones whose secretion depends on sympathetic or parasympathetic pathways. The pancreatic polypeptide responses to hypoglycaemia and eating have been used to test vagal integrity, and changes in plasma catecholamine levels in response to various stimuli to indicate sympathetic activity [1, 34]. However, assay of the hormones and interpretation of the results can be difficult, thus limiting their practical usefulness.

Management of autonomic neuropathy

General and preventative measures

As mentioned above, diabetic patients with symptomatic autonomic neuropathy pose particular anaesthetic hazards and great care must be taken during the perioperative period. Hypoglycaemic warning symptoms may be lost and the possibility of relaxing glycaemic control should be considered in such patients. Neurogenic bladder problems may be helped by encouraging regular bladder emptying, if necessary by using manual suprapubic pressure every 3–4 h. Long-term single or cyclical chemotherapy may be indicated for recurrent or persistent urinary tract infections. Bladder neck resection may need to be considered in cases with large residual urine volumes, but may cause incontinence.

Symptomatic treatment

Postural hypotension only needs treatment if it is symptomatic. Mild symptoms during the day can be treated by raising the head of the bed a few centimetres at night. In those with more marked symptoms, fludrocortisone is the drug of choice [49, 50] (Fig. 63.9). This acts directly to increase peripheral vascular tone and also increases blood volume [49]. Sometimes it is ineffective, when other drugs including pindolol, metoclopramide (either alone or in combination with flurbiprofen) and a combination of diphenhydramine and cimetidine can be tried. Antigravity suits and elastic tights are probably no longer necessary.

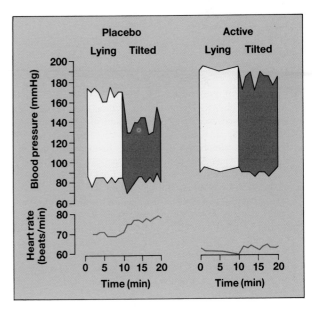

Fig. 63.9. Blood pressure and heart rate responses to tilting in a diabetic patient with autonomic neuropathy during placebo and fludrocortisone treatment periods. (Redrawn with permission from Campbell *et al.* 1975 [49].)

Profuse and socially embarrassing sweating may be limited by anticholinergic drugs such as propantheline hydrobromide or poldine methylsulphate. A prophylactic dose of either drug taken before a meal is often effective in preventing gustatory sweating. Side-effects, including urinary retention, often restrict the use of these agents.

Curative measures

As yet, no way has been found to limit or reverse autonomic neuropathy. There have been some encouraging accounts of slight improvement in the reflex abnormalities with improved glycaemic control, particularly CSII [8]. Some reports have suggested that treatment with the aldose reductase inhibitors may slightly improve certain cardiovascular test indices [51–54], but the clinical relevance of these results is uncertain. Such drugs administered long-term and before irreversible nerve damage has occurred may possibly prevent the morbid and mortal consequences of autonomic nerve damage.

DAVID J. EWING

References

1 Ewing DJ, Clarke BF. Diabetic autonomic neuropathy: present insights and future prospects. *Diabetes Care* 1986; **9**: 648–65.

2 Bannister R. Introduction and classification. In: Bannister R, ed. *Autonomic Failure. A Textbook of Clinical Disorders of the Autonomic Nervous System.* Oxford: Oxford University Press, 1988: 1–20.

3 O'Brien IAD, O'Hare JP, Lewin IG, Corrall RJM. The prevalence of autonomic neuropathy in insulin-dependent diabetes mellitus: a controlled study based on heart rate variability. *Q J Med* 1986; **61**: 957–67.

4 Krolewski AS, Warram JH, Cupples A, Gorman CK, Szabo AJ, Christlieb AR. Hypertension, orthostatic hypotension and the microvascular complications of diabetes. *J Chronic Dis* 1985; **38**: 319–26.

5 Pfeifer MA, Weinberg CR, Cook DL, Reenan A, Halter JB, Ensinck JW et al. Autonomic neural dysfunction in recently diagnosed diabetic subjects. *Diabetes Care* 1984; **7**: 447–53.

6 Masaoka S, Lev-Ran A, Hill LR, Vakil G, Hon EHG. Heart rate variability in diabetes: relationship to age and duration of the disease. *Diabetes Care* 1985; **8**: 64–8.

7 Young RJ, MacIntyre CCA, Martyn CN, Prescott RJ, Ewing DJ, Smith AF et al. Progression of subclinical polyneuropathy in young patients with Type 1 (insulin-dependent) diabetes: associations with glycaemic control and microangiopathy (microvascular complications). *Diabetologia* 1986; **29**: 156–61.

8 Jakobsen J, Christiansen JS, Kristoffersen I, Christensen CK, Hermansen K, Schmitz A et al. Autonomic and somatosensory nerve function after 2 years of continuous subcutaneous insulin infusion in Type 1 diabetes. *Diabetes* 1988; **37**: 452–5.

9 Guy RJC, Richards F, Edmonds ME, Watkins PJ. Diabetic autonomic neuropathy and iritis: an association suggesting an immunological cause. *Br Med J* 1984; **289**: 343–5.

10 Martyn CN, Young RJ, Ewing DJ. Is there a link between iritis and diabetic autonomic neuropathy? *Br Med J* 1986; **292**: 934.

11 Young RJ, Zhou YQ, Rodriguez E, Prescott RJ, Ewing DJ, Clarke BF. Variable relationship between peripheral somatic and autonomic neuropathy in patients with different syndromes of diabetic polyneuropathy. *Diabetes* 1986; **35**: 192–7.

12 Pfeifer MA, Weinberg CR, Cook DL, Reenan A, Halar E, Halter JB et al. Correlations among autonomic, sensory, and motor neural function tests in untreated non-insulin-dependent diabetic individuals. *Diabetes Care* 1985; **8**: 576–84.

13 Lilja B, Nosslin B, Bergstrom B, Sundkvist G. Glomerular filtration rate, autonomic nerve function and orthostatic blood pressure in patients with diabetes mellitus. *Diabetes Res* 1985; **2**: 179–81.

14 Winocour PH, Dhar H, Anderson DC. The relationship between autonomic neuropathy and urinary sodium and albumin excretion in insulin-treated diabetics. *Diabetic Med* 1986; **3**: 436–40.

15 Ewing DJ, Martyn CN, Young RJ, Clarke BF. The value of cardiovascular autonomic function tests: 10 years experience in diabetes. *Diabetes Care* 1985; **8**: 491–8.

16 Ewing DJ, Campbell IW, Clarke BF. The natural history of diabetic autonomic neuropathy. *Q J Med* 1980; **49**: 95–108.

17 Watkins PJ, Mackay JD. Cardiac denervation in diabetic neuropathy. *Ann Intern Med* 1980; **92**: 304–7.

18 Sala JMV, Saez JMG, Esteve RI, Hosselbarth AF, Uriach CV, Bertran MM et al. Mortalidad en la neuropatia vegetativa cardiovascular de la diabetes mellitus. *Med Clin (Barc)* 1983; **81**: 794–6.

19 Hasslacher C, Bassler G. Prognose der kardialen autonomen Neuropathie bei Diabetikern. *Münch Med Wschr* 1983; **125**: 375–7.

20 Page MMcB, Watkins PJ. Provocation of postural hypotension by insulin. *Diabetes* 1976; **25**: 90–5.

21 Takata S, Yamamoto M, Yagi S, Noto Y, Ikeda T, Hattori N. Peripheral circulatory effects of insulin in diabetes. *Angiology* 1985; **36**: 110–15.

22 Watkins PJ. Facial sweating after food; a new sign of diabetic autonomic neuropathy. *Br Med J* 1973; **1**: 583–7.

23 Archer AG, Roberts VC, Watkins PJ. Blood flow patterns in painful diabetic neuropathy. *Diabetologia* 1984; **27**: 563–7.

24 Edmonds ME, Archer AG, Watkins PJ. Ephedrine: a new treatment for diabetic neuropathic oedema. *Lancet* 1983; i: 548–51.

25 Page MMcB, Watkins PJ. Cardiorespiratory arrest and diabetic autonomic neuropathy. *Lancet* 1978; i: 14–16.

26 Ewing DJ, Borsey DQ, Travis P, Bellavere F, Neilson JMM, Clarke BF. Abnormalities of ambulatory 24 hour heart rate in diabetes mellitus. *Diabetes* 1983; **32**: 101–5.

27 Catterall JR, Calverley PMA, Ewing DJ et al. Breathing, sleep and autonomic neuropathy. *Diabetes* 1984; **33**: 1025–7.

28 Ewing DJ, Campbell IW, Clarke BF. Heart rate changes in diabetes mellitus. *Lancet* 1981; i: 183–6.

29 Hreidarsson AB. Pupil size in insulin-dependent diabetes. Relationship to duration, metabolic control, and long-term complications. *Diabetes* 1982; **31**: 442–8.

30 Hreidarsson AB, Gundersen HJG. Reduced pupillary unrest. Autonomic nervous system abnormalities in diabetes

mellitus. *Diabetes* 1988; **37**: 446–51.

31 Smith SE, Smith SA, Brown PM, Fox C, Sönksen PH. Pupillary signs in diabetic autonomic neuropathy. *Br Med J* 1978; **2**: 924–7.

32 Douglas NJ, Campbell IW, Ewing DJ, Clarke BF, Flenley DC. Reduced airway vagal tone in diabetic patients with autonomic neuropathy. *Clin Sci* 1981; **61**: 581–4.

33 Heaton RW, Guy RJC, Gray BJ, Watkins PJ, Costello JF. Diminished bronchial reactivity to cold air in diabetic patients with autonomic neuropathy. *Br Med J* 1984; **289**: 149–51.

34 Kennedy FP, Go VLW, Cryer PE, Bolli GE, Gerich JE. Subnormal pancreatic polypeptide and epinephrine responses to insulin-induced hypoglycemia identify patients with insulin-dependent diabetes mellitus predisposed to develop overt autonomic neuropathy. *Ann Int Med* 1988; **108**: 54–8.

35 Ballmann M, Conlon JM. Changes in the somatostatin, substance P and vasoactive intestinal peptide contents of the gastrointestinal tract following streptozotocin-induced diabetes in the rat. *Diabetologia* 1985; **28**: 355–8.

36 De Jong RN. The nervous system complications in diabetes mellitus with special reference to cerebrovascular changes. *J Nerv Ment Dis* 1950; **111**: 181–206.

37 Reske-Nielson E, Lundbaek K, Gregersen G, Harmsen A. Pathological changes in central and peripheral nervous system of young long-term diabetics. *Diabetologia* 1970; **6**: 98–103.

38 Franceschi M, Cecchetto R, Minicucci F, Smirne S, Baio G, Canal N. Cognitive processes in insulin-dependent diabetes. *Diabetes Care* 1984; **7**: 228–31.

39 Pozzessere G, Rizzo PA, Valle E *et al.* Early detection of neurological involvement in IDDM and NIDDM. Multimodal evoked potentials versus metabolic control. *Diabetes Care* 1988; **11**: 473–80.

40 Collier A, Reid W, McInnes A, Cull RE, Ewing DJ, Clarke BF. Somatosensory and visual evoked potentials in insulin-dependent diabetics with mild peripheral neuropathy. *Diabetes Res Clin Pract* 1988; **5**: 171–5.

41 Ewing DJ. Practical bedside investigation of diabetic autonomic failure. In: Bannister R, ed. *Autonomic Failure. A Textbook of Clinical Disorders of the Autonomic Nervous System.* Oxford: Oxford University Press, 1983: 371–405.

42 Consensus statement. Report and recommendations of the San Antonio Conference on diabetic neuropathy. *Diabetes* 1988; **37**: 1000–4.

43 Gilbey SG, Watkins PJ. Measurement by epigastric impedance of gastric emptying in diabetic autonomic neuropathy. *Diabetic Med* 1987; **4**: 122–6.

44 Vogelberg KH, Rathmann W, Helbig G. Sonographic examination of gastric motility in diabetics with autonomic neuropathy. *Diabetes Res* 1987; **5**: 175–9.

45 Low PA, Caskey PE, Tuck RR, Fealey RD, Dyck PJ. Quantitative sudomotor axon reflex test in normal and neuropathic subjects. *Ann Neurol* 1983; **14**: 573–80.

46 Kennedy WR, Sakuda M, Sutherland D, Goetz FC. The sweating deficiency in diabetes mellitus: methods of quantitation and clinical correlation. *Neurology (Cleveland)* 1984; **34**: 758–63.

47 Smith SA, Dewhurst RR. A simple diagnostic test for pupillary abnormality in diabetic autonomic neuropathy. *Diabetic Med* 1986; **3**: 38–41.

48 Martyn CN, Ewing DJ. Pupil cycle time: a simple way of measuring an autonomic reflex. *J Neurol Neurosurg Psychiatr* 1986; **49**: 771–4.

49 Campbell IW, Ewing DJ, Clarke BF. 9-alpha-fluorohydrocortisone in the treatment of postural hypotension in diabetic autonomic neuropathy. *Diabetes* 1975; **24**: 381–4.

50 Campbell IW, Ewing DJ, Clarke BF. Therapeutic experience with fludrocortisone in diabetic postural hypotension. *Br Med J* 1976; **1**: 872–4.

51 Jaspan JB, Herold K, Bartkus C. Effects of sorbinil therapy in diabetic patients with painful peripheral neuropathy and autonomic neuropathy. *Am J Med* 1985; **79** (suppl 5A): 24–37.

52 Fagius J, Brattberg A, Jameson S, Berne C. Limited benefit of treatment of diabetic polyneuropathy with an aldose reductase inhibitor: a 24-week controlled trial. *Diabetologia* 1985; **28**: 323–9.

53 Sundkvist G, Lilja B, Rosen I, Agardh C-D. Autonomic and peripheral nerve function in early diabetic neuropathy. Possible influence of a novel aldose reductase inhibitor on autonomic function. *Acta Med Scand* 1987; **221**: 445–53.

54 Young RJ, Martyn CN, Ewing DJ, Clarke BF. Improvement of nerve function with Statil (ICI 128436) in asymptomatic diabetic neuropathy: a six week controlled study. *Diabetic Med* 1986; **3**: 589A.

PART 13.4
DIABETIC NEPHROPATHY

64 Epidemiology and Natural History of Diabetic Nephropathy

Summary

• Diabetic nephropathy is defined by persistent albuminuria (albumin excretion rate (AER) >300 mg/day; Albustix-positive), declining glomerular filtration rate (GFR) and rising blood pressure.

• Established nephropathy follows several years of incipient nephropathy, characterized by worsening microalbuminuria (AER, 30–300 mg/day) which is Albustix-negative and detectable by, for instance, radioimmunoassay.

• The natural history of nephropathy differs between IDDM and NIDDM. In IDDM, nephropathy develops in about 35% of cases, especially in males and those whose diabetes presents before the age of 15 years. The incidence of nephropathy peaks after 15–16 years of diabetes and declines thereafter. In NIDDM, estimates of prevalence range from 3% to 16% and nephropathy often supervenes after a shorter known duration of diabetes than in IDDM.

• The incidence of diabetic nephropathy is falling, possibly due in part to improved diabetic management.

• GFR is often increased above normal ('hyperfiltration') from the onset of IDDM, due to increased renal blood flow, glomerular capillary hypertension and increased filtration surface area. The glomeruli are hypertrophied and the kidneys enlarged. These changes do not seem to occur in NIDDM.

• In both IDDM and NIDDM, GFR begins to decline irreversibly when AER has risen to 100–300 mg/day, at an average rate of 10 ml/min/1.73 m^2 per year. This is due to progressive reduction of the filtration surface area through mesangial expansion. Serum creatinine levels begin to rise when GFR falls below 50 ml/min/1.73 m^2 and end-stage renal failure follows after an average of 5 years.

• Blood pressure is normal at the onset of IDDM and generally remains so in patients with normoalbuminuria. In microalbuminuric subjects, however, blood pressure begins to rise when AER exceeds 50 mg/day.

• Albuminuria in diabetic nephropathy is due to glomerular capillary damage and reflects generalized damage to the microcirculation and large vessels. Nephropathic patients have an increased incidence of retinopathy and a tenfold increase in cardiovascular mortality which is the major cause of death in nephropathic NIDDM patients.

• Other concomitants of albuminuria include increased urinary IgG excretion, hyperlipidaemia and elevated fibrinogen levels.

• The rate of progression of incipient and established nephropathy can be slowed and the associated mortality reduced by aggressive antihypertensive treatment.

Diabetic nephropathy is an important complication of diabetes for a number of reasons. Firstly, it is relatively common, affecting about one in three of patients with IDDM. Secondly, the proteinuria which is its hallmark is only one consequence of widespread damage to small and large blood vessels, and is a marker for the cardiovascular disease which is a common cause of death in these patients. Thirdly, there is increasingly convincing and optimistic evidence that the progression of nephropathy and its associated mortality can be ameliorated by antihypertensive and other treatments if started at an early stage.

This section will describe the epidemiology and natural history of the condition and will set the scene for the detailed descriptions of the causes, pathological and clinical features, diagnosis and treatment of diabetic nephropathy in the following chapters.

Definitions

Diabetic nephropathy is characterized by persistent proteinuria, decreasing glomerular filtration rate (GFR) and increasing blood pressure. Persistent proteinuria is defined as a urinary protein excretion of > 0.5 g/day, a level detectable by routine dip-stick testing of random urine samples (e.g. with Albustix) in more than two consecutive urine samples in a diabetic patient without urinary infection, cardiac insufficiency or other renal diseases. The excretion of 0.5 g/day of total protein is equivalent to a urinary albumin excretion of about 300 mg/day or 200 µg/min. This stage is preceded by a long 'silent' phase of *incipient diabetic nephropathy* characterized by a subclinical increase in albumin excretion to above the normal range but below the limit defining diabetic nephropathy. This degree of albuminuria is known as *microalbuminuria* (30–300 mg/day or 20–200 µg/min) and, being below the threshold of detection by Albustix, must be measured by radioimmunoassay or other highly-sensitive methods (see Fig. 64.1).

The morphological changes seen in the diabetic kidney consist of diffuse and nodular glomerulosclerosis and arteriolohyalinosis. The term 'diabetic nephropathy' is not synonymous with glomerulosclerosis as diabetic glomerulosclerosis is found in almost all (> 90%) IDDM patients after 10 years of diabetes [1], whereas diabetic

nephropathy (with persistent proteinuria and declining renal function) will develop in only about 35–40% of diabetic patients [2, 3]. The correlation between morphological and functional abnormalities is therefore poor [4, 5] (see Chapter 66).

Prevalence and incidence

Diabetic nephropathy occurs in both IDDM and NIDDM but its natural history differs between the two. In IDDM, the prevalence of diabetic nephropathy is about 15–20% while a further 15–28% of patients are reported to show persistent microalbuminuria [6, 7]. The incidence of diabetic nephropathy reaches a peak of 3–5% of unaffected patients per year after about 15–16 years of diabetes. Thereafter, the incidence decreases and reaches a very low level after 35 years of diabetes (Figs 64.2 and 64.3) [2, 3, 8]. The incidence is higher in males than in females [2] and higher in patients who develop diabetes before the age of 15 than after this age [9]. The majority of IDDM patients, however, do not develop clinical nephropathy, the cumulative incidence being 35% after 40 years of diabetes [2, 3]. The incidence of diabetic nephropathy seems to depend to some extent upon the quality of metabolic control [3]. Improved diabetic care has been accompanied by and may have resulted in a 30% reduction in the incidence of diabetic nephropathy during the last 30 years [3, 9].

The epidemiology of diabetic nephropathy in NIDDM is less well-defined. The prevalence rates of clinical proteinuria reported in different studies vary from 3% to 16% [10, 11] and those of microalbuminuria from 15% to 59% [10, 12, 13]. The

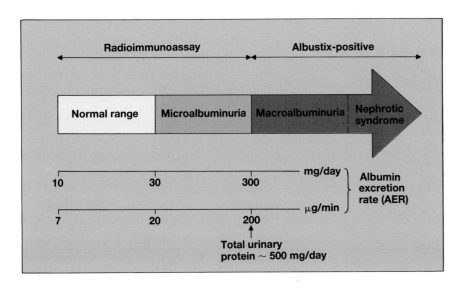

Fig. 64.1. Limits of normo-, micro- and macroalbuminuria.

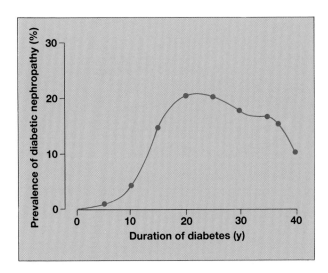

Fig. 64.2. Prevalence of diabetic nephropathy in IDDM. (Redrawn from [2].)

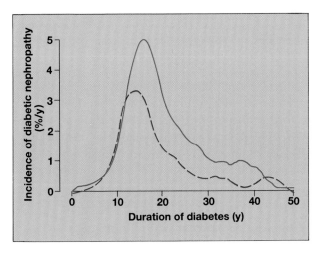

Fig. 64.3. Incidence of diabetic nephropathy in IDDM as a function of diabetes duration in women (blue), and men (red). (Redrawn from [8].)

incidence of diabetic nephropathy in NIDDM is not known. The interval from the clinical onset of diabetes to the development of clinical nephropathy tends to be shorter in NIDDM than in IDDM, probably because the former may be present for some years before diagnosis.

Natural history

The onset of persistent proteinuria is a late stage in a long-lasting process which in IDDM starts soon after the onset of diabetes. At this stage, when diabetes has been adequately controlled, urinary albumin excretion rate (AER) averages

about 10 mg/day. In those patients who will later develop persistent proteinuria, AER increases at an exponential rate of about 20% per year (Fig. 64.4). This means that most of these patients will exceed the upper level of normoalbuminuria (about 30 mg/day) some 5 years after the onset of diabetes. Thereafter, AER continues to increase within the Albustix-negative, microalbuminuric range [14]. It must be appreciated that AER shows great variability and that repeated estimations may be required to characterized a given patient [15, 16]. AER also rises during exercise [17] in normoalbuminuric diabetic subjects and to a greater extent in those with microalbuminuria [18].

As discussed below, albuminuria is due to capillary lesions in the glomerulus and is a manifestation of widespread vascular damage. Patients with persistent microalbuminuria display other abnormalities, within and beyond the kidney. There is an increased urinary IgG excretion rate [19]. They also have a relatively raised blood pressure [20, 21] and the incidence of retinopathy is considerably increased [22]. Exchangeable sodium [23], LDL, VLDL, triglycerides and fibrinogen [24] are increased while serum albumin is decreased [23, 24]. The transcapillary escape rate and the catabolic rate of fibrinogen and albumin are increased [25, 26]. In contrast to the glomerular defects, tubular function as assessed by urinary excretion of β2-microglobulin or retinol-binding protein appears to be normal [19]. The cause of albuminuria is unknown but might be due to

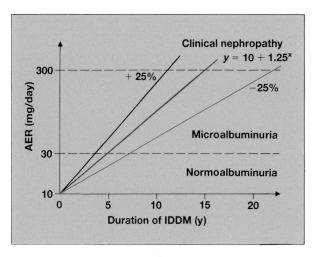

Fig. 64.4. Progression of microproteinuria and clinical nephropathy in IDDM, showing average rate and 25% confidence intervals for the increase in AER, plotted on a logarithmic scale. (Redrawn from [14].)

alterations in the metabolism of anionic compounds of the glomerular basement membrane (see Chapter 65).

Evolution of changes in GFR

Glomerular filtration rate is significantly increased from the onset of IDDM [27, 28]. This 'hyperfiltration' is due to a combination of hyperperfusion (i.e. increased renal blood flow), glomerular hypertension and increased filtration surface area [29, 30]. Not only are individual glomeruli enlarged but overall kidney size is increased from the onset of IDDM [29, 31]. Hyperfiltration and hyperperfusion probably play a role in the development of mesangial expansion although it has not been convincingly demonstrated that hyperfiltration is greater in diabetic patients who ultimately develop nephropathy than in those who do not [32−34]. The degree of hyperfiltration is considerably influenced by metabolic control and protein intake. In contrast to IDDM, glomerular hyperfiltration and renal enlargement do not seem to occur in NIDDM [35].

GFR starts to fall when AER is between 100 and 300 mg/day, at an average rate of about 10 ml/min/1.73 m^2 per year. This decline in GFR is caused by a reduction in the glomerular filtration surface area due to mesangial expansion [36]. Initially, mesangial expansion is compensated for by glomerular hypertrophy but in patients developing albuminuria, mesangial expansion becomes so marked that GFR cannot be maintained by this mechanism [37]. This results in an irreversible decline in GFR (Fig. 64.5). Once GFR is < 50 ml/min/1.73 m^2, serum creatinine concentration begins to rise, and there is an inexorable decline towards end-stage renal failure at a rate which is quite constant for a given patient but highly variable between patients.

Progression of hypertension

Blood pressure is normal at the onset of IDDM and remains so in patients with normal AER, despite chronic volume expansion and increased exchangeable sodium (see Chapter 69) [23]. In albuminuric patients, however, recent prospective studies have demonstrated that AER increases to about 50 mg/day before blood pressure begins to rise [21, 38]. The blood pressure increase in patients with persistent microalbuminuria seems to be of renal origin [23] and may be related to

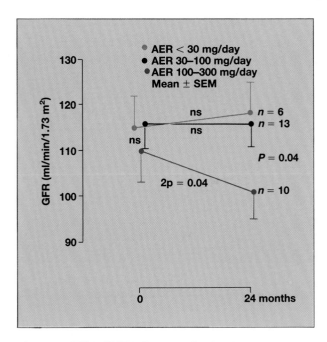

Fig. 64.5. GFR in IDDM. Patients who develop persistent albuminuria will demonstrate a decline in GFR after the onset of persistent microalbuminuria.

reduction in filtration capacity by mesangial expansion. Hypertension is associated with a further increase of extracellular sodium volume whereas plasma volume remains normal [23]. Plasma renin activity is low or normal and plasma aldosterone, angiotensin II and catecholamine concentrations are reduced [23].

Prognosis of patients with albuminuria

Increased AER not only indicates renal disease, but reflects universal vascular damage affecting large and small vessels [39, 40]. In patients with persistent proteinuria, the incidence of coronary heart disease is significantly higher than in patients without proteinuria and their relative cardiovascular mortality is increased about tenfold [40−43]. The incidence of proliferative retinopathy is also increased several-fold in proteinuric patients [22, 44, 45].

Without special care, about 50% of patients will die within 7 years of the onset of persistent proteinuria [2, 3]. The cause of death in these patients is not only uraemia but also cardiovascular diseases such as myocardial infarction, cardiac failure and cerebrovascular accidents [2, 43, 46, 47]. Among NIDDM patients with nephropathy, cardiovascular disease is the commonest cause of death, progression to end-stage renal failure being

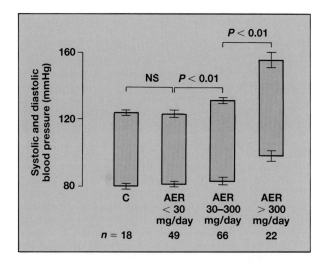

Fig. 64.6. Blood pressure among long-standing IDDM patients, showing progressively higher levels as AER increases. C=non-diabetic control population.

relatively unusual [48]. However, because NIDDM is more common than IDDM, nearly one-half of all diabetic patients receiving renal replacement therapy have NIDDM [48]. Indeed, most of the excess mortality among diabetic patients is associated with proteinuria [49]; those with normal AER have nearly normal survival. This consideration applies to both IDDM and NIDDM [12, 50, 51].

The prognosis of patients with incipient or established nephropathy can be altered by effective antihypertensive therapy. Case-control studies have recently demonstrated that aggressive antihypertensive therapy can slow the rate of decline in GFR and postpone the onset of uraemia by many years [52]. Overall mortality is also reduced by such treatment [53, 54]. The outlook for patients with diabetic nephropathy has therefore improved considerably in recent years.

Conclusions and practical implications

Persistent albuminuria in diabetic patients not only indicates renal disease but also signifies generalized vascular damage and identifies those subjects at high risk of premature cardiovascular death [55]. However, the outcome of this condition is becoming less gloomy. The incidence of diabetic nephropathy has declined during recent years and this may be due to improved metabolic control; moreover, mortality in diabetic people with proteinuria can be reduced by effective antihypertensive therapy, which also retards the

progression of nephropathy. These findings mean that the early identification of patients with incipient nephropathy (persistent microalbuminuria) is essential so that they can be offered appropriate therapy as soon as possible.

TORSTEN DECKERT

ANASUYA GRENFELL

References

1 Thomsen AC. *The Kidney in Diabetes Mellitus.* PhD Thesis, Munksgaard, Copenhagen, 1965.
2 Andersen AR, Christiansen JS, Andersen JK, Kreiner S, Deckert T. Diabetic nephropathy in Type 1 (insulin-dependent) diabetes: An epidemiological study. *Diabetologia* 1983; **25**: 496–501.
3 Krolewski AS, Warram JH, Christlieb AR *et al.* The changing natural history of nephropathy in type 1 diabetes. *Am J Med* 1985; **78**: 785–94.
4 Mauer SM, Steffes MW, Ellis EN, Sutherland DER, Brown DM, Goetz FC. Structural-functional relationship in diabetic nephropathy. *J Clin Invest* 1984; **74**: 1143–55.
5 Chavers BM, Bilous RW, Ellis EN, Steffes MW, Mauer SM. Glomerular lesions and urinary albumin excretion in type 1 diabetes without overt proteinuria. *N Engl J Med* 1989; **320**: 966–70.
6 Niazy S, Feldt-Rasmussen B, Deckert T. Microalbuminuria in insulin-dependent diabetes: Prevalence and practical consequences. *J Diabetic Compl* 1987; 76–80.
7 Parving H-H, Hommel E, Mathiesen E *et al.* Prevalence of microalbuminuria, arterial hypertension, retinopathy, and neuropathy in patients with insulin dependent diabetes. *Br Med J* 1986; **296**: 156–60.
8 Borch-Johnsen K, Andersen KP, Deckert T. The effect of proteinuria on relative mortality in Type 1 (insulin-dependent) diabetes mellitus. *Diabetologia* 1985; **28**: 590–6.
9 Kofoed-Enevoldsen A, Borch-Johnsen K, Kreiner S, Nerup J, Deckert T. Declining incidence of persistent proteinuria in type 1 (insulin-dependent) diabetic patients in Denmark. *Diabetes* 1987; **36**: 205–9.
10 Garancini P, Gallus G, Calori G *et al.* Microalbuminuria and its associated risk factors in a representative sample of Italian type II diabetics. *J Diabetic Compl* 1988; **2**: 12–15.
11 Fabré J, Balant LP, Dayer PG, Fox HM, Vernet AT. The kidney in maturity onset diabetes mellitus: A clinical study of 510 patients. *Kidney Int* 1982; **21**: 730–8.
12 Mogensen CE. Microalbuminuria predicts clinical proteinuria and early mortality in maturity onset diabetes. *N Engl J Med* 1984; **310**: 356–60.
13 Standl E, Rebell B, Steigler H *et al.* Prevalence and risk profile of incipient diabetic nephropathy in Type 2 (non-insulin dependent) diabetes mellitus. *Diabetologia* 1987; **30**: 584–5A.
14 Deckert T, Feldt-Rasmussen B, Borch-Johnsen K *et al.* Clinical assessment and prognosis of complications of diabetes. *Transplantation Proc* 1986; **18**: 1636–8.
15 Feldt-Rasmussen B, Mathiesen ER. Variability of urinary albumin excretion in incipient diabetic nephropathy. *Diabetic Nephropathy* 1984; **3**: 101–3.
16 Cohen DL, Close CF, Viberti GC. The variability of overnight urinary albumin excretion in insulin-dependent diabetic and normal subjects. *Diabetic Med* 1987; **4**: 437–40.

17 Viberti GC, Jarrett RJ, McCartney M, Keen H. Increased glomerular permeability to albumin induced by exercise in diabetic subjects. *Diabetologia* 1978; **14**: 293–300.

18 Feldt-Rasmussen B, Baker L, Deckert T. Exercise as a provocative test in early renal disease in Type 1 (insulin-dependent) diabetes: albuminuric, systemic, and renal haemodynamic responses. *Diabetologia* 1985; **28**: 389–96.

19 Deckert T, Feldt-Rasmussen B, Djurup R, Deckert M. Glomerular size and charge selectivity in insulin-dependent diabetes mellitus. *Kidney Int* 1988; **33**: 100–6.

20 Wiseman MJ, Viberti GC, Mackintosh D, Jarrett RJ, Keen H. Glycaemia, arterial pressure and microalbuminuria in Type 1 (insulin-dependent) diabetes mellitus. *Diabetologia* 1984; **26**: 401–5.

21 Mathiesen ER, Oxenbøll K, Johansen PAa, Svendsen PAå, Deckert T. Incipient nephropathy in Type 1 (insulin-dependent) diabetes. *Diabetologia* 1984; **26**: 406–10.

22 Barnett AH, Dallinger K, Jennings P *et al*. Microalbuminuria and diabetic retinopathy. *Lancet* 1985; i: 53–4.

23 Feldt-Rasmussen B, Mathiesen ER, Deckert T, Giese J, Christensen NJ, Bent-Hansen L, Nielsen MD. Central role for sodium in the pathogenesis of blood pressure changes independent of angiotensin, aldosterone and catecholamines in Type 1 (insulin-dependent) diabetes mellitus. *Diabetologia* 1987; **30**: 610–17.

24 Jensen T, Stender S, Deckert T. Abnormalities in plasma concentration of lipoproteins and fibrinogen in Type 1 (insulin-dependent) diabetic patients with increased urinary albumin excretion. *Diabetologia* 1988; **31**: 142–5.

25 Feldt-Rasmussen B. Increased transcapillary escape rate of albumin in Type 1 (insulin-dependent) diabetic patients with microalbuminuria. *Diabetologia* 1986; **29**: 282–6.

26 Bent-Hansen L, Deckert T. Metabolism of albumin and fibrinogen in type 1 (insulin-dependent) diabetes mellitus. *Diabetes Res* 1988; **7**: 159–64.

27 Christiansen JS, Gammelgaard J, Tronier B, Svendsen PA, Parving H-H. Kidney function and size in diabetics before and during initial insulin treatment. *Kidney Int* 1982; **21**: 683–8.

28 Wiseman MJ, Viberti GC, Keen H. Threshold effect of plasma glucose in the glomerular hyperfiltration of diabetes. *Nephron* 1984; **38**: 257–60.

29 Mogensen CE. Abnormal physiological processes in the kidney. In: Brownlee M, ed. *Handbook of Diabetes Mellitus*, 23–85. New York: Garland STMP Press, 1981.

30 Viberti GC, Wiseman MJ. The kidney in diabetes: significance of the early abnormalities. *Clin Endocrinol Metab* 1986; **15**: 753–82.

31 Wiseman MJ, Viberti GC. Glomerular filtration rate and kidney volume in Type 1 (insulin-dependent) diabetes mellitus revisited. *Diabetologia* 1982; **25**: 530.

32 Hostetter TH, Rennke HG, Brenner BM. The case for intra-renal hypertension in the initiation and progression of diabetic and other glomerulopathies. *Am J Med* 1982; **72**: 375–80.

33 Steffes MW, Brown DM, Mauer SM. Diabetic glomerulopathy following unilateral nephrectomy in the rat. *Diabetes* 1978; **27**: 35–41.

34 Mogensen CE. Early diabetic renal involvement and nephropathy. Can treatment modalities be predicted from identification of risk factors? *Diabetes Ann* 1987; **3**: 306–24.

35 Friedman EA, Sheih SD, Hirsch SR *et al*. No supranormal glomerular filtration (GFR) in type II (non-insulin-dependent) diabetes. *Am Soc Nephrol* 1981; **14**: 102A.

36 Ellis EN, Steffes MW, Goetz FC, Sutherland DER, Mauer SM. Glomerular filtration surface in type 1 diabetes mellitus. *Kidney Int* 1986; **29**: 889–94.

37 Østerby R, Gundersen HJG, Hørlyck A, Kroustrup JP, Nyberg G, Westberg G. Diabetic glomerulopathy. Structural characteristics of the early and advanced stages. *Diabetes* 1983; **32**: 79–82.

38 Mathiesen ER, Rønn B, Jensen T, Storm B, Deckert T. Relationship between blood pressure and urinary albumin excretion in development of microalbuminuria. *Diabetes* 1990; **39**: 245–9.

39 Gatling W, Mullee MA, Knight C, Hill RD. Microalbuminuria in diabetes. Relationship between urinary albumin excretion and diabetes related variables. *Diabetic Med* 1988; **5**: 348–51.

40 Jensen T, Borch-Johnsen K, Kofoed-Enevoldsen A, Deckert T. Coronary heart disease in young Type 1 (insulin-dependent) diabetic patients with and without diabetic nephropathy: Incidence and risk factors. *Diabetologia* 1987; **30**: 144–8.

41 Gonzalez-Carrillo M, Moloney A, Bewick M, Parsons V, Rudge CJ, Watkins PJ. Renal transplantation in diabetic nephropathy. *Br Med J* 1982; **285**: 1713–16.

42 Braun WE, Phillips DF, Vidt DG *et al*. Coronary artery disease in 100 diabetics with end stage renal failure. *Transplantation Proc* 1984; **16**: 603–7.

43 Borch-Johnsen K, Kreiner S. Proteinuria — a predictor of cardiovascular mortality in insulin dependent diabetes mellitus. *Br Med J* 1987; **294**: 1651–4.

44 Ramsay RC, Knobloch WH, Barbosa JJ, Sutherland DER, Kjellstrand CM, Najarian JS, Goetz FC. The visual status of diabetic patients after renal transplantation. *Am J Ophthalmol* 1979; **87**: 305–10.

45 Kofoed-Enevoldsen A, Jensen T, Borch-Johnsen K, Deckert T. Incidence of retinopathy in Type 1 (insulin-dependent) diabetes: Association with clinical nephropathy. *J Diabetic Compl* 1987; **3**: 96–9.

46 Moloney A, Tunbridge WMG, Ireland JT, Watkins PJ. Mortality from diabetic nephropathy in the United Kingdom. *Diabetologia* 1983; **25**: 26–30.

47 Kussman MJ, Goldstein HH, Gleason RE. The clinical course of diabetic nephropathy. *J Am Med Ass* 1976; **236**: 1861–3.

48 Friedman EA. Diabetes with kidney failure. *Lancet* 1986; i: 1285.

49 Borch-Johnsen K, Andersen KP, Deckert T. The effect of proteinuria on relative mortality in Type 1 (insulin-dependent) diabetes mellitus. *Diabetologia* 1985; **28**: 590–6.

50 Schmitz A, Vaeth M. Microalbuminuria: A major risk factor in non-insulin-dependent diabetes. A 10-year follow-up study of 503 patients. *Diabetic Med* 1988; **5**: 126–34.

51 Jarrett RJ, Viberti GC, Argyropoulos A *et al*. Microalbuminuria predicts mortality in non-insulin dependent diabetes. *Diabetic Med* 1984; **1**: 17–19.

52 Parving H-H, Andersen AR, Smidt UM, Hommel E, Mathiesen ER, Svendsen PA. Effect of anti-hypertensive treatment on kidney function in diabetic nephropathy. *Br Med J* 1987; **294**: 1443–7.

53 Parving H-H, Hommel E. Prognosis in diabetic nephropathy. *Br Med J* 1989; **299**: 230–3.

54 Mathiesen ER, Borch-Johnsen K, Jensen DV, Deckert T. Improved survival in patients with diabetic nephropathy. *Diabetologia* 1989; **32**: 884–6.

55 Deckert T, Feldt-Rasmussen B, Borch-Johnsen K, Jensen T, Kofoed-Enevoldsen A. Albuminuria reflects widespread vascular damage. The Steno hypothesis. *Diabetologia* 1989; **32**: 219–26.

65 Aetiology and Pathogenesis of Diabetic Nephropathy: Clues from Early Functional Abnormalities

Summary

- Functional abnormalities which occur early in the natural history of diabetic nephropathy include microalbuminuria and glomerular hyperfiltration. These features may help to identify a subset of patients at risk of developing clinical nephropathy, defined by persistent proteinuria and a progressive decline in renal function.
- *Microalbuminuria* is a subclinical increase in urinary albumin excretion rate (AER) in the range 30–300 mg/day. This is below the detection threshold of conventional methods for measuring protein in urine and so is detectable only by highly sensitive techniques such as radioimmunoassay. Persistent albuminuria detectable by dip-stick methods corresponds to an AER of over 250–300 mg/day and is termed *macroalbuminuria* or *clinical albuminuria*.
- The ratio of albumin:creatinine concentrations in a first morning urine sample is a useful screening test: values exceeding 2.0 mg/mmol indicate microalbuminuria.
- Microalbuminuria is due to increased permeability of the glomerular capillaries, probably because of raised glomerular capillary pressure and loss of negative charge on the glomerular basement membrane. Clinical albuminuria develops with further loss of membrane charge and an increase in membrane pore size.
- IDDM subjects with microalbuminuria have a 20-fold greater risk of ultimately developing clinical nephropathy than those with normal albumin excretion. Microalbuminuria also predicts clinical nephropathy and increased mortality in NIDDM.
- Diabetic nephropathy is closely associated with hypertension. Arterial blood pressure is elevated (although usually below the conventional threshold defining hypertension) in patients with microalbuminuria. Hypertension accelerates the rates at which albuminuria increases and glomerular filtration rate declines.
- The tendency to develop nephropathy may be partly genetically determined, as cases tend to cluster within families. A genetic predisposition to hypertension is suggested by the finding of increased blood pressure in the parents of diabetic patients with nephropathy.
- Sodium–lithium countertransport activity in red blood cells — which reflects physiologically important cation exchange mechanisms — is increased in nephropathic patients and their parents; increased activity is a marker for essential hypertension.
- *Glomerular hyperfiltration* is an increase in glomerular filtration rate (GFR) above the normal range, which occurs early in 20–40% of IDDM patients. Possible causes of hyperfiltration include increased renal plasma flow and filtration surface area in the glomerulus. Hyperglycaemia and disturbances in the balance between vasodilating and vasoconstricting prostaglandins may contribute to hyperfiltration.
- The relationship of glomerular hyperfiltration to the subsequent development of clinical nephropathy is uncertain.
- Strict glycaemic control can reduce microalbuminuria and lower glomerular hyperfiltration into the normal range. Effective antihypertensive treatment and restriction of dietary protein intake (to 45 g/day) can both reduce urinary albumin excretion. Whether these interventions influence the ultimate progression to clinical nephropathy is not known.

The term *diabetic nephropathy* describes a clinical state in which there are persistent proteinuria and a progressive decline in renal function, accompanied by retinopathy and arterial hypertension. By definition, other causes of renal disease are excluded.

Diabetic nephropathy is a major diabetic complication whose impact varies considerably in different diabetic populations. Clinically progressive renal disease develops in approximately 30% of IDDM patients and in approximately 15% of NIDDM patients of European origin [1–3]. In IDDM, the incidence of nephropathy reaches a peak after about 15 years duration of diabetes. In NIDDM, the condition may be detected sooner after diagnosis and, although nephropathy is rarer than in IDDM, the larger number of patients with NIDDM results in the absolute numbers of patients with nephropathy being similar in both types of diabetes [2]. Nephropathy may be commoner in NIDDM subjects of certain ethnic origins, especially in Asian and Afro-Caribbean people resident in Britain [4–6], who accounted for 48% of all NIDDM patients receiving renal replacement therapy in a recent series from King's College Hospital in London [5]. On the other hand, the frequency of end-stage renal failure in the Pima Indians of Arizona, in whom NIDDM is particularly common, is similar to that in the general IDDM population in North America [7].

Diabetic nephropathy is therefore an important problem. Attempts to trace its genesis can be made by investigating the earliest functional abnormalities seen in diabetic patients and in animal models of diabetes. This may eventually enable us to identify a subset of diabetic subjects at special risk of developing nephropathy and help to target preventative and therapeutic measures.

Microalbuminuria

Conventional methods for detecting protein in urine include the salicylsulphonic acid test and various acid–base colour-change indicators used in dip-stick methods such as Albustix. These methods are relatively insensitive and can reliably detect protein excretion rates in excess of about 250–300 mg/day. Albustix-positive proteinuria is termed *macroproteinuria*, or *clinical proteinuria*.

In 1963, a sensitive and specific radioimmunoassay was described which could detect human albumin at low concentrations in the urine [8]. This subclinical, Albustix-negative elevation in urinary albumin excretion has been termed *microalbuminuria*. The reported prevalence of microalbuminuria varies from 20% in a hospital clinic in Denmark to 5.7% in a community-based survey in England [9, 10].

Definition and measurement of microalbuminuria

The albumin excretion rate (AER) in healthy, non-diabetic individuals ranges from 2.5 to 26.0 mg/day with a geometric mean of 9.5 mg/day; 92% of the values fall below 18 mg/day [11]. Albumin in these subjects represents 11% of total urinary protein. This range of AER is defined as *normoalbuminuria*. Albumin excretion rates of 30–300 mg/day are termed *microalbuminuria*, whereas persistent *macroalbuminuria* (Albustix-positive) corresponds to an AER exceeding 300 mg/day. Albumin in microalbuminuric patients represents about 22% of the total urinary protein and some 50% in patients with clinical proteinuria. These arbitrary terms of definition serve as a useful broad clinical classification (Table 65.1), although the cut-off levels separating the different categories vary somewhat between centres.

Urinary albumin excretion in diabetic and non-diabetic subjects has an average day-to-day variation of 40–50% and is further influenced by urine flow, posture, exercise and diet [12–17]. It is higher during the day in the upright, ambulant position than at night in the recumbent position. In an attempt at standardization, the overnight urine collection has been suggested and adopted by many investigators [10, 18, 19]. Due to the wide intrinsic variation in AER, multiple collections are necessary in order to define accurately an individual's status; patients whose AER lies near one of the cut-off levels are likely to move into and out of different categories (Fig. 65.1).

Present evidence suggests that the albumin concentration in random urine samples has a linear relationship with the AER [19]. In order to improve precision in screening for an elevated AER, the urinary albumin:creatinine ratio (ACR) has been suggested [20–22]. An ACR of greater than 2.0 mg/mmol in a first morning urine sample has a sensitivity of 96% and a specificity of 100% for detecting an overnight AER of $>30\,\mu g$/min [10].

Table 65.1. Characteristics of urinary albumin excretion in different phases of diabetic nephropathy.

	Normo-albuminuria	Micro-albuminuria	Macro- (clinical) albuminuria
Albumin excretion rate (AER):			
mg/day	<30	30–300	>300
µg/min	<20	20–200	>200
Albumin/total urinary protein (%)	11%	22%	50%
Albustix reaction	−	−	+

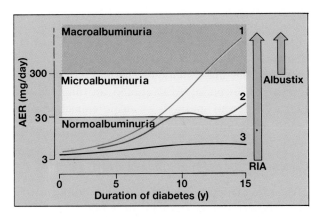

Fig. 65.1. Schematic time-courses of albumin excretion rate (AER) in IDDM patients, showing thresholds for normo-, micro- and macroalbuminuria and the detection limits of RIA and Albustix methods for measuring albumin concentrations in urine. About one-third of IDDM patients will ultimately develop clinical nephropathy with macroproteinuria (1). The remainder will stay within the microalbuminuric (2), or normoalbuminuric (3) ranges. Because of intrinsic variability in AER, individual subjects may move between one category and another.

Increasingly, clinical chemistry departments are able to offer routine urinary albumin concentration measurements as newer automated assays become more widely available [24]. Low concentrations of urinary albumin can now be measured semi-quantitatively as a side-room test, e.g. Albusure® (Cambridge Life Sciences) and Micro-bumintest® (Ames). These sensitive, specific and rapid tests are suitable for screening purposes [20]. The latter is a modified protein-error-of-indicators method and detects albumin concentrations above about 40 µg/ml. Other methods under development include laser turbidometry.

The origins of microalbuminuria

The barrier between the glomerular capillary and the urinary space of Bowman's capsule may be considered as a membrane perforated by pores of average size of 55 nm and coated with a negative electrical charge which is attributed to heparan sulphate and other proteoglycans [25]. Thus, both the size and charge of molecules will determine their passage across this membrane, in addition to the hydraulic and other dynamic forces controlling glomerular filtration. In early microalbuminuria, the clearances of albumin, a polyanion (pI 4.8, molecular weight 69 kDa) and IgG, a larger electrically neutral molecule (pI 7.5–7.8, molecular weight 160 kDa), are both increased. This is most likely to be due to an increase in the transglomerular pressure, which would favour increased filtration of proteins in general, irrespective of their charge [26]. As microalbuminuria increases, there is a disproportionate rise in albumin clearance and therefore a lower ratio of the clearances of IgG and albumin (the selectivity index). This may be due to loss of the electronegative glycosialoproteins and proteoglycans of the glomerular basement membrane, together with further haemodynamic abnormalities [26–28]. Subsequently, as the pore-size enlarges, microalbuminuria progresses to macroalbuminuria and the GFR begins to decline as the glomerular filtration barrier loses its size-selectivity (Figs 65.2 and 65.3).

The prognostic significance of microalbuminuria

Evidence is accumulating that microalbuminuria represents an early stage of diabetic renal disease which, in both IDDM and NIDDM, will tend to

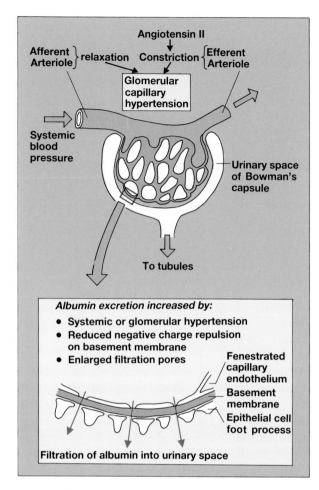

Fig. 65.2. Schematic diagram of glomerulus, indicating the main factors influencing excretion of albumin into the urine.

progress to clinically overt nephropathy (see Table 65.2). Three prospective studies in IDDM patients have identified a relationship between a raised AER and the subsequent development of clinical nephropathy [29–31]. IDDM subjects with an overnight or 24-h AER between 50 and 250 mg/day have a 20-fold greater risk of developing nephropathy than those with an AER below this level (Fig. 65.4) [29]. After initial stabilization of diabetes, microalbuminuria is found only rarely in the first 5 years of IDDM (see Fig. 65.1), suggesting that microalbuminuria may be a true sign of early disease rather than simply a marker of susceptibility [33].

In NIDDM patients, two studies have shown a raised AER to be associated with the later development of clinical proteinuria as well as increased mortality, especially from cardiovascular disease (Table 65.1) [3, 32]. The overall findings of these studies are remarkably similar and the different risk levels of AER quoted are likely to be due to different methods of urine collection and length of follow-up.

Concomitants of microalbuminuria

The immediate causes of microalbuminuria are not known but a number of clinical and biochemical associations have been identified. These are summarized in Table 65.3.

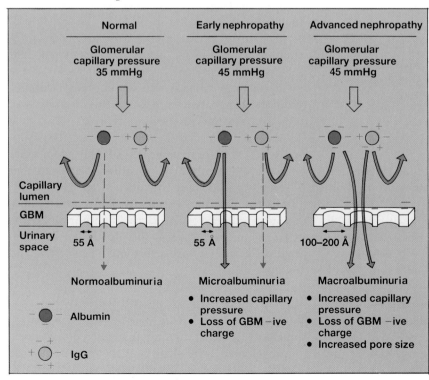

Fig. 65.3. The evolution of proteinuria in diabetes. Filtration of plasma proteins such as the polyanionic albumin and the larger electrically neutral IgG, is normally restricted by the resting negative charge on the glomerular basement membrane (GBM) and by the size of the filtration pores. Increased glomerular capillary pressure and loss of negative charge increase filtration of proteins, including albumin, in the early stage of microalbuminuria. With further loss of negative charge and enlargement of filtration pores in advanced nephropathy, albumin losses increase greatly and IgG is readily filtered.

Table 65.2. Values of urinary albumin excretion (microalbuminuria) which predict the development of clinical nephropathy and/ or mortality in diabetic patients.

Group	Type of diabetes	Predictive AER level	Urine collection method	Duration of follow-up (y)	Reference
Guy's Hospital	IDDM	30 μg/min	Overnight	14	29
Steno	IDDM	70 μg/min	24 h	6	30
Aarhus	IDDM	15 μg/min	1–2 h	6–14	31
Guy's Hospital	NIDDM	10 μg/min*	Overnight	14	32
Aarhus	NIDDM	30 μg/ml	Morning	10	3

Note the different units for AER used by the Aarhus group [3].
* Predictive of increased mortality, predominantly from cardiovascular disease.

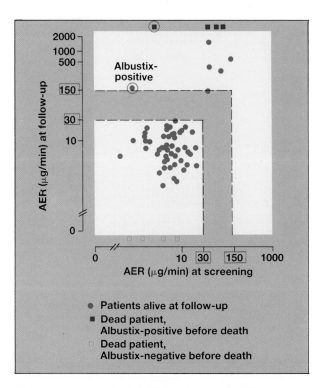

Fig. 65.4. Outcome in 63 IDDM patients with different levels of microalbuminuria at presentation, 55 of whom were followed up 14 years later. Only two cases with AER <30 μg/ min at screening had developed Albustix-positive proteinuria (ringed symbols), whereas seven out of the eight with initial AER >30 μg/min had become clinically proteinuric. The outer shaded area shows the threshold for Albustix-positivity and the inner segregates the patients who did not progress. (Redrawn from [29] with kind permission.)

BLOOD PRESSURE

The relationship between microalbuminuria and raised arterial blood pressure has aroused considerable interest. A positive, linear correlation exists between arterial pressure and AER [30, 34]. IDDM patients with microalbuminuria have mean systolic and diastolic blood pressures which are higher than those of a matched group of patients with normal AER, even though blood pressure generally remains within the 'normal' limits defined by WHO. As microalbuminuric patients have a normal or raised GFR (see below), it is improbable that the blood pressure elevation is simply a consequence of renal impairment. It is possible that hypertension *per se* causes microalbuminuria, which is found in non-diabetic hypertensive patients and is a predictor of cardiovascular disease in these subjects. An alternative hypothesis is that hypertension and microalbuminuria share a common determinant, which may be genetic. Recent evidence supports this possibility.

Possible genetic factors

The tendency to hypertension in nephropathic patients may be partly inherited, as after careful matching for age, sex and body mass index, blood pressure was found to be higher in the parents of IDDM patients with proteinuria than in the parents of non-proteinuric patients (Fig. 65.5) [35]. There was also a correlation between blood pressure in the proteinuric IDDM patients and their parents. The clustering of cases of diabetic nephropathy within families is further evidence of a genetic predisposition in at least a proportion of patients [36, 37].

The activity of cation-exchange pumps in cell membranes, which are essential to many metabolic processes including electrolyte homeostasis, may also be partly inherited. The pump most accessible to study is the sodium–lithium countertransport mechanism in red blood cell membranes. This is thought to reflect the physiological sodium–hydrogen ion antiporter, found in all cells, which regulates physiological functions such as cell growth and is also thought to be

Variable	Association with microalbuminuria
Sex	• Increased in males (2:1)
Duration of diabetes	• Very rare in first 5 years
Systemic BP	• Increased
Exercise	• May increase
Poor glycaemic control	• May increase
Acute glucose ingestion Insulin infusion Glucagon infusion Growth hormone injection Ketone bodies infusion	No effect

Table 65.3. Concomitants of microalbuminuria in IDDM.

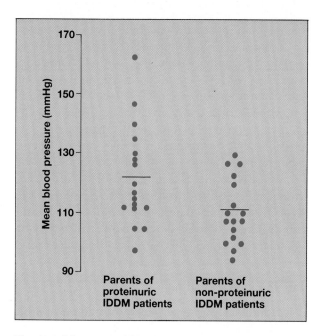

Fig. 65.5. Mean arterial blood pressure in the parents of proteinuric and non-proteinuric IDDM patients who were matched for age, sex and duration of diabetes. (Redrawn from [35], with kind permission of the Editor.)

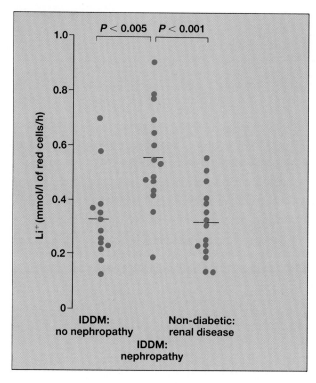

Fig. 65.6. Sodium−lithium countertransport activity in red blood cells of IDDM patients with nephropathy, compared with non-nephropathic IDDM patients and with non-diabetic subjects with other renal diseases. (Redrawn from [43], with kind permission of the Editor of the *New England Journal of Medicine*.)

important in determining sodium reabsorption from the proximal renal tubular cell. It is apparently a marker for essential hypertension [38]. Sodium−lithium countertransport activity aggregates in families and is largely genetically determined, even though a number of environmental factors may further affect it [39−41].

Two recent studies [42, 43] have demonstrated that red-cell sodium−lithium countertransport activity is increased in IDDM patients with either macroproteinuria or microproteinuria (see Fig. 65.6). Moreover, direct measurements of the sodium−hydrogen ion antiporter in fibroblasts have shown increased activity and enhanced cell

growth in nephropathic IDDM patients as compared with matched, normoalbuminuric control subjects [44]. Increased activity of this pump could be involved in the pathogenesis of diabetic nephropathy and may partly explain certain abnormalities, such as increased exchangeable sodium, previously demonstrated in IDDM patients with nephropathy [45].

As with hypertension, increased cation countertransport activity may be partly inherited.

Red blood cell sodium—lithium countertransport activity in the parents of IDDM patients with proteinuria has been found to be greater than in parents of IDDM patients with normoalbuminuria [46]. Furthermore, there is a significant correlation in countertransport activity between parents and offspring. A familial element therefore contributes to the elevation of the sodium—lithium countertransport activity seen in diabetic nephropathy. Prospective studies in normo- and microalbuminuric patients with increased activities are needed to clarify the specificity and sensitivity of this possible genetic marker.

Glomerular hyperfiltration

Abnormalities in GFR may precede microalbuminuria and may therefore be an even earlier indicator of diabetic renal disease. The theory that the GFR may be elevated in diabetes was first advanced in 1934 and current accurate measurements have shown that GFR is increased on average by 20–40% in children or adults with IDDM, compared with matched non-diabetic subjects (see Fig. 65.7) [47–49]. This abnormal increase in GFR is termed 'hyperfiltration'. Approximately 25% of insulin-dependent patients have a GFR exceeding the normal non-diabetic range (84–135 ml/min/1.73 m²) and even those with a GFR within the normal range may have a higher value than would be predicted if they were not diabetic [50].

Factors leading to glomerular hyperfiltration

GFR has four main determinants — renal plasma flow, glomerular transcapillary hydraulic pressure, afferent capillary oncotic pressure, and filtration surface area — which theoretically could contribute to hyperfiltration.

RENAL PLASMA FLOW (RPF)

RPF has been reported to be elevated in diabetes but in studies where both GFR and RPF have been measured simultaneously, the rise in RPF accounted for only 50–60% of that in GFR [50–52]. The finding of an increased filtration fraction (i.e. GFR/RPF) in IDDM has been taken to suggest that intraglomerular pressure may be elevated [53]. This proposition is supported by some, but not all, micropuncture studies in moderately hyperglycaemic diabetic rats which demonstrate an increase in the transglomerular pressure gradient [54–56]. This appears to be mediated by a reduction in total arteriolar resistance which is more marked at the afferent than efferent end of the arteriole [55]. In human diabetic subjects with glomerular hyperfiltration, a similar alteration in intraglomerular haemodynamics is indirectly suggested by the finding of a reduced renal vascular resistance [58]. Intraglomerular hypertension can be reduced and prevented, at least in diabetic rats, by angiotensin converting enzyme (ACE) inhibitors. These may act by relaxing the efferent arterioles which are thought to be particularly sensitive to the vasoconstrictor action of angiotensin II. As discussed below, ACE inhibitors have been the subject of several clinical trials in diabetic patients at various stages of nephropathy [58].

OTHER FACTORS

Oncotic pressure is thought to be normal in diabetes. This suggests that increased intracapillary pressure accounts for a further proportion of the rise in GFR.

Filtration surface area is increased in IDDM patients in proportion to the rise in GFR [60, 61]. The kidneys may be enlarged in diabetic patients and in animal models of diabetes, mainly through increased glomerular volume. Renal volume is also related to various other determinants of the GFR [52, 61].

Overall, the elevated GFR found in some dia-

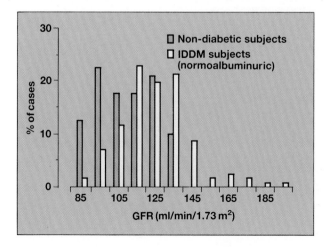

Fig. 65.7. Frequency histogram showing GFR in normoalbuminuric IDDM subjects and in age-matched non-diabetic controls (S.L. Jones, unpublished data).

betic patients is probably mediated by a combination of structural and functional changes. The relative contributions of these, and the extent to which they may vary between individuals, remain to be established [59, 60].

Possible metabolic and endocrine determinants of hyperfiltration

The principal metabolic and endocrine factors implicated in hyperfiltration are shown in Table 65.4.

GLYCAEMIC CONTROL

Hyperfiltration only occurs under conditions of moderate hyperglycaemia (>14 mmol/l). Diabetic patients with glomerular hyperfiltration show a further increase in GFR (by 10–15%) following an intravenous glucose challenge [53, 62]; this response does not occur in subjects with a normal GFR. Acute reduction of blood glucose levels by insulin infusion reduces the GFR within 30–60 min, but only by about 5% [63].

PROSTAGLANDINS

Prostaglandins affect many aspects of renal function and have a possible role in causing glomerular hyperfiltration. A recent study has found increased urinary excretion of 6-keto $PGF_{1\alpha}$ (a vasodilator prostaglandin derivative of vascular, possibly glomerular, origin) in hyperfiltering IDDM patients as compared with matched subjects whose GFR was normal. Urinary levels of PGE_2 (another vasodilator compound) and of thromboxane B_2 (a vasoconstrictor) were comparable in both diabetic groups and in non-diabetic subjects [64]. Another study found increased urinary excretion of both 6-keto $PGF_{1\alpha}$ and of PGE_2 in IDDM subjects [65]. Short-term improvements in blood glucose control which produce small reductions in GFR are accompanied by decreased urinary excretion of 6-keto $PGF_{1\alpha}$ and of PGE_2 [65, 66]. These findings suggest an imbalance between the vasodilating and vasoconstricting prostaglandins which could account for, or contribute towards, the hyperfiltration of diabetes.

Table 65.4. Possible metabolic and endocrine mediators of glomerular hyperfiltration.

Mediator	Increase in GFR when administered experimentally	Comment
Glucose	5–13%	• Only with moderate hyperglycaemia • Threshold level of 14–16 mmol/l • Effect more marked in hyperfiltering subjects
Ketone bodies	Up to 48%	• High physiological or pharmacological doses required
Glucagon	6%	• Supraphysiological levels required
Growth hormone	7%	• Requires several days of administration
Insulin	—	• Trivial effect at levels tested
Prostaglandins	?	• Elevation of 6-keto $PGF_{1\alpha}$ associated with hyperfiltration
Renin–angiotensin axis	?	• Controversial (see text)
Atrial natriuretic peptide	?	• Controversial. Possibly higher in hyperfiltration

RENIN−ANGIOTENSIN−ALDOSTERONE AXIS

The renin−angiotensin−aldosterone axis has also been investigated as a possible mediator of glomerular hyperfiltration but conflicting results have so far been obtained, with either small elevations or decreases in plasma renin activity being described in hyperfiltering patients [67, 68].

The prognostic significance of renal haemodynamic changes

Glomerular haemodynamic disturbances apparently influence the development of glomerular pathology in experimental models of diabetes [69]. In humans, the situation is less clear. Three studies, one retrospective [31] and two prospective, have attempted to address this question. Mogensen and colleagues [31] reported that patients with glomerular filtration showed a faster fall in GFR and that more progressed to clinical nephropathy than those whose GFR was initially normal. However, this finding may be difficult to interpret as some of the hyperfiltering patients also had microalbuminuria. The other two studies attempted to remove this confounding factor by investigating hyperfiltering patients with normal albumin excretion. In a 5-year prospective study, patients with glomerular hyperfiltration at the outset showed a faster fall in GFR than a matched group with initially normal GFR, although the number progressing to nephropathy (defined as the development of microalbuminuria) was not increased in the hyperfiltering group (S.L. Jones, unpublished observations). A recent 18-year follow-up study has also found no association between early glomerular hyperfiltration and follow-up AER [70].

On balance, glomerular hyperfiltration alone and in the absence of microalbuminuria does not appear at present to predict the later development of nephropathy.

Correction of early renal abnormalities: implications for the prevention and treatment of diabetic nephropathy

A number of studies attempting to correct microalbuminuria and glomerular hyperfiltration have helped to clarify the pathophysiological basis of these abnormalities and have highlighted the possible benefits of treatment at these early stages of nephropathy. Several strategies have been investigated.

Improved glycaemic control

Strict glycaemic control can reduce or normalize both microalbuminuria and glomerular hyperfiltration [71−73]. A 2-year randomized prospective study of patients with persistently elevated AER (30−300 mg/day) showed that improved metabolic control prevented a further rise in AER and the development of clinical proteinuria, but failed to lower albumin excretion [72]. A 4-year study involving patients with AER in the high normoalbuminuric range showed that a group treated with continuous subcutaneous insulin infusion (CSII) and obtaining a significant reduction in HbA_1 levels compared with a conventionally treated control group, reduced their AER during the treatment period. A group treated with multiple daily injections, achieving an HbA_1 level intermediate between the CSII group and the conventionally treated group, showed no reduction in AER, as was the case in the conventionally treated group [73]. The long-term significance of these results is still unclear but these preliminary findings suggest that strict glycaemic control may arrest or even reverse 'established' microalbuminuria and high-normal levels of albumin excretion.

The effects of improved glycaemic control on kidney size are less clear-cut. A reduction in renal volume has been reported after 3 months of insulin therapy and improved control in newly diagnosed IDDM subjects [74]. In another study, however, 6 months of improved glycaemic control had no effect on kidney volume in a group of hyperfiltering IDDM subjects, despite a reduction in GFR [75].

Antihypertensive treatment

The close clinical association between hypertension and diabetic nephropathy is described in Chapter 67, and the possible pathogenic effects of hypertension within the glomerulus have been discussed above. There is considerable debate as to whether hypertension precedes microalbuminuria or vice versa and therefore as to which is likely to be the prime mover [76−78].

Whatever the basis of the relationship, there is now no doubt that effective antihypertensive treatment can retard the progression of established nephropathy [79, 80], and recent studies have suggested similar benefits in the microalbuminuric stage. Various drugs have been used. In initial long-term studies, marginal blood pressure elevations in microalbuminuric patients were treated with diuretics and β-blockers, and a reversal in the steady increase in AER through the microalbuminuric range was seen (Fig. 65.8) [81]. Recently, attention has focused on the ACE inhibitors, largely because of their beneficial effects in reducing both intraglomerular hypertension and proteinuria in streptozotocin-diabetic rats [58]. In diabetic patients with various degrees of clinical nephropathy and macroproteinuria, ACE inhibitors reduced blood pressure, decreased urinary protein losses and slowed the rate of fall of GFR [80, 82, 83]. ACE inhibitors may also have beneficial effects in microalbuminuric patients, even when blood pressure is still below the accepted threshold for hypertension. In a small controlled trial, normotensive IDDM patients with microalbuminuria treated with enalapril showed a fall in AER and their blood pressure remained stable. By contrast, both AER and blood pressure rose in the untreated control group [84]. A reduction in the filtration fraction and fractional clearance of albumin in this study may suggest that these agents reduce intraglomerular pressure as well as systemic pressure, as in the animal model. However, the failure of enalapril to alter either GFR or RPF in a group of children with glomerular hyperfiltration, normal blood pressure and normal albumin excretion, may argue against this mechanism [85].

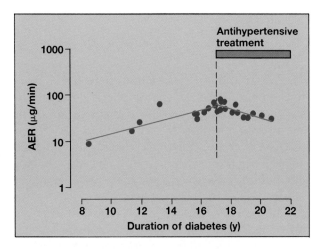

Fig. 65.8. Effect of antihypertensive treatment in reversing the steady increase in AER in an IDDM patient with microalbuminuria. (Redrawn from [81] with kind permission of the Editor of the *Journal of Diabetic Complications*.)

Dietary protein restriction

Intake of dietary protein has been found to influence renal haemodynamics and filtration selectivity. Short-term (3-week) controlled studies in diabetic patients have shown that a diet restricted to 45 g protein per day can significantly reduce microalbuminuria and GFR independently of changes in blood glucose concentration or blood pressure (Fig. 65.9) [17]. These findings complement studies in diabetic animals, in which dietary protein restriction protects the kidney against hyperfiltration, intraglomerular hypertension, albuminuria and the subsequent development of histological lesions [69].

Other agents

Preliminary reports have suggested that aldose reductase inhibitors given to diabetic rats cause a reduction in proteinuria [86]; results of controlled trials of these agents in man are awaited [87]. The recent discovery that the long-term deleterious effects of excessive glycosylation of structural membrane proteins may be prevented or even reversed by the administration of aminoguanidine (Chapter 54) opens up the possibility of influencing the biochemical steps which are thought responsible, at least in part, for the tissue damage of diabetes [88].

Screening for diabetic nephropathy

From the preceding discussion, it is clear that microalbuminuria is, at present, the most reliable indicator of early diabetic renal disease. In view of the preliminary studies suggesting that certain interventions can reduce AER and thus potentially delay, prevent or even reverse established diabetic nephropathy, screening for microalbuminuria is of considerable value.

For screening purposes, measurement of the urinary albumin concentration or albumin:creatinine ratio in the first morning urine sample is sufficient. This should ideally be carried out annually after 5 years of diabetes in IDDM patients (or sooner, if hypertension or retinopathy develop), and from the time of diagnosis in NIDDM patients. An albumin concentration exceeding 15 mg/l or an ACR of >2 mg/mmol should prompt timed overnight urine collections (probably at least three) and appropriate investigations should be carried out to exclude other

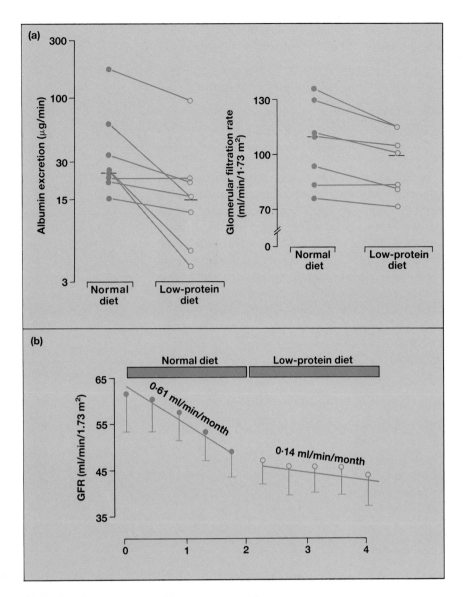

Fig. 65.9. (a) Effects of dietary protein restriction in microalbuminuric patients, showing falls in both albumin excretion rate and in GFR. (Redrawn from [17] with kind permission of the Editor.) In proteinuric IDDM patients, (b), a low-protein diet significantly reduced AER (not shown) and significantly slowed the rate of decline in GFR. (Redrawn from Walker JD et al, Lancet 1989; ii: 1411, with kind permission of the Editor).

causes of proteinuria, such as urinary tract infection and cardiac failure. As mentioned above, microalbuminuria has been defined by several criteria; our working definition is an AER of greater than 30 mg/day in least two out of three timed overnight collections. If persistent microalbuminuria is confirmed in a given patient, the following options are available to the clinician:

Glycaemic control

On the basis of present evidence, this should be optimized as far as possible.

Blood pressure control

Centile charts of blood pressure (see Fig. 69.4) [89] may help to decide whether an individual

has an acceptable blood pressure for his or her age. At present, there are no specific guidelines but the WHO criteria for the definition of hypertension are probably inadequate, given that many diabetic patients with microalbuminuria are young; the normal age- and sex-adjusted blood pressure may therefore be the appropriate treatment target. As discussed above, preliminary data suggest that ACE inhibitors reduce both blood pressure and AER and therefore may be of particular value in these patients. Treatment of hypertension is discussed further in Chapters 67 and 69.

Dietary protein

A reduction in dietary protein intake can effectively reduce AER in microalbuminuric diabetic patients, but the diet is unpalatable to many people and unlikely to meet with compliance.

Reducing other cardiovascular risk factors

Proteinuria is clearly the renal manifestation of a disease process affecting the entire vascular bed and is associated with both microvascular disease in other organs and macrovascular disease. The association with the latter, which may be attributable to lipid abnormalities, accounts for the fact that the additional mortality due to cardiovascular disease in diabetic patients is virtually confined to patients with proteinuria [91, 92]. These patients must therefore be carefully screened for coronary heart and peripheral vascular disease, which may be significant but often remain subclinical. Other risk factors — particularly smoking and lipid abnormalities which may be exacerbated by certain antihypertensive drugs — must be identified and treated as vigorously as possible.

Management of established clinical nephropathy

This is dealt with in detail in Chapter 67. The aim in this late phase is to retard the rate of decline of renal function. To date, the only therapies which are clearly established to slow the rate of decline in renal function are treatment of blood pressure and reduction in dietary protein intake.

Conclusions

The last few years have witnessed a steady broadening of our understanding of the events leading to diabetic nephropathy and, with this, the growing conviction that early identification and treatment may help to slow, prevent or even reverse the disease process. The increasing availability of simple screening tests for microalbuminuria will allow this hypothesis to be tested on a large scale in the next few years.

JAMES D. WALKER
GIAN CARLO VIBERTI

References

1 Andersen AR, Sandahl Christiansen J, Andersen JK, Kreiner S, Deckert T. Diabetic nephropathy in Type 1 (insulin-dependent) diabetes. An epidemiological study. *Diabetologia* 1983; **25**: 496–501.
2 Rettig B, Teutsch SM. The incidence of end-state renal disease in type I and type II diabetes mellitus. *Diabetic Nephropathy* 1984; **3**: 26–7.
3 Mogensen CE. Microalbuminuria predicts clinical proteinuria and early mortality in maturity-onset diabetes. *N Engl J Med* 1984; **310**: 356–60.
4 Grenfell A, Bewick M, Parsons V, Snowden S, Taube D, Watkins PJ. Non-insulin dependent diabetes and renal replacement therapy. *Diabetic Med* 1988; **5**: 172–6.
5 Allawi J, Rao PV, Gilbert R, Scott G, Jarrett RJ, Keen H, Viberti GC, Mather HM. Microalbuminuria in non-insulin-dependent diabetes: its prevalence in Indian compared with Europid patients. *Br Med J* 1988; **296**: 462–4.
6 Mather HM, Keen H. The Southall diabetes survey: prevalence of known diabetes in Asians and Europeans. *Br Med J* 1985; **291**: 1081–4.
7 Nelson RG, Newman JM, Knowler WC *et al.* Incidence of end-stage renal disease in Type 2 (non-insulin-dependent) diabetes mellitus in Pima Indians. *Diabetologia* 1988; **31**: 730–6.
8 Keen H, Chlouverakis C. An immunoassay for urinary albumin at low concentrations. *Lancet* 1963; ii: 913–16.
9 Parving HH, Hommel E, Mathiesen ER, Skott P, Edsberg B, Bahnser M *et al.* Prevalence of microalbuminuria, arterial hypertension, retinopathy and neuropathy in patients with insulin-dependent diabetes. *Br Med J* 1988; **296**: 156–60.
10 Gatling W, Knight C, Mullee MA, Hill RD. Microalbuminuria in diabetes: a population study of the prevalence and an assessment of three screening tests. *Diabetic Med* 1988; **5**: 343–97.
11 Viberti GC, Wiseman MJ, Redmond S. Microalbuminuria: its history and potential for prevention of clinical nephropathy in diabetes mellitus. *Diabetic Nephropathy* 1984; **3**: 70–82.
12 Cohen DL, Close CF, Viberti GC. The variability of overnight urinary albumin excretion in insulin-dependent diabetic and normal subjects. *Diabetic Med* 1987; **4**: 437–40.
13 Feldt-Rasmussen B, Mathiesen E. Variability of urinary albumin excretion in incipient diabetic nephropathy. *Diabetic Nephropathy* 1984; **3**: 101–3.
14 Viberti GC, Mackintosh D, Bilous RW, Pickup JC, Keen H. Proteinuria in diabetes mellitus: role of spontaneous and experimental variation of glycaemia. *Kidney Int* 1982; **21**: 714–20.
15 Viberti GC, Mogensen CE, Keen H *et al.* Urinary excretion of albumin in normal man: the effects of water loading. *Scand J Clin Lab Invest* 1982; **42**: 147–51.
16 Viberti GC, Jarrett RJ, McCartney M, Keen H. Increased glomerular permeability to albumin induced by exercise in diabetic subjects. *Diabetologia* 1978; **14**: 293–300.
17 Cohen DL, Dodds R, Viberti GC. Effect of protein restriction in insulin dependent diabetics at risk of nephropathy. *Br Med J* 1987; **294**: 795–8.
18 Rowe DJF, Bagga H, Betts PB. Normal variations in rate of albumin excretion and albumin to creatinine ratios in overnight and daytime urine collections in non-diabetic children. *Br Med J* 1985; **291**: 693–4.
19 Hutchinson AS, Paterson KR. Collecting urine for microalbumin assay. *Diabetic Med* 1988; **5**: 527–32.
20 Gatling W, Knight C, Hill RD. Screening for early diabetic nephropathy: which sample to detect microalbuminuria? *Diabetic Med* 1985; **2**: 451–5.
21 Marshall SM, Alberti KGMM. Screening for early diabetic nephropathy. *Ann Clin Biochem* 1986; **23**: 195–7.
22 Grenfell A. Screening for at risk microalbuminuria in Type 1 (insulin-dependent) diabetes mellitus. *Diabetologia* 1987; **30**: 525A.
23 Viberti GC, Wiseman MJ. The kidney in diabetes: signifi-

cance of the early abnormalities. In: Watkins PJ, ed. *Long-term Complications of Diabetes. Clin Endocrinol Metab* 1986; **15**: 753–82.

24 Close CF, Scott GS, Viberti GC. Rapid detection of urinary albumin at low concentration by an agglutination inhibition technique. *Diabetic Med* 1987; **4**: 491–2.

25 Myers BD, Winetz JA, Chui F, Michaels AS. Mechanisms of proteinuria in diabetic nephropathy: a study of glomerular barrier function. *Kidney Int* 1982; **21**: 633–41.

26 Viberti GC, Keen H. The patterns of proteinuria in diabetes mellitus. *Diabetes* 1984; **33**: 686–92.

27 Mogensen CE. Kidney function and glomerular permeability to macromolecules in early juvenile diabetes. *Scand J Clin Lab Invest* 1971; **28**: 79–90.

28 Partasarathy N, Spiro RG. Effect of diabetes on the glycosaminoglycan component of the human glomerular basement membrane. *Diabetes* 1982; **31**: 738–41.

29 Viberti GC, Hill RD, Jarrett RJ, Argyropoulos A, Mahmud U, Keen H. Microalbuminuria as a predictor of clinical nephropathy in insulin-dependent diabetes mellitus. *Lancet* 1982; i: 1430–2.

30 Mathiesen ER, Oxenbøll K, Johansen PAa, Svendsen PA, Deckert T. Incipient nephropathy in Type 1 (insulin-dependent) diabetes. *Diabetologia* 1984; **26**: 406–10.

31 Mogensen CE, Christensen CK. Predicting diabetic nephropathy in insulin-dependent patients. *N Engl J Med* 1984; **311**: 89–93.

32 Close CF, on behalf of the MCS Group. Sex, diabetes duration and microalbuminuria in Type 1 (insulin-dependent) diabetes mellitus. *Diabetologia* 1987; **30**: 508A.

33 Jarrett RJ, Viberti GC, Argyropoulos A et al. Microalbuminuria predicts mortality in non-insulin dependent diabetics. *Diabetic Med* 1984; **1**: 17–19.

34 Wiseman MJ, Viberti GC, Mackintosh D, Jarrett RJ, Keen H. Glycaemia, arterial pressure and microalbuminuria in Type 1 (insulin-dependent) diabetes mellitus. *Diabetologia* 1984; **26**: 401–5.

35 Viberti GC, Keen H, Wiseman M. Raised arterial pressure in parents of proteinuric insulin-dependent patients. *Br Med J* 1987; **295**: 515–7.

36 Seaquist ER, Goetz FC, Rich S, Barbosa J. Familial clustering of diabetic kidney disease. *N Engl J Med* 1989; **320**: 1161–5.

37 Pettitt DJ, Nelson RG, Saad MF, Knowler WC. Diabetic nephropathy in two generations of subjects with Type 2 diabetes mellitus. (Abstract). *Diabetes Res Clin Pract* 1988; **5**: 137.

38 Semplicini A, Mozato M-G, Sama B, Nosadini R, Fioretto P, Trevisan R et al. Na/H and Li/Na exchanger in red cells of normotensive and hypertensive patients with insulin-dependent diabetes mellitus. *Am J Hypertens* 1989; **2**: 174–7.

39 Boerwinkle E, Turner ST, Weinshilboum R, Johnson M, Richelson E, Sing CF. Analysis of the distribution of erythrocyte sodium–lithium countertransport in a sample representative of the general population. *Genet Epidemiol* 1986; **3**: 365–78.

40 Hilton PJ. Cellular sodium transport in essential hypertension. *N Engl J Med* 1986; **314**: 227–9.

41 Cooper R, Miller R, Trevisan M, Sempos C, Larbie E, Vestima H et al. Family history of hypertension and red cell cation transport in high school students. *J Hypertens* 1983; **1**: 145–52.

42 Krolewski AS, Canessa M, Rand LI, Warram JH, Christlieb AR, Knowler WC, Kahn CR. Genetic predisposition to hypertension as a major determinant of development of diabetic nephropathy. *N Engl J Med* 1988; **318**: 140–5.

43 Mangili R, Bending JJ, Scott GS, Li LK, Gupta A, Viberti GC. Increased sodium lithium countertransport activity in red cells of patients with insulin-dependent diabetes and nephropathy. *N Engl J Med* 1988; **318**: 146–9.

44 Trevisan R, Li LK, Walker JD, Viberti GC. Overactivity of the Na/H antiport and enhanced cell growth in insulin-dependent patients with nephropathy. *Diabetologia* 1989; **32**: 549A.

45 Feldt-Rasmussen B, Mathiesen ER, Deckert T, Giese J, Christensen NJ, Bent-Hansen L et al. Central role for sodium in the pathogenesis of blood pressure changes independent of angiotensin, aldosterone and catecholamines in Type 1 (insulin-dependent) diabetes mellitus. *Diabetologia* 1987; **30**: 610–17.

46 Walker JD, Tariq T, Viberti GC. Sodium–lithium countertransport activity in parents of Type I (insulin-dependent) diabetics with nephropathy. *Diabetologia* 1989; **32**: 555A.

47 Cambier P. Application de la théorie de Remberg à l'étude clinique des affections rénales et du diabète. *Ann Méd* 1934; **35**: 273–99.

48 Ditzel J, Schwartz M. Abnormal glomerular filtration rate in short term insulin treated diabetic subjects. *Diabetes* 1967; **16**: 264–7.

49 Mogensen CE. Glomerular filtration rate and renal plasma flow in short term and long term juvenile diabetes mellitus. *Scand J Clin Lab Invest* 1971; **28**: 91–100.

50 Christiansen JS, Gammelgaard J, Frandsen M, Parving HH. Increased kidney size, glomerular filtration rate, and renal plasma flow in short-term insulin-dependent diabetics. *Diabetologia* 1981; **20**: 451–6.

51 Ditzel J, Junker K. Abnormal glomerular filtration rate, renal plasma flow and renal protein excretion in recent and short term diabetics. *Br Med J* 1972; **2**: 13–19.

52 Mogensen CE, Andersen MJF. Increased kidney size and glomerular filtration rate in early juvenile diabetics. *Diabetes* 1972; **22**: 706–12.

53 Mogensen CE. Renal function changes in diabetics. *Diabetes* 1976; **25**: 872–9.

54 Deen WM, Satvat B. Determinants of glomerular filtration of proteins. *Am J Physiol* 1981; **241**: F162–70.

55 Hostetter TH, Troy JC, Brenner BM. Glomerular haemodynamics in experimental diabetes mellitus. *Kidney Int* 1981; **19**: 410–15.

56 Michels LD, Davidman M, Keane WF. Determinants of glomerular filtration and plasma flow in experimental diabetic rats. *J Lab Clin Med* 1981; **98**: 869–85.

57 Wiseman MJ, Mangili R, Alberetto M, Keen H, Viberti GC. Mechanisms of the glomerular response to glycaemic changes in insulin-dependent diabetic subjects. *Kidney Int* 1987; **31**: 1012–18.

58 Zatz R, Dunn R, Meyer TW, Anderson S, Rennke HG, Brenner BM. Prevention of diabetic glomerulopathy by pharmacological amelioration of glomerular capillary hypertension. *J Clin Invest* 1986; **77**: 1925–30.

59 Hirose K, Tsuschida H, Østerby R, Gunderson HJG. A strong correlation between glomerular filtration rate and filtration surface in diabetic kidney hyperfunction. *J Lab Invest* 1980; **43**: 434–7.

60 Østerby R, Parving HH, Nyberg G, Hommel E, Jørgensen HE, Løkkegaard H et al. A strong correlation between glomerular filtration rate and filtration surface in diabetic nephropathy. *Diabetologia* 1988; **31**: 265–70.

61 Wiseman MJ, Viberti GC. Glomerular filtration rate and kidney volume in Type 1 (insulin-dependent) diabetes mellitus revisited. *Diabetologia* 1982; **25**: 530.

62 Wiseman MJ, Viberti GC, Keen H. Threshold effect of

plasma glucose in the glomerular hyperfiltration of diabetes. *Nephron* 1984; **38**: 257−60.

63 Christiansen JS, Frandsen M, Parving HH. The effect of intravenous insulin infusion on kidney function in insulin-dependent diabetics. *Diabetologia* 1981; **20**: 199−204.

64 Viberti GC, Benigni A, Bognetti L, Remuzzi G, Wiseman MJ. Glomerular hyperfiltration and urinary prostaglandins in insulin-dependent diabetes mellitus. *Diabetic Med* 1989; **6**: 219−23.

65 Collier DA, Matthews DM, Bell G, Watson MC, Clarke BF. Increased urinary excretion of 6-keto $PGF_{1\alpha}$ and PGE_2 in male insulin dependent diabetics. *Diabetic Med* 1986; **3**: 358A.

66 Esmatjes E, Levy I, Gaya J, Rivera F. Renal excretion of prostaglandin E_2 and plasma renin activity in type 1 diabetes mellitus: relationship to normoglycemia achieved with artificial pancreas. *Diabetes Care* 1987; **10**: 428−31.

67 Esmatjes E, Fernandez MR, Halperin I *et al.* Renal hemodynamic abnormalities in patients with short-term insulin dependent diabetes mellitus: role of renal prostaglandins. *J Clin Endocrinol Metab* 1985; **60**: 1231−6.

68 Wiseman MJ, Drury PL, Keen H, Viberti GC. Plasma renin activity in insulin dependent diabetics with raised glomerular filtration rate. *Clin Endocrinol* 1984; **21**: 409−14.

69 Zatz R, Meyer TW, Rennke HG, Brenner BM. Predominance of hemodynamic rather than metabolic factors in the pathogenesis of diabetic glomerulopathy. *Proc Natl Acad Sci USA* 1985; **82**: 5963−7.

70 Lervang HH, Jensen S, Brochner-Mortensen J, Ditzel J. Early glomerular hyperfiltration and the development of late nephropathy in Type I (insulin-dependent) diabetes mellitus. *Diabetologia* 1988; **31**: 723−9.

71 The Kroc Collaborative Study Group. Blood glucose control and the evolution of diabetic retinopathy and albuminuria. *N Engl J Med* 1984; **311**: 365−72.

72 Feldt-Rasmussen B, Mathiesen ER, Deckert T. Effect of two years of strict metabolic control on progression of incipient nephropathy in insulin-dependent diabetics. *Lancet* 1986; ii: 1300−4.

73 Dahl-Jørgensen K, Hanssen KF, Kierulf P, Bjoro T, Sandvik L, Aageraes O. Reduction of urinary albumin excretion after 4 years of continuous subcutaneous insulin infusion in insulin-dependent diabetes mellitus. The Oslo study. *Acta Endocrinol (Copenhagen)* 1988; **117**: 19−25.

74 Mogensen CE, Andersen MJF. Increased kidney size and glomerular filtration rate in untreated juvenile diabetes: normalisation by insulin treatment. *Diabetologia* 1975; **11**: 221−4.

75 Wiseman MJ, Saunders AJ, Keen H, Viberti GC. Effect of blood glucose on glomerular filtration and kidney size in insulin-dependent diabetics. *N Engl J Med* 1985; **312**: 617−21.

76 Mathiesen ER, Ronn B, Jensen T, Storm B, Deckert T. Microalbuminuria precedes elevation in blood pressure in diabetic nephropathy. *Diabetologia* 1988; **31**: 519A.

77 Knowler WC, Bennett PH, Nelson RG, Saad MF, Pettit DJ. Blood pressure before the onset of diabetes predicts albuminuria in Type 2 (non-insulin dependent) diabetes. *Diabetologia* 1988; **31**: 509A.

78 Jensen T, Borch-Johnsen K, Deckert T. Changes in blood pressure and renal function in patients with type 1 (insulin-dependent) diabetes prior to clinical diabetic nephropathy. *Diabetes Res* 1987; **4**: 159−62.

79 Parving HH, Andersen AR, Smidt VM, Hommel E, Mathiesen ER, Svendsen PA. Effect of antihypertensive treatment on kidney function in diabetic nephropathy. *Br Med J* 1987; **294**: 1443−7.

80 Parving HH, Hommel E, Smidt VM. Protection of kidney function and decrease in albuminuria by captopril in insulin-dependent diabetics with nephropathy. *Br Med J* 1988; **297**: 1086−91.

81 Christensen CK, Mogensen CE. Antihypertensive treatment: long-term reversal of pressure of albuminuria in incipient diabetic nephropathy. A longitudinal study of renal function. *J Diabetic Compl* 1987; **1**: 45−52.

82 Hommel E, Parving HH, Mathiesen E, Edsberg B, Neilsen MD, Giese J. Effect of captopril on kidney function in insulin-dependent diabetic patients with nephropathy. *Br Med J* 1986; **293**: 467−70.

83 Björck S, Nyberg G, Mulec H, Granerus G, Herlitz H, Aurell M. Beneficial effects of angiotensin converting enzyme inhibitors on renal function in patients with diabetic nephropathy. *Br Med J* 1986; **293**: 471−4.

84 Marre M, Chatellier G, Leblanc H, Guyene TJ, Menard J, Passa P. Prevention of diabetic nephropathy with enalapril in normotensive diabetics with microalbuminuria. *Br Med J* 1988; **297**: 1092−5.

85 Drummond K, Levy-Marchal C, Laborde K. Enalapril does not alter renal function in normotensive, normoalbuminuric, hyperfiltering Type 1 (insulin-dependent) diabetic children. *Diabetologia* 1989; **32**: 255−60.

86 Beyer-Mears A, Cruz E, Edelist T, Varagiannis E. Diminished proteinuria in diabetes mellitus by Sorbinil, an aldose reductase inhibitor. *Pharmacology* 1986; **32**: 52−60.

87 Beyer-Mears A. The polyol pathway, sorbinil and renal dysfunction. *Metabolism* 1986; **35**: 46−54.

88 Brownlee M, Vlassara H, Kooney A, Cerami A. Inhibition of glucose-derived protein cross-linking and prevention of early diabetic changes in glomerular basement membrane by aminoguanidine. *Diabetes* 1986; **35**: 42A.

89 Acheson RM. Blood pressure in a national sample of U.S. adults: percentile distribution by age, sex and race. *Int J Epidemiol* 1973; **2**: 293−301.

90 Winocour PH, Durrington PN, Ishola M, Anderson DC, Cohen H. Influence of proteinuria on vascular disease, blood pressure, and lipoproteins in insulin dependent diabetes mellitus. *Br Med J* 1987; **294**: 1648−51.

91 Borch-Johnsen K, Kreiner S. Proteinuria: value as predictor of cardiovascular mortality in insulin dependent diabetes mellitus. *Br Med J* 1987; **294**: 1651−4.

92 Deckert T, Feldt-Rasmussen B, Borch-Johnsen K, Jensen T, Kofoed-Enevoldsen A. Albuminuria reflects widespread vascular damage. The Steno hypothesis. *Diabetologia* 1989; **32**: 219−26.

66 The Relationship between Structural and Functional Abnormalities in Diabetic Nephropathy

Summary

• The characteristic histopathological features of the diabetic kidney occur in the glomerulus.
• The major abnormalities are: increased glomerular volume secondary to basement membrane thickening and mesangial enlargement; hyaline deposits (of uncertain significance); and global glomerular sclerosis due to mesangial expansion or ischaemia, or both.
• GFR is closely correlated with the surface area of the glomerular capillary basement membrane (the filtration surface), itself determined by the number of glomeruli at diagnosis, the extent of mesangial expansion, the capacity for expansion and the number of sclerosed glomeruli.
• Urinary albumin excretion is related to the filtration slit pore length.
• Microalbuminuria is not always associated with abnormalities of glomerular structure.

The focus of microvascular injury in the kidney is the glomerulus and, accordingly, this has been the subject of intensive histological study. This chapter will briefly describe the pathological appearances of the glomerulus and other renal structures in diabetes, and will present the current understanding of the glomerular structural correlates of changes in glomerular filtration rate (GFR) and albuminuria. Finally, the indications for renal biopsy in diabetic patients will be discussed.

Normal glomerular histology

The renal glomerulus comprises a tuft of 20–40 capillary loops arising from an afferent and drained by an efferent arteriole [1]. The loops are arranged in lobules (Fig. 66.1) which are supported by mesangial tissue which has both cellular and acellular (matrix) components. Electron microscopy has shown that each loop is made up of a basement membrane lined by a fenestrated endothelium and covered by parietal epithelium. These epithelial cells are highly specialized 'podocytes' which do not lie entirely on the basement membrane, but possess foot processes which interdigitate along the membrane, leaving small gaps — the filtration slits or pores — between them. No two adjacent foot processes arise from the same podocyte [2]. The basement membrane is an amorphous, acellular structure whose average width is 383 nm in normal men and 326 nm in women [3]. It has a central lamina densa sandwiched between the less electron dense lamina rara interna and externa. The lamina densa is continuous with the mesangial matrix and both contain Type IV collagen, proteoglycan, laminin and fibronectin. The glomerular tuft is enclosed by Bowman's capsule which is continuous with the tubular basement membrane and defines the urinary space. It is lined by flattened visceral epithelial cells. Filtration takes place from within the capillary, across the endothelium (probably via the fenestrae), the basement membrane, the epithelium (probably via the filtration slit pores), into the urinary space and thus into the proximal tubule.

Pathology of the kidney in diabetes

Renal hypertrophy

Enlargement of the whole kidney and of individual glomeruli has been recognized at diagnosis of

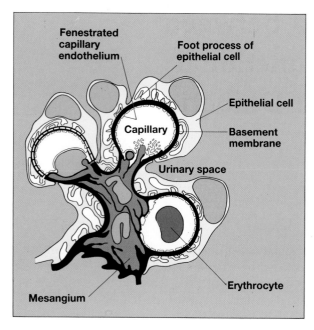

Fig. 66.1. Schematic representation of glomerular capillary tuft. Note continuity of glomerular basement membrane with mesangial matrix material (solid lines). (Adapted from Mauer *et al.* 1984 [10] with permission of the *Journal of Clinical Investigation.*)

diabetes [4], and enlarged glomeruli have been described in many cases of advanced nephropathy [5]. The early increase in glomerular volume is probably secondary to an increase in production of basement membrane material and an enlargement of the filtration surface area [6]. Later glomerular enlargement may represent an accommodation of an expanding mesangium or a response to nephron loss from global sclerosis [6]. As the glomeruli represent only 1% of total renal volume, most of the observed increase in total

kidney volume must be of tubular or interstitial origin [8].

Basement membrane

Basement membrane thickening in diabetes was first described in 1959 and is considered one of the pathological hallmarks of the disease [9]. The membrane width is normal at diagnosis of diabetes, but significant thickening can be detected within 2 years [4], and after 10 years or more the vast majority of patients have marked thickening [10], irrespective of the severity of other diabetic complications (Fig. 66.2). Similar increases in basement membrane width have been demonstrated in normal kidneys transplanted into diabetic recipients [11]. It is thought that basement membrane is produced by the epithelium and metabolized by mesangial cells [12]; whether the observed increase in membrane width is due to overproduction, or impaired clearance, or both is not clear. The increased basement membrane thickness is mostly uniform both within and between glomeruli in the same patient, but thinner irregular segments have been described in some patients with established nephropathy and these may represent either new capillary growth or microaneurysm formation [13].

Mesangium

Diffuse mesangial enlargement is a further pathological feature of diabetic glomerulosclerosis [14] (Fig. 66.2) and, like basement membrane thickening, can be detected after only 2 years of diabetes [4]. However, in contrast to basement

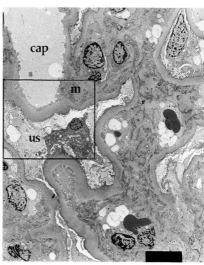

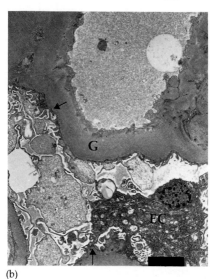

Fig. 66.2. Photomicrographs showing glomerular basement membrane thickening and mesangial expansion in the kidney of a diabetic patient. (a) ×1700; m = mesangial cell and matrix; us = urinary space; cap = capillary lumen. (b) ×4300, enlargement of boxed area in (a). G = glomerular basement membrane; EC = epithelial cell. Foot processes can be clearly seen (arrow). (Courtesy of Dr A. Morley, Department of Pathology, Medical School, University of Newcastle upon Tyne.)

(a)   (b)

membrane thickening, careful study has shown that mesangial volume is by no means always increased and may be normal after 25 years of diabetes [10]. What is certain, however, is that patients with established nephropathy always have marked mesangial expansion [10]. Most of the enlargement is secondary to an increase in periodic acid Schiff—positive (PAS—positive) matrix material, but cellular elements are also increased. Nodular lesions, which were the first glomerular changes to be described and are almost pathognomonic of diabetes [15], comprise ovoid accumulations of PAS-positive material which may be lamellated, and often occupy the central mesangium of a lobule (Fig. 66.3). They are by no means invariably present in patients with established nephropathy, and often coexist with diffuse changes [14]. Some workers consider that the nodules represent obliterated microaneurysms.

Electron microscopic studies in patients with nephropathy have suggested that the expanding mesangium gradually encroaches along the peripheral basement membrane, thus leading to a reduction in filtration surface area.

Hyaline lesions

Collections of eosinophilic, acellular hyaline are characteristic but not specific for diabetes and their precise significance is unclear. They can occur on the inside of Bowman's capsule ('capsular drop'), or within a capillary loop between the endothelial cell and basement membrane ('fibrin cap'). Hyaline deposition in afferent arterioles is an extremely common and non-specific pathological finding, but efferent arteriolar hyaline is thought to be pathognomonic of diabetes [11].

Other glomerular changes

Podocyte and endothelial structure are remarkably well preserved even in advanced nephropathy. Foot process width is probably increased, however, but not as markedly as in other nephropathies [16]. Abnormalities in endothelial fenestrae reported in diabetic animals have not yet been confirmed in man. Thickening and splitting of Bowman's capsule is a common feature of advanced nephropathy [14] and new capillary growth has been demonstrated within the thickened capsule. Global glomerular sclerosis or occlusion [5, 7, 10] due to either internal glomerular obliteration by unrestrained mesangial expansion, or ischaemia secondary to afferent arteriolar occlusion, is a feature of patients with a declining glomerular filtration rate (GFR). In support of the ischaemia hypothesis is the observation of clustering of occluded glomeruli in lines perpendicular to the surface of the kidney and parallel to the course of the interlobular arteries [17].

Tubular and interstitial changes

The first renal pathological abnormality to be described in diabetic man was the Armanni—Ebstein lesion of glycogen-containing vacuoles in the

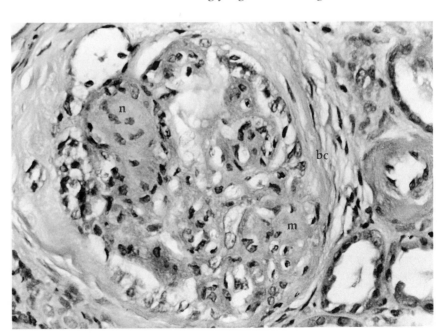

Fig. 66.3. Nodular glomerulosclerosis in a patient with diabetic nephropathy. Note thickened and split Bowman's capsule (bc) and obvious nodule (n). There is also a diffuse mesangial expansion (m) (×600). (Courtesy of Dr A. Morley, Department of Pathology, Medical School, University of Newcastle upon Tyne.)

proximal tubular cells [15]. Since the advent of insulin treatment, this lesion is now rarely seen in man. Tubular basement membrane width also increases and parallels the changes seen in the glomerulus. Tubular atrophy and interstitial changes are probably secondary to glomerular occlusion, and not, as previously thought, to an increased incidence of pyelonephritis [10].

Immunopathology

The immunopathological appearances are thought to represent secondary protein entrapment or accumulation in the basement membrane, rather than a primary cause of glomerulosclerosis. The most commonly described abnormality is a linear deposition of immunoglobulins and albumin, which is entirely non-specific [15].

Glomerular structure and GFR

The surface area of the glomerular capillary basement membrane in diabetic patients (also called the filtration surface — see Fig. 66.1) is closely related to GFR, whether estimated by creatinine clearance [18] or by radioisotopic methods [7] (Fig. 66.4). However, there does not appear to be any strict relationship between basement membrane thickness and GFR.

The total filtering surface area per kidney is the product of the filtration surface per glomerulus and the number of glomeruli per kidney, and the

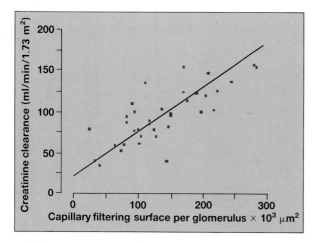

Fig. 66.4. Linear correlation ($r = 0.79$, $P < 0.01$) between GFR (in this case estimated by creatinine clearance) and filtration surface per glomerulus. Note wide range of filtration surface area for any given GFR reflecting the role of other factors such as glomerular number and per cent sclerosed glomeruli (see text). (Adapted from Østerby *et al.* 1986 [7], with permission.)

filtration surface per glomerulus has been shown to be determined by the degree of mesangial expansion and the volume of the glomerular tuft in which it is accommodated [18]. Put simply, a larger glomerulus would accommodate a considerable increase in mesangial tissue before any appreciable loss of filtration surface occurs.

Glomerular enlargement is known to be a feature of established nephropathy [5, 7, 10, 18] and we have shown that diabetic patients with nephropathy after 24−26 years of diabetes have larger glomeruli than those with nephropathy developing after 14−16 years [19]. Thus a capacity for glomerular enlargement may be a modifying factor of the rate of development of nephropathy in those patients destined to develop this complication. Glomerular number, on the other hand, is dependent upon the original number of glomeruli in the kidney (said to vary from 350 000 to 1 100 000 between individuals) (Bendtsen and Nyengaard, personal communications) and the number of those obliterated by glomerulosclerosis. These various factors can all influence filtration surface area and thus GFR (Table 66.1) and it is perhaps not surprising that significant correlations have been described between GFR and mesangial volume [10] and the percentage of sclerosed glomeruli [7] in diabetic patients. Thus, the combination of fewer glomeruli at outset, the development of severe mesangial expansion and a limited capacity for glomerular enlargement with significant glomerular occlusion would lead to a rapidly declining GFR. Although it has yet to be shown that fewer or smaller glomeruli at diagnosis of diabetes represent risk factors for the later development of

Table 66.1. Renal structural factors affecting GFR in diabetes. *Positive* = positive effect on maintenance and preservation of GFR. *Negative* = negative effect on maintenance and preservation of GFR.

1 *Total number of glomeruli at diagnosis*: Probably genetically determined. *Positive.*

2 *Percentage of totally sclerosed glomeruli*: Secondary to factor **4**, possible ischaemic component, ? both. *Negative.*

3 *Mean glomerular volume*: Probably genetically determined at diagnosis. May be influenced by glycaemic control. Late enlargement possibly secondary to factor **2**. *Positive.*

4 *Mesangial volume for glomerulus*: Possibly related to glycaemic control or blood pressure. *Negative.*

nephropathy, preliminary study of postmortem tissue has revealed fewer numbers of glomeruli in those patients dying with nephropathy compared with age- and duration-matched diabetic controls without clinical proteinuria (Bendtsen and Nyengaard, personal communication).

Near-normal glycaemic control can reverse glomerular and mesangial enlargement in diabetic animals [20], and pancreas transplantation might do the same in man [21]. There is, therefore, the intriguing possibility of baseline renal structure and glycaemic control operating as joint risk factors for the development of diabetic nephropathy.

Glomerular structure and albuminuria

Heavy albuminuria is often associated with diminished GFR and thus severe glomerulosclerosis. Significant correlations between podocyte foot process width, filtration slit pore length per glomerulus and the extent of urinary albumin excretion rate (AER) over the normal to nephrotic range have been recently described [16]. These observations lend support to the hypothesis that filtration of macromolecules occurs mainly through the filtration slit pore. As with GFR, there is no significant relationship between AER and basement membrane width.

The intense interest in the phenomenon of microalbuminuria, variously defined as an AER of >30 µg/min [22], 40 mg/24 h [23], 70 µg/min [24] or 15 µg/min [25] depending upon the method of collection used, but always <300 mg/l, derives from the association between microalbuminuria and the later development of nephropathy (Chapters 64 and 65). Detailed morphometric analysis has, however, failed to show any correlation between glomerular structure and microalbuminuria (>20 mg/24 h) in patients with normal blood pressure and GFR [26]. However, if patients with an AER of 40–200 mg/24 h and hypertension are selected, a significant association with increased mesangial volume is observed [26]. Thus, microalbuminuric patients with hypertension probably have established, albeit early, nephropathy. However, microalbuminuria alone does not automatically imply a particular severity of glomerular lesion. Furthermore, analysis of glomeruli from patients with normal AER reveals a wide range of mesangial volumes, suggesting that normoalbuminuria does not exclude underlying glomerulopathy [26]. Prospective studies are necessary to determine the long-term significance of these glomerular lesions in normoalbuminuric patients.

Indications for renal biopsy in diabetic patients

As diabetes is a common condition, the presence of non-diabetic causes of renal failure and proteinuria must always be borne in mind. If a patient has significant proteinuria or haematuria with normal retinal fundoscopy, then renal biopsy might reveal a potentially treatable glomerular disease [27], although many such patients will turn out to have diabetic glomerulosclerosis with a dissociation between renal and retinal complications [28]. Renal biopsy of diabetic patients is important and necessary from both clinical and research standpoints. The techniques for quantitative assessment of renal biopsy material are well described, provide reliable and reproducible data, and are relatively easy to perform [5, 10, 29, 30]. It is only when prospective studies of renal function are combined with renal biopsy, and the glomerular structural counterparts of the changes in GFR and AER are demonstrated, that the pathophysiology of this most serious complication of diabetes will be understood and rational interventions can be undertaken to prevent or modify its natural history.

RUDOLF W. BILOUS

References

1 Tisher CC. Anatomy of the kidney. In: Brenner BM, Rector FC, eds. *The Kidney*. Vol 11. Philadelphia: WB Saunders, 1981: 3–75.
2 Rodewald R, Karnovsky MJ. Porous substructure of the glomerular slit diaphragm in the rat and mouse. *J Cell Biol* 1974; **60**: 423–33.
3 Steffes MW, Barbosa J, Basgen JM, Sutherland DER, Najarian JS, Mauer SM. Quantitative glomerular morphology of the normal human kidney. *Lab Invest* 1983; **49**: 82–6.
4 Mogensen CE, Østerby R, Gundersen HJG. Early functional and morphologic vascular renal consequences of the diabetic state. *Diabetologia* 1979; **17**: 71–6.
5 Østerby R, Gundersen HJG, Nyberg G, Aurell M. Advanced diabetic glomerulopathy. Quantitative structural characterisation of non-occluded glomeruli. *Diabetes* 1987; **36**: 612–19.
6 Østerby R, Gundersen HJG. Fast accumulation of basement membrane material and the rate of morphological changes in acute experimental diabetic glomerular hypertrophy. *Diabetologia* 1980; **18**: 493–500.
7 Østerby R, Parving H-H, Nyberg G, Hommel E, Jørgensen HE, Løkkegaard H, Svalander C. A strong correlation between glomerular filtration rate and filtration surface in diabetic nephropathy. *Diabetologia* 1988; **31**: 265–70.

8 Seyer-Hansen K, Hansen J, Gundersen HJG. Renal hypertrophy in experimental diabetes. A morphometric study. *Diabetologia* 1980; **18**: 501−5.

9 Bergstrand A, Bucht H. The glomerular lesions of diabetes mellitus and their electron microscopic appearance. *J Pathol Bacteriol* 1959; **77**: 231−42.

10 Mauer SM, Steffes MW, Ellis EN, Sutherland DER, Brown DM, Goetz FC. Structural−functional relationships in diabetic nephropathy. *J Clin Invest* 1984; **74**: 1143−55.

11 Mauer SM, Barbosa J, Vernier RL, Kjellstand CM, Buselmeier TJ, Simmons RL, Najarian JS, Goetz FC. Development of diabetic vascular lesions in normal kidneys transplanted into patients with diabetes mellitus. *N Engl J Med* 1976; **295**: 916−20.

12 Walker F. The origin, turnover and removal of glomerular basement membrane. *J Pathol* 1973; **110**: 233−44.

13 Østerby R, Nyberg G. New vessel formation in the renal corpuscles in advanced diabetic glomerulopathy. *J Diabetic Comp* 1987; **1**: 122−7.

14 Gellman DD, Pirani CL, Soothill JF, Muehrke RC, Kark RM. Diabetic nephropathy: a clinical and pathological study based on renal biopsies. *Medicine (Baltimore)* 1959; **38**: 321−67.

15 Morley AR. Renal vascular disease in diabetes mellitus. *Histopathology* 1988; **12**: 343−58.

16 Ellis EN, Steffes MW, Chavers BM, Mauer SM. Observations of glomerular epithelial cell structure in patients with type 1 diabetes mellitus. *Kidney Int* 1987; **32**: 736−41.

17 Hørlyck A, Gundersen HJG, Østerby R. The cortical distribution pattern of diabetic glomerulopathy. *Diabetologia* 1986; **29**: 146−50.

18 Ellis EN, Steffes MW, Goetz FC, Sutherland DER, Mauer SM. Glomerular filtration surface in type 1 diabetes mellitus. *Kidney Int* 1986; **29**: 889−94.

19 Bilous RW, Mauer SM, Sutherland DER, Steffes MW. Mean glomerular volume and rate of development of diabetic nephropathy. *Diabetes* 1989; **38**: 1142−7.

20 Steffes MW, Brown DM, Basgen JM, Mauer SM. Amelioration of mesangial volume and surface alterations following islet transplantation in diabetic rats. *Diabetes* 1980; **29**: 509−15.

21 Bilous RW, Mauer SM, Sutherland DER, Najarian JS, Goetz FC, Steffes MW. The effects of pancreas transplantation on the glomerular structure of renal allografts in patients with insulin-dependent diabetes. *N Engl J Med* 1989; **321**: 80−5.

22 Viberti GC, Jarrett RJ, Mahmud U, Hill RD, Argyropoulos A, Keen H. Microalbuminuria as a predictor of clinical nephropathy in insulin-dependent diabetes mellitus. *Lancet* 1982; ii: 1430−2.

23 Parving H-H, Oxenbøll B, Svendsen PAå, Christiansen JS, Andersen AR. Early detection of patients at risk of developing diabetic nephropathy. A longitudinal study of urinary albumin excretion. *Acta Endocrinol* 1982; **100**: 550−5.

24 Mathiesen ER, Oxenbøll B, Johansen K, Svendsen PAå, Deckert T. Incipient nephropathy in Type 1 (insulin-dependent) diabetes. *Diabetologia* 1984; **25**: 406−10.

25 Mogensen CE, Christensen CK. Predicting diabetic nephropathy in insulin-dependent patients. *N Engl J Med* 1984; **311**: 89−93.

26 Chavers BM, Bilous RW, Ellis EN, Steffes MW, Mauer SM. Glomerular lesions and urinary albumin excretion in type 1 diabetes without overt proteinuria. *N Engl J Med* 1989; **320**: 966−70.

27 Hommel E, Carstensen H, Skøtt P, Larsen P, Parving H-H. Prevalence and causes of microscopic haematuria in Type 1 (insulin-dependent) diabetic patients with persistent proteinuria. *Diabetologia* 1987; **30**: 627−30.

28 Bilous RW, Viberti GC, Sandahl-Christiansen J, Parving H-H, Keen H. Dissociation of diabetic complications in insulin-dependent diabetes: a clinical report. *Diabetic Nephr* 1985; **4**: 73−6.

29 Ellis EN, Basgen JM, Mauer SM, Steffes MW. Kidney biopsy technique and evaluation. In: Clarke WL, Larner J, Pohl SL, eds. *Methods of Diabetes Research. Clinical Methods*, Vol 11. New York: J Wiley and Sons, 1986: 633−47.

30 Gundersen HJG, Bagger P, Bendtsen TF *et al.* The new stereological tools: disector, fractionator, nucleator and point sampled intercepts and their use in pathological research and diagnosis. *Acta Pathol Microbiol Immunol Scand* 1988; **96**: 857−81.

67 Clinical Features and Management of Established Diabetic Nephropathy

Summary

- Proteinuria develops in 40% of IDDM patients, of whom two-thirds will develop renal failure. Nephropathy is rarer in NIDDM, but due to the relatively high prevalence of NIDDM, 50% of diabetic patients entering end-stage renal failure in Britain each year are non-insulin-dependent.

- Non-diabetic renal disease accounts for proteinuria in up to 8% of diabetic patients. Alternative diagnoses are suggested by acute renal impairment, absence of retinopathy, haematuria, or short duration of IDDM (<5 years), and must be excluded by renal biopsy.

- Blood pressure is generally above normal in the early microalbuminuric stage of nephropathy. Hypertension affects virtually all patients with persistent proteinuria and tends to worsen as renal function declines. Supine hypertension and orthostatic hypotension (due to autonomic neuropathy) may coexist.

- Early effective control of blood pressure may delay the advent of end-stage renal failure by over 20 years. Angiotensin converting enzyme inhibitors may have an additional beneficial effect in reducing intraglomerular pressure.

- Extensive, severe cardiovascular disease develops early in diabetic patients with nephropathy. Coronary heart disease is often asymptomatic but electrocardiographic and angiographic abnormalities are common. Peripheral vascular disease includes widespread multisegmental atheromatous lesions and medial arterial calcification in hands and feet; digital ischaemia and gangrene are common.

- Neuropathic foot ulceration affects one-quarter of diabetic patients with nephropathy, but Charcot joints are relatively uncommon. Tests of sensory and autonomic function are abnormal in most patients. Symptoms vary considerably.

- Retinopathy is virtually always present in nephropathy and is proliferative in about 70% of cases. Untreated retinopathy often deteriorates together with renal function, possibly through worsening hypertension and fluid retention.

- GFR, serum creatinine, urea and electrolytes must be monitored regularly in proteinuric patients. The interval to end-stage renal failure may be estimated by linear extrapolation of plots of inverse creatinine or GFR. Urine must be cultured regularly to exclude infection, especially in patients with incomplete bladder emptying. Infection, dehydration and radiographic contrast media may precipitate acute-on-chronic renal failure.

- Insulin requirements fall (often by 50%) in renal failure due to reduced renal elimination of insulin. Metformin and most sulphonylureas are also cleared through the kidneys and accumulate in uraemia, causing hypoglycaemia and toxicity: transfer to insulin treatment is therefore recommended.

- Moderate dietary protein restriction (45 g/day) may slow the rate of decline in GFR if started early in diabetic nephropathy (before GFR falls below 15 ml/min).

- Renal replacement therapy — renal transplantation, haemodialysis or continuous ambulatory peritoneal dialysis (CAPD) — should be offered as freely to diabetic as to non-diabetic patients as their survival rates are now nearly comparable.

- Renal transplantation, ideally from a live related donor, is the treatment of choice in patients under 60 years of age. Transplantation is recommended when the serum creatinine reaches about 500 μmol/l. 5-year survival now exceeds 60% for cadaver grafts at most centres. Transplanted kidneys generally develop histological features of diabetic nephropathy but this is not known to have caused graft failure as yet.

• Chronic haemodialysis may be complicated in diabetic patients by difficult vascular access, postural hypotension and poor metabolic control and was previously associated with rapidly worsening retinopathy, causing blindness in 40% of cases. Haemodialysis may need to be started relatively early (serum creatinine 500–600 μmol/l) because of the tendency to fluid retention. 5-year survival is now about 45% and only 3% of cases now suffer visual loss; prognosis is poorer in patients over 60 years. Common causes of death are cardiovascular disease, sepsis and uraemia following withdrawal from dialysis.

• CAPD is inexpensive, avoids rapid volume fluctuations and allows patients to be independent. It is suitable for elderly patients and those with ischaemic heart disease, severe autonomic neuropathy or visual impairment. Insulin (at about twice the usual subcutaneous dose) can be added directly to the dialysis fluid and is absorbed into the portal system. Peritonitis is no more common than in non-diabetic patients. 3-year survival is now about 60%.

• Coexistent vascular disease, retinopathy and foot problems must be identified and treated if possible before undertaking renal replacement therapy, and carefully monitored thereafter. Coronary heart disease is the major cause of death in the first few years after starting renal replacement therapy, accounting for 50–65% of deaths (10 times the rate in non-diabetic patients); patients receiving haemodialysis are particularly at risk. Strokes, digital and limb gangrene are also common.

Proteinuria was first recognized in diabetic patients over 150 years ago but its true importance as indicating a severe and often fatal complication of diabetes was not realized until the 1930s [1]. Most of the excess mortality of diabetes occurs in patients with proteinuria (Fig. 67.1) [2, 3]. About 40% of IDDM patients will develop proteinuria; two-thirds of these will develop renal failure whereas the rest will die of cardiovascular disease (Table 67.1) [2–5]. Nephropathy also affects NIDDM patients and although most die from cardiovascular disease [6, 7], the relatively high prevalence of NIDDM means that nearly 50% of the diabetic patients entering end-stage renal failure are non-insulin-dependent [8–11].

Diabetic patients with renal failure are now accepted for renal replacement therapy in steadily increasing numbers (Fig. 67.2) [12], accounting for up to 25% of new patients in some countries [8, 13, 14]. In Britain, however, relatively few of the 600 diabetic patients estimated to develop end-stage renal failure each year enter renal replacement programmes [15], probably because of the outdated impression that diabetic patients fare badly with dialysis or transplantation [16, 17]. In

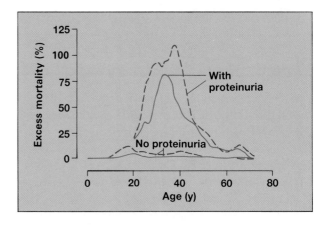

Fig. 67.1. Relative mortality of diabetic patients with and without persistent proteinuria, in men (——) and women (– – – –) as a function of age. Mortality is greatly increased at all ages in proteinuric patients. (Redrawn from [2], with kind permission of the Editor of *Diabetologia*.)

Table 67.1. Causes of death in diabetic nephropathy.

	UK study 1983 [5]	Steno [4]	Joslin [28]	UK study 1985 [92]
Renal failure	60%	66%	59%	50%
Cardiovascular disease	25%	24%	36%	25%

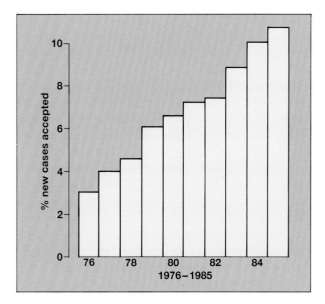

Fig. 67.2. Percentages of diabetic nephropathic patients entering end-stage renal failure who were accepted for renal replacement therapy in Europe in 1976–1985. (Redrawn from [12], with kind permission of Martinus Nijhoff Publishing, Boston.)

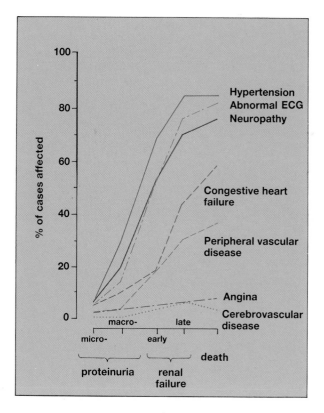

Fig. 67.3. Frequency of other diabetic complications at various stages of diabetic nephropathy. (Redrawn from [28], with kind permission of the Editor of the *Journal of the American Medical Association*.)

fact, the results of renal replacement therapy in diabetic patients have improved considerably during the past 10 years and in some centres are now comparable with those in non-diabetic patients [18, 19].

Renal disease is often accompanied by widespread vascular disease, severe retinopathy and neuropathy (Fig. 67.3) [20], all complications which limit the success of renal replacement therapy. Successful management requires a joint approach by diabetes and renal specialists with an understanding of the natural history of diabetic nephropathy.

This chapter will describe the clinical features and management of established diabetic nephropathy and end-stage renal failure.

Clinical features of diabetic nephropathy

Proteinuria is usually the first manifestation of diabetic nephropathy and may be intermittent for many years before becoming persistent (see Chapter 64). Once persistent proteinuria has developed, renal function declines gradually but progressively, reaching end-stage renal failure on average within 7 years (see Figs 64.4 and 64.5) [4, 21]. Proteinuria increases as diabetic nephropathy progresses but only rarely reaches nephrotic proportions; however, fluid retention is common

and occurs earlier than in non-diabetic patients [22].

Some elevation of blood pressure is usually present from the early, microalbuminuric stage of diabetic nephropathy (Fig. 67.4) [23–27], and almost all patients with persistent proteinuria have hypertension which continues to worsen as GFR falls (Figs 67.5 and 67.6). This may be masked by the postural hypotension of autonomic neuropathy, which is universal in such patients, if blood pressure is measured only in the sitting position; blood pressure must therefore be recorded both lying and standing to assess both the degree of hypertension and the effect of treatment. Hypertension in diabetic nephropathy is exquisitely volume-sensitive and this becomes more apparent as renal failure progresses.

Cardiovascular disease is common and extensive in diabetic nephropathy patients, even those in their 20s and 30s, but is often asymptomatic [28–30]. Angina is reported by only 10–20% of cases [5, 30, 31] and previous myocardial infarction is rare, but abnormal electrocardiograms are found in 50–70% of cases and radiographic evidence of cardiomegaly in 50% [28, 30, 32].

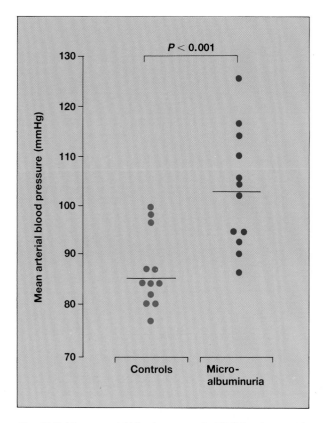

Fig. 67.4. Mean arterial blood pressure in IDDM patients with microalbuminuria (urinary albumin excretion 32–91 µg/min) and in matched diabetic patients with normal albumin excretion (2–10 µg/min). (Adapted from [25] with kind permission of the Editor of *Diabetologia*.)

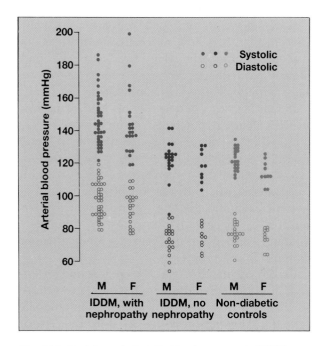

Fig. 67.5. Systolic and diastolic blood pressure in IDDM patients with and without nephropathy and in non-diabetic controls. All groups are age-matched. (Redrawn from [24] with kind permission of the Editor of *Diabetologia*.)

Coronary angiography has shown the presence of significant coronary occlusive disease in 20–100% of patients, depending on selection and diagnostic criteria [29, 30, 33]. Even in the absence of significant coronary artery disease, diffuse myocardial dysfunction is frequent [34]. Left ventricular hypertrophy is common and usually severe in patients with advanced nephropathy (Fig. 67.7) [35, 36], probably reflecting long-standing and inadequately treated hypertension.

Peripheral vascular disease in patients with advanced nephropathy affects hands as well as feet, complicating vascular access for haemodialysis and leading to a high amputation rate especially after transplantation [37–41]. Among patients being considered for renal transplantation, 10–20% have absent foot pulses, claudication or gangrene and about 1–2% have had amputations [42, 43]. Atheromatous lesions in these patients are often multisegmental, bilateral and distal and involve the vessels below the knee [44]. Striking medial arterial calcification is frequently seen on radiographs and involves both large and small vessels, including the digital arteries of the hands and feet (Fig. 67.8) [32, 45]. This is partly related to the neuropathy which

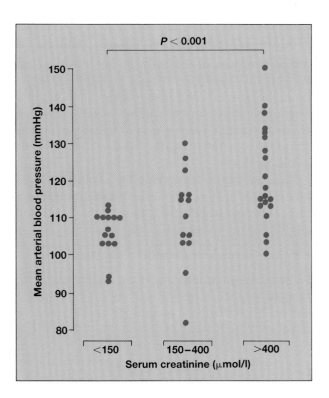

Fig. 67.6. Mean arterial blood pressure in three groups of diabetic nephropathic patients subdivided according to serum creatinine level (A. Grenfell, unpublished observations).

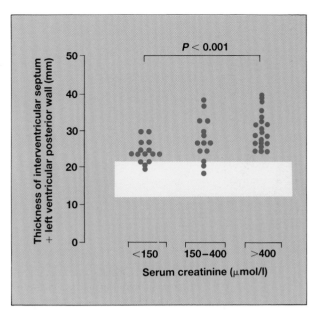

Fig. 67.7. Left ventricular wall thickness in patients with diabetic nephropathy subdivided according to serum creatinine level, showing increasing left ventricular hypertrophy with worsening renal impairment. Yellow area represents normal adult range. (Redrawn from [35] with kind permission of the Editor of *Diabetic Medicine*.)

affects these patients but is usually more extensive than in patients with neuropathy alone [46]. Digital arterial calcification is associated with the digital gangrene common in these patients (Fig. 67.9) but its precise aetiological role is uncertain [45].

Neuropathy affects most patients with advanced diabetic nephropathy to a variable extent [30, 32, 47], some being completely asymptomatic whereas others suffer severe features of somatic and autonomic neuropathy. Various reports suggest that 40–100% of patients receiving renal transplants have some degree of somatic neuropathy [30, 47, 48]. Neuropathic ulceration is the most important consequence, occurring in up to one-quarter of patients with diabetic nephropathy. Charcot joints are much rarer, affecting only 3% of a series of diabetic patients with renal failure at King's College Hospital (A. Grenfell, unpublished observations).

Autonomic neuropathy is almost invariable in those with established nephropathy, although symptoms are very variable. Postural hypotension is usually mild but may complicate antihypertensive therapy. Gustatory sweating and diarrhoea

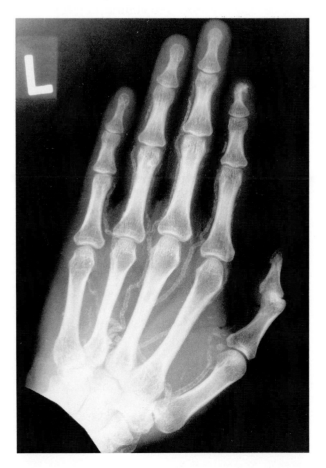

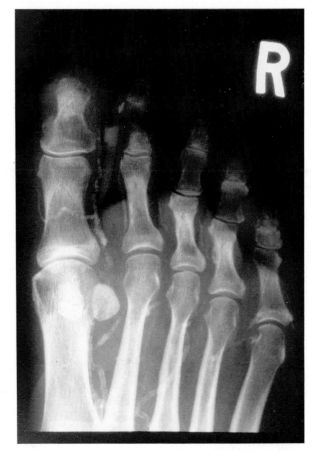

Fig. 67.8. Medial calcification of digital arteries of hands and feet in a patient with renal failure due to diabetic nephropathy.

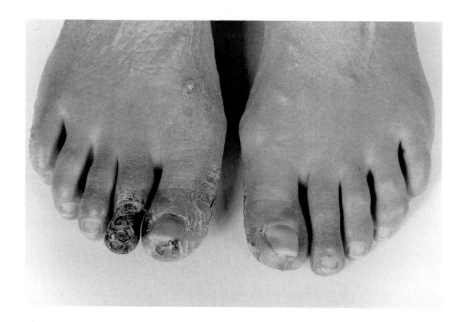

Fig. 67.9. Digital gangrene in a diabetic nephropathic patient with renal failure.

are relatively common and occur in about 50% of patients. Incomplete bladder emptying is rare: only 10% of patients assessed with micturating cystography at King's College Hospital had a significant residual urine volume (>50 ml). Vomiting due to gastroparesis is rare but can be devastating and refractory to treatment. Vomiting is difficult to assess in uraemic patients: a barium meal is often unhelpful and more sophisticated tests of stomach emptying may be required [49] (see Chapter 71). Respiratory arrests associated with sedative drugs or anaesthesia occur in occasional patients with autonomic neuropathy [50].

Retinopathy is virtually always present in established diabetic nephropathy [20, 51]; its absence suggests that the renal disease is not due to diabetes. Proliferative retinopathy is reported in 70% of cases, with roughly one-third being registered blind and another one-third having severely impaired vision [32, 42, 48]. As renal failure develops, retinopathy tends to deteriorate, probably due to a combination of hypertension and fluid retention, especially if previously untreated [52].

Diagnosis of diabetic nephropathy

Renal disease other than diabetic nephropathy may occur in diabetic patients [53, 54] and may account for proteinuria in 3–8% of cases [4, 55]. Of the 163 patients treated at King's College Hospital, 17% had a non-diabetic renal disease, being found more often among NIDDM (27%) than IDDM patients (10%). The distinction is

crucial as other renal diseases may need specific treatment and may carry a different prognosis.

The diagnosis of diabetic nephropathy is straightforward in the presence of a typical history and clinical features. Proteinuria developing in an IDDM patient of 10–20 years standing who has other complications, especially retinopathy, needs few investigations. Urine should be examined for red cells and casts, and cultured to exclude infection. Ultrasound examination is important to demonstrate renal size. This is usually normal or even large in diabetic nephropathy [56], although biopsy-proven glomerulosclerosis has been observed in small kidneys [57]. Bladder ultrasound examination will exclude obstruction and urinary retention due to a neuropathic bladder. Immunological tests to exclude systemic lupus erythematosus and other glomerulonephritides should be performed as indicated.

Features suggestive of an alternative diagnosis (Table 67.2) [58] include a rapid deterioration in renal function from normal, sudden development of nephrotic syndrome, absence of retinopathy, the presence of haematuria [59] (although red cell casts occur rarely in diabetic nephropathy [60]),

Table 67.2. Features suggesting an alternative cause of renal impairment in diabetic patients.

- Rapid deterioration in renal function from normal
- Sudden development of nephrotic syndrome
- Presence of haematuria
- Short duration (<5 years) of IDDM

and short duration of otherwise uncomplicated IDDM. Renal biopsy should be performed if there is any doubt as to the diagnosis.

Monitoring renal function

Renal function must be monitored in patients with diabetic nephropathy, both to estimate the time to end-stage renal failure and to determine the effects of intervention. Serum creatinine concentration does not reflect glomerular filtration rate (GFR) in the early stages of nephropathy and only rises when GFR is reduced by 50–70% (Fig. 67.10). GFR should therefore be measured, ideally using isotopic methods, during the early stages (Fig. 67.11). Serial plots of inverse creatinine (1000/creatinine in μmol/l) generally show a linear decline which, if extrapolated, may predict when end-stage renal failure is likely to occur (Fig. 67.12); this method is only useful when the serum creatinine concentration exceeds 200 μmol/l [61]. The quantity of proteinuria and serum albumin levels should also be monitored. Urine should be cultured regularly to detect infection.

Certain circumstances, notably sepsis and dehydration, may cause an acute deterioration in patients with diabetic nephropathy [62]. Diabetic patients are particularly prone to septicaemia, especially arising from urinary tract infections, and to the serious complication of papillary

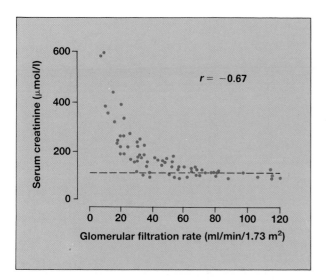

Fig. 67.10. Glomerular filtration rate (GFR) measured by ^{51}Cr-EDTA clearance, plotted against serum creatinine concentration in 73 subjects at various stages of diabetic nephropathy. Dashed line represents upper limit of normal serum creatinine concentration. (Redrawn from [61] with kind permission of the Editor of the *American Journal of Medicine*.)

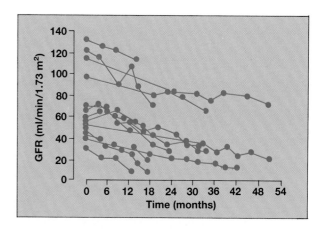

Fig. 67.11. Progressive and generally linear decline in GFR (measured by ^{51}Cr-EDTA clearance) in 13 diabetic patients with nephropathy. (Redrawn from [61] with kind permission of the Editor of the *American Journal of Medicine*.)

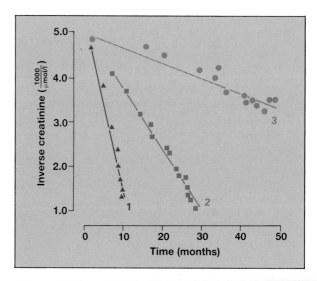

Fig. 67.12. Serial plots of inverse creatinine values (1000/serum creatinine concentration in μmol/l) in three representative diabetic nephropathic patients. Inverse serum creatinine declines linearly with time, at a fixed rate for each individual patient (fastest for patient 1 (▲) and slowest for patient 3 (●)). (Adapted from Jones *et al. Lancet* 1979; i: 1105–6, with kind permission of the Editor.)

necrosis [63]. Urinary retention due to autonomic neuropathy is rare but must be actively excluded; it is usually asymptomatic and commonly leads to recurrent urinary tract infections which aggravate renal impairment [64].

Radiographic contrast media should be avoided if possible, especially in patients whose serum creatinine exceeds 200 μmol/l, as renal function often declines acutely [65]; newer contrast agents with lower osmolarity are less nephrotoxic. Essential investigations (e.g. coronary angiography)

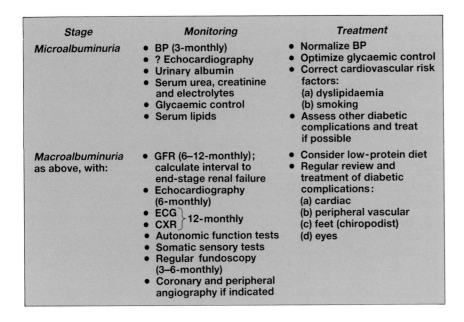

Stage	Monitoring	Treatment

Microalbuminuria	• BP (3-monthly)
	• ? Echocardiography
	• Urinary albumin
	• Serum urea, creatinine and electrolytes
	• Glycaemic control
	• Serum lipids
		• Normalize BP
		• Optimize glycaemic control
		• Correct cardiovascular risk factors:
		  (a) dyslipidaemia
		  (b) smoking
		• Assess other diabetic complications and treat if possible

Macroalbuminuria as above, with:	• GFR (6–12-monthly); calculate interval to end-stage renal failure
	• Echocardiography (6-monthly)
	• ECG ⎱ 12-monthly
	• CXR ⎰
	• Autonomic function tests
	• Somatic sensory tests
	• Regular fundoscopy (3–6-monthly)
	• Coronary and peripheral angiography if indicated
		• Consider low-protein diet
		• Regular review and treatment of diabetic complications:
		  (a) cardiac
		  (b) peripheral vascular
		  (c) feet (chiropodist)
		  (d) eyes

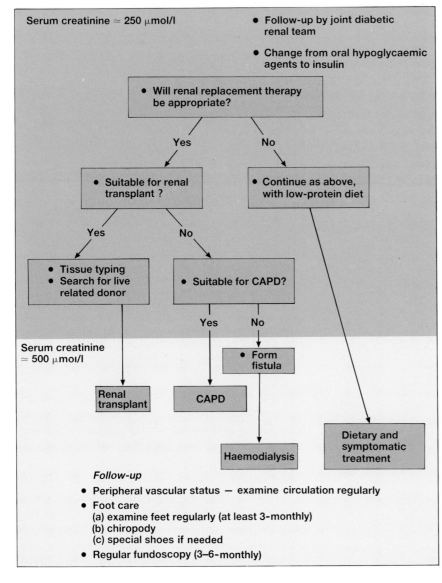

Fig. 67.13. Flow-chart illustrating the management of patients with diabetic nephropathy, before the onset of renal failure (upper panel) and with renal failure (lower panel).

should ideally be performed as early as possible and the patient should be well hydrated with intravenous fluids and mannitol [66]. Patients with significant renal impairment are best established on dialysis before investigation. Other nephrotoxic drugs (such as aminoglycosides, especially if used concurrently with loop diuretics) should similarly be avoided.

Management of established diabetic nephropathy

Patients with persistent proteinuria should be followed up at least 3-monthly and every effort made to achieve good glycaemic control and a normal blood pressure and to correct any other risk factors (particularly smoking and dyslipidaemia) for the cardiovascular disease which will remain a serious threat to their lives.

Renal function should be monitored as above and, after GFR has been falling for some months, its rate of decline should be calculated and the likely interval to end-stage renal failure estimated. Once serum creatinine has reached 250 μmol/l, the patient is best managed by a joint team of diabetologist, renal physician and transplant surgeon, together with the diabetes specialist nurse, dietitian, and ultimately the renal replacement specialist nurse. Current policy in many centres is to aim for renal transplantation or long-term dialysis before the serum creatinine is much over 500 μmol/l; many preparations (e.g. tissue typing and searching for an appropriate live related donor) will need to be made before then. Patients with symptomatic uraemia will need to be seen at least every 1–3 months, and should have access to specialist advice in case of acute complications. A suggested management flow chart is shown in Fig. 67.13. The treatment of specific problems is described below.

Control of hypertension

In 1976, Mogensen first demonstrated a positive correlation between diastolic blood pressure and the rate of decline of GFR [23]. Several studies have subsequently demonstrated that effective antihypertensive therapy can reduce the rate of decline, sometimes to less than one-fifth of pretreatment values (Fig. 67.14) [67–71]. The most favourable results suggest that the progression from normal GFR to end-stage renal failure may take up to 30 years, rather than the average of 7

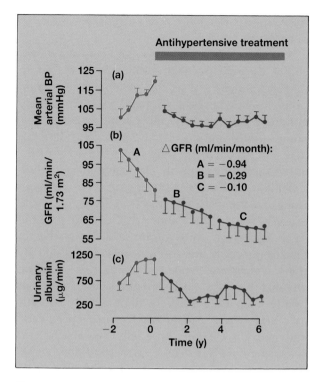

Fig. 67.14. Effects of antihypertensive treatment on mean arterial blood pressure (a), GFR (b) and urinary albumin excretion (c) in IDDM patients with nephropathy. Rate of decline in GFR and albumin excretion were both significantly reduced. Error bars are SEM. (Reproduced from [68] with kind permission of the Editor of the *British Medical Journal*.)

years in inadequately treated patients. Hypertension must therefore be discovered and treated early; all too often, lack of effective treatment initially may lead to a loss in GFR of several ml/min.

The optimal blood pressure and therapeutic target in nephropathic patients are uncertain (see Chapter 69). The WHO criteria may be too lax for this relatively young population and a more appropriate target may be the age-related norms (Fig. 69.4) [72]. However, higher supine levels may have to be accepted if postural hypotension is a problem.

Many drugs, particularly β-blockers and diuretics, have been used to control blood pressure in patients with diabetic nephropathy but have not been adequately compared in controlled studies. Accordingly, no specific drug or combination of drugs can be regarded as first choice, although certain recommendations can be made. The aim should be to reduce blood pressure satisfactorily using drugs and other means acceptable to the patient (see Chapter 69), and in most cases this can be achieved. Important features of the main antihypertensive drugs used are shown in Table 69.3.

A diuretic is usually necessary and a rational choice as exchangeable sodium is increased in diabetic patients [73, 74] and oedema is a common problem. Blood pressure appears to be particularly volume-sensitive, especially when serum creatinine concentrations start to rise; loop diuretics may be needed at this stage. Selective β_1-adrenoceptor blockers are also useful despite their potential problems, notably delayed recovery from and impaired awareness of hypoglycaemia, exacerbation of lipid abnormalities and possibly hyperglycaemia. Most of these are probably of limited practical importance, as is suggested by their widespread and successful use. Calcium channel blockers such as nifedipine are often poorly tolerated by diabetic nephropathy patients as they often cause troublesome peripheral oedema. Vasodilators, especially hydralazine and prazosin, have been used as second-line agents in diabetic patients but commonly exacerbate postural hypotension.

Angiotensin-converting enzyme (ACE) inhibitors are now promoted as first-line agents for treating diabetic nephropathy. As well as their systemic hypotensive action, these drugs are thought to reduce intraglomerular pressure by specifically relaxing efferent glomerular arterioles and so may further help to preserve renal function in the diabetic patient [75]. ACE inhibitors undoubtedly reduce the rate of decline of renal function in diabetic nephropathy [69]; whether this simply reflects effective blood pressure control or a specific action on glomerular haemodynamics is undetermined, as alternative antihypertensive drugs have achieved similar results. ACE inhibitors are well tolerated by diabetic patients and are useful first- or second-line agents when other drugs are unsuitable or blood pressure control is inadequate.

Glycaemic control

The importance of hyperglycaemia in the progression of established diabetic nephropathy has been addressed by several studies [76–78] but remains unclear. Two controlled studies from Guy's Hospital showed no influence of strict metabolic control (imposed by CSII) on the rate of decline of GFR or fractional clearance of protein in diabetic patients with persistent or intermittent proteinuria [76, 77]. Both studies can be criticized

for their small size (six patients in each group), inadequate control of hypertension (which is probably a more important factor than hyperglycaemia), and the fact that metabolic control may have been suboptimal. In patients with established nephropathy and tightly controlled blood pressure, progression of GFR has been reported to relate to the degree of metabolic control as assessed by HbA_1 [78].

As renal failure progresses, insulin clearance and degradation by the kidneys decreases and insulin requirements gradually fall in most patients, often by up to 50%. Frequent home blood glucose monitoring is therefore essential to direct any changes in the insulin regimen.

Most of the oral hypoglycaemic agents, particularly chlorpropamide, glibenclamide, tolbutamide and metformin, are normally metabolized or cleared by the kidneys and so accumulate in uraemic patients, increasing the risks of hypoglycaemia and toxicity. Some second-generation sulphonylureas such as gliclazide are cleared predominantly through the liver and may be relatively safer in renal failure. However, many specialist centres prefer to transfer all patients receiving oral agents to insulin when serum creatinine concentration reaches 250 μmol/l.

Dietary protein intake

Dietary protein intake is known to influence renal function [79] and a low-protein diet prevents the progression of both experimental and human chronic renal failure [80, 81]. In diabetic renal failure, low-protein diets (20–30 g/day) were used initially to relieve the symptoms of advanced uraemia but did not apparently delay the progression to end-stage renal failure [82]. A cross-sectional study of IDDM patients found no correlation between protein intake and the presence of nephropathy or its rate of decline [83].

Studies of moderate protein restriction in early diabetic renal failure have yielded inconclusive and conflicting results [83–86]. In a study from Guy's Hospital [84], one year of treatment with a low protein diet slowed the rate of decline of GFR and reduced total urinary protein excretion in a group of 20 IDDM patients as a whole (see Fig. 65.9). However, individual responses varied considerably, GFR remaining stable or declining less rapidly in one half of the subjects but continuing to decline at the same rate in the rest.

Equivocal results are also reported in a separate but similar study from the same centre [85]. By contrast, an Italian study found that a low-protein, low-phosphate diet supplemented with essential amino acids and ketoanalogues apparently slowed the fall in creatinine clearance and urinary protein excretion in all eight patients studied during a 17-month period [86].

Longer-term, larger-scale controlled studies are needed to clarify the role of dietary protein, although some sensible suggestions can be made [87]. Severe protein restriction (20–25 g/day) is inadvisable because it runs the risk of malnutrition and is unacceptable to most patients. Moderate protein restriction (45 g/day, 0.5–0.6 g/kg/day) if started before renal impairment is too advanced (GFR > 15 ml/min) may be useful and is nutritionally adequate for long periods. However, such diets are unpalatable for many patients and long-term compliance is likely to be poor.

In the past, carbohydrate-restricted diabetic diets have had a high protein content which may have had a deleterious effect on the kidneys. Pending clearer evidence regarding protein restriction, diabetic patients should be advised to eat more unrefined carbohydrate and therefore less protein, in line with recent guidelines [88].

Assessment and management of other diabetic complications

Complications which commonly accompany diabetic nephropathy should be assessed carefully and at an early stage, in order to pre-empt the problems which in the past have placed diabetic patients with end-stage renal failure at such a high risk.

Cardiovascular examination is mandatory early in the course of diabetic nephropathy. Hypertension must be treated energetically, especially if causing left ventricular hypertrophy. This can be measured accurately and monitored using echocardiography, which should probably be performed at the microalbuminuric stage and then repeated every 3–6 months; effective antihypertensive therapy will reverse left ventricular hypertrophy.

Coronary angiography may be required, as non-invasive methods such as thallium stress testing do not seem to provide adequate information on myocardial status [89]. Future work will establish whether coronary angiography helps to select patients for renal replacement and whether coronary artery bypass or angioplasty will influence its outcome.

Peripheral vascular disease must be assessed and treated as necessary. The absence of foot pulses predicts poor healing of foot lesions which are common in these patients [90]. Plain radiography of the hands and feet will demonstrate medial arterial calcification (Fig. 67.8), which causes spuriously high systolic pressures. Arteriography should be performed to resolve any doubts about the circulation. Angioplasty is used increasingly and may accelerate the healing of foot lesions, but amputation should be considered for widespread vascular disease, particularly if complicated by infection or non-healing foot lesions and especially if transplantation is being considered.

Testing vibration perception threshold and thermal discrimination may identify feet at risk of neuropathic ulceration and this should be repeated regularly as sensation may only become impaired later in the course of nephropathy. Autonomic function tests are abnormal in virtually all nephropathic patients, but symptoms are very variable. The important manifestations are postural hypotension (which may complicate antihypertensive therapy) and incomplete bladder emptying. The latter should be assessed with ultrasound scanning or micturating cystography and may require regular self-catheterization.

Foot care is critical to the management of patients with diabetic nephropathy before, during and after renal replacement therapy and demands close liason between chiropodist, shoe fitter, physician and surgeon [90]. Removal of callus and provision of special shoes to off-load weight-bearing areas avoids many problems but infection must be treated promptly and vigorously, with intravenous antibiotics if cellulitis is suspected. Early surgical drainage of abscesses and removal of necrotic tissue may prevent osteomyelitis or gangrene; limited ray amputation often successfully treats these complications [91].

Retinopathy, usually proliferative, almost always accompanies diabetic nephropathy and tends to deteriorate as renal failure progresses. With early regular ophthalmological review and prompt treatment as necessary, fewer patients should become blind before renal failure develops.

Renal replacement therapy

Dialysis and renal transplantation are now accepted as appropriate for diabetic patients. In

Europe the proportion of diabetic patients entering end-stage renal failure who were offered renal replacement therapy increased steadily from only 3% in 1976 to 10.7% in 1985 and reached 30% in some Scandinavian countries (Fig. 67.2) [12]; in the UK in 1985, the proportion was 11.4% [15], indicating a considerable shortfall in treatment. A recent British survey showed that, despite increasing use of renal replacement therapy for diabetic renal failure, one-third of these patients died without receiving renal support, half of whom died directly from renal failure [92]. In Britain, diabetes accounts for some 20–25% of cases requiring renal replacement [93]. The patient populations accepted for renal replacement differ considerably between countries, IDDM patients being treated virtually exclusively in Sweden, Finland and Norway and those with NIDDM predominating in Austria, Denmark and the Federal Republic of Germany [94]. About 20% of British diabetic patients treated for renal failure are non-insulin-dependent. These different patterns may be partly explained by the high frequency of IDDM in Sweden, Finland and Norway and possibly by an accelerated progression of the disease in these countries.

The methods of renal replacement therapy chosen for diabetic patients differ from those for other primary renal diseases (Fig. 67.15) and also show geographical variation. Peritoneal dialysis, especially continuous ambulatory peritoneal dialysis (CAPD), is a relatively common initial and maintenance treatment for diabetic patients

[94]. Renal transplantation is chosen more commonly as first-line treatment for IDDM patients than for those with NIDDM or other primary renal diseases. In Scandinavia particularly, many IDDM patients receive renal transplantation whereas surgeons in France and Germany still apparently resist transplanting patients with diabetic nephropathy (Fig. 67.16). In the UK in 1985, 46% of diabetic patients alive on renal replacement therapy were treated with CAPD while 34% had had a renal transplant [12].

Selection criteria

Selection policies for renal replacement therapy vary considerably but until recently were stricter for diabetic than for non-diabetic patients. Older and more complicated diabetic patients are now being treated.

Age is an important selection criterion for renal replacement. Older patients (>60 years) have a much poorer prognosis [95] and therefore tend to be treated by dialysis alone and not referred for transplantation. However, age restrictions have recently been relaxed considerably, as is shown by the increasing number and greater age of NIDDM patients treated [10, 96].

Cardiovascular disease is probably the most important factor to consider in selecting patients for renal replacement therapy. Patients with severe symptomatic coronary artery disease, severe cardiac failure and/or marked cardiomegaly generally fare badly [43] and should probably

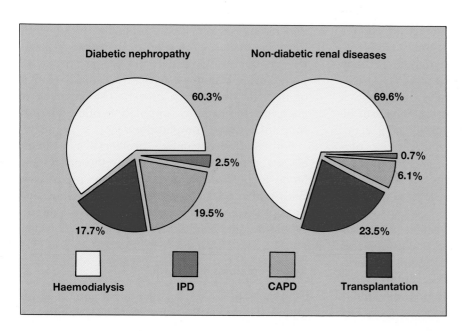

Fig. 67.15. Methods of renal replacement used to treat patients with diabetic nephropathy and other primary renal diseases throughout Europe in 1985. IPD and CAPD = intermittent and continuous ambulatory peritoneal dialysis respectively. (Redrawn from [12] with kind permission of Martinus Nijhoff Publishing, Boston.)

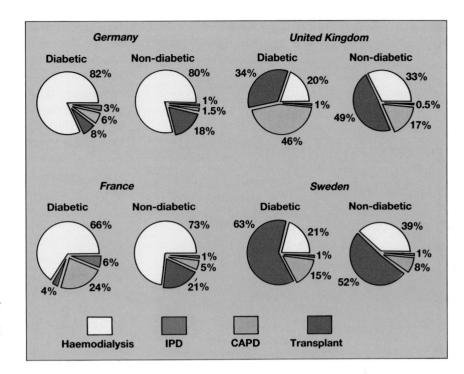

Fig. 67.16. Methods of renal replacement used to treat patients with diabetic nephropathy and other primary renal diseases in four different European countries in 1985. (Redrawn from [12] with kind permission of Martinus Nijhoff Publishing, Boston.)

be referred for dialysis rather than transplantation. Peripheral vascular disease does not contraindicate treatment but may limit vascular access for haemodialysis. Incipient or established gangrene and sepsis are contraindications for transplantation because of the risks of infection during immunosuppression.

Autonomic neuropathy may exacerbate hypotension during haemodialysis whereas a neuropathic bladder is a relative contraindication to transplantation. The presence of retinopathy should not influence decisions about renal replacement therapy. Deterioration of vision during haemodialysis is now rare with better treatment of hypertension and fluid overload and with early and more effective laser treatment. Blind patients usually manage well with all forms of treatment, including CAPD [97].

Timing of renal replacement

Previously, diabetic patients were often referred very late or treated according to the criteria used for non-diabetic patients. However, diabetic patients are now recognized to have symptoms (especially of fluid overload) at lower creatinine levels than non-diabetic subjects. Earlier treatment is therefore now recommended. In Minneapolis, for example, transplantation is advised when serum creatinine levels reach about

500 μmol/l, an approach made possible by a large number of live related donors [19]. However, a period of uraemia is thought to help to prevent rejection by inducing a degree of immunosuppression; transplantation should therefore not be performed too early. Aggressive treatment of hypertension and fluid overload may make this compromise possible.

Transplantation

Renal transplantation has been available as a routine treatment for diabetic patients with end-stage renal failure in some centres for over 15 years and is considered by many to be the treatment of choice. The criteria identifying patients suitable for transplantation are outlined in Table 67.3.

The early results of renal transplantation in diabetic patients [16, 17, 43], although not as good as for non-diabetic patients, were considerably better than for chronic haemodialysis [98, 99]. Subsequent reports emphasized the value of renal transplantation for diabetic patients with renal failure [30, 38, 42, 47] and their considerably improved survival (Fig. 67.17). At some centres, the survival of diabetic patients who receive grafts from living donors is now the same as for non-diabetic subjects [18, 19]. Results of cadaver transplantation are less favourable but have

Table 67.3. Criteria for renal transplantation.

- Age <65 years
- Absence of severe cardiac disease
- Absence of sepsis
- Suitable donor available

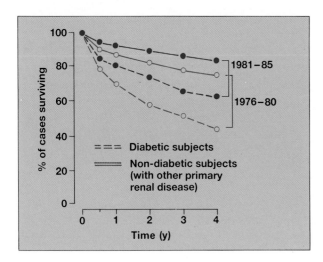

Fig. 67.17. Patient survival after first cadaver graft, for diabetic subjects and patients with other primary renal diseases, showing the improved survival of diabetic patients transplanted in 1981–85 (●) as compared with 1976–80 (○). (Adapted from [12] with kind permission of Martinus Nijhoff Publishing, Boston.)

nonetheless improved markedly. Factors underlying these improved results include the use of pretransplant blood transfusions, earlier acceptance and treatment of diabetic patients, better pretransplant management of hypertension and fluid overload, improved immunosuppression regimens with cyclosporin and lower steroid dosages, and better management of diabetes using intensive insulin regimens.

Preparation of the diabetic patient for transplantation is similar to that for non-diabetic subjects but also requires the careful assessment and treatment of diabetic complications. Transplantation, if possible, should be performed before dialysis is needed, especially in patients with live related donors.

Careful diabetic control during and after transplantation is important. Perioperatively, all patients should be treated with continuous intravenous insulin infusion (see Chapter 81) until able to eat and drink (usually within 24 h). The use of steroids following transplantation usually demands an increase in insulin dose (often exceeding 50%) in IDDM patients and

transfer to insulin in NIDDM patients. A regimen of soluble insulin before each meal and an intermediate-acting insulin before bed is suitable immediately postoperatively while insulin requirements are being established. Intravenous methylprednisolone for treating rejection episodes always causes severe hyperglycaemia which is best treated with a continuous intravenous insulin infusion started with the first pulse of steroid [100]. Increased oral steroids can usually be covered by increased doses of subcutaneous insulin.

Excellent rehabilitation is possible for diabetic patients following renal transplantation [13, 42]. At King's College Hospital, 80% of diabetic transplant patients were fit (although only half of these were in full-time work) and 20% of those transplanted between 1974–1987 have survived for longer than 5 years (range, 6–14 years) with good rehabilitation; the Minneapolis group have reported 26 patients surviving for over 10 years [101].

Histological changes compatible with diabetic nephropathy can be detected in most transplanted kidneys after about 4 years [102, 103] but vary considerably from minimal to severe changes. No transplanted kidney has yet been reported to have failed due to diabetic nephropathy *per se*.

Haemodialysis

Despite the high transplant rates of some renal units and some countries, dialysis is the only treatment available for most patients [12, 92, 104]. Dialysis is indicated in patients unsuitable for transplantation, while awaiting transplantation or following graft failures. The early results of chronic haemodialysis in diabetic patients were very poor, with 2-year survival rates of only 20–40% and a high morbidity rate [105, 106]. Improved dialysis techniques and earlier dialysis, together with effective management of hypertension, metabolic state and nutrition, have made dialysis a viable long-term treatment option for the diabetic patient [40, 107].

Diabetic patients need careful preparation for haemodialysis. Dialysis may need to be started at lower serum creatinine levels (about 500 μmol/l) than in non-diabetic subjects because of the tendency to fluid retention and volume-dependent hypertension. Haemodialysis poses special problems in diabetic patients (Table 67.4). Vascular access should be created 3–6 months in

Table 67.4. Problems of haemodialysis in diabetic patients.

- Difficult vascular access and failure of A–V fistulae
- Haemodynamic instability
- Erratic glycaemic control
- Progression of retinopathy
- Poor rehabilitation

advance, as technical problems due to arteriosclerosis and medial calcification are commoner and maturation of fistulae slower than in non-diabetic patients.

Arteriovenous fistulae also tend to fail prematurely: about 67% remain functional at 1 year compared with 83% in non-diabetic patients [108]. Bovine or PTFE grafts appear to survive better. Distal ischaemia causing pain and/or digital necrosis may supervene, sometimes requiring closure of the fistula or graft and occasionally amputation [109].

Satisfactory metabolic control during dialysis may be hard to achieve [110]. It is often difficult to impose fluid restriction on patients with thirst due to hyperglycaemia and to maintain adequate nutrition. Dialysate containing glucose (5–8 mmol/l) should be used to prevent hypoglycaemia and minimize protein catabolism and ketone body production. Insulin requirements may be very variable, depending on the patient's appetite, physical activity and other medical problems. With worsening renal failure, insulin requirements generally fall due to reduced renal clearance of insulin. On starting dialysis, insulin requirements increase, often to twice the pre-dialysis level.

Chronic haemodialysis in diabetic patients was previously associated with rapid progression of retinopathy, leading to blindness in 40% of cases [111]. With earlier dialysis, improved treatment of hypertension and fluid overload and above all, active treatment of diabetic eye disease before beginning dialysis, only 3% of cases now suffer visual loss [40]. Indeed, vision may improve after starting dialysis due to loss of retinal oedema.

Significant postural hypotension due to autonomic neuropathy may make it impossible to remove enough fluid at haemodialysis to achieve the patient's optimal 'dry' weight, which is an important factor in the successful control of hypertension. Certain antihypertensive drugs aggravate the problem but can often be omitted while excess body fluid is gradually decreased over several weeks by progressive ultrafiltration. If blood pressure falls during dialysis before optimum weight has been achieved, it may be better to use hypertonic rather than normal saline to expand the intravascular volume as smaller volumes of fluid are required.

The prognosis of diabetic patients receiving haemodialysis has improved dramatically during the past 20 years. The 1- and 5-year survival figures of 85% and 45% respectively are now similar to those for cadaver transplants and many patients have survived for over a decade [107, 112]. In those over the age of 60 years, however, survival is much poorer. An important cause of death is withdrawal from dialysis by patients [107]. Prognosis and rehabilitation are worse in patients treated by haemodialysis than following transplantation, partly because older, high-risk patients are selected for dialysis [107]. Long-term survivors (>4 years) seem to have better rehabilitation [104].

Peritoneal dialysis

Peritoneal dialysis, and particularly continuous ambulatory peritoneal dialysis (CAPD), offers specific benefits to the diabetic patient as well as its general advantages of independence and low cost (Table 67.5). Vascular access is not required. Extracellular fluid volume and blood pressure do not fluctuate rapidly, which benefits patients with ischaemic heart disease or severe autonomic neuropathy. Another major advantage of CAPD is that insulin may be administered intraperitoneally, which can provide a simple, physiological and very effective method of metabolic control. Intraperitoneal insulin is absorbed mainly by diffusion across the visceral peritoneum into the portal venous circulation and directly through the capsule of the liver, thereby acting preferentially on the liver and avoiding peripheral hyperinsulinaemia. Insulin is absorbed fastest when administered into an empty peritoneal cavity but most patients add insulin to their peritoneal

Table 67.5. Advantages of continuous ambulatory peritoneal dialysis (CAPD).

- Vascular access not required
- Haemodynamic instability rare
- Good metabolic control with intraperitoneal insulin
- Better rehabilitation

dialysis bags, which produces peak insulin levels 90–120 min later [113]. Insulin absorption continues throughout the dwell time (6–8 h) but amounts only to about 50% of the total insulin administered. As peritoneal dialysis fluid contains glucose as an osmotic agent, which is partly absorbed and further increases insulin requirements, the daily intraperitoneal insulin dose is usually about twice the previous subcutaneous dose. The estimated daily requirement should be divided equally between the number of dialysis bags used (usually four); a reduced dose may be needed in the overnight bag to avoid nocturnal hypoglycaemia. Higher insulin doses, often double those used in isosmotic ('weak') bags, are required when hypertonic ('strong') bags of higher glucose concentration are used. CAPD exchanges containing insulin should be timed for 30–40 min before meals to match peak insulin action with food absorption and so minimize postprandial glycaemic swings. Excellent control can be achieved and insulin requirements often remain remarkably stable [114, 115].

Visual impairment is not a contraindication to CAPD [93]. With good education and support, blind patients can achieve excellent results [97]. Injection aids are available, or insulin can be injected into the dialysis bag by a nurse or partner up to 24 h before use without significant adsorption of the insulin on to the plastic bags [116]. Blood glucose monitors and other equipment designed for visually impaired patients are described in Chapter 60.

The most important complication of CAPD is peritonitis, occurring at very similar rates (1–2 episodes per patient per year) in non-diabetic and diabetic patients [93, 14, 117]. The commonest organisms causing peritonitis in both groups of patients are skin bacteria, notably *Staphylococcus epidermidis*, accounting for about 40% of bacterial peritonitis. Other organisms isolated include *Staphylococcus aureus*, *Streptococcus viridans*, Gram-negative enteric organisms and very rarely anaerobic organisms. Peritonitis is occasionally caused by fungi. Treatment is the same for both diabetic and non-diabetic patients. Most episodes are mild and can be treated at home by the patient injecting antibiotics into the dialysis bags. Occasional severe episodes require hospital admission and parenteral antibiotics. The majority recover without complications but occasionally the dialysis catheter has to be removed due to persistent infection. Recurrent infections require

a period of about a month off CAPD, when temporary haemodialysis is needed. During episodes of peritonitis, insulin requirements are usually increased [118]. The inflamed peritoneum increases absorption of both insulin and glucose, and the latter may lead to fluid retention, requiring additional exchanges or more frequent use of hypertonic dialysis fluid.

Long-term survival with CAPD is possible (Table 67.6) [93, 119]. Although experience is still limited, the outcome is probably somewhat worse for patients with diabetic nephropathy than with non-diabetic renal disease.

Progression of complications following renal replacement therapy

Following renal replacement therapy, diabetic patients have a higher mortality (especially from cardiovascular disease) and morbidity than non-diabetic patients, because of coexistent diabetic complications.

Cardiovascular disease is the major determinant of outcome during renal replacement in both diabetic and non-diabetic subjects. Most early deaths in diabetic patients treated with dialysis or transplantation are due to pre-existing cardiovascular disease [107]. Long-term survivors tend to be relatively free of cardiovascular disease at the time of starting renal replacement therapy [112], but this remains the most important cause of morbidity and mortality: of those surviving for over 10 years after transplantation by the Minneapolis group, 20% have suffered myocardial infarcts and 15% strokes [101]. Of the 163 patients treated at King's College Hospital between 1974–1987, 15% suffered new cardiac events; three-quarters of these have died, most from myocardial infarction. Patients receiving haemodialysis appear to have the highest cardiovascular

Table 67.6. Actuarial survival (%) of diabetic patients treated by CAPD.

| Study | Year | Years of CAPD | | |
		1	2	3
Legrain *et al.* [41]	1984	85	68	62
Rottembourg *et al.* [118]	1985	85	63	58
Grefberg *et al.* [119]	1984	80	57	—
Amair *et al.* [114]	1982	92	81	—
Berisa *et al.* [93]	1988	88	71	47

mortality (50–65%), although this may largely reflect selection bias [40, 112].

Amputation is disturbingly common in diabetic patients receiving renal replacement. The higher rate after renal transplantation [37, 47] may be because many dialysis patients die before the need for amputation arises. The Minneapolis group have reported that following renal transplantation, 17% of diabetic patients underwent amputations (mostly of the lower limb), of whom two-thirds had more than one amputation [37]; 70% of amputations occurred 2 years or more after transplantation and 30% of patients surviving for over 10 years had undergone amputation [101]. Overall amputation rates reported by other groups range from 7% at King's College Hospital (A. Grenfell, unpublished observations) to 25% in Scandinavia [13]. Digital gangrene is particularly common and in some cases may be related to difficulties with vascular access. Patients receiving either CAPD or haemodialysis apparently have amputation rates of about 5–10% [40, 93, 95].

Neuropathic ulceration is a considerable problem during renal replacement therapy, affecting up to 20–25% of patients. Sepsis may spread rapidly to threaten the limb, especially in immunosuppressed patients, and may ultimately require ray excision or extensive amputation. Motor and sensory nerve conduction measurements show little change 1–2 years after transplantation [120], which is in contrast to reports of striking improvement in muscle weakness following transplantation [30, 47, 120]. Patients with severe somatic neuropathy show little symptomatic improvement after transplantation [47], but some autonomic symptoms may improve, notably gustatory sweating [32], postural hypotension [13], vomiting and diarrhoea.

As mentioned above, modern practice generally prevents significant deterioration in retinopathy and visual acuity often remains stable, especially in those with good vision before treatment [30, 47]. The frequency of blindness during haemodialysis has fallen dramatically [95], for the reasons discussed above rather than due to changes in heparinization [121], and is now comparable with that in transplanted patients [122]. However, retinopathy does progress: one-third of patients with background retinopathy at transplantation subsequently developed proliferative retinopathy [122]. About 30% of patients are blind 3–10 years after starting treatment, although most had been blind before renal replacement therapy:

only one of the 26 patients surviving longer than 10 years after renal transplantation by the Minneapolis group became blind during this period [101].

Recent advances in laser therapy and microsurgery (see Chapter 59), together with more effective treatment of hypertension, should mean that fewer diabetic patients with nephropathy will become blind in the future, either before or after renal replacement therapy. Regular fundoscopy and testing of visual acuity are crucial.

Rehabilitation is obviously affected by severe visual impairment or blindness, but there is no evidence that the outcome of renal replacement therapy is adversely affected. One report suggesting that visually impaired patients had a poor prognosis following renal transplantation is probably explicable by the association with severe cardiac disease [43].

Causes of death following renal replacement therapy

Cardiovascular disease and sepsis are the commonest causes of death in patients undergoing renal replacement therapy, whether diabetic or not. Among diabetic patients, cardiovascular deaths are particularly frequent, accounting for 50–65% of deaths [30–32, 40, 41, 43, 93, 107]. Fatal coronary heart disease is about 10 times commoner in young diabetic patients receiving renal replacement therapy than in comparable patients with other diseases. Cerebrovascular disease is also common: strokes account for about 10–12% of deaths in dialysed patients and for somewhat fewer in transplant recipients (6%).

Sepsis, sometimes arising from gangrenous lesions, is a common and serious complication responsible for between 30–50% of deaths [123]. Fatal sepsis is about twice as frequent in transplanted patients as in those receiving dialysis (presumably because of immunosuppressive treatment in the former), but relatively high rates are reported with increasing duration of dialysis [112].

Withdrawal from treatment may account for as many as 24% of deaths in diabetic dialysis patients [40, 112]. Patients with diabetes withdraw from dialysis about 4–5 times more commonly than non-diabetic patients, probably because of coexistent severe medical complications [124].

Conclusions

The last decade has seen many improvements in the management of diabetic nephropathy. The conviction is now growing that the evolution of the early stages of the disease, which can now be identified relatively easily, can be favourably modified by effective antihypertensive therapy and perhaps by other measures including a moderately restricted protein intake.

There is now no doubt that renal replacement therapy by transplantation, haemodialysis or CAPD is virtually as successful in diabetic as in non-diabetic people; it is no longer acceptable to regard end-stage diabetic nephropathy as untreatable.

ANASUYA GRENFELL

References

1 Joslin EP, Root HF, White P, Marble A. *The Treatment of Diabetes Mellitus*. Philadelphia: Lea & Febiger, 1959.
2 Borch-Johnsen K, Andersen PK, Deckert T. The effect of proteinuria on relative mortality in Type 1 (insulin-dependent) diabetes mellitus. *Diabetologia* 1985; **28**: 590−6.
3 Borch-Johnsen K, Kreiner S. Proteinuria: value as predictor of cardiovascular mortality in insulin dependent diabetes mellitus. *Br Med J* 1987; **294**: 1651−4.
4 Andersen AR, Christiansen JS, Andersen JK, Kreiner S, Deckert T. Diabetic nephropathy in Type 1 (insulin dependent) diabetes: An epidemiological study. *Diabetologia* 1983; **25**: 496−501.
5 Moloney A, Tunbridge WMG, Ireland JT, Watkins PJ. Mortality from diabetic nephropathy in the United Kingdom. *Diabetologia* 1983; **25**: 26−30.
6 Mogensen CE. Microalbuminuria predicts clinical proteinuria and early mortality in maturity-onset diabetes. *N Engl J Med* 1984; **310**: 356−60.
7 Jarrett RJ, Viberti GC, Argyropoulos A, Hill RD, Mahmud U, Murrels TJ. Microalbuminuria predicts mortality in non-insulin dependent diabetes. *Diabetic Med* 1984; **2**: 17−19.
8 Rettig B, Teutsch SM. The incidence of end-stage renal disease in type I and type II diabetes mellitus. *Diabetic Nephropathy* 1984; **3**: 26−7.
9 Grenfell A, Bewick M, Parsons V, Snowden S, Taube D, Watkins PJ. Non-insulin dependent diabetes and renal replacement therapy. *Diabetic Med* 1988; **5**: 172−6.
10 Cameron JS, Challah S. Treatment of end-stage renal failure due to diabetes in the United Kingdom 1975−1984. *Lancet* 1986; ii: 962−6.
11 Ordonez JD, Hiatt RA. Comparison of type II and type I diabetics treated for end-stage renal disease in a large prepaid health plan population. *Nephron* 1989; **51**: 524−9.
12 Challah S, Brunner FP, Wing AJ. Evolution of the treatment of patients with diabetic nephropathy by renal replacement therapy in Europe over a decade: Data from the EDTA registry. In: Mogensen CE, ed. *The Kidney and Hypertension in Diabetes Mellitus*. Boston: Martinus Nijhoff Publishing, 1988; 365−77.
13 Jervell J, Dahl BO, Fauchold P et al. Clinical results of renal transplantation in diabetic patients. *Transplant Proc* 1984; **16**: 599−602.
14 Shyh T-P, Beyer MM, Friedman EA. Treatment of the uremic diabetic. *Nephron* 1985; **40**: 129−38.
15 Working Party Report. Renal failure in diabetics in the UK: Deficient provision of care in 1985. *Diabetic Med* 1988; **5**: 79−84.
16 Barnes BA, Bergan JJ, Braun WE et al. The 12th report of the human renal transplant registry. Prepared by the Advisory Committee to the Renal Transplant Registry. *J Am Med Ass* 1975; **233**: 787−96.
17 Kjellstrand CM, Simmons RL, Goetz FC et al. Renal transplantation in patients with insulin dependent diabetes. *Lancet* 1973; ii: 4−8.
18 Brynger H, Nyberg G, Larsson O. Renal transplantation, the optimal treatment for renal failure in diabetic patients. *Transplant Proc* 1986; **18**: 1713−14.
19 Sutherland DER, Canafax DM, Goetz FC, Najarian JS. Renal transplantation in diabetic patients: the treatment of choice. In: Mogensen CE, ed. *The Kidney and Hypertension in Diabetes Mellitus*. Boston: Martinus Nijhoff Publishing, 1988; 341−7.
20 Grenfell A, Watkins PJ. Clinical diabetic nephropathy. Natural history and complications. *Clin Endocrinol Metab* 1986; **15**: 783−805.
21 Krowleski AS, Warram JH, Christlieb AR et al. The changing natural history of nephropathy in type 1 diabetes. *Am J Med* 1985; **78**: 785−94.
22 Viberti GC, Keen H. The patterns of proteinuria in diabetes mellitus. *Diabetes* 1984; **33**: 686−92.
23 Mogensen CE. High blood pressure as a factor in the progression of diabetic nephropathy. *Acta Med Scand* 1976; **602** (suppl): 29−32.
24 Parving H-H, Andersen AR, Smidt VM, Oxenbøll B, Edsberg B, Christiansen JS. Diabetic nephropathy and arterial hypertension. *Diabetologia* 1983; **24**: 10−12.
25 Wiseman M, Viberti GC, Mackintosh D, Jarrett RJ, Keen H. Glycaemia, arterial pressure, and microalbuminuria in Type 1 (insulin-dependent) diabetes mellitus. *Diabetologia* 1984; **26**: 401−5.
26 Mathiesen ER, Oxenbøll K, Johansen PAa, Svendsen PA, Deckert T. Incipient nephropathy in Type 1 (insulin-dependent) diabetes. *Diabetologia* 1984; **26**: 406−10.
27 Sampson MJ, Chambers J, Spriggings D, Drury PJ. Echocardiographic evidence of relative left ventricular hypertrophy in Type 1 (insulin-dependent) diabetic patients with microalbuminuria. *Diabetologia* 1988; **31**: 539A.
28 Knussman MJ, Goldstein HH, Gleason RE. The clinical course of diabetic nephropathy. *J Am Med Assoc* 1976; **236**: 1861−3.
29 Bennett WM, Kloster F, Rosch J, Barry J, Porter GA. Natural history of asymptomatic coronary arteriographic lesions in diabetic patients with end-stage renal disease. *Am J Med* 1978; **65**: 779−84.
30 Libertino JA, Zinman L, Salerno R, D'Elia J, Kaldany A, Weinrauch LA. Diabetic renal transplantation. *J Urol* 1980; **124**: 593−5.
31 Rohrer RJ, Madras PN, Sahyoun AI, Monaco AP. Renal transplantation in the diabetic. *World J Surg* 1986; **10**: 397−403.
32 Gonzalez-Carrillo M, Moloney A, Bewick M, Parsons V, Rudge CJ, Watkins PJ. Renal transplantation in diabetic nephropathy. *Br Med J* 1982; **285**: 1713−16.

33 Braun WE, Phillips DF, Vidt DG *et al*. Coronary artery disease in 100 diabetics with end-stage renal failure. *Transplant Proc* 1984; **16**: 603–7.

34 D'Elia JA, Weinrauch LA, Healy RN, Libertino JA, Bradley RF, Leland OS. Myocardial dysfunction without coronary artery disease in diabetic renal failure. *Am J Cardiol* 1979; **43**: 193–9.

35 Grenfell A, Monaghan M, Watkins PJ, McCleod AA. Left ventricular hypertrophy in diabetic nephropathy: An echocardiographic study. *Diabetic Med* 1988; **5**: 840–4.

36 Shapiro LM. A prospective study of heart disease in diabetes mellitus. *Q J Med* 1984; **209**: 55–68.

37 Peters C, Sutherland DER, Simmons RL, Fryd DS, Najarian JS. Patient and graft survival in amputated versus non-amputated diabetic primary renal allograft recipients. *Transplantation* 1981; **32**: 498–503.

38 Wilczek H, Gunnarsson R, Lundgren G, Ost L. Improved results of renal transplantation in diabetic nephropathy. *Transplant Proc* 1984; **16**: 623–7.

39 Rao VK, Andersen RC. The impact of diabetes on vascular complications following cadaver renal transplantation. *Transplantation* 1987; **43**: 193–7.

40 Shapiro FL. Haemodialysis in diabetic patients. In: Keen H, Legrain M, eds. *Prevention and Treatment of Diabetic Nephropathy*. Lancaster: MTP Press, 1983; 247–59.

41 Legrain M, Rottembourg J, Bentchikou A *et al*. Dialysis treatment of insulin dependent diabetic patients: ten year experience. *Clin Nephrol* 1984; **21**: 72–81.

42 Najarian JS, Sutherland DER, Simmons RL *et al*. Ten year experience with renal transplantation in juvenile onset diabetics. *Ann Surg* 1979; **190**: 487–500.

43 Jervell J, Dahl BO, Flatmark A *et al*. Renal transplantation in insulin dependent diabetics. A joint Scandinavian report. *Lancet* 1978; ii: 915–17.

44 Strandness DE Jr, Priest RE, Gibbons GE. Combined clinical and pathological study of diabetic and non-diabetic peripheral arterial disease. *Diabetes* 1964; **13**: 366–72.

45 Gilbey SG, Grenfell A, Edmonds ME, Archer A, Watkins PJ. Vascular calcification, autonomic neuropathy, and peripheral blood flow in patients with diabetic nephropathy. *Diabetic Med* 1989; **6**: 37–42.

46 Edmonds ME, Morrison N, Laws JW, Watkins PJ. Medial arterial calcification and diabetic neuropathy. *Br Med J* 1982; **284**: 928–30.

47 Khauli RB, Novick AC, Braun WE *et al*. Improved results of cadaver renal transplantation in the diabetic patient. *J Urol* 1983; **130**: 867–70.

48 Traeger J, Dubenard JM, Bosie E *et al*. Patient selection and risk factors in organ transplantation in diabetics: experience with kidney and pancreas. *Transplant Proc* 1984; **16**: 577–82.

49 Horowitz M, Collins PJ, Shearman DJC. Disorders of gastric emptying in humans and the use of radionuclide techniques. *Arch Intern Med* 1985; **145**: 1467–72.

50 Page MMcB, Watkins PJ. Cardiorespiratory arrest and diabetic autonomic neuropathy. *Lancet* 1978; i: 14–16.

51 Ramsay RC, Knoblach WH, Barbosa JJ, Sutherland DER, Kjellstrand CM, Najarian JS *et al*. The visual status of diabetic patients after renal transplantation. *Am J Ophthalmol* 1979; **87**: 305–10.

52 Kohner E, Chahal PS. Retinopathy in diabetic nephropathy (a preliminary report) In: Keen M, Legrain M, eds. *Prevention and Treatment of Diabetic Nephropathy*. Lancaster: MTP Press, 1983; 191–6.

53 Kasinath BS, Mujais SK, Spargo BH, Katz AI. Non-diabetic renal disease in patients with diabetes mellitus. *Am J Med* 1983; **75**: 613–17.

54 Yum M, Maxwell DR, Hamburger R, Kleit SA. Primary glomerulonephritis complicating diabetic nephropathy: a report of 7 cases and review of the literature. *Hum Pathol* 1984; **15**: 921–7.

55 Fabre J, Balant LP, Dayer PG, Fox HM, Vernet AT. The kidney in maturity onset diabetes mellitus: A clinical study of 510 patients. *Kidney Int* 1982; **21**: 730–8.

56 Ellis EN, Steffes MW, Goetz FC, Sutherland DER, Mauer SM. Relationship of renal size to nephropathy in Type 1 (insulin-dependent) diabetes. *Diabetologia* 1985; **28**: 12–15.

57 Etz J, Ritz E, Hasslacher C, Gotz R. Renal size in diabetics with endstage renal failure. *Diabetic Nephropathy* 1985; **4**: 77–9.

58 Wass JAH, Watkins PJ, Dische FE, Parsons V. Renal failure, glomerular disease and diabetes mellitus. *Nephron* 1978; **21**: 289–96.

59 Hommel E, Carstensen H, Skøtt P *et al*. Prevalence and causes of microscopic haematuria in Type 1 (insulin-dependent) diabetic patients with persistent proteinuria. *Diabetologia* 1987; **30**: 627–30.

60 O'Neill WM, Wallim JD, Walker PD. Hematuria and red cell casts in typical diabetic nephropathy. *Am J Med* 1983; **74**: 381–95.

61 Viberti GC, Bilous RW, Mackintosh D, Keen H. Monitoring glomerular function in diabetic nephropathy. A prospective study. *Am J Med* 1983; **74**: 256–64.

62 Grenfell A. Acute renal failure in diabetics. In: Mogensen CE, ed. *The Kidney and Hypertension in Diabetes Mellitus*. Boston: Martinus Nijhoff Publishing, 1988; 243–50.

63 Eknoyan G. Renal papillary necrosis in diabetic patients. In: Mogensen CE, ed. *The Kidney and Hypertension in Diabetes Mellitus*. Boston: Martinus Nijhoff Publishing, 1988; 259–67.

64 Medina M, Tomasula JR, Cohen LS, Laungani GB, Butt KMH, Friedman EA. Diabetic cystopathy. In: Mogensen CE, ed. *The Kidney and Hypertension in Diabetes Mellitus*. Boston: Martinus Nijhoff Publishing, 1988; 269–81.

65 Manis T, Friedman EA. Contrast media induced nephropathy in diabetic nephropathy. In: Mogensen CE, ed. *The Kidney and Hypertension in Diabetes Mellitus*. Boston: Martinus Nijhoff Publishing, 1988; 251–8.

66 Anto HR, Chou SY, Porush JG, Schapiro WB. Infusion intravenous pyelography and renal function: effects of hypertonic mannitol in patients with chronic renal insufficiency. *Arch Intern Med* 1981; **141**: 1652–6.

67 Mogensen CE. Long term anti-hypertensive treatment inhibiting progression of diabetic nephropathy. *Br Med J* 1982; **285**: 685–8.

68 Parving H-H, Andersen AR, Smidt UM, Hommel E, Mathiesen ER, Svendsen PAå. Effect of anti-hypertensive treatment on kidney function in diabetic nephropathy. *Br Med J* 1987; **294**: 1443–7.

69 Björck S, Nyberg G, Mulec H, Granerus G, Herlitz H, Aurell M. Beneficial effects of angiotensin converting enzyme inhibition on renal function in patients with diabetic nephropathy. *Br Med J* 1986; **293**: 471–4.

70 Christensen CK, Mogensen CE. Antihypertensive treatment: long term reversal of progression of albuminuria in incipient diabetic nephropathy. A longitudinal study of renal function. *J Diabetic Compl* 1987; **1**: 45–52.

71 Marre M, Chatellier G, Leblanc H *et al*. Prevention of diabetic nephropathy with enalapril in normotensive diabetics with microalbuminuria. *Br Med J* 1988; **297**: 1092–5.

72 Acheson RM. Blood pressure in a national sample of US adults: percentile distribution by age, sex, and race. *Int J Epidemiol* 1973; **2**: 293–301.

73 Weidman P, Beretta-Piccoli C, Keusch G *et al.* Sodium-volume factor, cardiovascular reactivity and hypotensive mechanism of diuretic therapy in mild hypertension associated with diabetes mellitus. *Am J Med* 1979; **67**: 779–84.

74 O'Hare JA, Ferriss JB, Brady D, Twomey B, O'Sullivan DJ. Exchangeable sodium and renin in hypertensive diabetic patients with and without nephropathy. *Hypertension* 1985; **7** (suppl 2): II43–8.

75 Anderson S, Brenner BM. Pathogenesis of diabetic glomerulopathy: Haemodynamic considerations. *Diabetes Metab Rev* 1988; **4**: 163–77.

76 Viberti GC, Bilous RW, Mackintosh D, Bending JJ, Keen H. Long term correction of hyperglycaemia and progression of renal failure in insulin dependent diabetes. *Br Med J* 1983; **286**: 598–602.

77 Bending JJ, Viberti GC, Watkins PJ, Keen H. Intermittent clinical proteinuria and renal function in diabetes: evolution and the effect of glycaemic control. *Br Med J* 1986; **292**: 83–6.

78 Nyberg G, Blohme G, Norden G. Impact of metabolic control in progression of clinical diabetic nephropathy. *Diabetologia* 1987; **3**: 82–6.

79 Brenner BM, Meyer TW, Hostetter TH. Dietary protein intake and the progressive nature of kidney disease. *N Engl J Med* 1982; **307**: 652–60.

80 Hostetter TH, Meyer TW, Rennke HG, Brenner BM. Chronic effects of dietary protein in the rat with intact and reduced renal mass. *Kidney Int* 1986; **30**: 509–17.

81 Rosman JB, Ter Wee PM, Meyer S, Piers-Becht TPM, Sluiter WJ, Dohker AJM. Prospective randomised trial of early dietary protein restriction in chronic renal failure. *Lancet* 1984; ii: 1291–6.

82 Attman PO, Bucht H, Larsson O, Uddebom G. Protein reduced diet in diabetic renal failure. *Clin Nephrol* 1983; **19**: 217–20.

83 Nyberg G, Norden G, Attman PO *et al.* Diabetic nephropathy: is dietary protein harmful? *J Diabetic Compl* 1987; **1**: 37–40.

84 Bending JJ, Dodds R, Keen H, Viberti GC. Lowering protein intake and progression of diabetic renal failure. *Diabetologia* 1986; **29**: 516A.

85 Walker JD, Bending JJ, Dodds RA, Mattock MB, Murrell TJ, Keen H, Viberti GC. Restriction of dietary protein and progression of renal failure in diabetic nephropathy. *Lancet* 1989; ii: 1411–15.

86 Barsotti G, Ciardella F, Morelli E, Cupisti A, Mantovanelli A, Giovanetti S. Nutritional treatment of renal failure in type 1 diabetic nephropathy. *Clin Nephrol* 1988; **29**: 280–7.

87 Levine SE, D'Elia JA, Bistrian B *et al.* Protein-restricted diets in diabetic nephropathy. *Nephron* 1989; **52**: 55–61.

88 Nutrition Sub-Committee of the Medical Advisory Committee of the British Diabetic Association. *Dietary recommendation for diabetics in the 1980s.* The British Diabetic Association, London, 1982.

89 Morrow CE, Schwartz JS, Sutherland DER *et al.* Predictive value of thallium stress testing for coronary and cardiovascular events in uremic diabetic patients before renal transplantation. *Am J Surg* 1983; **146**: 331–5.

90 Edmonds ME, Blundell MP, Morris HE *et al.* Improved survival of the diabetic foot: the role of a special foot clinic. *Q J Med* 1986; **232**: 763–71.

91 Edmonds ME. The diabetic foot: pathophysiology and treatment. *Clin Endocrinol Metab* 1986; **15**: 889–916.

92 Joint Working Party on Diabetic Renal Failure of the British Diabetic Association, Renal Association and the Research Unit of the Royal College of Physicians. Treatment of and mortality from diabetic renal failure in patients identified in the 1985 United Kingdom Survey. *Br Med J* 1989; **299**: 1135–6.

93 Berisa F, McGonigle R, Beaman M, Adu D, Michael J. The treatment of diabetic renal failure by continuous ambulatory peritoneal dialysis. *Diabetic Med* 1989; **6**: 67–70.

94 Brunner FP, Brynger H, Challah S *et al.* Renal replacement therapy in patients with diabetic nephropathy 1980–1985. Report from the European Dialysis and Transplant Association Registry. *Nephrol Dial Transplant* 1988; **3**: 585–95.

95 Whitley KY, Shapiro FL. Hemodialysis for end-stage diabetic nephropathy. In: Friedman EA, L'Esperance FA, eds. *Diabetic Renal–Retinal Syndrome 3.* New York: Grune and Stratton 1986; 349–62.

96 Cowie CC, Port FK, Wolfe RA, Savage PJ, Moll PP, Hawthorne VM. Disparities in incidence of diabetic end-stage renal disease according to race and type of diabetes. *N Engl J Med* 1989; **321**: 1074–9.

97 Flynn CT. Why blind diabetics with renal failure should be offered treatment. *Br Med J* 1983; **287**: 1177–8.

98 Totten MA, Izenstein B, Gleason RE, Kassissieh SD, Libertino JA, D'Elia JA. Chronic renal failure in diabetes: survival with hemodialysis versus transplantation. *Kidney Int* 1977; **12**: 492A.

99 Kjellstrand CM. Cadaver transplantation versus hemodialysis. *Trans Am Soc Artif Intern Organs* 1980; **26**: 611–24.

100 O'Donovan R, Devlin P, Bennet-Jones D, Parsons V, Bewick M, Weston M *et al.* The use of intravenous insulin in the treatment of diabetes during rejection episodes. *Transplant Proc* 1984; **16**: 643–4.

101 Sutherland DER, Bentley FR, Mauer SM *et al.* A report of 26 diabetic renal allograft recipients alive with functioning grafts at 10 or more years after primary transplantation. *Diabetic Nephropathy* 1984; **3**: 39–43.

102 Mauer SM, Goetz FC, McHugh LE, Sutherland DER, Barbosa J, Najarian JS *et al.* Long term study of normal kidneys transplanted into patients with type-1 diabetes. *Diabetes* 1989; **38**: 516–23.

103 Bohman S-O, Wilczek H, Jaremko G, Tyden G. Recurrence of diabetic nephropathy in renal transplants. In: Mogensen CE, ed. *The Kidney and Hypertension in Diabetes Mellitus.* Boston: Martinus Nijhoff Publishing, 1988; 395–402.

104 Jacobson SH, Fryd D, Sutherland DER, Kjellstrand CM. Treatment of the diabetic patient with end-stage renal failure. *Diabetes Metab Rev* 1988; **4**: 191–200

105 Ghavamian M, Gutch C, Kopp F, Kolff WJ. The sad truth about hemodialysis in diabetic nephropathy. *J Am Med Ass* 1972; **222**: 1386–9.

106 Shapiro FL, Leonard A, Comty CM. Mortality, morbidity, and rehabilitation. Results in regularly dialysed patients with diabetes mellitus. *Kidney Int* 1974; **6** (suppl 1): 8–14.

107 Matson M, Kjellstrand CM. Long-term follow-up of 369 diabetic patients undergoing dialysis. *Arch Intern Med* 1988; **148**: 600–4.

108 Aman LC, Levin NW, Smith DW. Hemodialysis access site morbidity. *Proc Clin Dial Transplant Forum* 1980; **10**: 277–82.

109 Buselmeier TJ, Najarian JS, Simmons RL. A–V fistulas

and the diabetic: ischemia and gangrene may result in amputation. *Trans Am Soc Artif Intern Organs* 1973; **19**: 49–52.

110 Levitz CS, Hirsch S, Ross JM *et al*. Lack of blood glucose control in hemodialyzed and renal transplantation diabetics. *Trans Am Soc Artif Intern Organs* 1980; **26**: 362–5.

111 Leonard A, Comty C, Raij L. The natural history of regularly dialysed diabetics. *Trans Am Soc Artif Intern Organs* 1973; **19**: 282–6.

112 Kjellstrand CM, Lins L-E. Hemodialysis in type 1 and type 2 diabetic patients with end-stage renal failure. In: Mogensen CE, ed. *The Kidney and Hypertension in Diabetes Mellitus*. Boston: Martinus Nijhoff Publishing, 1988; 323–30.

113 Schade DS, Eaton RP, Davis T *et al*. The kinetics of peritoneal insulin absorption. *Metabolism* 1981; **30**: 149–55.

114 Amair P, Khanna R, Leibel B *et al*. Continuous ambulatory peritoneal dialysis in diabetics with end-stage renal disease. *N Engl J Med* 1982; **306**: 625–30.

115 Madden MA, Zimmerman SW, Simpson DP. CAPD in diabetes mellitus: the risks and benefits of intraperitoneal insulin. *Am J Nephrol* 1982; **2**: 133–9.

116 Twardowski ZJ, Nolph KD, McGary TJ, Moore HL. Influence of temperature and time on insulin absorption to plastic bags. *Am J Hosp Pharm* 1983; **40**: 583–6.

117 *Report of the National CAPD registry*. A publication of the National CAPD Registry of the National Institute of Arthritis, Diabetes and Digestive and Kidney Disease. Bethesda MD, 1986, 25–36.

118 Rottembourg J, Remaoun M, Maiga K *et al*. Continuous ambulatory peritoneal dialysis in diabetic patients. *Diabetes Hypertension* 1985; **7** (suppl 11): 125–30.

119 Grefberg N, Danielson BG, Nilsson P. Continuous ambulatory peritoneal dialysis in the treatment of end-stage diabetic nephropathy. *Acta Med Scand* 1984; **215**: 427–34.

120 Barbosa J, Burke B, Busselmeier TJ *et al*. Neuropathy, retinopathy, and biopsy findings in transplanted kidney in diabetic patients. *Kidney Int* 1974; **6** (suppl 1): S32–6.

121 Diaz-Buxo JA, Burgess WP, Greenman M. Visual function in diabetics undergoing dialysis: comparison of peritoneal and hemodialysis. *Int J Artif Organs* 1984; **7**: 257–62.

122 Ramsay RC, Knobloch WH, Cantrill HL *et al*. Visual status in transplanted and dialysed diabetic patients. In: Friedman EA, L'Espérance FA, eds. *Diabetic Renal–Retinal Syndrome 2*. New York: Grune and Stratton, 1982, 427–35.

123 Sagalowsky AI, Gailiunas P, Helderman JH *et al*. Renal transplantation in diabetic patients: the end result does justify the means. *J Urol* 1983; **129**: 253–5.

124 Neu S, Kjellstrand CM. Stopping long-term dialysis. *N Engl J Med* 1986; **314**: 14–20.

PART 13.5
MACROVASCULAR DISEASE
AND HYPERTENSION

68 The Heart and Macrovascular Disease in Diabetes Mellitus

Summary

• Deaths from cardiovascular disease predominate in patients with diabetes of over 30 years' duration and in those diagnosed after 40 years of age. Patients with proteinuria have a greatly increased risk of fatal cardiovascular disease.

• The frequency of coronary heart disease (CHD) in diabetes is related to that in the background population (e.g. it is low in diabetic patients in China and Japan).

• General risk factors for cardiovascular disease include smoking, obesity, hyperlipidaemia, hypertension, insulin resistance, haemostatic and platelet abnormalities, lack of exercise and a positive family history. Specific diabetes-related risk factors may include hyperglycaemia (especially for peripheral vascular disease) and hyperinsulinaemia.

• CHD in diabetic patients is associated with increased plasma cholesterol levels, with reduced HDL-cholesterol in NIDDM patients, and possibly with increased triglyceride levels.

• The most common lipid abnormality in diabetes is raised triglyceride levels due to excess VLDL concentrations, caused by reduced clearance via the insulin-sensitive enzyme lipoprotein lipase and (in NIDDM) by increased VLDL production. Triglyceride levels often fall with intensified insulin treatment.

• LDL levels are also increased in poor metabolic control, due to decreased clearance by LDL receptors which are stimulated by insulin and have a lower affinity for glycosylated apoprotein B.

• HDL levels are reduced in NIDDM, in proportion to increased triglyceride and VLDL levels, but are relatively normal in IDDM; glycosylated HDL may be cleared more rapidly from the circulation.

• Hyperlipidaemia can be assessed from measurements of fasting plasma total cholesterol, HDL-cholesterol and triglyceride levels and calculation of LDL-cholesterol.

• Hyperlipidaemia is managed by improving metabolic control, dietary modification, stopping smoking and specific lipid-lowering drugs.

• A high-carbohydrate, low-fat (20–30% of total calories, 50% being unsaturated fat), low-cholesterol diet may lower cholesterol levels in IDDM. In NIDDM, weight reduction frequently lowers triglyceride concentrations and raises HDL.

• Lipid-lowering drugs suitable for use in diabetes include the fibrates (bezafibrate, gemfibrozil) for hypertriglyceridaemia or mixed hyperlipidaemia, and the resins (e.g. cholestyramine) and HMG CoA reductase inhibitors ('statins', e.g. simvastatin) for hypercholesterolaemia.

• Mortality from CHD in diabetic patients is increased about two and four times respectively for males and females, compared with the non-diabetic population.

• Acute myocardial infarction carries twice the mortality of that in the general population. Contributory factors may include coexistent diabetic cardiomyopathy, blunting of cardiac reflexes by autonomic neuropathy, and adverse cardiac and metabolic effects of increased non-esterified fatty acid levels.

• Acute myocardial infarction in diabetic patients should be managed with tight control of blood glucose and potassium levels and prompt

Table 68.1. Percentage cause of death according to age at diagnosis and duration of diabetes. (Modified from Marks and Krall 1971 [2].)

Age at onset:	<20				20–39				40–59				>60			
Duration (years)	<10	10–19	20–9	>30	<10	10–19	20–9	>30	<10	10–19	20–9	>30	<10	10–19	20–9	>30
Cause of death																
Macrovascular (total)	13	17	29	56	30	51	66	74	62	73	75	73	69	75	74	75
Cardiac	3	15	23	46	23	44	58	61	52	58	57	49	51	52	46	75
Cerebral	10	2	5	9	2	5	7	9	8	12	15	19	14	18	17	—
Other	—	—	1	1	5	2	1	3	2	3	3	5	4	5	11	—
Nephropathy	5	55	46	22	3	17	10	4	1	3	2	—	1	1	1	—
Other causes	82	28	25	22	67	32	24	22	37	24	23	27	30	24	25	25
All causes	100	100	100	100	100	100	100	100	100	100	100	100	100	100	100	100

treatment of cardiac failure; the role of thrombolytic drugs is not yet established and they should be avoided in proliferative retinopathy.

• The symptoms of angina may be masked in diabetes by autonomic neuropathy.

• Angina may be treated by nitrates, calcium channel antagonists or β-blockers; other diabetic complications may influence the choice of drug.

• Coronary artery atherosclerosis may be more diffuse and severe than in non-diabetic subjects but the frequency of inoperable vessels is no higher, and the results and survival after coronary artery bypass grafting are now comparable with those in the general population. Coronary artery surgery or angioplasty should therefore be considered if medical treatment of angina is ineffective.

• Breathlessness and exercise intolerance in a diabetic patient is often due to heart failure, in which physical examination and chest X-ray may be normal. Possible causes include diabetic cardiomyopathy with microvascular disease and interstitial fibrosis and defective myosin and actinomyosin ATPases; autonomic neuropathy may also contribute.

• Management of cardiac failure involves improved glycaemic control, treatment of hypertension and the use of nitrates, calcium channel antagonists, loop diuretics and angiotensin converting enzyme inhibitors.

• Half of all lower-limb amputations are performed in diabetic patients. However, proximal and distal bypass grafting now often achieve good results.

Microvascular disease is an important cause of morbidity in diabetes, but diseases of the larger arteries and the heart are responsible for well over half of all deaths in diabetic patients. There is an association between micro- and macrovascular disease, as is demonstrated by the large excess of cardiovascular deaths in patients with proteinuria [1]. Although small vessel disease is specific to diabetes, arterial and cardiac diseases are also the commonest cause of death in the general population; the increased risk associated with diabetes is shared by those with impaired glucose tolerance (IGT).

Epidemiology

Atherosclerotic arterial disease may be manifested clinically as coronary heart disease (CHD), cerebrovascular disease or peripheral vascular disease. The effect of diabetes on atherosclerosis is different at each of these sites. The relative risk of arterial disease also varies widely with gender, age, geographical location, type and duration of diabetes.

Mortality data from the Joslin Clinic [2] have been analysed according to age of onset and duration of diabetes (Table 68.1). In those diagnosed before the age of 20 years, there is a preponderance of renal deaths during the second and third decades of diabetes, but beyond 30 years from diagnosis, cardiovascular deaths predominate. In those diagnosed over the age of 40 years, renal disease only accounts for 1–2% of all deaths, and cardiovascular disease for 50–75%. In this group, the proportion of deaths attributable to CHD, but not to cerebral or peripheral arterial disease, is not related to the duration of diabetes.

These figures underline important differences between IDDM and NIDDM, which are often considered together in epidemiological studies.

NIDDM, which predominates in the age group where cardiovascular disease is common, accounts for most of the differences described below.

Coronary heart disease

In population studies, male diabetic patients have about twice, and females about 4 times, the CHD mortality rate of age- and sex-matched controls [3]. The mortality ratio is higher in young women: premenopausal non-diabetic females are at relatively low risk of CHD compared with males, but this protection is lost in diabetes. Non-fatal manifestations follow a similar pattern.

The Whitehall study of male civil servants has demonstrated twice the control rate of CHD mortality in subjects whose blood glucose concentration 2 h after a 50-g oral glucose load exceeded the 95th centile for the population (5.4 mmol/l) [4]. There was no trend in mortality at lower blood glucose levels, and the suggestion of a threshold effect for glucose has been supported by a number of other studies [3].

The frequency of CHD in diabetes depends on its frequency in the background population. In Japan and China, where the overall prevalence of CHD is low, angina and electrocardiographic (ECG) abnormalities are also uncommon in diabetic patients, although still commoner than in the background population [5]. Japanese migrants to Hawaii have a much higher CHD mortality than in Japan (presumably due to dietary differences), which is higher still in diabetic migrants [6]. If changes in diet can raise the risk of CHD, then the high risk in Western populations should be amenable to reduction by dietary manipulation.

In parts of Africa, large vessel disease is extremely rare in Black diabetic patients [7] despite a high prevalence of hypertension. This is not explicable by differences in serum lipid levels or adiposity [8], and is not restricted to malnutrition-associated diabetes.

Cerebrovascular disease

Cerebrovascular mortality is increased about two- to fourfold in diabetes in Western populations, and here sex differences in relative mortality are less marked than in CHD [9]. In Japan, where cerebrovascular disease is the most frequent cardiovascular cause of death, strokes are predominantly haemorrhagic. Only a slight excess mortality is conferred by diabetes, the risk ratio being 1.15 [5], but the proportion of occlusive strokes is higher, suggesting an increased thrombotic tendency. The Whitehall study [10] again showed evidence of a threshold effect of blood glucose, with the relative risk of strokes, like myocardial infarction, being higher in the group above the 95th centile of the glucose distribution.

Peripheral vascular disease

Diabetes confers a particularly high relative risk of peripheral vascular disease: about half of all lower limb amputations performed are on diabetic patients. The relative risk of amputation is highest below age 45, although the absolute risk increases with age [11]. These amputation figures include patients with microvascular disease and neuropathy, but in the 20-year Framingham study, the incidence of intermittent claudication was increased 3.8-fold in men and sixfold in women with diabetes as compared with non-diabetic subjects [12]. Loss of arterial foot pulses, unlike the manifestations of CHD, appears to be related to the duration of diabetes in both NIDDM and IDDM [9].

Risk factors and prevention

The high prevalence of arterial disease in diabetes is partly explained by the increased frequency of conventional risk factors together with some additional interrelated factors associated with diabetes (Table 68.2). In practice, the important factors are those whose correction can be shown to reduce cardiovascular risk. This section will discuss the role of the various risk factors, and highlight the possible scope for their prevention (Table 68.2). Hypertension is discussed in full elsewhere (Chapter 69).

SMOKING

This seems to influence atherosclerosis similarly in diabetic and non-diabetic subjects [13], and little difference has been reported in smoking habits between the two groups [14]. The direct advice of a doctor is the most important single factor in motivating smokers to stop, and this should be a routine part of diabetic education.

OBESITY

Obesity adversely affects blood pressure, insulin

(a) Risk factors for coronary heart disease	
General	Diabetes-related
Smoking	Hyperglycaemia
Hypertension	Hyperinsulinaemia
Hyperlipidaemia	Proteinuria
Hypercoagulability	Microalbuminuria
Obesity	Both sexes affected equally
Lack of exercise	
Male sex	
Family history	
Oestrogen treatment	
(b) Approaches to risk reduction	
Stop smoking	
Optimize diabetic control	
Seek and treat hypertension	
Seek and treat hyperlipidaemia	
Give dietary advice	
• Optimizing control	
• Maintaining ideal body weight	
• Lowering lipids	
Encourage aerobic exercise	

Table 68.2. Risk factors and reductions for coronary heart disease.

sensitivity, blood glucose control and lipoprotein patterns, and weight reduction is an important aspect of diabetic treatment. However, epidemiological studies relating obesity to cardiovascular risk in diabetes have yielded conflicting results, with some finding a positive association [13], and others finding no link [9, 15].

EXERCISE

No direct information is available about the effects of physical exercise on the development of atherosclerosis in diabetes. However, aerobic exercise reduces obesity and plasma insulin levels and increases high-density lipoprotein (HDL) cholesterol, all of which are theoretically beneficial. Cardiovascular status and the presence of other complications should be considered when giving advice about exercise (see Chapter 78).

HAEMOSTATIC FUNCTION

Haemostatic abnormalities, particularly raised fibrinogen and factor VII levels, are strongly predictive of CHD in non-diabetic subjects [16]. Preliminary evidence suggests that similar associations also apply in diabetes [17]. Fibrinogen levels are raised in both IDDM and NIDDM, and are higher in those with cardiovascular complications. Fibrinolytic activity is lower in NIDDM than IDDM and may be associated with ECG ab-

normalities. However, factor VII levels are highest in diabetic patients with retinopathy and nephropathy, and have not been shown to be associated with large-vessel disease. Clotting factors may nonetheless be an important link between large- and small-vessel complications.

In addition to their role in thrombus formation, platelets are involved in atherogenesis through their release of platelet-derived growth factor and chemotactic factors which stimulate cellular proliferation in the atheromatous plaque. Measurements of platelet activity in diabetes have sometimes yielded conflicting results [18]. However, in vitro aggregation of platelets in reponse to ADP and collagen is increased in diabetes and is highest in those with complications. In vivo platelet activity, assessed from plasma levels of β-thromboglobulin and platelet factor 4, is elevated in non-diabetic subjects with vascular disease and in uncomplicated diabetes, and is further raised in those with retinopathy. Thromboxane production is increased in non-diabetic subjects with CHD; amongst diabetic patients, it is also highest in those with macrovascular complications.

The relationship between diabetic control and haemostatic function is not yet clear. Continuous subcutaneous insulin infusion has not led to consistent improvements in clotting factors or measures of platelet function in several studies in IDDM. However, fibrinolytic activity may improve after initiation of treatment for NIDDM [19]. Hypoglycaemia increases platelet activity through the action of catecholamines released as a counter-regulatory response, and this may partly account for the variable results obtained in studies of the effect of improved control on platelet function. Sulphonylureas appear to reduce platelet activity, but whether this is attributable to the improved blood glucose control or the drugs themselves is subject to debate.

BLOOD INSULIN LEVELS

Diabetic patients with arterial disease have higher fasting levels of C peptide, and higher circulating insulin levels (both fasting and after oral glucose challenge) than those without [20]. In non-diabetic subjects, exaggerated insulin reponses to oral glucose are seen in subjects with cerebral, peripheral and coronary artery disease, and some prospective epidemiological studies have found significant associations between blood insulin concentration and subsequent development of ischaemic heart disease [21]. This association may partly be explained by the interactions between hyperinsulinaemia and hypertension, obesity and hypertriglyceridaemia, which may be related to insulin resistance. However, insulin stimulates proliferation of arterial smooth muscle cells *in vitro*, and lipid synthesis in the arterial wall in animals [20], suggesting that insulin could be directly involved in atherogenesis. High circulating insulin levels are seen both in NIDDM and in treated IDDM, and levels can be reduced by avoidance of obesity and by regular physical exercise. The relationship between hyperinsulinaemia and hypertension is discussed further in Chapter 69.

BLOOD GLUCOSE LEVELS

In a large study of several diabetic populations [22], no relationship was found between fasting glycaemia and ECG abnormalities, but there was a weak association with stroke and a strong association with peripheral vascular disease (especially amputation). A similar pattern was seen when duration of diabetes was considered in the same population. Further work is needed to examine IDDM specifically.

ADVANCED GLYCOSYLATION END-PRODUCTS

Prolonged exposure of proteins to glucose leads to reversible non-enzymatic glycosylation of amino groups, and subsequent covalent cross-linking of the proteins by complex modification of the glucose-derived groups (see Chapter 54) [23]. Collagen modified in this way shows increased binding of low-density lipoprotein (LDL) *in vitro* [24]. Modification of the structural proteins of the vessel wall and basement membrane may in itself contribute to luminal narrowing [23]. Moreover, macrophages recognizing modified proteins release various cytokines, which promote cellular proliferation [25]. These observations may provide a link between large- and small-vessel disease.

TREATMENT EFFECTS

Oral hypoglycaemic agents were found to be associated with increased cardiovascular mortality in the University Group Diabetes Program trial, which compared different treatment regimens [26]. These findings have been reviewed in the light of other data [9] and have not been confirmed (see Chapter 48).

Lipoprotein abnormalities

The major lipoprotein classes can be separated by ultracentrifugation, and their characteristics and effects on atheroma are outlined in Table 68.3. Each comprises a hydrophobic core of triglycerides and cholesterol esters, surrounded by a coat containing polar phospholipids, free cholesterol and apoproteins. Their major metabolic pathways are outlined in Figs 68.1–3.

Data from the Framingham study suggest that plasma cholesterol has a similar influence on CHD in diabetic as in non-diabetic subjects [13]. A number of cross-sectional studies have demonstrated an inverse relationship between HDL-cholesterol and arterial disease in NIDDM, but reports in IDDM have been inconsistent [9]. Raised triglyceride levels have also been associated with CHD in cross-sectional studies [22]. The impact of lipid-lowering therapy on CHD in non-diabetic subjects is well established [27–29], and detection and treatment of hyperlipidaemia should be a key part of the routine management of cardiovascular risk factors (Table 68.2).

EFFECTS OF DIABETES ON LIPOPROTEINS

The commonest abnormality in diabetes is hyper-triglyceridaemia due to an excess of very low

Table 68.3. Lipoprotein classification.

	Chylomicrons	VLDL	IDL	LDL	HDL
Diameter (nm)	80–500	30–80	25–35	20	10
Electrophoresis	Origin	Pre-beta	Broad beta	Beta	Alpha
Principal core lipid	Exogenous triglyceride	Triglyceride Cholesterol esters	Cholesterol esters Triglyceride	Cholesterol esters Triglyceride	Cholesterol esters
Effect on atheroma	Nil	+	++	+++	Protects
Major apoproteins	AI and II B48 CII and III E	B100 CII and III E	B100 E	B100	AI and II CIII
Dietary and drug treatment	Diet Drugs ineffective	Fibrates Nicotinic acid ω-3 (N-3) fish oils	Fibrates Nicotinic acid	Resins Nicotinic acid Fibrates Probucol	Fibrates Nicotinic acid ω-3 (N-3) fish oils Resins raise HDL Probucol lowers HDL

Notes: VLDL: very low density; IDL: intermediate density; LDL: low-density; and HDL: high-density lipoproteins. +, ++, +++: moderate, strong and very strong associations.

density lipoprotein (VLDL) [30]. Lipoprotein lipase depends for its full activity on insulin (Fig. 68.1), and VLDL clearance is reduced in poorly controlled patients with IDDM. In NIDDM patients, there is also overproduction of VLDL and apoprotein (apo) B. Insulin deficiency or resistance increases production of non-esterified fatty acids from adipose tissue by the action of hormone-sensitive lipase, and these provide a substrate for hepatic triglyceride synthesis. Hypertriglyceridaemia in diabetes therefore usually responds to intensified insulin treatment.

LDL levels are also raised in association with poor glycaemic control, but a substantial improvement in blood glucose is required to lower LDL [31]. Insulin stimulates LDL receptor activity (Fig. 68.2) [32], increasing LDL clearance, while non-enzymatic glycosylation of apo B reduces its affinity for the receptor, thereby slowing LDL removal [33].

HDL levels vary inversely with VLDL, since reduced lipoprotein lipase activity impairs catabolism of VLDL and hence transfer of lipids and apoproteins to HDL (Fig. 68.3). In NIDDM, HDL levels are low, especially in association with hypertriglyceridaemia, whereas in IDDM the levels are normal. Glycosylation of HDL occurs *in vivo*,

and in animal studies glycosylated HDL is removed faster from the circulation [34].

ASSESSMENT

Initial screening is by measurement of plasma cholesterol, triglyceride and HDL cholesterol after a 12-h overnight fast. The LDL cholesterol can then be calculated (in mmol/l) from the Friedewald formula [35]:

$$\text{LDL cholesterol} = \text{total cholesterol} - \text{HDL cholesterol} - \frac{\text{triglyceride}}{2.19}$$

(This should not be used when the triglyceride level is over 5 mmol/l.)

Cholesterol levels are not significantly changed postprandially, but triglycerides may rise. A non-fasting sample may therefore be used for screening, but should be repeated fasting if the triglycerides are elevated.

MANAGEMENT

The European Atherosclerosis Society has recently published guidelines for management of hyper-

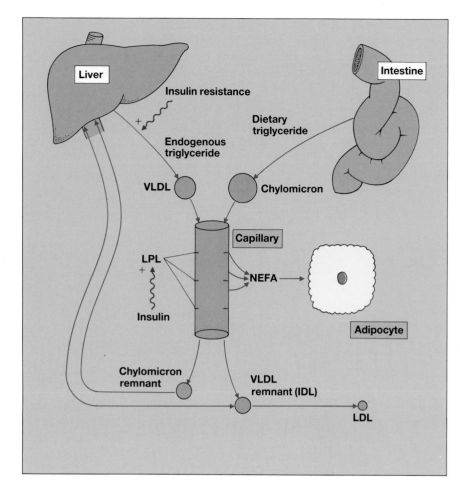

Fig. 68.1. Very low density lipoprotein (VLDL), containing endogenous triglyceride, and chylomicrons, containing dietary triglyceride, are catabolized by the endothelial enzyme lipoprotein lipase (LPL), releasing non-esterified fatty acids (NEFA) for use as fuel or storage in adipose tissue. The resulting remnant particles may be taken up by the liver, and the VLDL remnant (intermediate-density lipoprotein or IDL), containing all its original cholesterol, may be further catabolized to produce low-density lipoprotein (LDL).

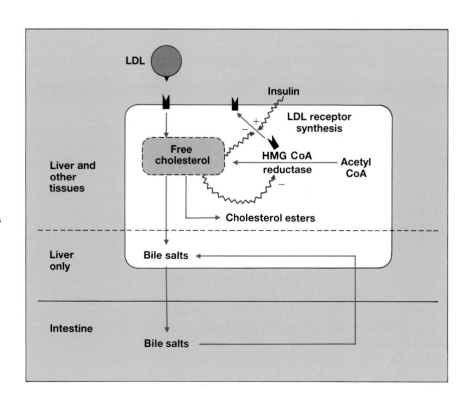

Fig. 68.2. Low-density lipoprotein (LDL) is taken up predominantly via a receptor recognizing apoprotein B100. Free cholesterol is released into the cytoplasmic pool, which also receives endogenously synthesized cholesterol. The cholesterol is used in membrane and bile-salt synthesis or stored as cholesterol ester. The free cholesterol inhibits both LDL receptor synthesis and the activity of HMG CoA reductase, the rate-limiting enzyme in cholesterol synthesis, thus regulating its own concentration.

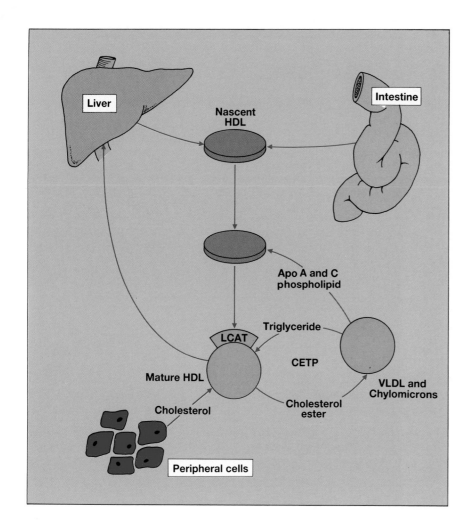

Fig. 68.3. High-density lipoprotein (HDL) is produced as a lipid-poor disc. It receives apoproteins and phospholipids from triglyceride-rich lipoproteins, and the enzyme lecithin:cholesterol acyltransferase (LCAT) is activated by apo AI. It can then receive cholesterol from peripheral cells, esterify it and transport it to the liver either directly or by transferring it to other lipoproteins via cholesterol ester transfer protein (CETP).

lipidaemia which are outlined in Table 68.4 [36]. The same therapeutic goals are recommended in diabetes, but management should be guided by the fact that diabetes itself puts the patient into a high-risk group and therefore demands aggressive treatment. A management scheme is suggested in Fig. 68.4.

Initial treatment is by optimizing body weight and glucose control, and by dietary adjustment. In IDDM, a high-carbohydrate, low-saturated-fat, low-cholesterol diet has been shown to lower cholesterol without a deterioration in glucose control or triglyceride levels [37], and the diet currently recommended for diabetes provides about 35% of energy as fat, with partial substitution of polyunsaturated for saturated fats [38]. The American Heart Association has published dietary recommendations for the treatment of hyperlipidaemia [39], with gradual introduction of the phases in Table 68.5; phase I is most commonly used in the UK.

In NIDDM, weight reduction is accompanied by a fall in triglycerides and a rise in HDL-cholesterol. A lowering of LDL depends on the dietary fat composition, but does not result from weight reduction alone. Dietary fibre, especially soluble gums and pectins found in pulses and legumes, is also important in lowering cholesterol (see Chapter 104).

Patients unresponsive to diet and intensified control may have an underlying primary hyperlipidaemia or another cause of secondary hyperlipidaemia (Table 68.6). They should be reassessed for these and dietary compliance checked before proceeding to drug treatment.

DRUG THERAPY

In *hypertriglyceridaemia* or *combined hyperlipidaemia*, bezafibrate and gemfibrozil are the drugs of choice. They elevate HDL, which may have an additional protective effect [29]. Bezafibrate [40] may also improve glycaemic control. Nicotinic acid is also effective, but frequently causes flushing, pruritus and gastrointestinal side-effects. Its newer analogues such as acipimox are better tolerated.

Table 68.4. Guidelines for management of hyperlipidaemia. Adapted from the guidelines of the European Atherosclerosis Society [36].

Group	Lipid level (mmol/l)	Assessment	Treatment
A	Cholesterol 5.2–6.5 Triglyceride <2.3	Assess overall risk of CHD	Restrict food energy if overweight; give nutritional advice and correct other risk factors. If high risk, monitor as in B
B	Cholesterol 6.5–7.8 Triglyceride <2.3	Assess overall risk of CHD	Restrict food energy if overweight; prescribe lipid-lowering diet and monitor response and compliance. If cholesterol remains high, consider lipid-lowering drugs
C	Cholesterol <5.2 Triglyceride 2.3–5.6	Seek underlying cause	Restrict food energy if overweight; treat underlying causes if present. Prescribe and monitor lipid-lowering diet. Monitor response and compliance
D	Cholesterol 5.2–7.8 Triglyceride 2.3–5.6	Assess overall risk of CHD Seek underlying cause	Proceed as for group C above. If response is inadequate and overall CHD risk is high, consider lipid-lowering drugs
E	Cholesterol >7.8, or Triglyceride >5.6	Make full diagnosis	Consider referral to lipid clinic or specialized physician for investigation and treatment

Table 68.5. American Heart Association lipid-lowering dietary phases [39].

Phase I	30% calories as fat; equal proportions of saturated, monounsaturated and polyunsaturated; under 300 mg cholesterol
Phase II	25% calories as fat; equal proportions of fatty acid types; 200–250 mg cholesterol
Phase III	20% calories as fat; equal proportions of fatty acid types; 100–150 mg cholesterol

Table 68.6. Causes of secondary hyperlipidaemia.

Dietary	Alcohol
Hypothyroidism	Drugs:
Obesity	Thiazide diuretics
Chronic renal failure	β-blockers
Nephrotic syndrome	Oral contraceptives
Dysglobulinaemia	Isotretinoin

For *hypercholesterolaemia*, the bile-acid-sequestering resins, cholestyramine and colestipol, are effective [27, 28], although unpleasant to swallow and subject to gastrointestinal side-effects. By preventing the enterohepatic recirculation of bile, these agents cause the hepatocyte to synthesize more bile acids from cholesterol and to increase the number of cell-surface LDL receptors to keep pace with the increased demand (Fig. 68.2). They may worsen any coexisting hypertriglyceridaemia because of a compensatory increase in hepatic VLDL secretion. Combined therapy with a fibrate and a resin avoids the adverse rise in triglycerides and has an additional cholesterol-lowering effect.

The inhibitors of 3-hydroxymethyl 3-glutaryl coenzyme A (HMG CoA) reductase, now known as stains (Fig. 68.2), are very effective cholesterol-lowering agents and the first of these, lovastatin, is available in the US. It inhibits intracellular cholesterol synthesis at its rate-limiting step, reducing the cytoplasmic pool of cholesterol, and thereby stimulating production of more LDL receptors. It has recently been shown to be effective in diabetes [41] and simvastatin, a related drug, is available in the UK.

Heart disease

The major clinical manifestations of CHD are heart failure, angina pectoris and myocardial infarction. The following discussion emphasizes their management in diabetes.

Heart failure

PATHOPHYSIOLOGY

The origin of heart failure in diabetes is multifactorial. In a series of patients dying of heart

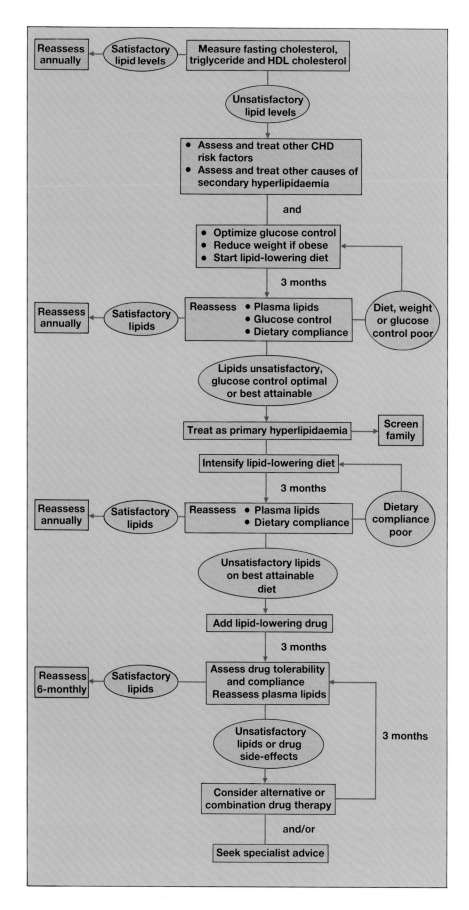

Fig. 68.4. Management of hyperlipidaemia.

failure of unknown cause [42], most were diabetic and showed multiple non-transmural infarcts at post-mortem examination. Non-invasive studies of resting left ventricular function have demonstrated abnormalities both of contraction and relaxation of the ventricle in diabetic patients without ischaemic heart disease or hypertension. About a quarter of such patients were affected in one study [43], the majority having evidence of microvascular disease (retinopathy of nephropathy). These findings have supported the concept of a specific diabetes-associated cardiomyopathy. In the diabetic heart, collagen and periodic acid-Schiff-(PAS) -positive staining material are deposited around blood vessels and between the muscle fibres [44], a process accelerated by coexisting hypertension, both in humans [45] and in animal models [46]. The microvascular abnormalities seen in the diabetic heart are similar to those described elsewhere in the body, with capillary microaneurysms and thickening of the capillary basement membranes. A milder degree of basement membrane thickening has been observed in IGT. There is no evidence for ischaemia at a microvascular level [44], although leakage of protein from abnormally permeable capillaries may stimulate interstitial fibrosis. Abnormal cardiac function after exercise has recently been described in children and adolescents with diabetes [47], and an apparent association with finger contractures may suggest a generalized fibrotic process. Diabetic children have an exaggerated pressor response to exercise [48], which could both affect the pattern of ventricular contraction and also contribute to myocardial damage. Functionally, the fibrosis reduces ventricular compliance, impairing both filling and emptying. The inability of the myocardium to distend may reduce contractility by blunting the Starling reflex, and autonomic neuropathy may further impair the ability of the ventricle to respond to stress.

Metabolic changes associated with diabetes can cause reversible myocardial dysfunction. In NIDDM, improvement of control by diet or insulin therapy may be accompanied by improved ventricular function and exercise tolerance [49]. Diabetic animals show changes in the activity and type of actinomyosin and myosin ATPases [50] which result in defective activation of the contractile proteins. In normal subjects, injection of insulin has a small immediate positive inotropic action which precedes hypoglycaemia and its

catecholamine response [51], but the mechanism of this is not known.

ASSESSMENT AND MANAGEMENT

In any diabetic presenting with breathlessness or exercise intolerance, heart failure should be suspected, and the diagnosis cannot be excluded by a normal ECG and chest X-ray. Non-invasive assessment of myocardial contraction by radionuclide ventriculography or echocardiography will detect resting abnormalities, and the echocardiogram will also give valuable information about the heart valves and pericardium. After exercise, the ejection fraction should increase, and combining an exercise ECG with radionuclide ventriculography may reveal a fall in ejection fraction or regional akinesia due to silent reversible ischaemia.

Optimizing glucose control is important in the treatment of heart failure, first because of the effects on myocardial function described above, and secondly because glucose may contribute to osmotic gradients resulting in pulmonary oedema [52]. Detection and treatment of hypertension may prevent further deterioration as well as reducing the cardiac workload. Similarly, treatment of reversible ischaemia with nitrates and calcium channel antagonists may improve exercise tolerance.

Thiazide diuretics may worsen diabetic control and aggravate hyperlipidaemia (see Chapter 69); loop diuretics are therefore preferred, but hypokalaemia must be avoided as it impairs insulin secretion and predisposes to arrhythmias. The potassium-sparing diuretics, triamterene and amiloride, may also worsen control in poorly controlled diabetic patients and paradoxically increase plasma potassium levels after a glucose load [53]. Plasma potassium and glucose concentrations must therefore be carefully monitored during diuretic therapy.

Angiotensin converting enzyme (ACE) inhibitors are effective second-line therapy, and have been shown to improve the prognosis in non-diabetic subjects with severe heart failure [54]. They are less effective than diuretics when used alone [55], but as diuretics activate the renin—angiotensin system, the combination of ACE inhibitors and diuretics is particularly effective. Blood pressure should be monitored when starting treatment because of first-dose hypotension (see Chapter 69), and plasma potassium levels monitored during treatment.

Myocardial infarction

The mortality rate following myocardial infarction in diabetic patients is about twice that of the general population, and a review of published figures since 1929 [56] has revealed no sign of improvement with time, although the mortality (both in diabetic and control subjects) has varied widely. A concomitant prospective analysis showed that the proportions of deaths attributable to heart failure, sudden death and arrhythmias were similar to those in non-diabetic subjects, and that the principal cause of death was pump failure.

Infarct size is an important determinant of mortality and correlates with the degree of stress hyperglycaemia in non-diabetic cases [57]. However, most studies have not found larger infarcts in diabetic than in control populations [58]. Ischaemia of the surviving myocardium due to multivessel disease and pre-existing ventricular dysfunction due to cardiomyopathy, hypertension, or previous infarction will reduce the heart's ability to compensate for the loss of infarcted muscle. Compensatory reflexes are also blunted by autonomic neuropathy. Cardiac pain sensation may be impaired in autonomic neuropathy, although a recent study of in-patients revealed no evidence of delayed referral [58].

Ischaemia inhibits both glycolysis and the oxidation of non-esterified fatty acids (NEFA), the principal source of energy in the myocardium [59, 60]. At the same time, the stress hormone response and suppression of insulin secretion raises plasma levels of glucose and NEFA and reduces glucose entry into the myocardium. These metabolic abnormalities are exaggerated in diabetes by insulin deficiency and/or resistance.

NEFA inhibit ATP generation in the mitochondria, and in experimental infarction have been shown to increase infarct size, reduce myocardial contractility and increase oxygen requirements [61]. In man, serum NEFA levels correlate with the risk of postinfarction arrhythmias [62]. They also increase platelet aggregability and reduce the synthesis of prostacyclin in the endothelium [61].

Postinfarct blood glucose levels are of prognostic significance both in diabetic patients [58] and in stress hyperglycaemia [57], but it is not clear whether the raised blood glucose contributes to the increased mortality or is simply consequent upon the stress response and therefore an indicator of poor outcome. Careful metabolic control using an intravenous insulin infusion has not

been consistently beneficial [63, 64], but normoglycaemia is only achieved some hours after admission when the damage is probably already complete. In dogs with experimental infarction, glucose—insulin—potassium infusions have been shown to reduce infarct size and to improve the metabolic derangement around the infarct zone [65], but trials in humans have produced conflicting results, and their use has not been accepted.

Diabetic ketoacidosis complicates only some 3% of myocardial infarcts in diabetic patients but is obviously important in affected individuals [56].

MANAGEMENT OF MYOCARDIAL INFARCTION

Several points specific to diabetes should supplement normal coronary care. First, blood glucose levels should be carefully controlled, where necessary by intravenous insulin infusion. A successfully used regimen is given in Table 68.7 [66]. Hypokalaemia should be avoided, since this predisposes to ventricular arrhythmias, and the plasma potassium level should be kept above 4 mmol/l. Secondly, heart failure should be sought and treated aggressively; there is an argument for early invasive monitoring by Swan—Ganz catheter to allow optimal therapy, since cardiovascular reflexes may be impaired. Thirdly, in view of the increased numbers of diabetic patients presenting with reinfarction, secondary prevention is important, and risk factor management, β-blockade and suitability for bypass surgery should all be considered.

Table 68.7. Intravenous insulin infusion and glycaemic monitoring schedule suggested for diabetic patients with acute myocardial infarction. (Adapted from Gwilt et al. 1982 [66] with permission from the British Medical Journal.)

(a) Infusion regimen	
Blood glucose (mmol/l)	Infusion rate (U/h)
<4	0
4—8	1
8—12	2
>12	4
(b) Monitoring regimen	
Time (h)	Monitor glucose
0—4	Hourly
4—24	4-hourly
>24	Before meals

The treatment of myocardial infarction has recently undergone major changes, with the widespread use of intravenous thrombolytic therapy and aspirin [67]. If myocardium is to be salvaged in diabetic patients, the early correction of metabolic control may become especially important. Reperfusion arrhythmias have not been a problem in general, but separate studies in diabetic patients are needed. In view of their hypercoagulable state, diabetic subjects may respond differently to thrombolysis, and more information is required before they can gain maximum benefit from this treatment. Thrombolysis is contraindicated by proliferative retinopathy because of the risk of haemorrhage.

Angina pectoris

Symptoms of angina may be masked in diabetes by autonomic neuropathy, and breathlessness may be the only symptom of silent reversible ischaemia. Non-invasive techniques to confirm the diagnosis include exercise electrocardiography, ^{201}Thallium ventricular perfusion scanning and exercise radionuclide ventriculography.

The sensitivity and specificity of these techniques depends on the study population and there is little information on their reliability as compared with coronary angiography in diabetic patients. The effects of hypertension and cardiomyopathy may produce non-specific changes, and glucose ingestion can cause both ST depression and T-wave inversion [68]. The specificity of the exercise ECG may be increased, with some loss of sensitivity, by choosing 1.5- or 2-mm ST depression as the criterion for a positive test [69]. The diagnosis must be made after consideration of all the available iinformation rather than relying on a single result.

Nitrates, calcium antagonists and β-blockers may be used in the normal way in the treatment of angina, but certain features of diabetes may influence the choice. Nitrates can cause postural hypotension in patients whose baroreceptor reflexes are impaired by autonomic neuropathy; this problem can be minimized by advising patients to spit out the sublingual tablet as soon as pain is relieved.

Non-selective β-blockade impairs insulin release and hence may worsen diabetic control in NIDDM. It can mask the warning symptoms of hypoglycaemia, and also impairs catecholamine-mediated glycogenolysis and gluconeogenesis,

slowing recovery from hypoglycaemia. In addition, β-blockers may adversely affect plasma lipids, exacerbate heart failure and ischaemia of the lower limb and cause impotence. In spite of all this, they are used successfully in many diabetic patients, and one long-term study [70] failed to demonstrate an increase in severe hypoglycaemic episodes with β-blockade in IDDM. Cardioselective agents such as atenolol, metoprolol and acebutolol should be used to minimize non-cardiac side-effects, and these points should be considered when selecting treatment and monitoring response.

Calcium channel antagonists have also been reported to worsen blood glucose control in large doses and in acute studies, but this does not seem to be a problem in NIDDM patients with hypertension [71]. There are significant differences between the available drugs in their suppression of sinoatrial node function, atrioventricular conduction and myocardial contractility. Verapamil has the most pronounced effects on the heart and may exacerbate heart failure, whereas the cardiac effects of nifedipine are slight, although reflex tachycardia may result. The effects of diltiazem are intermediate and it is a useful single agent for angina prophylaxis.

Coronary artery surgery and angioplasty

Surgical treatment of coronary disease should be considered either when medical treatment has failed to relieve symptoms adequately or when the prognosis may be improved by surgery. Coronary angiography is normally only undertaken when this is considered.

There has been debate as to whether the pattern of coronary atherosclerosis in diabetes is more diffuse, or simply more severe than in non-diabetic patients. This point is clearly important when coronary surgery or angioplasty are contemplated. In one angiographic study, diabetic patients had more severe and extensive disease than carefully matched non-diabetic controls [72]. The number of stenosed segments per vessel was significantly greater in the diabetic group, but did not affect operability, the number of inoperable vessels being similar in the two groups.

The exercise ECG is a valuable prognostic indicator in selecting patients for angiography. In non-diabetic subjects, poor prognosis is associated with ST depression at a low workload or heart rate (stage 3 of the Bruce protocol or 120 beats/min), failure of the systolic pressure to rise above

130mmHg or a fall in blood pressure indicating impaired ventricular function [69]. There is no evidence that the absence of chest pain confers a better prognosis than symptomatic ischaemia of equivalent severity.

In non-diabetic subjects, prognosis is improved by surgery in patients with disease affecting the left main coronary artery, three-vessel disease or two-vessel disease in which the left anterior descending artery is involved [73]. The use of internal mammary grafts improves long-term results. The effect of percutaneous transluminal coronary angioplasty (PTCA) on prognosis is not known, but its success and safety are increasing with a mortality rate of around 1% in spite of its increasing use in multivessel disease [74].

The in-hospital mortality of diabetic patients undergoing coronary artery bypass grafting (CABG) has been about twice that of controls. In a review of long-term results of surgery, initial symptomatic relief was similar in diabetic and non-diabetic subjects, but 15-year survival was 53% in non-diabetics, 43% in diabetic patients treated by diet alone, 33% in those on oral hypoglycaemic agents and 19% in those on insulin [75]. Late graft patency was similar in all groups. With improved technique and postoperative care, a more recently operated series [76] showed no significant excess in perioperative morbidity or mortality in diabetic patients, even though they had twice the control rate of previous infarction and hypertension. Survival and symptomatic relief in the medium term were also comparable. There are no longer any grounds for denying the benefit of this treatment to people with diabetes.

PTCA is suited mainly to localized stenoses and may therefore be less appropriate for diabetic patients in whom widespread disease is common, although PTCA is increasingly used in multivessel disease [74]. In one large series, the slightly higher mortality seen in diabetic patients was attributable to the worse pattern of their disease [77], and patients should be selected with this in mind. The long-term results in diabetes are uncertain, but one small series [78] has reported that restenosis is more frequent; further information is clearly needed.

Given the poor prognosis of CHD in diabetes and the demonstrable prognostic benefits of surgery in selected non-diabetic cases, it seems reasonable to pursue an active policy to detect those diabetic patients who may benefit from surgery in the same way. Until the situation has been clarified, angioplasty should be reserved for symptomatic relief or for localized disease in diabetes. A suggested scheme of selection is given in Fig. 68.5.

Peripheral arterial disease

Intermittent claudication may present as numbness or weakness, especially if the limb is already affected by neuropathy. As ischaemia worsens, it may progress to pain or discomfort at rest, especially at night, and finally to necrosis. Surgery is directed either to the symptoms of claudication and rest pain, or to the jeopardized limb which may otherwise require amputation; its prophylactic use in mild claudication is not justified.

Clinical assessment involves palpation of the aorta and iliac vessels in the abdomen as well as the limb pulses, and auscultation for bruits. The skin must also be examined for signs of poor nutrition, sites of possible trauma and disordered sweating. The latter is useful in assessing the potential value of sympathectomy, since loss of sweating indicates that the sympathetic nerves are already affected by neuropathy [79].

Conservative treatment involves careful diabetic control, prohibition of smoking, weight reduction where necessary and meticulous foot care. Drugs designed to improve blood flow are disappointing, but venesection to reduce blood viscosity has been shown to improve walking distance in selected patients [80] and merits further evaluation in diabetic patients, whose blood viscosity is raised.

When reconstruction is contemplated, arteriographic assessment must include the distal vessels which are often affected by both atheroma and medial sclerosis with calcification (Fig. 67.8 and 68.6) in diabetes. Aorto-iliac and aorto-femoral grafts are technically as successful as in non-diabetic cases. In one series, all patients survived with patent grafts, and patency at 5 years was 94% in both groups. However, at 4 years one-third of the diabetic patients were dead and the diabetic survivors showed more progression of distal arterial disease [79]. Comparable good results have been obtained with femoro-popliteal grafts.

Distal arterial surgery is only indicated for rest pain or limb salvage. Grafts from the femoral or popliteal vessels to arteries at ankle level are technically demanding, but can save limbs. In one recent report of 26 patients (25 diabetic) undergoing distal grafts using the saphenous vein *in situ* [81], only one major amputation was re-

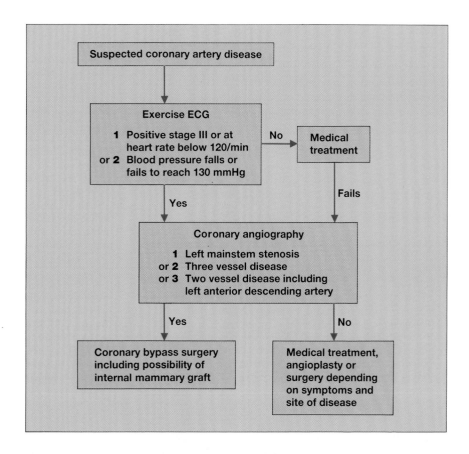

Suspected coronary artery disease

↓

Exercise ECG

1 Positive stage III or at
heart rate below 120/min
or **2** Blood pressure falls or
fails to reach 130 mmHg

→ No → **Medical treatment**

↓ Yes   ↓ Fails

Coronary angiography

1 Left mainstem stenosis
or **2** Three vessel disease
or **3** Two vessel disease including
left anterior descending artery

↓ Yes   ↓ No

Coronary bypass surgery including possibility of internal mammary graft

Medical treatment, angioplasty or surgery depending on symptoms and site of disease

Fig. 68.5. Management of coronary artery disease.

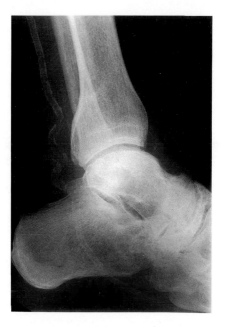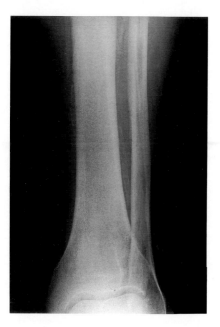

Fig. 68.6. Radiographic calcification accompanying medial sclerosis involving the distal lower limb arteries.

quired, but three patients died in the first month from myocardial infarction and seven required minor amputations. This reflects the severity of disease in this group of patients.

Percutaneous transluminal balloon angioplasty is best suited to dilating discrete stenoses in proximal vessels, which may sometimes improve perfusion in the difficult problem of distal disease. The initial success rate of angioplasty is reduced in diabetic patients but, as with PTCA, this is due to the pattern of disease encountered rather than the presence of diabetes itself [82].

The restenosis rate after angioplasty in diabetes is not certain. Ankle systolic pressures have been observed to fall during the first year following successful angioplasty of iliac or superficial femoral artery stenoses in diabetic patients, although there was no concomitant deterioration in symptoms [83].

ROGER H. JAY
D. JOHN BETTERIDGE

References

1 Borch-Johnsen K, Kreiner S. Proteinuria: value as a predictor of cardiovascular mortality in insulin dependent diabetes mellitus. *Br Med J* 1987; **294**: 1651–4.
2 Marks HH, Krall LP. Onset, course, prognosis and mortality in diabetes mellitus. In: Marble A, White P, Bradley RF, Krall LP, eds. *Joslin's Diabetes Mellitus* 11th edn. Philadelphia: Lea and Febiger, 1971: 209–54.
3 Jarrett RJ. The epidemiology of coronary heart disease and related factors in the context of diabetes mellitus and impaired glucose tolerance. In: Jarrett RJ, ed. *Diabetes and Heart Disease*. Amsterdam: Elsevier Science Publishers BV, 1984: 1–23.
4 Fuller JH, Shipley MJ, Rose G, Jarrett RJ, Keen H. Coronary heart disease risk and impaired glucose tolerance: the Whitehall study. *Lancet* 1980; i: 1373–6.
5 Sasaki A, Kamado K, Horiuchi N. A changing pattern of causes of death in Japanese diabetics. Observations over fifteen years. *J Chron Dis* 1978; **31**: 433–44.
6 Kawate R, Yamakido M, Nishimoto Y, Bennett PH, Hamman RF, Knowler WC. Diabetes mellitus and its vascular complications in Japanese migrants on the island of Hawaii. *Diabetes Care* 1979; **2**: 161–70.
7 Seftel HC, Walker ARP. Vascular disease in South African Bantu diabetics. *Diabetologia* 1966; **2**: 286–90.
8 Krut LH, Dubb A, Mangera C. Serum lipid levels in black diabetics in Baragwaneth Hospital. *S Afr Med J* 1980; **57**: 350–4.
9 Pyörälä K, Laakso M, Uusitupa M. Diabetes and atherosclerosis: an epidemiologic view. *Diabetes/Metab Rev* 1987; **3**: 464–524.
10 Fuller JH, Shipley MJ, Rose G, Jarrett RJ, Keen H. Mortality from coronary heart disease and stroke in relation to the degree of hyperglycaemia: the Whitehall study. *Br Med J* 1983; **287**: 867–70.
11 Most RS, Sinnock P. The epidemiology of lower extremity amputations in diabetic individuals. *Diabetes Care* 1983; **6**: 87–91.
12 Kannel WB, McGee DL. Diabetes and glucose tolerance as risk factors for cardiovascular disease: the Framingham Study. *Diabetes Care* 1979; **2**: 120–6.
13 Kannel WB, McGee DL. Diabetes and cardiovascular risk factors: the Framingham study. *Circulation* 1979; **59**: 8–13.
14 Kesson CM, Slater SD. Smoking in diabetics. *Lancet* 1979; i: 504–5.
15 Hayward RE, Lucena BC. An investigation into the mortality of diabetics. *J Inst Actuaries* 1965; **91**: 286–315.
16 Meade TW, Brozovic M, Chakrabarti RR et al. Haemostatic function and ischaemic heart disease: principal results of the Northwick Park Heart Study. *Lancet* 1986; ii: 533–7.
17 Fuller JH. The haemocoagulation system and macroangio-

18 Betteridge DJ. Platelets and diabetes mellitus. In: Taylor KG, ed. *Diabetes and the Heart*. Tunbridge Wells: Castle House Publications, 1987: 79–119.
19 Bedi HK, Vyas BR, Bomb BS, Agarival ML, Bedi T. Fibrinogen content and fibrinolytic activity of blood in diabetics before and after antidiabetic drugs. *J Ass Phys India* 1977; **25**: 181–5.
20 Stout RW. Insulin and atheroma — an update. *Lancet* 1987; i: 1077–9.
21 Jarrett RJ. Is insulin atherogenic? (editorial). *Diabetologia* 1988; **31**: 71–5.
22 West KM, Ahuja MMS, Bennett PH et al. The role of circulating glucose and triglyceride concentrations and their interactions with other "risk factors" as determinants of arterial disease in nine diabetic population samples from the WHO multinational study. *Diabetes Care* 1983; **6**: 361–9.
23 Brownlee M, Cerami A, Vlassara H. Advanced products of nonenzymatic glycosylation in the pathogenesis of diabetic vascular disease. *Diabetes Metab Rev* 1988; **4**: 437–51.
24 Brownlee M, Vlassara H, Cerami A. Nonenzymatic glycosylation products on collagen covalently trap low-density lipoprotein. *Diabetes* 1985; **34**: 938–41.
25 Vlassara H, Brownlee M, Manogue K et al. Cachectin/TNF and IL-1 induced by glucose-modified proteins: role in normal tissue remodelling. *Science* 1988; **240**: 1546–8.
26 University Group Diabetes Program. A study of the effects of hypoglycemic agents on vascular complications in patients with adult-onset diabetes: V. Evaluation of phenformin therapy. *Diabetes* 1975; **24** (suppl 1): 65–184.
27 Lipid Research Clinics Program. The Lipid Research Clinics Coronary Primary Prevention Trial results I. Reduction in the incidence of coronary heart disease. *J Am Med Ass* 1984; **251**: 351–64.
28 Lipid Research Clinics Program. The Lipid Research Clinics Coronary Primary Prevention Trial results. II. The relationship of reduction in incidence of coronary heart disease to cholesterol lowering. *J Am Med Ass* 1984; **251**: 365–74.
29 Frick MH, Elo O, Haapa K et al. Helsinki Heart Study: primary-prevention trial with gemfibrozil in middle-aged men with dyslipidemia; safety of treatment, changes in risk factors and incidence of coronary heart disease. *N Engl J Med* 1987; **317**: 1237–45.
30 Albrink MJ. Dietary and drug treatment of hyperlipidemia in diabetics. *Diabetes* 1974; **23**: 913–18.
31 Pietri A, Dunn FL, Raskin P. The effect of improved diabetic control on plasma lipid and lipoprotein levels. A comparison of conventional therapy and continuous subcutaneous insulin. *Diabetes* 1980; **29**: 1001–5.
32 Chait A, Bierman EL, Albers JJ. Low density lipoprotein receptor activity in cultured fibroblasts: mechanism of insulin-induced stimulation. *J Clin Invest* 1979; **64**: 1309–19.
33 Steinbrecher UP, Witztum JL. Glucosylation of low density lipoproteins to an extent comparable to that seen in diabetes slows their catabolism. *Diabetes* 1984; **33**: 130–4.
34 Witztum JL, Fischer M, Pietro T, Steinbrecher UP, Elam RL. Non-enzymatic glycosylation of high density lipoprotein accelerates its catabolism in guinea pigs. *Diabetes* 1982; **31**: 1029–32.
35 Friedewald WT, Levy RI, Fredrickson DS. Estimation of the concentration of low-density lipoprotein cholesterol in plasma without use of the preparative ultracentrifuge. *Clin Chem* 1972; **18**: 499–502.

36 Study Group of the European Atherosclerosis Society. The recognition and management of hyperlipidaemia in adults: a policy statement of the European Atherosclerosis Society. *Eur Heart J* 1988; **9**: 571−600.

37 Stone DB, Connor WE. The prolonged effects of a low cholesterol, high carbohydrate diet upon the serum lipids in diabetic patients. *Diabetes* 1963; **12**: 127−35.

38 British Diabetic Association. Dietary recommendations for diabetics in the 1980s — a policy statement by the British Diabetic Association. *Hum Nutr Appl Nutr* 1982; **36A**: 378−94.

39 Ad Hoc Committee to Design a Dietary Treatment of Hyperlipoproteinemia. Recommendations for treatment of hyperlipidemia in adults. A joint statement of the nutrition committee and the council on arteriosclerosis. *Circulation* 1984; **69**: 1065A−90A.

40 Wahl P, Hasslacher CL, Lang PD *et al*. Lipid-lowering effect of bezafibrate in patients with diabetes mellitus and hyperlipidaemia. In: Greten H, Lang PD, Schettler G, eds. *Lipoproteins and Coronary Heart Disease: New Aspects in the Diagnosis and Therapy of Disorders of Lipid Metabolism*. Baden-Baden: Gerhard Witztrock, 1980: 154−8.

41 Garg A, Grundy SM. Lovastatin for lowering cholesterol levels in non-insulin-dependent diabetes mellitus. *N Engl J Med* 1988; **318**: 81−6.

42 Boucher CA, Fallon JT, Johnson RA, Yurchak PM. Cardio-myopathic syndrome caused by coronary artery disease. III: prospective clinicopathological study of its prevalence among patients with clinically unexplained chronic heart failure. *Br Heart J* 1979; **41**: 613−20.

43 Shapiro LM. A prospective study of heart disease in diabetes mellitus. *Q J Med* 1984; **209**: 55−68.

44 Regan TJ, Lyons MM, Levinson GE *et al*. Evidence for cardiomyopathy in familial diabetes mellitus. *J Clin Invest* 1977; **60**: 885−99.

45 Factor SM, Minase T, Sonnenblick EH. Clinical and mor-phological features of human hypertensive diabetic cardio-myopathy. *Am Heart J* 1980; **99**: 446−58.

46 Fein FS, Capasso JM, Aronson RS *et al*. Combined reno-vascular hypertension and diabetes in rats: a new prep-aration of congestive cardiomyopathy. *Circulation* 1984; **70**: 318−30.

47 Baum VC, Levitsky LL, Englander RM. Abnormal cardiac function after exercise in insulin-dependent diabetic chil-dren and adolescents. *Diabetes Care* 1987; **10**: 319−23.

48 Karlefors T. Circulatory studies during exercise with par-ticular reference to diabetics. *Acta Med Scand* 1966; **180** (suppl 449).

49 Uusitupa M, Mustonen J, Laakso M, Pyörälä K. Left ventri-cular dysfunction in diabetes: evidence for the impact of metabolic factors. *Diabetologia* 1987; **30**: 193−4.

50 Dillman WH. Diabetes mellitus induces changes in cardiac myosin in the rat. *Diabetes* 1980; **29**: 579−82.

51 Fisher BM, Gillen G, Dargie HJ, Inglis GC, Frier BM. The effects of insulin-induced hypoglycaemia on cardiovascular function in normal man: studies using radionuclide ventriculography. *Diabetologia* 1987; **30**: 841−5.

52 Axelrod L. Response of congestive heart failure to correction of hyperglycemia in the presence of diabetic nephropathy. *N Engl J Med* 1975; **293**: 1243−5.

53 Walker BR, Capuzzi DM, Alexander F *et al*. Hyperkalaemia after triamterene therapy in diabetic patients. *Clin Pharmacol Ther* 1972; **13**: 643−51.

54 The CONSENSUS Trial Study Group. Effects of enalapril on mortality in severe congestive heart failure. Results of the Cooperative North Scandinavian Enalapril Survival

Study (CONSENSUS). *N Engl J Med* 1987; **316**: 1429−35.

55 Richardson A, Bayliss J, Scriven AJ, Parameshwar J, Poole-Wilson PA, Sutton GC. Double-blind comparison of captopril alone against frusemide plus amiloride in mild heart failure. *Lancet* 1987; ii: 709−11.

56 Gwilt DJ. Why do diabetics die after myocardial infarction? *Practical Diabetes* 1984; **1**: 36−9.

57 Oswald GA, Smith CCT, Betteridge DJ, Yudkin JS. Deter-minants and importance of stress hyperglycaemia in non-diabetic patients with myocardial infarction. *Br Med J* 1986; **293**: 917−22.

58 Yudkin JS, Oswald GA. Determinants of hospital admission and case fatality in diabetic patients with myocardial in-farction. *Diabetes Care* 1988; **11**: 351−8.

59 Opie LH. Metabolism of free fatty acids, glucose, and catecholamines in acute myocardial infarction. *Am J Cardiol* 1975; **36**: 938−53.

60 Liedtke AJ. Alterations of carbohydrate and lipid meta-bolism in the acutely ischaemic heart. *Prog Cardiovasc Dis* 1981; **23**: 321−6.

61 Gwilt DJ, Pentecost BL. The heart in diabetes. In: Nattrass M, ed. *Recent Advances in Diabetes 2*. Edinburgh: Churchill Livingstone, 1986: 177−94.

62 Oliver MF, Kurien VA, Greenwood TW. Relation between serum free fatty acids and arrhythmias and death after myocardial infarction. *Lancet* 1968; i: 710−15.

63 Gwilt DJ, Petri M, Lamb P, Nattrass M, Pentecost BL. Effect of intravenous insulin infusion on mortality among diabetic patients after myocardial infarction. *Br Heart J* 1984; **51**: 626−31.

64 Clark RS, English M, McNeill GP, Newton RW. Effect of intravenous infusion of insulin in diabetics with acute myocardial infarction. *Br Med J* 1985; **291**: 303−5.

65 Dalby AJ, Bricknell OL, Opie LH. Effect of glucose−insulin−potassium infusions on epicardial ECG changes and on myocardial metabolic changes after coronary artery ligation in dogs. *Cardiovasc Res* 1981; **15**: 588−98.

66 Gwilt DJ, Nattrass M, Pentecost BL. Use of low-dose insulin infusions in diabetics after myocardial infarction. *Br Med J* 1982; **285**: 1402−4.

67 ISIS-2 (Second International Study of Infarct Survival) Collaborative Group. Randomised trial of intravenous streptokinase, oral aspirin, both or neither among 17,187 cases of suspected acute myocardial infarction. *Lancet* 1988; ii: 349−60.

68 Riley CG, Oberman A, Sheffield LT. Electrocardiographic effects of glucose ingestion. *Arch Intern Med* 1972; **130**: 703−7.

69 Crean PA, Fox KM. Exercise electrocardiography in coronary artery disease. *Q J Med* 1987; **237**: 7−13.

70 Barnett AH, Leslie D, Watkins PJ. Can insulin-treated dia-betics be given beta-adrenergic blocking drugs? *Br Med J* 1980; **280**: 976−8.

71 Whitcroft I, Thomas J, Davies IB, Wilkinson N, Rawthorne A. Calcium antagonists do not impair long term glucose control in hypertensive non-insulin diabetics (NIDDs). *Br J Clin Pharmacol* 1986; **22**: 208P.

72 Dortimer AC, Shenoy PN, Shiroff RA *et al*. Diffuse coronary artery disease in diabetic patients. Fact or fiction? *Circulation* 1978; **57**: 133−6.

73 Oakley CM. Surgery and prognosis in coronary heart disease. *Q J Med* 1986; **231**: 637−41.

74 Detre K, Holubkov R, Kelsey S *et al*. Percutaneous trans-luminal coronary angioplasty in 1985−1986 and 1977−1981. The National Heart, Lung and Blood Institute Registry. *N Engl J Med* 1988; **318**: 265−70.

75 Lawrie GM, Morris GC, Glaeser DH. Influence of diabetes mellitus on the results of coronary bypass surgery. Follow-up of 212 diabetic patients ten to 15 years after surgery. *J Am Med Ass* 1986; **256**: 2967−71.

76 Devineni R, McKenzie FN. Surgery for coronary artery disease in patients with diabetes mellitus. *Can J Surg* 1985; **28**: 367−70.

77 Ellis SG, Roubin GS, King SB *et al*. In-hospital cardiac mortality after acute closure after coronary angioplasty: analysis of risk factors from 8,207 procedures. *J Am Coll Cardiol* 1988; **11**: 211−16.

78 Margolis JL, Krieger J, Glemser E. Coronary angioplasty: increased restenosis rate in insulin-dependent diabetics. *Circulation* 1984; **70** (suppl 2): 175.

79 Wheelock FC, Gibbons GW, Marble A. Surgery in diabetes. In: Marble A, Krall LP, Bradley RF, Christlieb AR, Soeldner JS, eds. *Joslin's Diabetes Mellitus*, 12th edn. Philadelphia: Lea and Febiger, 1985: 712−32.

80 Ernst E, Matrai A, Kollar L. Placebo-controlled, double-blind study of haemodilution in peripheral arterial disease. *Lancet* 1987; i: 1449−51.

81 Rhodes GR, Rollins D, Sidawy AN, Skudder P, Buchbinder D. Popliteal-to-tibial *in situ* saphenous vein bypasses for limb salvage in diabetic patients. *Am J Surg* 1987; **154**: 245−7.

82 Johnston KW, Rae M, Hogg-Johnston SA *et al*. 5-year results of a prospective study of percutaneous transluminal angioplasty. *Ann Surg* 1987; **206**: 403−13.

83 Burnett JR, Walshe JA, Howard PR *et al*. Transluminal balloon angioplasty in diabetic peripheral vascular disease. *Aust NZ J Surg* 1987; **57**: 307−9.

69   Hypertension in Diabetes Mellitus

Summary

- Hypertension affects over 30% of European diabetic patients and is twice as common as in the non-diabetic population.
- Diabetes may predispose to hypertension by promoting sodium retention, increasing vascular tone and by contributing to nephropathy. Hypertension in NIDDM may, like the commonly associated hyperlipidaemia, be partly a consequence of insulin resistance and hyperinsulinaemia.
- The presence of hypertension in diabetic patients increases mortality four- to fivefold, largely through coronary heart disease and stroke. Women and Afro-Caribbean patients are particularly at risk.
- Hypertension may also be an aetiological factor in diabetic nephropathy (to which it may determine susceptibility) and retinopathy.
- Initial investigations of the hypertensive diabetic patient must exclude rare causes of secondary hypertension, assess vascular and renal damage, and identify other cardiovascular risk factors.
- General measures such as dietary advice and reducing alcohol intake may themselves normalize blood pressure. Other cardiovascular risk factors — particularly smoking and hyperlipidaemia — must be treated energetically.
- First-line antihypertensive drugs in diabetic patients include: diuretics at low dosage, to avoid adverse metabolic effects due to potassium depletion; cardioselective β-blockers, which may worsen metabolic control; calcium channel blockers, which do not affect metabolic control and have useful anti-anginal and anti-arrhythmic effects; and ACE inhibitors, which have no metabolic side-effects and can reduce albumin excretion in diabetic nephropathy. Second-line drugs include vasodilators and centrally acting agents.
- Patients failing to respond to general measures should receive a single suitable first-line drug. Treatment failures should be given, in sequence: another suitable first-line drug; a logical combination of two first-line drugs; and then triple therapy with another first-line drug or a vasodilator.
- Only 5% of patients will fail to respond to triple therapy; possible underlying causes of hypertension should be investigated and addition of a fourth drug (e.g. clonidine) may be helpful.

Hypertension in diabetes represents an important health problem as the combination of the two diseases is common, carries significant morbidity and mortality, and is frequently difficult to treat.

Epidemiology

These two common conditions will frequently be associated by chance alone, but diabetes apparently predisposes to hypertension and, conversely, hypertensive people are more likely to develop diabetes.

The reported prevalence of hypertension in diabetic people varies widely, but is probably 1.5−2 times higher than in the general population. As many as 30−50% of the European diabetic population aged 35−54 years may be hypertensive, with even higher frequencies in women and Afro-Caribbean patients [1−3]. Many newly diagnosed NIDDM patients are found to be hypertensive, whereas hypertension generally appears later in

IDDM, predominantly associated with nephropathy: after 30 years of IDDM, 50% of patients have hypertension and most of these have nephropathy [4] (see Fig. 69.1).

Hypertensive patients show an increased prevalence of impaired glucose tolerance and diabetes, predominantly NIDDM. This is sometimes present when hypertension is diagnosed but more often appears subsequently, possibly in part because certain antihypertensive drugs are diabetogenic [5].

Aetiology of hypertension in diabetes

As shown in Table 69.1, diabetes and hypertension are occasionally associated in specific endocrine syndromes (acromegaly, Cushing's and Conn's syndromes, phaeochromocytoma) or as a result of treatment with the oral contraceptive pill or glucocorticoids (see Chapters 28 and 79). These rare possibilities must always be considered, as both hypertension and diabetes may be cured by treating the underlying problem. Hypertension in diabetes may also be due to nephropathy, renal scarring following repeated urinary tract infections, or coincidental renal disease.

Diabetes in general predisposes to hypertension. Postulated mechanisms are shown in Fig. 69.2. Hyperglycaemia promotes reabsorption of glucose in the proximal convoluted tubule, causing obligatory sodium reabsorption, increased total body sodium content (usually by about 10%) and expansion of the extracellular fluid (ECF) volume;

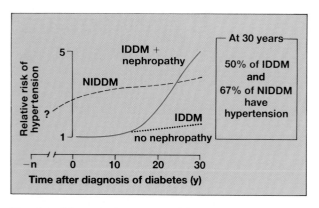

Fig. 69.1. Schematic time-course of development of hypertension in NIDDM patients, and in IDDM patients with and without nephropathy. The majority of hypertensive IDDM subjects are those with nephropathy.

however, this occurs in normotensive as well as hypertensive diabetic subjects [6–9]. The activity of the renin–angiotensin–aldosterone system in diabetic man and animals is generally decreased or normal [9, 10]; as a decrease would be expected with ECF expansion, 'normal' levels may in fact be inappropriately increased. Circulating renin activity may, however, be increased in volume-depleted patients with ketoacidosis [11]. Circulating catecholamine levels are increased in poorly controlled diabetes [12] but essentially normal in most patients [13]. Peripheral resistance may be increased through enhanced vascular sensitivity to various vasoconstrictor agents, including noradrenaline and angiotensin II [7, 8, 14].

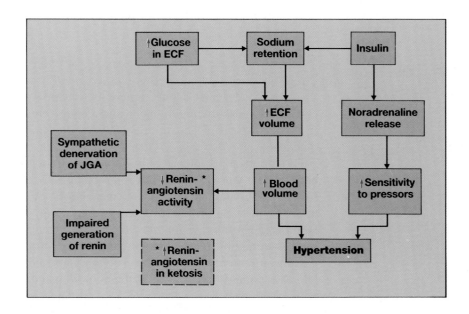

Fig. 69.2. Metabolic factors which may contribute to hypertension in diabetes. Sodium retention (due to both hyperglycaemia and high insulin levels) increases extracellular fluid (ECF) volume. Hyperinsulinaemia (in NIDDM, or during insulin treatment) also stimulates noradrenaline release, which together with enhanced vascular sensitivity to pressors, may increase peripheral resistance. Renin–angiotensin–aldosterone axis activity is generally suppressed by increased ECF volume and sodium load but is increased by volume depletion in ketoacidosis. Renin biosynthesis and release from the juxtaglomerular apparatus (JGA) may also be impaired in diabetes (see Simonson 1988 [4] for review).

Table 69.1. Possible associations of diabetes with hypertension.

Endocrine diseases causing both hypertension and diabetes
Acromegaly
Cushing's syndrome
Conn's syndrome
Phaeochromocytoma

Drugs causing both hypertension and diabetes
Oral contraceptives (combined preparations)
Glucocorticoids

Antihypertensive drugs causing diabetes
Potassium-losing diuretics (especially chlorthalidone)
β-blockers
Diazoxide

Hypertension secondary to diabetic complications
Nephropathy
Renal scarring following recurrent urinary tract infections
Isolated systolic hypertension due to atherosclerosis

Hypertension associated with NIDDM, insulin resistance and
  hyperlipidaemia ('Syndrome X') [24]

Hypertension associated with intensified insulin treatment

Coincidental hypertension in diabetic patients
Essential hypertension
Isolated systolic hypertension

Hypertension and diabetic nephropathy are intimately interrelated (see Chapters 64 and 65). Advanced nephropathy occurs more often in IDDM than in NIDDM, perhaps because the latter appears later in life and many NIDDM patients die from other causes before renal failure can develop. None the less, some two-thirds of North American diabetic patients with end-stage nephropathy have NIDDM [4]. The risk of NIDDM patients progressing to renal failure appears to be greater in Afro-Caribbean and Asian people than in Caucasians [15]. Blood pressure is already slightly but significantly elevated at the early stage of microalbuminuria, although there is debate as to whether blood pressure or urinary albumin excretion rises first [16, 17]. Almost all IDDM patients with macroproteinuria are hypertensive by WHO criteria (see below) and blood pressure rises further as renal function deteriorates. Hypertension is a major determinant of the rate of fall of glomerular filtration rate (GFR), and effective antihypertensive treatment is one of the few factors known to delay the otherwise inexorable decline towards renal failure, as illustrated in Fig. 69.3 [18–20] (see Chapters 64 and 65). There is growing evidence that treatment with angiotensin converting enzyme (ACE) inhibitors during the microalbuminuric stage [21–23], even in normotensive individuals [23], may slow the progression to macroproteinuria. It is not yet clear whether this action is due to a fall in systemic blood pressure or to a selective reduction in intraglomerular hypertension [19] (see Chapter 65).

NIDDM is commonly associated with hypertension, obesity, hyperinsulinaemia, insulin resistance and hyperlipidaemia. Insulin resistance may play a central role in causing this constellation of interdependent factors [24], which act in concert to increase the risks of large-vessel atheroma and death from coronary heart disease or stroke. Obesity and hyperinsulinaemia may both contribute to hypertension, but hyperinsulinaemia is apparently the more important. Circulating insulin concentrations correlate closely with blood pressure across a broad population spectrum [25] and acute fasting — which reduces plasma insulin levels but not weight — significantly lowers blood pressure [26]. Hyperinsulinaemia may raise blood pressure by stimulating proximal tubular sodium reabsorption [27] and by activating the sympathetic nervous system, causing a rise in plasma noradrenaline [28] which is also reversed by fasting [26]. Exogenous insulin may exert similar effects and intensifying insulin treatment may significantly raise blood pressure [29].

A further causal link between hypertension and diabetes is that several antihypertensive drugs — notably the potassium-losing diuretics — may worsen glucose tolerance [30] (see Chapter 79). Thiazide diuretics are among the drugs most widely prescribed in the elderly and an important iatrogenic cause of diabetes, which may be cured by stopping unnecessary diuretic treatment, using lower dosages or changing to alternative medication.

Morbidity and mortality of hypertension in diabetes

The major threat posed by the combination of hypertension and diabetes (especially with hyperlipidaemia) is accelerated, severe atherosclerosis of the large arteries. Coronary heart disease and peripheral vascular disease are commoner in diabetes and even more so when associated with hypertension [31]. Myocardial infarction and stroke are the major excess causes of death in NIDDM [32], and the overall mortality in diabetic patients with hypertension (systolic BP

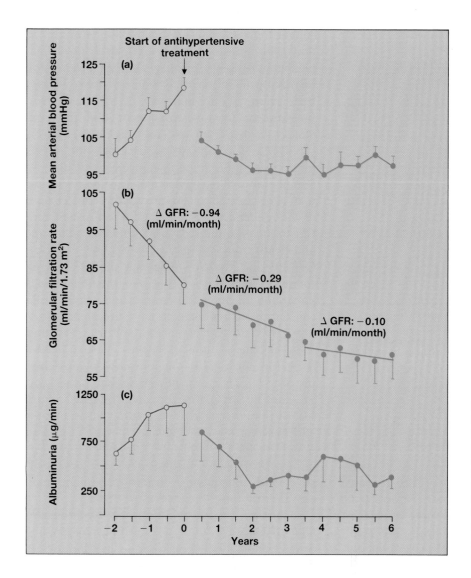

Fig. 69.3. Effects of antihypertensive therapy on blood pressure (a), GFR (b), and urinary albumin excretion (c), in hypertensive patients with diabetic nephropathy. Various combinations of β-blockers, diuretics, vasodilators and centrally acting agents were used. (Redrawn from Parving *et al.* 1987 [18], with kind permission of the Editor of the *British Medical Journal*.)

>160 mmHg) is 4 times greater in males and 5 times greater in females than in matched normotensive diabetic people [3, 33]. Diabetic hypertensive women also lose the protection against atheroma which they usually enjoy before the menopause [3, 33]. Mortality is particularly high in Afro-Caribbean populations [34].

As well as its incontrovertible role in *macro*vascular disease, hypertension has also been implicated in the pathogenesis of the *micro*vascular diabetic complications. Epidemiological studies have reported significant associations between hypertension and nephropathy [17–20] and retinopathy [35]. The beneficial effects of antihypertensive treatment in nephropathy have already been mentioned, and some preliminary evidence suggests that this may also delay the development of retinopathy [35].

It has been suggested that susceptibility to

nephropathy in IDDM is determined by an inherited predisposition to hypertension, as manifested by two putative markers for essential hypertension — having parents with hypertension, and increased lithium–sodium countertransport activity in red blood cells [36, 37]. The latter abnormality may reflect abnormal renal tubular cation exchange which could lead to sodium retention. However, the significance of these findings has been debated [17].

Screening and diagnosis of hypertension in diabetes

Because the two conditions coexist so commonly, patients known to have diabetes must be screened regularly for hypertension and vice versa. Hypertensive patients, especially if obese or treated with potentially diabetogenic drugs (see below), should be tested for diabetes at diagnosis and during follow-up. In this event, treatment should be changed to drugs which do not impair glucose tolerance (e.g. ACE inhibitors or calcium entry blockers), when normoglycaemia may be restored.

All diabetic patients must have their blood pressure checked at diagnosis and at least annually thereafter. This is vitally important in patients with other cardiovascular risk factors, nephropathy (especially macroproteinuria, which is associated with a several-fold increase in cardiovascular mortality [38]), or poor diabetic control.

Blood pressure must be measured using an accurate sphygmomanometer and a cuff of an appropriate size (i.e. wider for NIDDM patients with fat arms). The WHO criteria in general use define hypertension as a blood pressure exceeding 160/95 and borderline hypertension as being below these limits but above 140/90 mmHg [1]. Hypertension is diagnosed when readings consistently exceed 160/95 mmHg for several weeks, or when the pressure is very high (diastolic pressure >110 mmHg), or when there is clinical evidence of tissue damage due to long-standing hypertension. The WHO thresholds may be too high in diabetic patients because of their additional risk of vascular disease [39]; this argument may be supported by the apparent benefits of treating 'normotensive', microalbuminuric patients [23]. Age-related centile charts of systolic and diastolic blood pressure in different populations have been produced (Fig. 69.4) but there are not yet any clear guidelines for their use in diagnosing hypertension in clinical practice.

Investigation of hypertension in diabetes

The initial investigation of the hypertensive diabetic patient (Table 69.2) must aim to exclude the rare causes of secondary hypertension; to assess the extent of tissue damage due to hypertension and diabetes; and to identify other potentially-treatable risk factors of vascular disease.

The major points in the history and examination are shown in Table 69.2. The urine must be tested for protein, using 'Albustix' dip-sticks for macro-proteinuria or preferably the simple screening procedures now available for microalbuminuria (see Chapter 65). A fresh sample should be examined microscopically for red and white blood cells, casts and other signs of renal disease; microscopic haematuria can occasionally occur in IDDM patients, particularly children, in the apparent

absence of significant renal dysfunction but co-existent renal disease must always be excluded [40]. Blood urea, creatinine, electrolytes (especially potassium) and fasting lipid concentrations should be checked. If the serum creatinine concentration is raised, glomerular filtration rate should be measured, ideally by a formal clearance method.

Secondary hypertension may be indicated by clinical findings of endocrine or renal disease, significant hypokalaemia (plasma potassium <3.5 mmol/l, without previous diuretic treatment), failure of hypertension to respond to standard treatment, or a sudden decline in renal function after starting treatment with ACE inhibitors (suggestive of renal artery stenosis).

Management of hypertension in diabetes

Treatment targets

Treatment should lower blood pressure to a level where the additional morbidity and mortality attributable to hypertension are eliminated. This threshold in diabetic people is unknown, but reduction of severe hypertension (diastolic pressure >115 mmHg, or that accompanied by hypertensive tissue damage) to below 140/90 significantly diminishes cardiovascular mortality in non-diabetic populations [41]. The criteria for treating mild hypertension (diastolic pressures, 90–110 mmHg) are less clear-cut: the British Medical Research Council study (in non-diabetic patients) showed that the incidence of stroke was halved but that mortality due to coronary heart disease — the main cause of death in NIDDM — was unaffected [42].

While awaiting more precise information, and given the increased hazards of diabetes at all grades of hypertension [32], it seems reasonable to treat mild hypertension (>160/95 mmHg) in diabetic patients and probably to aim for the WHO target pressures (140/90 mmHg). Reducing blood pressure to 'normal' levels may theoretically increase mortality from coronary artery disease, especially in the elderly with pre-existing myocardial ischaemia. However, patients with nephropathy, and perhaps other significant micro- or macrovascular complications, should probably be treated to normalize their blood pressure as far as possible [18–22]. Appropriate target levels in these cases may be the age-related population mean values (see the centile charts in Fig. 69.4).

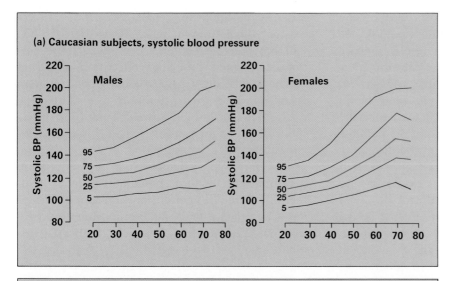

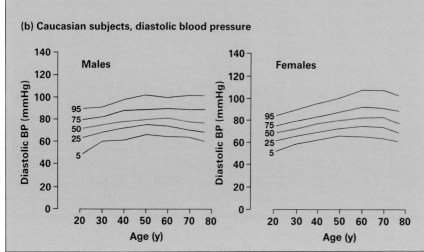

Fig. 69.4. Centile charts showing age-related distribution of systolic and diastolic blood pressures in healthy American Caucasian (a) and (b), and Negro (c) and (d) populations.

General measures

Modification of the patient's lifestyle often markedly reduces blood pressure, and may avoid the need for drug treatment.

EDUCATION

Hypertension is almost always asymptomatic and yet another burden for a person with diabetes. Its significance and the need for treatment must therefore be fully explained, without using 'threats' to try to win co-operation. Overall compliance with antihypertensive medication is probably less than 50% but may be improved by involving the patient in making decisions about his own treatment [43].

DIET, DRINK AND EXERCISE

Current dietary guidelines for diabetes (Chapter 41) should generally be followed. Overweight patients should have a formal weight-reducing diet prescribed and reviewed periodically by a dietitian. Moderate sodium restriction (i.e. not adding salt to food) has a definite hypotensive action [44] and a high-fibre, low-fat, low-sodium diet can lower blood pressure as much as antihypertensive drugs and also improves HbA_1 and triglyceride concentrations [45]. Nephropathic patients should probably be given a moderately low-protein diet, which may slow the rate of decline in renal function [17] (see Chapter 67).

Alcohol, a potent cause of 'refractory' hypertension, should be restricted to 20 U/week in men and 12 U/week in women, and excluded altogether if the blood pressure is difficult to control. Regular exercise is probably beneficial, and a gradually increasing programme within the patient's capacity should be encouraged.

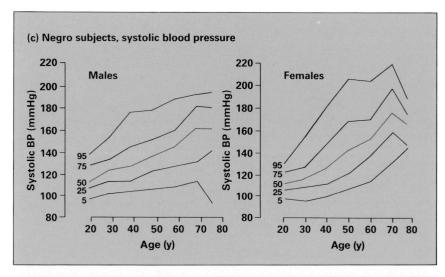

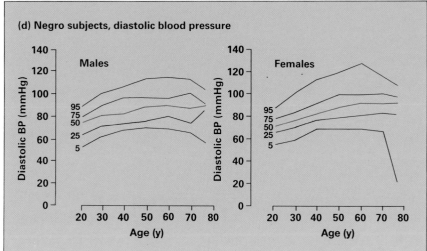

Fig. 69.4. (cont'd) (Redrawn from Acheson RM. *International Journal of Epidemiology* 1973; **2**: 293–301, with kind permission from the Editor.)

SMOKING

Smoking is one of the most important risk factors for macrovascular disease, increasing 10-year mortality by 20% in non-diabetic people but by a staggering 120% in diabetic subjects [46] (Fig. 69.5). Smoking has also been implicated in the pathogenesis of retinopathy [47] and nephropathy [48]. All diabetic patients must therefore be questioned about smoking and strongly urged to stop. They may be encouraged by the information that stopping smoking has a greater effect on reducing mortality in hypertension than antihypertensive drugs.

HYPERLIPIDAEMIA

Well-controlled IDDM patients are generally normolipaemic but NIDDM patients, particularly those with hypertension, have an atherogenic lipaemic profile (see Chapter 68) which may be exacerbated by antihypertensive treatment [49]. Hyperlipidaemia may respond to weight loss, stopping smoking, reducing alcohol intake, improved glycaemic control or a change in antihypertensive drugs (avoiding thiazide diuretics and β-blockers). Some patients may require specific lipid-lowering drugs such as a fibrate, cholestyramine or a statin (see Chapters 68 and 104). Omega-3 fish oils improve the lipaemic profile in NIDDM, but aggravate glycaemic control and are therefore not currently recommended [50].

Antihypertensive drugs

Many antihypertensive drugs present particular problems in diabetes; there is no 'ideal' drug for diabetic hypertension and no general agreement

Table 69.2. Investigation of the diabetic patient with hypertension.

	Questions to be answered
History Cardiovascular symptoms Previous urinary disease Smoking and alcohol use Medication Family history of hypertension or cardiovascular disease	*Is hypertension significant?* *Does hypertension have an underlying cause?* ● Renal ● Endocrine ● Drug-induced

Examination
Blood pressure erect and supine
Left ventricular hypertrophy?
Cardiac failure?
Peripheral pulses (including renal bruits
    and radio-femoral delay)
Fundal changes
Evidence of underlying endocrine or renal
    disease
	Has hypertension caused tissue damage?
	● Left ventricular hypertrophy
	● Ischaemic heart disease
	● Cardiac failure
	● Peripheral vascular disease
	● Renal impairment
	● Fundal changes

ECG Left ventricular hypertrophy Ischaemic changes Rhythm	*Are other cardiovascular risk factors present?* ● Smoking ● Hyperlipidaemia ● Poor glycaemic control ● Positive family history
Chest radiograph Cardiac shadow size Left ventricular failure	
Blood tests Urea, creatinine, electrolytes Fasting lipids	

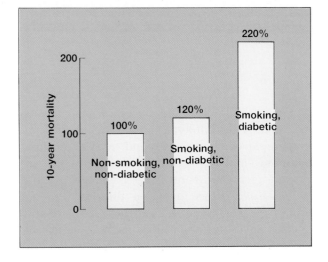

Fig. 69.5. Risks of smoking in non-diabetic and diabetic populations. Smoking more than doubles the 10-year mortality in diabetic people. (Adapted from [46].)

about treatment regimens [51]. The current first-line drugs are diuretics, cardioselective β-adrenergic blockers, calcium channel blockers and ACE inhibitors (see Table 69.3).

DIURETICS

Diuretics are often effective antihypertensive agents in diabetes, in which the total body sodium load is increased and the extracellular fluid volume expanded [7–9]. However, diuretics which increase urinary potassium losses can worsen glucose tolerance, as insulin secretion is impaired by potassium depletion: the use of thiazide diuretics may increase the risk of non-diabetic hypertensive patients developing diabetes by up to 3 times [30]. Potassium depletion is particularly severe with chlorthalidone (which should therefore be avoided), less with frusemide and bendrofluazide and apparently trivial with indapamide [52]. This mechanism is irrelevant to C-peptide-negative IDDM patients who are totally dependent on exogenous insulin. Diuretics may precipitate hyperosmolar, non-ketotic coma and should be avoided or used at the lowest effective dose in patients with a history of this complication.

Thiazides may aggravate hyperlipidaemia [53], although low dosages probably carry a small risk [48, 54]. Thiazides have also been associated with impotence and may be best avoided in diabetic men with erectile failure.

Table 69.3. Antihypertensive drugs used in diabetes.

Group	Examples	Dosage	Relative indications	Relative contraindications	Precautions
Diuretics	Bendrofluazide	1.25–2.5 mg o.d.	Cardiac failure	Hyperosmolar coma	Give with potassium supplements or ACE inhibitors
	Hydrochlorothiazide	25 mg o.d.	Renal failure (frusemide)	Impotence	Monitor blood potassium
	Indapamide	2.5–5 mg o.d.		Gout	Check blood glucose and lipids
	Frusemide	40–80 mg o.d.		Hyperlipidaemia	
β-blockers (cardio-selective)	Atenolol	50–100 mg o.d.	Angina	Cardiac failure	Warn about loss of hypoglycaemic awareness
	Metoprolol	50–100 mg b.d.	Previous myocardial infarction	Heart block	Monitor blood glucose and lipids
				Peripheral vascular disease	
				Impotence	
				Asthma, chronic airflow obstruction	
				Hyperlipidaemia	
ACE inhibitors	Captopril	12.5–50 mg b.d (6.25 mg initially)	Cardiac failure	Renal artery stenosis	First-dose hypotension (use small starting dose at night)
	Enalapril	10–40 mg o.d. (2.5–5 mg initially)	Proteinuria	Renal impairment	Monitor renal function
					Monitor plasma potassium (risk of hyperkalaemia)
Calcium entry blockers	Nifedipine	20 mg b.d. (sustained release)	Angina	Significant cardiac failure	
	Diltiazem	60–120 mg t.d.s.	Arrhythmias	Treatment with digoxin + β-blocker (verapamil)	
	Verapamil	120–240 mg b.d. (sustained release)			
Other agents	Labetolol	50–1200 mg b.d.	Hypertensive crisis		First-dose hypotension (prazosin)
	Prazosin	0.5–5 mg t.d.s.	Impotence		Use with diuretics and β-blockers
	Hydralazine	25–50 mg b.d.	Renal failure		
	Clonidine	50–400 mg t.d.s.	Migraine		

Note: Dosage schedules: o.d., one daily; b.d., twice daily; t.d.s., thrice daily.

Combination	Specific benefits	Disadvantages
Diuretic + ACE inhibitor	ACE inhibitors prevent activation of angiotensin-aldosterone system due to diuretic-induced ECF volume contraction, and help to retain potassium	High risk of 'first-dose' hypotension with ACE-inhibitor in patients overtreated with diuretics
Diuretic + atenolol	—	Possibly aggravate hyperglycaemia in NIDDM
Diuretic + nifedipine	Diuretic reduces mild ankle swelling due to nifedipine	—
Atenolol + nifedipine	Atenolol counteracts tachycardia due to nifedipine's vasodilator action; effective anti-anginal therapy	May aggravate or provoke cardiac failure (both are negative inotropes)

Table 69.4. 'Logical' double-drug antihypertensive therapy.

Notes: Diuretics should be used in the lowest possible dose and combined with potassium supplements (or an ACE inhibitor) to minimize potassium depletion. Atenolol and nifedipine are used as examples of a β-blocker and a calcium channel blocker suitable for use in diabetic patients.

Diuretics suitable for use in diabetic hypertension include bendrofluazide, hydrochlorothiazide and indapamide. Low dosages (Table 69.3) should be used, in combination with potassium supplements (or an ACE inhibitor). If ineffective, diuretics should be combined with another first-line drug (e.g. an ACE inhibitor), rather than given at increased dosage. Frusemide can be used instead in patients with renal impairment or stubborn oedema. Plasma urea, creatinine and potassium should be checked initially and 3- to 6-monthly thereafter; dangerous *hyper*kalaemia can develop in diabetic patients with renal impairment.

β-ADRENERGIC BLOCKING AGENTS

β-blockers may significantly lower blood pressure in diabetic hypertension, even though renin release (one of these agents' major targets) is generally already reduced in diabetes. These drugs are often ineffective in Afro-Caribbean patients, who have a particular tendency to low-renin hypertension [34].

Like diuretics, β-blockers may aggravate both hyperglycaemia and hyperlipidaemia [30, 53]. Their hyperglycaemic effect is attributed to inhibition of β2-adrenergic-mediated insulin release [55], and has been estimated to increase the risks of a non-diabetic person developing the disease by 6-fold and by 15-fold if given together with thiazides [30]. However, recent studies suggest that the hazards of both hyperglycaemia and hyperlipidaemia have been exaggerated [34, 56]. The metabolic side-effects of β-blockers can be reduced by using low dosages combined with other agents, particularly the calcium entry blockers (Table 69.5).

β-blockers have other side-effects relevant to diabetes. They may interfere with the counter-regulatory effects of catecholamines secreted during hypoglycaemia, blunting perception of anxiety, tachycardia and tremor and delaying recovery from hypoglycaemia. In clinical practice, however, this rarely presents a serious problem, especially when cardioselective β1-blockers are used [57]. β-blockers may also aggravate impotence, and are generally contraindicated in significant cardiac failure, second- or third-degree heart block, peripheral vascular disease, asthma or chronic airflow obstruction.

Atenolol is a useful drug as it is cardioselective, water-soluble (which reduces central nervous system side-effects and renders its metabolism and dosage more predictable) and effective as a single daily dose, which probably encourages compliance.

CALCIUM ENTRY (SLOW VOLTAGE-DEPENDENT CHANNEL) BLOCKERS

These useful vasodilator agents do not worsen metabolic control when used at currently accepted dosages [34, 58]. Calcium entry blockers have a slight negative inotropic effect and are contra-indicated in significant cardiac failure, although the mild ankle oedema often associated with their use is probably due to relaxation of the precapillary sphincter rather than to right ventricular failure.

Because of their other cardiac actions, they are particularly indicated in hypertensive patients who also have angina (nifedipine and diltiazem especially) or supraventricular tachycardia (verapamil). Their vasodilator properties may also be beneficial in peripheral vascular disease. Calcium entry blockers may usefully be combined with diuretics or β-blockers, but the specific combination of verapamil and β-blockers (especially with digoxin) must be avoided because of the risk of conduction block and asystole.

Sustained-release nifedipine, given twice daily, is a convenient preparation for general use.

ANGIOTENSIN-CONVERTING ENZYME (ACE) INHIBITORS

ACE inhibitors are useful in diabetic hypertension, even though renin–angiotensin–aldosterone axis activity is not generally increased [10]. When used alone, however, these agents have a limited hypotensive action in many Black patients [59]. They have no adverse metabolic effects, and may be particularly beneficial in diabetic nephropathy, by reducing albuminuria and possibly the progression of the condition [21–23, 60, 61]. Their antiproteinuric effect may be due specifically to relaxation of the efferent arteriole in the glomerulus (which is highly sensitive to vasoconstriction by angiotensin II), so reducing the intraglomerular hypertension which has been postulated to favour albumin filtration [17, 19], although the importance of this mechanism remains controversial [62]. This selective effect may not be shared by other antihypertensive drugs, such as the calcium channel blockers [61]. ACE inhibitors are also indicated in cardiac failure, in combination with relatively low dosages of diuretics (see Chapter 68).

ACE inhibitors may occasionally precipitate acute renal failure, particularly in the elderly, those taking non-steroidal anti-inflammatory agents and patients with renal artery stenosis. Other side-effects (rashes, neutropenia, taste disturbance) are unusual with the low dosages currently recommended but are more prominent in renal failure. Because of their tendency to potassium retention, potassium-sparing diuretics or potassium supplements should not be taken concurrently. Blood creatinine and potassium levels should be monitored regularly, especially in patients with renal failure, in whom hyperkalaemia may occasionally reach dangerous levels.

Captopril, enalapril and lisinopril are all suitable for use in diabetic patients; enalapril and lisinopril are given once daily for hypertension. The first dose of an ACE inhibitor should be small (e.g. 6.25 mg of captopril) and given just before bedtime to minimize postural hypotension, which may be profound in subjects overtreated with diuretics, although rarely symptomatic.

SECOND-LINE AGENTS

Should the above drugs be ineffective or contra-indicated, others can be used, usually in conjunction with one or more first-line agents.

Direct vasodilators (e.g. the α_1-blocker, *prazosin*, and *hydralazine*) cause tachycardia and sodium retention and can logically be combined with a β-blocker and/or a diuretic. Hydralazine is useful in renal failure as it does not accumulate to toxic levels. Prazosin has been recommended in diabetic hypertension as it is effective, devoid of metabolic side-effects and not associated with impotence [63].

Labetolol, a racemate which blocks both α- and β-adrenoceptors (properties of its D- and L-isomers respectively), is useful in hypertensive crisis and in phaeochromocytoma.

Clonidine, a central α_2-agonist, has obtrusive side-effects (drowsiness, dry mouth, depression and postural hypotension) but it is specifically indicated in patients who also suffer from migraine, in which it has a prophylactic effect.

Alpha-methyldopa and *ganglion blockers* cause numerous side-effects (including impotence) and are now little used.

Treatment strategy

Antihypertensive treatment is simply one aspect of a multipronged attack on cardiovascular risk factors. Any drugs must be chosen carefully to minimize any adverse effects on the patient's diabetic control, cardiovascular risks or quality of life. A treatment schedule is suggested below and summarized in Fig. 69.6.

1 *General measures.* When the diagnosis has been confirmed and secondary hypertension excluded, general measures alone can be tried for 2–3 months in most patients. However, those with severe hypertension (defined as above) are un-

likely to respond and will also require antihypertensive drugs from the outset. General measures should be continued indefinitely.

2 *Single-drug therapy.* If general measures alone are ineffective, a single first-choice drug should be selected from Table 69.3, according to the patient's individual needs (angina, cardiac failure, hyperlipidaemia, etc.). The drug's action and possible side-effects must be fully explained. Weight, cardiovascular status, glycaemic control, renal function and blood lipid levels should be monitored.

3 *Alternative single-drug therapy.* If hypertension persists for a further 2–3 months and compliance

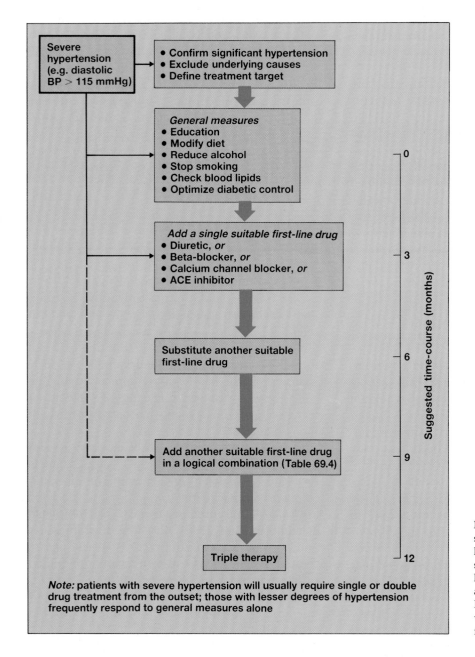

Fig. 69.6. Suggested management scheme for diabetic patients with hypertension. Drug treatment should be started as shown if hypertension remains uncontrolled after 3 months of general measures. Patients with severe hypertension will generally need drug treatment from the outset.

seems satisfactory, another suitable first-line drug should be substituted.

4 *Double-drug therapy.* If single-drug therapy fails, another first-line drug should be added to give a 'logical' combination (Table 69.4).

5 *Triple-drug therapy.* Should double-drug therapy prove ineffective after 2–3 months, a third drug (e.g. another first-line agent or a vasodilator) should be added.

6 *Management of resistant hypertension.* About 95% of hypertensive patients will respond to triple-drug therapy. In resistant cases, the possibility of secondary hypertension should be reconsidered and compliance reinforced if possible. All other risk factors must be minimized, although adherence to advice about diet, smoking and alcohol is often poor in this group. The addition of a fourth drug (e.g. clonidine) may be helpful.

The duration of antihypertensive treatment is controversial, as blood pressure may remain normal for some time after stopping effective treatment. Antihypertensive drugs may be withdrawn for a trial period in those patients who have been well-controlled for several months. Those who remain normotensive without treatment should be encouraged to continue the general measures and be reviewed to ensure that hypertension does not recur.

GARETH WILLIAMS

References

1 World Health Organization Multinational Study. Prevalence of small vessel and large vessel disease in diabetic patients from 14 centres. *Diabetologia* 1985; **28** (suppl): 615–40.
2 Drury PL. Hypertension. In: Nattrass M, Hale PJ, eds. *Non-Insulin Dependent Diabetes. Clin Endocrinol Metab* 1988; **2**: 375–9.
3 Jarrett RJ, ed. *Diabetes and Heart Disease.* Amsterdam: Elsevier, 1984; 1–23.
4 Simonson DC. Etiology and prevalence of hypertension in diabetic patients. *Diabetes Care* 1988: **11**: 821–7.
5 Lundgren H, Björkman L, Keiding P, Lundmark S, Bengtsson C. Diabetes in patients with hypertension receiving pharmacological treatment. *Br Med J* 1988; **297**: 1512–13.
6 Feldt-Rasmussen B, Mathiesen ER, Deckert T *et al.* Central role for sodium in the pathogenesis of blood pressure changes independent of angiotensin, aldosterone and catecholamines in Type 1 (insulin-dependent) diabetes mellitus. *Diabetologia* 1987; **30**: 610–17.
7 Weidmann P, Beretta-Piccoli C, Keusch G, Gluck Z, Mujagic M, Grimm M, Meier A, Ziegler WH. Sodium-volume factor, cardiovascular reactivity and hypotensive mechanism of diuretic therapy in mild hypertension associated with diabetes mellitus. *Am J Med* 1979; **67**: 779–84.
8 Weidmann P, Beretta-Piccoli C, Trost BN. Pressor factors and responsiveness in hypertension accompanying diabetes mellitus. *Hypertension* 1985; **7** (suppl II): 33–42.
9 DeChatel R, Weidmann P, Flammer J, Ziegler WH, Beretta-Piccoli C, Vetter W, Reubin FC. Sodium, renin, aldosterone, catecholamines and blood pressure in diabetes mellitus. *Kidney Int* 1977; **12**: 412–21.
10 Christlieb AR, Kaldany A, D'Elia JA. Plasma renin activity and hypertension in diabetes mellitus. *Diabetes* 1976; **25**: 969–74.
11 Christlieb AR, Assal J-P, Katsilambros N, Williams GH, Kozak GP, Suzuki T. Plasma renin activity and blood volume in uncontrolled diabetes: ketoacidosis, a state of secondary aldosteronism. *Diabetes* 1975; **24**: 190–3.
12 Christensen NJ. Plasma norepinephrine and epinephrine in untreated diabetes, during fasting and after insulin administration. *Diabetes* 1974; **23**: 1–8.
13 Christensen NJ. Plasma catecholamines in long-term diabetes with and without neuropathy and in hypophysectomized subjects. *J Clin Invest* 1972; **51**: 779–87.
14 Christlieb AR, Janka H-U, Kraus B, Gleason RE, Icasas-Cabral EA, Aiello LM, Cabral BV, Solano A. Vascular reactivity to angiotensin II and to norepinephrine in diabetic subjects. *Diabetes* 1976; **25**: 268–74.
15 Grenfell A, Watkins PJ. Clinical diabetic nephropathy: natural history and complications. In: Watkins PJ, ed. *Long-term Complications of Diabetes. Clin Endocrinol Metab* 1986; **15**: 783–806.
16 Wiseman MJ, Viberti GC, Mackintosh D, Jarrett RJ, Keen H. Glycaemia, arterial pressure and microalbuminuria in Type 1 (insulin-dependent) diabetes mellitus. *Diabetologia* 1984; **26**: 401–5.
17 Deckert T, Feldt-Rasmussen B, Borch-Johnsen K, Jensen T, Kofoed-Enevoldsen A. Albuminuria reflects widespread vascular damage. The Steno hypothesis. *Diabetologia* 1989; **32**: 219–26.
18 Parving H-H, Andersen AR, Smidt UM, Hommel E, Mathiesen ER, Svendsen PAå. Effect of antihypertensive treatment on kidney function in diabetic nephropathy. *Br Med J* 1987; **294**: 1443–52.
19 Anderson S, Brenner BM. Influence of antihypertensive therapy on development and progression of diabetic glomerulopathy. *Diabetes Care* 1988; **11**: 846–9.
20 Parving H-H, Hommel E. Prognosis in diabetic nephropathy. *Br Med J* 1989; **299**: 230–3.
21 Björck S, Nyberg G, Mulec H *et al.* Beneficial effects of angiotensin converting enzyme inhibition on renal function in patients with diabetic nephropathy. *Br Med J* 1986; **293**: 471–4.
22 Parving H-H, Hommel E, Smidt UM. Protection of kidney function and decrease in albuminuria by captopril in insulin dependent diabetics with nephropathy. *Br Med J* 1988; **297**: 1086–91.
23 Marre M, Chatellier G, Leblanc H, Guyene TT, Menard J, Passa P. Prevention of diabetic nephropathy with enalapril in normotensive diabetics with microalbuminuria. *Br Med J* 1988; **297**: 1092–6.
24 Reaven GM. Role of insulin resistance in human disease. *Diabetes* 1988; **37**: 1596–1607.
25 Manicardi V, Camellini L, Bellode G, Coscelli C, Ferranini E. Evidence for an association of high blood pressure and hyperinsulinemia in obese man. *J Clin Endocrinol Metab* 1986; **62**: 1302–4.
26 Landsberg L. Insulin and hypertension: lessons from obesity. *N Engl J Med* 1987; **317**: 378–9.
27 Baum M. Insulin stimulates volume absorption in the

rabbit proximal convoluted tubule. *J Clin Invest* 1987; **79**: 1104–9.

28 Rowe JW, Young JB, Minaker KL, Stevens AL, Pallotta J, Landsberg J. Effect of insulin and glucose infusions on sympathetic nervous system activity in normal man. *Diabetes* 1981; **30**: 219–25.

29 Murray DP, Ferriss JB, O'Sullivan DJ. Is good diabetic control bad for blood pressure? *Clin Sci* 1988; **74** (suppl 17): 58.

30 Struthers AD. The choice of anti-hypertensive therapy in the diabetic patient. *Postgrad Med J* 1985; **61**: 563–9.

31 Kannel WB, McGee DL. Diabetes and glucose tolerance as risk factors for cardiovascular disease. The Framingham study. *Diabetes Care* 1979; **2**: 120–6.

32 Fuller JH. Epidemiology of hypertension associated with diabetes mellitus. *Hypertension* 1985; **7** (part II): 3–7.

33 Dupree EA, Meyer MB. Role of risk factors in the complications of diabetes mellitus. *Am J Epidemiol* 1980; **112**: 100–12.

34 Cruikshank JK, Anderson NMcF, Wadsworth J *et al.* Treating hypertension in black compared with white non-insulin-dependent diabetics: a double blind trial of verapamil and metoprolol. *Br Med J* 1988; **297**: 1155–9.

35 Teuscher A, Schnell H, Wilson PWF. Incidence of diabetic retinopathy and relationship to baseline plasma glucose and blood pressure. *Diabetes Care* 1988; **11**: 246–51.

36 Krolewski AS, Canessa M, Warram JH, Laffel LMB, Christlieb AR, Knowler WC, Rand LI. Predisposition to hypertension and susceptibility to renal disease in insulin-dependent diabetes mellitus. *N Engl J Med* 1988; **318**: 140–5.

37 Mangili R, Bending JJ, Scott G, Li LK, Gupta A, Viberti GC. Increased sodium–lithium counter-transport activity in red cells of patients with insulin-dependent diabetes and nephropathy. *N Engl J Med* 1988; **318**: 146–50.

38 Borch-Johnsen K, Kreiner S. Proteinuria — A predictor of cardiovascular mortality in insulin-dependent diabetes mellitus. *Br Med J* 1987; **294**: 1651–4.

39 Drury PL, Tarn AC. Are the WHO criteria for hypertension appropriate in young insulin-dependent diabetics? *Diabetic Med* 1985; **2**: 79–82.

40 Hommel E, Carstensen H, Skøtt P, Larsen S, Parving H-H. Prevalence and causes of microscopic haematuria in Type 1 (insulin-dependent) diabetic patients with persistent proteinuria. *Diabetologia* 1987; **30**: 627–30.

41 World Health Organization. The 1986 guidelines for the treatment of mild hypertension. *Hypertension* 1986; **8**: 957–61.

42 Collins R, Peto R, MacMahon S *et al.* Blood pressure, stroke, and coronary heart disease. Part 2. *Lancet* 1990; **335**: 827–38.

43 Mühlhauser I, Sawicki P, Didjurgeit V, Jörgens V, Berger M. Uncontrolled hypertension in type 1 diabetes: Assessment of patients' desires about treatment and improvement of blood pressure control by a structured treatment and teaching programme. *Diabetic Med* 1988; **5**: 693–8.

44 Dodson PM, Beevers M, Hallworth R, Webberley MJ, Fletcher RF, Taylor KG. Sodium restriction and blood pressure in hypertensive type II diabetics: randomized blind controlled and crossover studies of moderate sodium restriction and sodium supplementation. *Br Med J* 1989; **298**: 227–30.

45 Pacy PJ, Dodson PM, Kubicki AJ, Fletcher RF, Taylor KG. Comparison of the hypotensive and metabolic effects of bendrofluazide therapy with a high fibre, low sodium, low fat diet in diabetic subjects with mild hypertension. *J Hypertens* 1984; **2**: 215–20.

46 Saurez L, Barrett-Connor E. Interaction between cigarette smoking and diabetes mellitus in the prediction of death attributed to cardiovascular disease. *Am J Epidemiol* 1984; **120**: 670–5.

47 Mühlhauser I, Sawicki P, Berger M. Cigarette-smoking as a risk factor for macroproteinuria and proliferative retinopathy in Type 1 (insulin-dependent) diabetes. *Diabetologia* 1986; **29**: 500–3.

48 Telmer S, Christiansen JS, Andersen AR, Nerup J, Deckert T. Smoking habits and prevalence of clinical diabetic microangiopathy in insulin-dependent diabetics. *Acta Med Scand* 1984; **215**: 613–18.

49 Dall'Aglio E, Strata A, Reaven G. Abnormal lipid metabolism in treated hypertensive patients with non-insulin-dependent diabetes mellitus. *Am J Med* 1988; **84**: 899–903.

50 Glauber H, Wallace P, Griver K, Brechtel G. Adverse metabolic effect of omega-3 fatty acids in non-insulin dependent diabetes mellitus. *Ann Intern Med* 1988; **108**: 663–8.

51 Kaplan NM. Critique of recommendations from Working Group on Hypertension in Diabetes. *Am J Kidney Dis* 1989; **13**: 38–40.

52 Osei K, Holland G, Falko JM. Indapamide — effects on apoprotein, lipoprotein, and glucoregulation in ambulatory diabetic patients. *Arch Int Med* 1986; **146**: 1973–7.

53 MacMahon SW, Macdonald GJ. Antihypertensive treatment and plasma lipoprotein levels. The associations in data from a population study. *Am J Med* 1987; **80** (suppl 2A): 40–7.

54 Prince MJ, Stuart CA, Padia M, Bandi Z, Holland OB. Metabolic effects of hydrochlorothiazide and enalapril during treatment of the hypertensive diabetic patient. Enalapril for hypertensive diabetics. *Arch Int Med* 1988; **148**: 2363–8.

55 Wright AD, Barber SG, Kendall MJ, Poole PH. Beta-adrenoceptor-blocking drugs and blood sugar control in diabetes mellitus. *Br Med J* 1979; **1**: 159–64.

56 Marengo C, Marena S, Renzetti A, Mossino M, Pagano G. Beta-blockers in hypertensive non-insulin-dependent diabetes: comparison between penbutolol and propranolol on metabolic control and response to insulin-induced hypoglycaemia. *Acta Diabetol Lat* 1988; **25**: 141–7.

57 Lager I, Blohme G, Smith U. Effect of cardioselective and nonselective beta-blockade on the hypoglycaemic response in insulin-dependent diabetics. *Lancet* 1979; i: 458–62.

58 Trost BN, Weidmann P. Effects of calcium antagonists on glucose homeostasis and serum lipids in non-diabetic and diabetic subjects: a review. *J Hypertens* 1987; **5** (suppl 4): 81–104.

59 Burr AJ, Hay J. Captopril and hypertension in black diabetics. *Br Med J* 1989; **299**: 458–9.

60 Taguma Y, Kitamoto Y, Futaki G, Ueda H, Monma H, Ishizaki M, Takahishi H, Sekino H, Sasaki Y. Effect of captopril on heavy proteinuria in azotemic diabetics. *N Engl J Med* 1985; **313**: 1617–20.

61 Mimran A, Insua A, Ribstein J, Monnier L, Bringer J, Mirouze J. Contrasting effects of captopril and nifedipine in normotensive patients with incipient diabetic nephropathy. *J Hypertens* 1988; **6**: 919–23.

62 Bank N, Klose R, Áynedjian HS, Nguyen D, Sablay LB. Evidence against increased glomerular pressure initiating diabetic nephropathy. *Kidney Int* 1987; **31**: 898–905.

63 Lipson LG. Treatment of hypertension in diabetic men: problems with sexual dysfunction. *Am J Cardiol* 1984; **53**: 46A–50A.

PART 13.6
OTHER DIABETIC
COMPLICATIONS

70   The Diabetic Foot

Summary

- Both neuropathy and ischaemia, frequently acting in combination and often complicated by infection, predispose to ulceration in the diabetic foot.
- The 'neuropathic' foot is numb, warm and dry, with palpable pulses; complications include neuropathic ulcers, Charcot arthropathy and (rarely) neuropathic oedema.
- Neuropathic ulcers occur at points of high pressure loading, especially on the soles or at sites of deformity; pressure damage leads progressively to callosity formation, autolysis and finally ulceration. Secondary infection is common. Treatment involves removing skin callosities to drain the ulcer, reducing pressure loading by special shoes or total-contact plaster casting, and appropriate antibiotics.
- Charcot arthropathy usually involves the metatarso-tarsal joints, frequently follows minor trauma, and presents as warmth, swelling and redness, sometimes with pain. Bone scans allow early diagnosis and radiographs later show disorganization of the joint and new bone formation. Treatment is by immobilizing and unloading the limb, with non-steroidal anti-inflammatory drugs for pain.
- Neuropathic oedema may be due to microcirculatory disturbances following autonomic denervation; ephedrine treatment is often effective.
- The 'ischaemic' foot is cold and pulseless and subject to rest pain, ulceration and gangrene.
- Ischaemic ulceration usually affects the foot margins. Medical treatment alone is often effective; focal stenoses of the iliac, femoral or even popliteal arteries are often amenable to angioplasty or bypass grafting; amputation must be avoided if at all possible.
- The management of diabetic foot ulceration is best guided by determining the relative contributions of neuropathy, ischaemia and infection. Collaborative teamwork involving the chiropodist, orthotist (shoe fitter), nurse, physician and surgeon is most effective.
- Effective education is essential in the prevention of diabetic foot problems.

Three factors predispose to tissue damage in the diabetic foot, namely neuropathy, peripheral vascular disease and infection. Infection is rarely a sole factor but often complicates neuropathy and ischaemia.

From the practical point of view, the diabetic foot can generally be considered as one of two entities, the 'neuropathic foot' and the 'ischaemic foot'. In the neuropathic foot, somatic and autonomic nerve fibres have been damaged but the circulation is intact and the pulses palpable, resulting in a warm, numb, dry foot [1]. The neuropathic foot has three main complications: the neuropathic ulcer, the neuropathic (Charcot) joint and neuropathic oedema. The ischaemic foot suffers predominantly from its reduced blood supply, but usually also shows a variable degree of neuropathy and so should strictly be termed the 'neuro-ischaemic' foot. Blood flow is reduced because of atherosclerosis in the major leg arteries, particularly in the calf vessels; the possible role of 'small vessel' (arteriolar) disease has received much attention in the past but there is no strong evidence to show that it plays an important part in tissue necrosis [2]. The neuro-ischaemic foot is usually cold and pulseless and may be complicated by rest pain, ulceration due to localized pressure necrosis, and ultimately gangrene.

Neuropathic and neuro-ischaemic feet are therefore distinguished by characteristic lesions, which need specific management. The following sections will describe the clinical features of diabetic feet, simple bedside investigations (vibration perception threshold and ankle blood pressure measurements) which may help to identify the cause of tissue damage, and the various treatments available. Finally, the organization of diabetic foot care will be discussed.

The neuropathic foot

The neuropathic ulcer

PRESENTATION

This characteristically occurs at sites of high mechanical pressure on the plantar surface of the foot (Fig. 70.1). The presence of neuropathy (even in its earliest stage, with relatively mild sensory defects) may itself disturb the posture of the foot and so predispose to local increases in pressure [3], which are also commonly caused by deformities such as claw or hammer toes, pes cavus, Charcot joints and previous ray amputations [4]. The situation is exacerbated by wearing tight, ill-fitting shoes, especially in the presence of oedema. If the foot is deformed, the high vertical and shear forces under the plantar surface of the metatarsal heads lead to the formation of callosities (Figs

70.1 and 70.2) [5], of which the patient is often unaware. Repetitive mechanical forces lead to inflammatory autolysis and subkeratotic haematomas, which eventually break through to the skin surface, forming an ulcer (Figs 70.2 and 70.3). The pressures to which localized areas of the sole are subjected under normal walking conditions can be measured accurately by pressure transducers worn in the shoes, or by the 'optical paedabarograph' (Fig. 70.4). Pressures over the metatarsal heads in neuropathic feet are often increased several-fold.

Ulcers are often infected by staphylococci, streptococci, coliforms or anaerobes [4]. Streptococci and staphylococci may act synergistically, the streptococci producing hyaluronidase which facilitates the spread of the necrotizing toxins released by staphylococci. In severe cases, this can result in thrombotic arterial occlusion and gangrene. In the deep tissues of the foot, aerobic organisms may act synergistically with microaerophilic or anaerobic organisms to produce necrotizing infection, which often generates subcutaneous gas (Fig. 70.5) or spreads to involve the bones (Fig. 70.6). Extensive tissue loss and gangrene may finally result.

MANAGEMENT OF THE NEUROPATHIC ULCER

Excess callus tissue should be pared away with a scalpel (but only by a trained chiropodist) to expose and drain the ulcer base [6]. Oral antibiotics,

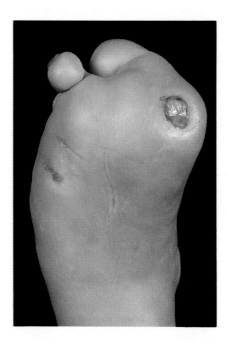 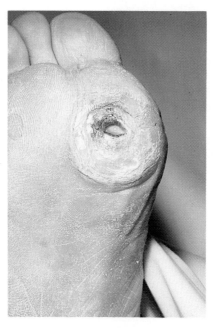

Fig. 70.1. Typical 'punched-out' neuropathic ulcers arising in heavily calloused skin underlying the first metatarsal head. Note previous amputations (left) and particularly thick callosities (right). (Left panel reproduced by kind permission of Dr Ian Casson, Broadgreen Hospital, Liverpool.)

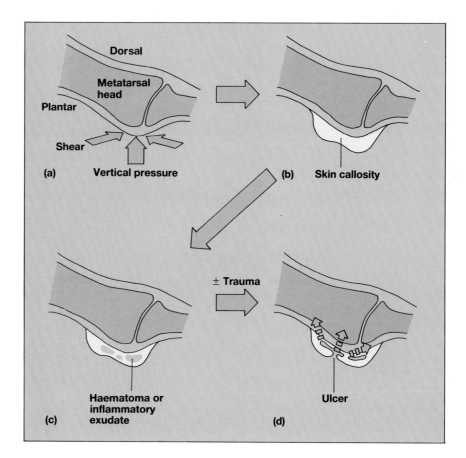

Fig. 70.2. Formation of a neuropathic pressure ulcer. (a) Abnormal foot posture and loss of sensation, both due to neuropathy, increase vertical pressure and tangential shear forces applied to vulnerable areas such as the metatarsal heads. (b) Increased pressure and shear forces cause hyperkeratosis and ultimately callosity formation. (c) Haematomas and inflammatory exudate (initially sterile) form within the callosity, finally breaking through to the surface to form an ulcer (d). Trauma accelerates the process. Secondary infection may spread to cause soft-tissue necrosis or osteomyelitis.

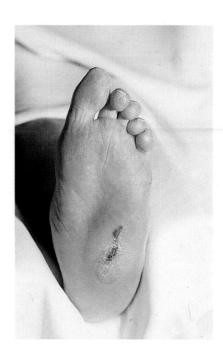

Fig. 70.3. Large subcutaneous haematoma following trauma to a neuropathic foot which subsequently broke through the skin to form an ulcer. (Reproduced by kind permission of Mr Patrick Laing, Royal Liverpool Hospital.)

appropriate to the organisms isolated from a swab of the ulcer base, should be given until the ulcer has healed. Suitable antibiotics include phenoxymethyl penicillin (500 mg 6-hourly) for streptococcal infections, flucloxacillin (500 mg 6-hourly) for staphylococci and metronidazole (400 mg 8-hourly) for anaerobic infections. If the ulcer is superficial and there is no cellulitis, out-patient

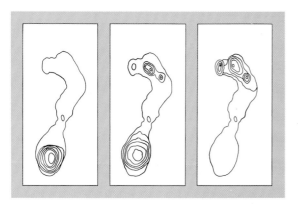

Fig. 70.4. Map of pressure distribution over the sole of a diabetic patient with peripheral neuropathy measured by the optical paedabarograph, at three successive stages during normal walking. Note the high pressures (>10 kg/cm²) generated under the first and second metatarsal heads, which are considerably greater than in subjects without neuropathy and with normal foot posture. (Reproduced by kind permission of Dr Andrew Boulton, Manchester Royal Infirmary.)

Table 70.1. Treatment of sepsis in the neuropathic foot.

- Admit to hospital
- Bedrest
- Antibiotics: 'general cover' regimen or specific, if organisms known:
  cefuroxime 1.5 g 8-hourly i.v. }
  flucloxacillin 500 mg 6-hourly i.v. 'general cover' regimen
  metronidazole 1 g 8-hourly rectally
- Urgent surgical drainage of pus and debridement of dead tissue
- Send pus and tissue for culture; adjust antibiotics accordingly
- Consider ray amputation of digit if bone is destroyed
- Ensure tight glycaemic control, using i.v. insulin if necessary (see Chapter 81)

treatment is adequate. If cellulitis is present, however, the limb is potentially threatened and the patient should be hospitalized immediately and treated strictly by the regimen described in Table 70.1.

Reduction of weight-bearing forces is necessary both in the acute phase and also in long-term management. In the presence of sepsis, bedrest is indicated but foam wedges must be used to protect the heels against pressure damage. In the short term, a light-weight, total-contact plaster cast which entirely encases the foot (including the ulcerated area) can be applied to unload pressure from the ulcer and reduce shear forces on vulnerable parts of the foot (Fig. 70.7) [7]. In the long term, weight-bearing forces can be redistributed more equally over the sole by using special footwear and insoles made of energy-absorbing material such as Plastozote® or microcellular rubber [1, 8].

Certain cases may need shoes constructed specifically by the orthotist, but extra-depth stock shoes will be adequate for many patients. These shoes are made in standard sizes but are deeper to allow insertion of either sponge rubber cushions or of purpose-made insoles or foot cradles.

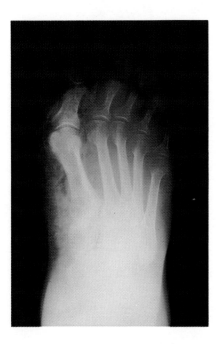

Fig. 70.5. Extensive soft-tissue infection with gas formation arising from a neuropathic ulcer in a diabetic foot. (Reproduced by kind permission of Dr Ian MacFarlane, Walton Hospital, Liverpool.)

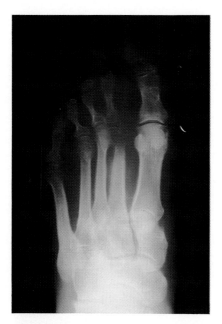

Fig. 70.6. Osteomyelitis destroying the head of the second metatarsal. The infection spread from an underlying neuropathic ulcer. (Reproduced by kind permission of Dr Ian MacFarlane, Walton Hospital, Liverpool.)

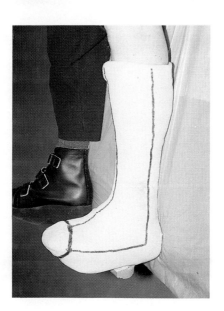

Fig. 70.7. Total-contact plaster cast used to treat neuropathic ulcer. Weight is taken by the plastic rocker, off-loading pressure from the ulcerated area. Lines show where the cast is cut for removal. (Reproduced by kind permission of Mr Patrick Laing, Royal Liverpool Hospital.)

Neuropathic (Charcot) arthropathy

PRESENTATION

The precipitating event is often surprisingly minor trauma such as tripping, which results in a swollen, erythematous, hot and sometimes painful foot (Figs 70.8 and 70.9). Initial radiological examination is usually normal, but subsequent films show evidence of fracture, osteolysis and fragmentation of bone, followed by new bone formation and finally subluxation and disorganization of the joint (Fig. 70.10). Bone scans are more

sensitive indicators of new bone formation than radiography and should be used to confirm the diagnosis (Fig. 70.11). This destructive process often takes place over only a few months, and can lead to considerable deformity of the foot. The tarso-metatarsal joints are most commonly involved [9].

Early diagnosis is essential and is suggested by three features:

1 A history of trauma, often minor.
2 The presence of unilateral warmth and swelling.
3 Positive radiographic or bone scan findings.

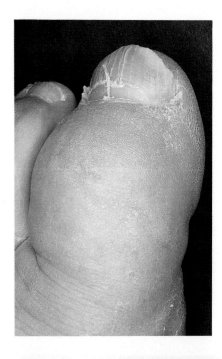

Fig. 70.8. Acute Charcot arthropathy affecting the interphalangeal joint of the great toe. Sudden onset of pain, redness and swelling with no obvious preceding trauma initially suggested a diagnosis of acute gout. (Reproduced by kind permission of Dr Geoffrey V. Gill, Arrowe Park Hospital, Wirral.)

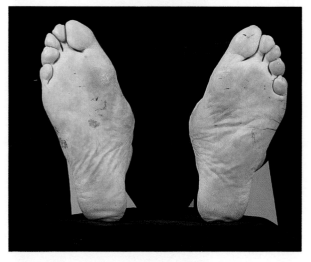

Fig. 70.9. Advanced Charcot arthropathy of both feet, showing gross disorganization. (Reproduced by kind permission of Dr Ian Casson, Broadgreen Hospital, Liverpool.)

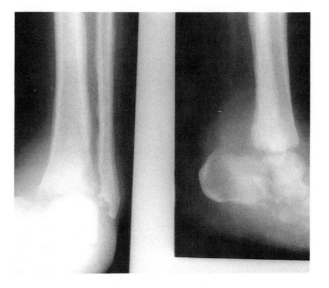

Fig. 70.10. Radiograph of advanced Charcot arthropathy, showing destruction of the ankle and foot joints, with widespread bone resorption, soft tissue swelling and a large effusion.

MANAGEMENT

Initial management comprises immobilization and unloading of the injured limb, such as by non-weight-bearing crutches or a total-contact plaster cast [10]. This is continued until oedema and warmth have subsided, when the foot should be gradually mobilized using a moulded insole in a custom-fitted shoe. Non-steroidal anti-inflammatory drugs may be useful in painful cases.

Neuropathic oedema

PRESENTATION

Neuropathic oedema is fluid accumulation in the feet and lower legs which is associated with severe peripheral neuropathy and is not explicable by other causes such as cardiac failure or hypo-albuminaemia. It is extremely uncommon. Its pathogenesis may be related to abnormal vaso-

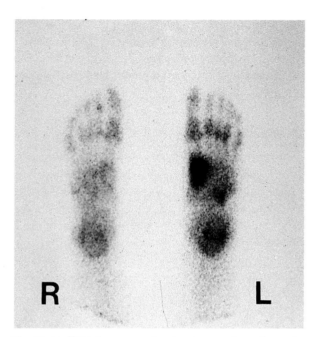

Fig. 70.11. ^{99m}Tc bone scan showing increased uptake in the region of the base of the first metatarsal and the metatarso-cuneiform joint, indicating new bone formation in early Charcot arthropathy (L). At this stage, plain radiography showed no definite abnormality.

motor function following autonomic denervation, causing arterio-venous shunting and disturbances in hydrostatic pressure in the microcirculation (see Chapter 55).

MANAGEMENT

The sympathomimetic drug, ephedrine (30 mg 8-hourly), has been shown to be useful, probably by reducing peripheral blood flow and by increasing urinary sodium excretion [11].

The neuro-ischaemic foot

Presentation

REST PAIN

Pain is continuous in the foot, often worse at night and characteristically relieved by dependency; it may be reduced by elevating the head of the bed. At this stage, the foot is often pink because of capillary dilatation in response to hypoxia but, in contrast to the neuropathic foot, it is cold.

ULCERATION

Gangrene and ulcers in the ischaemic foot usually result from continuous excessive pressure on the margins of the foot (Fig. 70.12); ulceration of the plantar surface is rare because its pressure loading is intermittent. The most important precipitating factor is the wearing of tight shoes, which is exacerbated by deformity and oedema [4]. Digital ischaemia and gangrene are also common in patients with diabetic nephropathy, who frequently have extensive medial calcification of the digital and limb arteries (see Figs 67.8 and 67.9). Ulceration is often complicated by secondary infection, commonly with both aerobic and anaerobic bacteria.

MANAGEMENT

Medical management. This is indicated if the ulcer is small, shallow and of recent onset (within the previous month), and is the mainstay of treatment for patients in whom reconstructive surgery is not feasible because of widespread vascular disease.

It is important to eradicate infection promptly with specific antibiotic therapy. Cardiac failure, which accounted for foot oedema in two-thirds of cases in one series [4], must also be treated, but with care to avoid dehydration. The provision of suitable shoes is simpler than for the purely neuropathic foot. Deep, widely fitting shoes are needed to protect the margins of the foot and accomodate any deformity, and can often be obtained ready-made. Regular chiropody should be performed to debride ulcers and, in the case of subungual ulcers, to cut back the nail to encourage free drainage of pus.

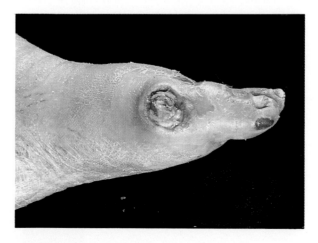

Fig. 70.12. Ulceration over the medial margin of the first metatarsal head in a neuro-ischaemic foot.

Surgical treatment. If the ulcer does not respond to medical management within 4 weeks, angiography should be carried out to identify any stenoses which might be amenable to angioplasty or other reconstructive surgery.

The lesions most suitable for angioplasty are focal stenoses of less than 4 cm long and occlusions shorter than 10 cm long. Angioplasty is indicated for localized stenoses in the iliac or femoral arteries. At present, iliac artery angioplasties have a higher general success rate than those in the femoral or popliteal vessels [12]. Diabetic patients show a predilection to stenosis in the branches of the popliteal artery; experience with popliteal artery dilatation is very limited, but fewer than 50% of reconstructions remain patent after 2 years [13].

The relative roles of angioplasty and bypass surgery are currently being assessed. They are likely to be complementary measures, but angioplasty is particularly useful for patients unfit for major arterial reconstruction. If a block in the femoral artery is not amenable to angioplasty, reversed saphenous-vein grafts may successfully bypass the femoral to the popliteal artery and have resulted in high rates of limb salvage, even in elderly diabetic patients [14]. More distal stenoses in the branches of the popliteal artery are now treated by bypass grafts bridging the femoral to distal tibial or peroneal arteries and by percutaneous transluminal angioplasty [13]. Methods using the saphenous vein '*in situ*' have been developed, thus preserving the vasa vasorum and minimizing endothelial injury [15].

Sympathectomy generally fails to promote ulcer healing but may occasionally ameliorate rest pain [16]. In many cases, neither angioplasty nor arterial reconstruction are possible, when digitial necrosis in the ischaemic foot is often best managed with the conservative methods described above. Amputation of the foot should be avoided if at all possible as rehabilitation is often poor. Limited surgery, such as 'ray' excision of the affected digit may sometimes be successful and the patient's ability to walk and balance may be little impaired if the great toe is preserved (Fig. 70.13) but this option should also only be considered if conservative methods fail [17].

Assessment of the foot

Neuropathy, ischaemia, deformity and oedema are all important factors which may lead to ulceration in the diabetic foot. When assessing the foot, the relative contribution of each of these factors must be determined in order to plan rational management.

Integrated examination of the diabetic foot

INSPECTION AND PALPATION

The key points are shown in Table 70.2. All areas of the foot, including the dorsum, sole, back of the heel and between the toes, should be first inspected and then palpated. The pulses and temperature and moisture of the skin should be assessed and the presence of oedema and regions of tenderness noted.

NEUROLOGICAL EXAMINATION

Perception of pinprick, light touch and vibration should be determined and the knee and ankle tendon reflexes examined, with and without reinforcement.

BEDSIDE INVESTIGATIONS

Bacteriological swabs should be taken from the base of any ulcers. Physical examination can be complemented by two other simple tests, measurement of vibration perception threshold and the determination of the ankle−brachial pressure index.

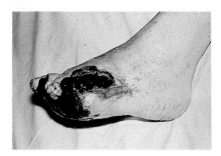

(a)

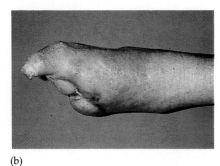

(b)

Fig. 70.13. Distal gangrene in a neuro-ischaemic foot (a). After ray excision (b), the great toe is preserved and the foot remains able to maintain balance and walking.

Table 70.2. Examination of the foot in a diabetic patient.

Colour:
- Red foot (cellulitis or early Charcot arthropathy)
- Pale or cyanotic foot (ischaemia)
- Pink foot associated with pain and absent pulses (severe ischaemia)

Deformity:
- Claw toe, hammer toe, hallux valgus, hallux varus
- Pes cavus, prominent metatarsal heads
- Charcot arthropathy

Oedema:
- Bilateral may be due to cardiac failure, fluid overload or neuropathy
- Unilateral may indicate sepsis or Charcot arthropathy

Nails:
- Atrophic in neuropathy and ischaemia
- Discoloured in fungal infection and subungual ulceration

Skin callosities:
- In the neuropathic foot, found on the plantar surface of the metatarsal heads and apices of toes

Tissue breakdown: ulcers:
- Neuropathic typically on soles
- Neuro-ischaemic typically on foot margins

Tissue breakdown: fissures, blisters

Foot pulses:
- Posterior tibial and dorsalis pedis are weak or absent in ischaemic feet, often strong in neuropathic feet

Skin temperature:
- Neuropathic feet are usually warm, ischaemic feet are cold

Skin moisture:
- Neuropathic feet are dry

Signs of infection:
- Crepitus, fluctuation, deep tenderness

VIBRATION PERCEPTION THRESHOLD (VPT)

VPT can be measured using a hand-held Biothesiometer [18]. The vibrating tactor is applied to the test site (e.g. medial malleolus or tip of the big toe) and the amplitude of vibration increased from zero until the patient first perceives the sensation of vibration. The threshold is usually taken as the mean of three values, expressed in arbitrary voltage units (which are related to the amplitude of vibration). The vibration threshold increases with age, and values must always be compared with age-adjusted nomograms. As discussed in Chapter 62, VPT values may vary considerably with time and site.

ANKLE—BRACHIAL PRESSURE INDEX

The pressure index [19] is calculated by dividing the systolic blood pressure at the ankle by the brachial systolic pressure (measured in the conventional way). The ankle systolic pressure is measured by applying a 12-cm sphygmomanometer cuff just above the ankle. The cuff is inflated to obliterate the posterior tibial pulse and is then slowly released. The systolic pressure is indicated by the return of flow.

In normal subjects, the pressure index is usually greater than 1.0. Some 5—10% of diabetic patients have stiff, non-compressible peripheral vessel walls (probably due to medial calcification), which artificially elevate the systolic pressure. Nonetheless, the pressure index can be a useful guide to the state of the peripheral arteries: values below 0.6 in diabetic patients indicate a severely compromised circulation.

The results of the clinical examination and bedside investigation should lead to a rational management plan, based on the treatment approaches outlined above.

Organization of foot care for diabetic patients

No single individual can handle every diabetic foot problem. The care of the diabetic foot depends crucially on close liaison between chiropodist, shoe-fitter, nurse, physician and surgeon, ideally in the forum of the diabetic foot clinic [4]. This should provide routine chiropodial care, specific treatment for ulcers and an open access service for emergencies, with the ultimate goal of preventing diabetic foot problems.

This aim will only be achieved through education of the patient in practical aspects of foot care. It is important to emphasize simple advice (Table 70.3). The early recognition of danger signs is important (Table 70.4) and special advice should be given about selection of shoes (Table 70.5). Tissue damage is always potentially serious in the diabetic foot and provision of an emergency service which allows rapid self-referral of the patient, even for apparently trivial lesions, is an important part of preventative care [20].

Many disasters can still befall the diabetic foot but fortunately, most are preventable with adequate education, routine foot care and attention

Table 70.3. Simple foot care advice for the diabetic patient.

Do
- Wash feet daily with mild soap and warm water
- Check feet daily
- Seek urgent treatment of any problems
- See a chiropodist regularly
- Wear sensible shoes

Don't
- Use corn cures
- Use hot water bottles
- Walk barefoot (except children and adolescents)
- Cut corns or callosities
- Treat foot problems yourself

Table 70.4. Danger signs in the diabetic foot.

Check your feet every morning
Come to the clinic *immediately* if you notice:
- Swelling
- Colour change of a nail, toe or part of a foot
- Pain or throbbing
- Thick hard skin or corns
- Breaks in the skin, including cracks, blisters or sores

Table 70.5. Simple footwear advice for diabetic patients.

For everyday use, especially when on the feet for long periods:
- Wear a lace-up shoe, with plenty of room for the toes, and either flat or low heeled
- Never wear slip-on or court shoes, except for special occasions
- Don't wear slippers at home

to footwear. Early detection followed rapidly by specific treatment of neuropathic and neuro-ischaemic lesions provide the best opportunity for a favourable outcome.

MICHAEL E. EDMONDS

ALI V.M. FOSTER

References

1 Edmonds ME. The diabetic foot: pathophysiology and treatment. In: Watkins PJ, ed. *Long-term Complications of Diabetes.* *Clin Endocrinol Metab.* London: WB Saunders 1986; **15:** 889–916.

2 Logerfo FW, Coffman JD. Vascular and microvascular disease of the foot in diabetes. *N Engl J Med* 1984; **311:** 1615–19.

3 Boulton AJM. The importance of abnormal foot pressures and gait in the causation of foot ulcers. In: Connor H, Boulton AJM, Ward JD, eds. *The Foot in Diabetes.* Chichester: John Wiley & Sons, 1987; 11–21.

4 Edmonds ME, Blundell MP, Morris HE, Thomas EM, Cotton LT, Watkins PJ. Improved survival of the diabetic foot: the role of a specialised foot clinic. *Q J Med* 1986; **232:** 736–71.

5 Delbridge L, Ctercteko G, Fowler C, Reeve TS and Le Quesne LP. The aetiology of diabetic neuropathic foot ulceration. *Br J Surg* 1985; **72:** 1–6.

6 Edmonds ME. The diabetic foot. *Med Int* 1985; **13:** 551–3.

7 Coleman WC, Brand PW, Burke JA. The total contact cast. *J Am Podiatry Ass* 1984; **74:** 548–51.

8 Tovey FI. Establishing a diabetic shoe service. *Practical Diabetes* 1985; **2:** 5–8.

9 Sinha S, Munichoodappa CS, Kozak GP. Neuroarthropathy (Charcot joints) in diabetes mellitus. *Medicine (Baltimore)* 1972; **51:** 191–210.

10 Frykberg RG, Kozak GP. The diabetic Charcot foot. In: Kozak GP, Hoar SC, Rowbotham JL *et al.*, eds. *Management of Diabetic Foot Problems.* Philadelphia: WB Saunders, 1984; 103–12.

11 Edmonds ME, Archer AG, Watkins PJ. Ephedrine: A new treatment for diabetic neuropathic oedema. *Lancet* 1983; i: 548–51.

12 Nieman HL, Brabdt TD, Greenberg M. Percutaneous transluminal angioplasty: an angiographer's viewpoint. *Arch Surg* 1981; **116:** 821–8.

13 Sprayregen S, Sniderman KW, Sos TA *et al.* Popliteal artery branches: percutaneous transluminal angioplasty. *Am J Roentgenol* 1980; **135:** 945–50.

14 Reinhold RB, Gibbons GW, Wheelock FC, Hoar CS. Femoral–popliteal bypass in elderly diabetic patients. *Am J Surg* 1979; **137:** 549–55.

15 Leather RP, Shah DM, Karmody AM. Infrapopliteal bypass for limb salvage: increased patency and utilization of the saphenous vein used 'in situ'. *Surgery* 1981; **90:** 1000–8.

16 Cotton LT, Cross FW. Lumbar sympathectomy for arterial disease. *Br J Surg* 1985; **72:** 678–83.

17 Foster AVM, Gibby D, Nelson M, Nash C, Edmonds ME. Successful management of digital necrosis by autoamputation: avoidance of surgery in the diabetic ischaemic foot. *Diabetic Med* 1988; Vol **5** (suppl): 5.

18 Guy RJC, Clark CA, Malcolm PN, Watkins PJ. Evaluation of thermal and vibration sensation in diabetic neuropathy. *Diabetologia* 1985; **28:** 131–7.

19 Foster AVM, Edmonds ME. Examination of the diabetic foot. Part II. *Practical Diabetes* 1987; **4:** 153–4.

20 Foster AVM, Edmonds ME. Diabetic foot emergencies: A strategy for their care. *Diabetic Med* 1987; **4:** 555A–6A.

71 Gastrointestinal Problems in Diabetes Mellitus

Summary

• Impaired gut motility, largely attributed to autonomic (especially vagal) neuropathy, is common in diabetic patients.

• Diabetic gastrointestinal involvement is usually asymptomatic; diabetic patients with significant gastrointestinal symptoms must be fully investigated to exclude other pathology.

• Disordered gut motility may be identified by manometry, scintigraphy of isotope-labelled meals or barium studies, but abnormalities often correlate poorly with symptoms.

• Oesophageal dilatation and hypomotility are occasionally associated with heartburn and dysphagia.

• Gastric emptying of both solids and liquids is delayed and uncoordinated. Severe gastroparesis may cause severe vomiting, weight loss and unstable diabetic control.

• Diabetic diarrhoea is often intermittent, worse at night, urgent and watery and does not usually cause malabsorption or weight loss. Incontinence due to anorectal dysfunction may also occur.

• Upper gastrointestinal symptoms may respond to prokinetic drugs such as metoclopramide, domperidone or cisapride, and diabetic diarrhoea may be helped by α_2-adrenergic agonists such as clonidine.

Problems relating to the gastrointestinal system are commonly encountered in patients with diabetes mellitus. Newer techniques of assessment have demonstrated, even in patients who are entirely asymptomatic, impairment of smooth muscle function with decreased motility throughout most of the gut. Symptoms, when present, are usually mild and intermittent but, in a minority of patients, can be severe enough to cause considerable disability and interfere with the patient's usual lifestyle.

The diagnosis of specific diabetic gastrointestinal involvement is usually made by excluding other disorders which commonly affect the gut in diabetic and non-diabetic patients alike. The typical gastrointestinal symptom complexes usually occur in long-standing IDDM patients and are associated with clinical neuropathy, but can sometimes develop shortly after diagnosis and may affect NIDDM patients.

Because of the often vague and non-specific nature of the symptoms, together with a lack of suitable screening methods, the prevalence of gastrointestinal problems in diabetic patients remains uncertain. However, this may be much higher than previously suspected. When a careful history was taken, 76% of 136 unselected diabetic out-patients had one or more gastrointestinal symptoms [1]. Recent reports emphasize the high proportion of asymptomatic diabetic patients in whom abnormal gut motility can be demonstrated. In a scintigraphic study of unselected IDDM patients, the transit of a solid bolus through the oesophagus was delayed in 42% of patients and gastric emptying was delayed in 56% [2]. Another study, also using scintigraphy, found abnormal oesophageal motility in 38% of 40 asymptomatic IDDM patients [3].

Pathophysiology

The pathophysiology of the gut motility disturbance in diabetes is probably multifactorial but considerable evidence suggests that autonomic neuropathy plays a dominant role [4]. Several

745

studies have found that disturbed gastrointestinal motility is associated with abnormal cardiac autonomic function tests [3–6]. Damage to the efferent nerve supply impairs the tone and contractility of gut smooth muscle. Autonomic nerve morphology in human diabetes has been little studied and the precise extent of involvement of the extrinsic and intrinsic (myenteric plexus) nerve supply and the relative contributions of parasympathetic and sympathetic damage at the various levels of the gut have not yet been determined. The possible effects of afferent sensory denervation on gut reflex activity and awareness of symptoms are also largely unknown.

Other factors may contribute to the abnormal gut motility in diabetes. A primary disturbance of smooth muscle function is unlikely, since the hypotonic gut muscle still responds when adequately stimulated by prokinetic drugs [7]. The possible role of disturbances in the secretion of the various gut regulatory peptides, which influence gut motility, digestion and absorption and whose secretion is partly modulated by the autonomic nervous system [8], has not yet been systematically studied.

In recent years, a variety of techniques including manometry and radionuclide scintigraphy have helped to clarify the defects in gut motility in diabetes. Manometry is more sensitive than traditional radiographic methods but requires intubation and is time-consuming. On the other hand, scintigraphic imaging of fluid and solid markers labelled with gamma-emitting radioisotopes is simple, quick, non-invasive, as sensitive as manometry and involves less radiation dosage than radiography. Evaluation of gut motility using such techniques is, however, generally restricted to specialist centres. The evaluation of prokinetic drugs such as metoclopramide and domperidone has also added impetus to the understanding of gastrointestinal disorders in diabetes.

Abnormalities in specific parts of the gut will now be described in greater detail.

Clinical features of gastrointestinal involvement

Oesophageal dysfunction

Impaired oesophageal smooth muscle function can be frequently demonstrated in asymptomatic patients, but symptoms — consisting of heartburn and dysphagia for solids — are uncommon. Diabetic patients who develop significant oeso-phageal symptoms therefore require a barium swallow or endoscopy to exclude alternative causes, especially hiatus hernia, reflux oesophagitis, moniliasis and malignancy. Oesophageal symptoms may also indicate an underlying psychiatric illness such as anxiety or an affective disorder [9].

Barium swallow studies in diabetic patients may show a variety of abnormalities, including mild dilatation, decreased or absent primary peristaltic waves, sporadic tertiary contractions, prolonged transit and delayed emptying of the contrast, together with gastro-oesophageal reflux. The most characteristic manometric features are those of hypomotility with decreased amplitude, frequency and velocity of the peristaltic waves in the distal oesophagus following swallowing. Reduced resting pressure and uncoordinated function of the lower sphincter are also seen. Multiphasic, multipeaked oesophageal peristaltic pressure waves in diabetic patients with neuropathy have been regarded as pathognomonic of the disease [10], but other changes are now considered non-specific. Certain oesophageal contraction abnormalities, such as increased distal wave amplitude and triple-peaked waves, are independent of diabetic neuropathy and correlate more with the psychiatric state of the patient [9].

Radionuclide scintigraphy allows quantification of the delayed oesophageal transit of liquid and solid food boluses [5, 11] and time–activity curves in the different segments of the oesophagus [3]. A solid food bolus is probably more useful than liquid in detecting abnormal oesophageal emptying [12].

Oesophageal motor dysfunction probably results from vagal neuropathy. The motility changes are similar to those following surgical vagotomy and scintigraphic abnormalities correlate with the results of vagally mediated cardiovascular tests of autonomic function [3, 5].

Diabetic gastroparesis

Diabetic gastroparesis (or gastropathy) is a well-recognized complication of diabetes and is characterized by hypomotility of gastric smooth muscle. When present, symptoms are non-specific and include early satiety and upper abdominal fullness during or immediately after eating. Patients who are more severely affected may complain of anorexia or may lose weight, symptoms which, in young diabetic women, must be distinguished from anorexia nervosa. Diabetic control may become difficult, with frequent and severe hypoglycaemic episodes because insulin injections and carbohydrate absorption are no longer in phase. Less commonly, some patients develop intermittent bouts of nausea and vomiting lasting for a few days, and rarely, vomiting may become persistent and intractable. The vomitus may contain material ingested several hours previously and occasionally altered blood ('coffee grounds') from Mallory—Weiss tears. A gastric splash may be elicited, or noticed by the patient, several hours after taking fluids. Diabetic gastroparesis, like surgical vagotomy, can predispose to the formation of bezoars, which can obstruct gastric outflow and also give rise to nausea, vomiting and abdominal distension [13]. Patients with symptomatic gastroparesis invariably have other clinical features of autonomic neuropathy such as postural hypotension, abnormal sweating and bladder dysfunction. They require frequent hospital admissions, become malnourished and are often depressed, and generally have a poor prognosis [14].

Diabetic patients complaining of gastric symptoms should always undergo routine investigation including upper gastrointestinal radiography and endoscopy to exclude an ulcer, pyloric stenosis or malignancy. In gastroparesis, barium meal examination characteristically shows a dilated stomach with food and fluid residues still present in the fasting state (Fig. 71.1). Following the meal, absent or ineffective peristalsis, delayed gastric emptying and atony of the duodenal bulb are seen. Radionuclide scintigraphy can demonstrate the individual progress of the liquid and solid components labelled by different isotopes of the test meal. The normal stomach empties solids and liquids by different mechanisms, at different rates and in different patterns. Several distinctive abnormal emptying patterns have been observed in patients with gastroparesis. Gastric emptying of both liquid and solid tends to be slower in diabetic patients (either symptomatic or asymptomatic), with loss of the normal differentiation between the two components [15, 1]. This abnormality is in keeping with impaired distal stomach (antral) motor function in diabetic patients. Gastric motility abnormalities correlate poorly with upper gastrointestinal symptoms and some severely symptomatic patients unexpectedly show nearly normal emptying of liquids and digestible solids [16]. Moreover, some patients display rapid early gastric emptying [17], which may result from impaired

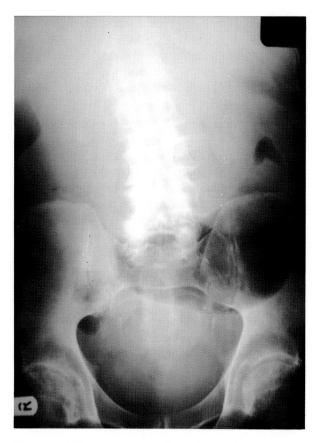

Fig. 71.1. Plain abdominal radiograph showing gastric dilatation.

receptive relaxation of the proximal stomach (fundus) and may represent a milder degree of neuropathy before gastric stasis has supervened. The use of solid radiopaque markers as a measure of the progress of indigestible substances may be a more sensitive indicator of gastric motor dysfunction than radionuclide scintigraphy [16]. In the normal stomach, digestible solids empty during the postprandial period whereas indigestible material empties later during the interdigestive (fasting) period. Patients with symptomatic gastroparesis will usually show delayed gastric transit of indigestible solid markers as a result of the decreased antral motor activity. The delayed emptying of indigestible solids may contribute to nausea and vomiting and also encourage bezoar formation.

The underlying cause of gastroparesis is probably vagal neuropathy, as is suggested by these patients' impaired acid secretion in response to insulin-induced hypoglycaemia [18] or sham feeding [19]. Furthermore, the gastric motility changes in diabetic patients are similar to those following truncal vagotomy. In diabetic patients with abnormal parasympathetic tests of cardiac function, the mean gastric emptying rate (assessed by scintigraphy) is significantly impaired [6]. There have been few histological studies of the vagus nerve from patients with gastroparesis, but one case showed severe loss of unmyelinated axons in the gastric branch of the vagus nerve [20].

The underlying mechanism of gastroparesis is still unclear. Manometric pressure measurements show diminished smooth muscle activity in both fundus and antrum. In symptomatic patients, myo-electric activity is especially reduced in the antral smooth muscle, with decreased phase II and absent interdigestive phase III motor complexes [7, 21, 22]. Similar myo-electric abnormalities are found in patients with postvagotomy gastroparesis [7]. The interdigestive motor complexes are considered to play an integral role in the clearing of undigestible debris from the stomach and upper small intestine. It has recently been observed, using quantitative manometry, that diabetic patients with nausea and vomiting have increased tonic activity of the pyloric smooth muscle [23]. This 'autonomic pylorospasm' is somewhat unexpected in view of the generalized hypomotility of the gut, but may explain the difficulty often encountered in passing a Crosby capsule into the duodenum in patients with gastroparesis.

The possible role of gut hormone disturbances in gastroparesis remains unclear. Diabetic patients with gastroparesis have higher than normal plasma concentrations of motilin, a peptide which is widely distributed throughout the upper gut and whose experimental administration causes contraction of the stomach and duodenum. However, this association may be merely coincidental, since metoclopramide can improve gastric motor activity without normalizing plasma motilin levels [22]. It has been speculated that hyperglycaemia, by a mechanism as yet undetermined, may also be a contributory factor [2] and may account for the intermittency of abnormal gastric emptying [24].

Gall-bladder dysfunction

Enlargement and poor contraction of the gall-bladder following a fatty meal, so-called 'diabetic cholecystopathy', is sometimes observed in diabetic patients. The finding is usually made by chance during ultrasonography or, more frequently, cholecystography [25]. There are no symptoms and there does not appear to be a higher frequency of associated gallstones. A similar abnormality of gall-bladder function can be seen following bilateral vagotomy.

Diabetic diarrhoea

Diabetic diarrhoea is a well-recognized complication of diabetes but remains poorly understood. Those affected usually have long-standing, poorly controlled IDDM and clinical evidence of somatic and autonomic neuropathy. The typical symptoms are intermittent bouts of diarrhoea, with the passage of upwards of 20 stools daily, often preceded by urgency. Although characteristically frequent at night, diarrhoea also continues during the day, occurring especially shortly after meals which may suggest, perhaps surprisingly, an exaggerated gastrocolic reflex. The bouts may persist for a few days or weeks and are then followed by spontaneous remission for a variable period. The stools vary in consistency but are frequently watery. Between episodes, the bowel habit often returns to normal and the patient may even complain of constipation. Fortunately, the symptoms are usually only mildly troublesome but a few patients suffer severely disabling diarrhoea which may force them to become housebound. Body weight and nutrition are usually maintained, even in those severely affected. Weight loss in a patient with diabetic diarrhoea is more likely to be due to associated gastroparesis.

There are no pathognomonic tests for diabetic diarrhoea and it is important to remember that the diagnosis must be made by exclusion. Diarrhoea associated with steatorrhoea may be the result of chronic pancreatic disease, which should respond to exocrine pancreatic replacement treatment. A further possibility is coeliac disease, which may resemble diabetic diarrhoea in its intermittency and nocturnal predilection. Coeliac disease will usually cause weight loss with clinical and biochemical features of malabsorption; an abnormal jejunal biopsy will support the diagnosis and the symptoms should respond to a gluten-free diet.

Diabetic diarrhoea is suggested by the typical clinical features, the lack of other positive findings and the almost invariable presence of diabetic peripheral neuropathy. Cardiovascular autonomic function tests are usually, but not always, abnormal at the time of onset of the symptoms. Routine assessment of small intestinal absorption (including serum iron, folate and vitamin B12 concentrations, the D-xylose tolerance and Shilling tests) should be entirely normal. There are no characteristic abnormalities in the barium meal follow-through examination and the jejunal biopsy in patients with diabetic diarrhoea shows normal histology.

The pathogenesis of diabetic diarrhoea is unclear and may be multifactorial. In some patients, the small intestinal motility disturbance which leads to stasis of gut contents may allow abnormal bacterial overgrowth. Excess bacterial activity has been demonstrated in a few patients with diarrhoea by the ^{14}C−glycocholate test. This might explain the prompt improvement in the diarrhoea which sometimes follows treatment with a broad-spectrum antibiotic.

Manometric pressure studies of gut motility in patients with diabetic diarrhoea are lacking. However, a disturbance of small intestinal motility involving both parasympathetic and sympathetic innervation can be demonstrated in patients with autonomic neuropathy [1] and with gastroparesis [21]. A possible role of autonomic neuropathy is supported by the observations that both truncal vagotomy and sympathectomy in non-diabetic patients may cause diarrhoea. The streptozotocin-diabetic rat frequently displays lower gut dysmotility associated with both parasympathetic and sympathetic denervation [26]. Chronic streptozotocin-diabetic rats develop impaired ileal and colonic absorption of fluid and electrolytes which results from denervation of α_2-adrenergic receptors on enterocytes [27]. There are some preliminary reports of the α_2-adrenergic agonists, limidine [28] and clonidine [29], being effective in some patients with diabetic diarrhoea.

Impaired bile acid absorption, which could lead to increased fluid and electrolyte load in the colon and so to watery diarrhoea, has been implicated in the pathogenesis of both postvagotomy and diabetic diarrhoea [30]. However, the failure of bile acid-binding agents such as cholestyramine to improve symptoms argues against bile acid malabsorption as an important factor in diabetic diarrhoea.

Colonic dysfunction

Constipation is a common gastrointestinal symptom in diabetic patients and results from large intestinal hypomotility. The prevalence of this complaint rises with increasing severity of symptomatic neuropathy, reaching 88% in one series [1]. The constipation may vary from mild to severe, the latter patients having two or fewer bowel actions per week. In some patients, constipation may be intermittent and can alternate with diabetic diarrhoea. Routine investigation of constipation in diabetic patients should include rectal examination, procto-sigmoidoscopy and testing for occult blood. It is usually necessary, especially in older patients, to exclude colonic carcinoma by performing a barium enema, which may show marked colonic dilatation (megacolon or megasigmoid).

Colonic dysfunction is associated with other clinical features of autonomic neuropathy but its precise pathogenesis remains poorly understood. Diabetic patients with severe constipation have an absent gastrocolic response to eating as assessed by measurements of distal colonic myo-electrical and motor activity. These motility abnormalities can be improved by intramuscular neostigmine or intravenous metoclopramide [31].

Anorectal dysfunction

Loss of anal sphincter control with faecal incontinence is a distressing symptom experienced by some diabetic patients with neuropathy. It is often, but not always, associated with diabetic diarrhoea. The symptom is liable to occur not only during sleep but also during the day.

Anorectal manometry in patients with faecal incontinence has shown reduced internal sphincter tone but with preservation of voluntary sphincter contraction, suggesting that external sphincter tone remains relatively normal [32]. However, another study in similar patients demonstrated impaired external sphincter function [33]. Some patients with faecal incontinence also have an increased threshold for conscious rectal sensation which suggests impaired afferent nerve function as another contributory factor [34].

Treatment of gastrointestinal problems

To date, there is no convincing evidence that intensified glycaemic control with either conventional insulin injections or continuous subcutaneous insulin infusion can reverse the clinical features of established diabetic gastrointestinal involvement. Likewise, several carefully conducted trials have failed to show any clear beneficial effect of aldose reductase inhibitors such as sorbinil on clinical autonomic neuropathy or the gut manifestations [4]. Once the various gastro-intestinal symptom complexes have become apparent clinically, the treatment is primarily symptomatic.

Oesophageal dysfunction

Oesophageal motor dysfunction is usually asymptomatic and treatment is seldom required. If heartburn or dysphagia are troublesome and other causes have been excluded, the patient can be given a trial of treatment with a prokinetic drug such as metoclopramide, domperidone or cisapride to increase oesophageal contractions. The oesophagus may, however, be more resistant to treatment with prokinetic drugs than gastric emptying [11].

Gastroparesis

Gastric symptoms of nausea and vomiting may respond to metoclopramide, a dopamine antag-onist and cholinergic agonist which probably increases smooth muscle tone and contractility by enhancing the local effect of acetylcholine and also acts centrally as an anti-emetic. The usual dosage is 10 to 20 mg taken about 30 min before each meal and at bedtime. Side-effects occasionally limit its use. Domperidone, like metoclopramide, is also a potent dopamine antagonist but lacks cholinergic activity, and may also help symp-toms [35]. There is some evidence, however, that long-term administration of metoclopramide or domperidone may reduce their gastrokinetic properties [35, 36]. Cisapride is a more recent prokinetic drug which stimulates oesophageal, gastric and intestinal motility in general [24], probably by promoting acetylcholine release in the myenteric plexus. Unlike metoclopramide and domperidone, cisapride has no dopamine antag-onist properties. Cisapride can improve the rate of gastric emptying of both solids and liquids [12] but a few patients may develop marked stool fre-quency as a result of increased small bowel and colonic motility.

Patients experiencing more severe gastric symptoms present a difficult problem. Acute bouts of vomiting may require hospital admission for both intravenous fluid replacement and control of the diabetes. Intranasal gastric suction should be carried out to decompress the stomach and metoclopramide given intravenously. Eating

should be re-introduced as frequent, small semi-fluid feeds. In the longer term, patients should probably avoid high-fibre foods. Surgical drainage procedures will need to be considered for the few patients with vomiting which has become refractory to conventional measures. Surgical experience is limited, with only a few reports in the literature, and it may not always relieve symptoms. To reduce the tendency to postoper-ative biliary reflux vomiting and gastritis, a Roux-en-Y gastrojejunostomy has been recom-mended [20].

An alternative to gastric surgery for refractory gastroparesis is the use of jejunostomy with direct enteral feeding which has been described in a small number of severely affected patients [37]. Gastric bezoars, when identified, should be treated by endoscopic fragmentation [14].

Diabetic diarrhoea

The treatment of this condition is often unsatis-factory and difficult to evaluate as the episodes of diarrhoea may be self-limiting. Mild symptoms are best managed by opiate derivatives such as codeine phosphate and loperamide hydrochloride. If a disturbance of bowel flora is suspected, tetra-cycline or other broad-spectrum antibiotics may rapidly abolish symptoms and can then be given intermittently for 1 week in every 4. For more resistant cases, especially where the diarrhoea is watery, a specific α_2-adrenergic agonist such as limidine [28] or clonidine [29] may be tried on the basis that adrenergic innervation of intestinal enterocyte receptors has a role in fluid and elec-trolyte absorption. The use of bile acid-binding agents such as cholestyramine, although helpful in postvagotomy diarrhoea, has proved dis-appointing in diabetic patients.

Diabetic constipation

The treatment of constipation in diabetic patients is often neglected. If constipation is not improved by routine laxatives, treatment with one of the prokinetic group of drugs may be helpful [38].

Faecal incontinence

This distressing condition is difficult to treat and the patient may have to resort to the use of ab-sorbent pads. Treatment by means of biofeedback has been described in a limited number of patients [34].

Other gastrointestinal disorders in diabetes mellitus

Diabetic patients may develop the same gastrointestinal disorders that occur in the general population. Although these conditions are not directly related to diabetes, their prevalence and clinical features may in some circumstances be modified by the presence of the disease.

Oral infections

Both their increased tendency to infection and microangiopathy may make diabetic patients more prone to gingival and periodontal disease, although prevalence data are lacking. Diabetic patients have a high carrier rate of *Candida albicans* [39] and, especially if taking long-term antibiotic treatment such as for foot problems, may be more liable to pharyngeal and oesophageal moniliasis. The latter can be confirmed by examination of material recovered at endoscopy. Oropharyngeal and oesophageal moniliasis should usually respond to oral nystatin, ketoconazole, amphotericin, or fluconazole.

Atrophic gastritis

Atrophy of the gastric mucosa and impaired gastric acid secretion following histamine have been reported to be more common in diabetic patients. The diminished gastric acid secretion may result in part from vagal neuropathy but may also be due to autoimmune gastritis. Through its association with other organ-specific autoimmune diseases, the prevalences of gastric parietal cell and intrinsic factor antibodies and of pernicious anaemia are relatively high in IDDM [40].

Gastric and duodenal ulceration

The prevalence of gastric ulcers in diabetic patients is probably similar to that in the general population. Earlier reports of a lower prevalence of duodenal ulceration have remained unconfirmed, although this might be expected in diabetic patients because of the decreased gastric acid secretion. There is some evidence that bleeding from duodenal ulcers may have more severe consequences in diabetic patients because of vascular changes. The clinical features of gastric outlet obstruction due to peptic ulceration and scarring may be accentuated in diabetic patients because of coexistent vagal neuropathy.

Gallstones and cholecystitis

Diabetic patients might be expected to be at increased risk of developing gallstones since many are overweight and have abnormal lipid metabolism which could lead to alterations in bile composition. Moreover, autonomic neuropathy could lead to delayed gall-bladder emptying. The prevalence of gallstones and gall-bladder disease in diabetic patients has not so far been satisfactorily assessed.

Diabetic patients who develop cholecystitis suffer higher morbidity and mortality following both emergency and elective biliary tract surgery [41]. Diabetic patients must therefore be monitored very closely for complications, especially infection, in the postoperative period. Careful bacteriological examination, including culture of the bile duct during surgery and of the T-tube postoperatively, is recommended and it is probably best to continue antibiotic treatment after surgery. Prophylactic cholecystectomy was previously recommended in asymptomatic diabetic patients but this policy has recently been questioned [42].

Steatorrhoea

Chronic pancreatitis may be associated with secondary diabetes. Where pancreatic exocrine function is insufficient, steatorrhoea will result and may resemble diabetic diarrhoea. Although coeliac disease was considered to occur more frequently in IDDM, it has been claimed that this condition is no more common than in the general population [43]. As described above, coeliac disease may resemble diabetic diarrhoea clinically but the two conditions can be easily distinguished.

BASIL F. CLARKE

References

1 Feldman M, Schiller LR. Disorders of gastrointestinal motility associated with diabetes mellitus. *Ann Intern Med* 1983; **98**: 378–84.
2 Horowitz M, Harding PE, Maddox A, Madden GJ, Collins PJ, Chatterton BE, Wishart J, Shearman DJC. Gastric and oesophageal emptying in insulin-dependent diabetes mellitus. *J Gastroenterol Hepatol* 1986; **1**: 97–113.
3 Westin L, Lilja B, Sundkvist G. Oesophagus scintigraphy

in patients with diabetes mellitus. *Scand J Gastroenterol* 1986; **21**: 1200–4.

4 Ewing DJ, Clarke BF. Diabetic autonomic neuropathy: present insights and future prospects. *Diabetes Care* 1986; **9**: 648–65.

5 Channer KS, Jackson PC, O'Brien I, Corrall RJM, Coles DR, Davies ER, Virjee JP. Oesophageal function in diabetes mellitus and its association with autonomic neuropathy. *Diabetic Med* 1985; **2**: 378–82.

6 Buysschaert M, Moulart M, Urbain JL, Pauwels S, Roy LD, Ketelslegers JM, Lambert AE. Impaired gastric emptying in diabetic patients with cardiac autonomic neuropathy. *Diabetes Care* 1987; **10**: 448–52.

7 Malagelada JR, Rees WDW, Mazzotta L, Gu VLW. Gastric motor abnormalities in diabetic and post-vagotomy gastroparesis: effect of metoclopramide and bethanicol. *Gastroenterology* 1980; **78**: 286–93.

8 Smith PH, Madson KL. Interactions between autonomic nerves and endocrine cells of the gastroenteropancreatic system. *Diabetologia* 1981; **20**: 314–24.

9 Clouse RE, Lustman PJ, Reidel WL. Correlation of esophageal motility abnormalities with neuropsychiatric status in diabetics. *Gastroenterology* 1986; **90**: 1146–54.

10 Loo FD, Dodds WJ, Soergel KH, Arndorfer RC, Helm JF, Hogan WJ. Multipeaked esophageal peristaltic pressure waves in patients with diabetic neuropathy. *Gastroenterology* 1985; **88**: 485–91.

11 Maddern GJ, Horowitz M, Jamieson GG. The effect of domperidone on oesophageal emptying in diabetic autonomic neuropathy. *Br J Clin Pharmacol* 1985; **19**: 441–4.

12 Horowitz M, Maddox A, Harding PE, Maddern GJ, Chatterton BE, Wishart J, Shearman DJC. Effect of cisapride on gastric and esophageal emptying in insulin-dependent diabetes mellitus. *Gastroenterology* 1987; **92**: 1899–1907.

13 Brady PG, Richardson R. Gastric bezoar formation secondary to gastroparesis diabeticorum. *Arch Int Med* 1977; **137**: 1729.

14 Ewing DJ, Campbell IW, Clarke BF. The natural history of diabetic autonomic neuropathy. *Q J Med* 1980; **49**: 95–108.

15 Campbell IW, Heading RC, Tothill P, Buist AS, Ewing DJ, Clarke BF. Gastric emptying in diabetic autonomic neuropathy. *Gut* 1977; **18**: 462–7.

16 Feldman M, Smith HJ, Simon TR. Gastric emptying of solid radiopaque markers: studies in healthy subjects and diabetic patients. *Gastroenterology* 1984; **87**: 895–902.

17 Loo FD, Palmer DW, Soergel KH, Kalbfleisch JH, Wood CM. Gastric emptying in patients with diabetes mellitus. *Gastroenterology* 1984; **86**: 485–94.

18 Hosking DJ, Moony F, Stewart IM, Atkinson M. Vagal impairment of gastric secretion in diabetic autonomic neuropathy. *Br Med J* 1975; **2**: 588–90.

19 Feldman M, Corbett DB, Ramsey EJ, Walsh JH, Richardson CT. Abnormal gastric function in longstanding insulin-dependent diabetic patients. *Gastroenterology* 1979; **77**: 12–17.

20 Guy RJC, Dawson JL, Garrett JR, Laws JW, Thomas PK, Sharma AK, Watkins PJ. Diabetic gastroparesis from autonomic neuropathy: surgical considerations and changes in vagus nerve morphology. *J Neurol Neurosurg Psychiatr* 1984; **47**: 686–91.

21 Camilleri M, Malagelada JR. Abnormal intestinal motility in diabetics with the gastroparesis syndrome. *Eur J Clin Invest* 1984; **14**: 420–7.

22 Achem-Karam SR, Funakoshi A, Vinik AI, Owyang C. Plasma motilin concentration and interdigestive migrating motor complexes in diabetic gastroparesis: effect of metoclopramide. *Gastroenterology* 1985; **88**: 492–9.

23 Mearin F, Camilleri M, Malagelada JR. Pyloric dysfunction in diabetics with recurrent nausea and vomiting. *Gastroenterology* 1986; **90**: 1919–25.

24 Feldman M, Smith JH. Effect of cisapride on gastric emptying of indigestible solids in patients with gastroparesis diabeticorum. *Gastroenterology* 1987; **92**: 171–4.

25 Marumo K, Fujii S, Seki J, Wada M. Studies on gallbladder dysfunction in patients with diabetes mellitus. In: Goto Y, Horiuchi A, Kogurie K, eds. *Diabetic Neuropathy*, International Congress Series No 581. Amsterdam: Excerpta Medica, 1982: 284–9.

26 Schmidt RE, Nelson JS, Johnson EM. Experimental diabetic autonomic neuropathy. *Am J Pathol* 1981; **103**: 210–25.

27 Chang EB, Bergenstal RM, Field M. Diarrhea in streptozotocin treated rats. *J Clin Invest* 1985; **75**: 1666–70.

28 Goff JS. Diabetic diarrhea and limidine. *Ann Intern Med* 1984; **101**: 874–5.

29 Fedorak RN, Field M, Chang EB. Treatment of diabetic diarrhea with clonidine. *Ann Intern Med* 1985; **102**: 197–9.

30 Molloy AM, Tomkin GH. Altered bile in diabetic diarrhoea. *Br Med J* 1978; **2**: 1462–3.

31 Battle WM, Snape WJ, Alavi A, Cohen S, Braunstein S. Colonic dysfunction in diabetes mellitus. *Gastroenterology* 1980; **79**: 1217–21.

32 Schiller LR, Santa Ana CA, Schmulen AC, Hendler RS, Harford WV, Fordtran JS. Pathogenesis of fecal incontinence in diabetes mellitus: evidence for internal anal sphincter dysfunction. *N Engl J Med* 1982; **307**: 1666–71.

33 Tunuguntla AK, Wald A. Comparison of anorectal function in diabetics and non-diabetics with fecal incontinence. *Gastroenterology* 1984; **86**: 1285.

34 Wald A, Tunuguntla AK. Anorectal sensorimotor dysfunction in fecal incontinence and diabetes mellitus. Modification with biofeedback therapy. *N Engl J Med* 1984; **310**: 1282–7.

35 Horowitz M, Harding PE, Chatterton BE, Collins PJ, Shearman DJC. Acute and chronic effects of domperidone on gastric emptying in diabetic autonomic neuropathy. *Digest Dis Sci* 1985; **30**: 1–9.

36 Schade RR, Dugas MC, Lhotsky DM, Gavaler JS, Van Thiel DH. Effect of metoclopramide on gastric liquid emptying in patients with diabetic gastroparesis. *Digest Dis Sci* 1985; **30**: 10–15.

37 Jacober SI, Narayan A, Strodel WE, Vinik AI. Jejunostomy feeding in the management of gastroparesis diabeticorum. *Diabetes Care* 1986; **9**: 217–19.

38 Snape WJ, Battle WM, Schwartz SS, Braunstein SN, Goldstein HA, Alavi A. Metoclopramide to treat gastroparesis due to diabetes mellitus. A double-blind controlled trial. *Ann Intern Med* 1982; **96**: 444–6.

39 Tapper-Jones LM, Aldred MJ, Walker DM, Hayes TM. Candidal infections and populations of candida albicans in mouths of diabetics. *J Clin Pathol* 1981; **34**: 706–11.

40 Irvine WJ, Clarke BF, Scarth L, Cullen DR, Duncan LJP. Thyroid and gastric autoimmunity in patients with diabetes. *Lancet* 1970; **ii**: 163–8.

41 Sandler RS, Maule WF, Baltus ME. Factors associated with postoperative complications in diabetics after biliary tract surgery. *Gastroenterology* 1986; **91**: 157–62.

42 Pellegrini CA. Asymptomatic gallstones. Does diabetes mellitus make a difference? *Gastroenterology* 1986; **91**: 245–6.

43 Walsh CH, Cooper BT, Wright AD, Malins JM, Cooke WT. Diabetes mellitus and coeliac disease: a clinical study. *Q J Med* 1978; **47**: 89–100.

72   The Skin in Diabetes Mellitus

Summary

- Various skin conditions occur frequently in diabetes, although common lesions may be associated by chance.
- Necrobiosis lipoidica diabeticorum consists of non-scaling plaques with atrophic epidermis and thick, degenerating collagen in the dermis, usually in the pretibial region.
- Granuloma annulare is an annular or arciform lesion with a raised papular border and flat centre, usually found on the dorsum of the hands and arms. Histologically, there is mid-dermal collagen degeneration and abundant mucin.
- Diabetic dermopathy consists of bilateral pigmented pretibial patches ('shin spots') which mostly affect older male diabetic patients.
- 'Diabetic thick skin' includes both the rare scleroedema (affecting the neck, upper back and arms) and the common diabetic hand syndrome (Dupuytren's contractures, sclerosing tenosynovitis, knuckle pads and carpal tunnel syndrome).
- Acanthosis nigricans forms brown, velvety hyperkeratotic plaques in the axilla or back of the neck, often associated with insulin resistance. Histologically, the epidermis is extensively folded with increased melanocytes.
- Bullosis diabeticorum usually occurs in patients with long-standing neuropathy and consists of tense blisters on a non-inflamed base which appear suddenly on the feet or hands.
- Cutaneous complications of diabetic treatment include reactions to sulphonylurea drugs (especially first generation), insulin allergy and injection-site lipodystrophy.
- The rare glucagonoma syndrome (associated with an A-cell pancreatic tumour) presents with a migratory erythematous eruption, with peripheral scaling and vesiculation leading to erosions and ulceration. The characteristic sites are perioral, genital and perianal.

Skin disorders affect about 30% of diabetic patients [1]. These conditions fall into four general categories (see Table 72.1). This chapter will concentrate principally on disorders regarded as cutaneous markers of diabetes and the dermatological complications of treatment; other rarer associations are reviewed elsewhere [2].

Certain cutaneous disorders clearly occur commonly in diabetes, but it is often difficult to define the exact nature of their association with the disease. First, the mechanisms responsible for the skin lesions are poorly understood and have no obvious biological links with the disease process of diabetes. Secondly, conclusions drawn from a highly selected group of patients referred to a dermatological practice may not apply to the general diabetic population. Thirdly, if both conditions are common, they will often be associated by chance alone and not necessarily causally related. Various 'cutaneous manifestations' of diabetes have been described in the older literature, but their relative frequencies in IDDM and NIDDM and precise relationship to glucose metabolism need to be clarified. An example is generalized pruritus, previously widely regarded as a marker of diabetes. A recent study of 300 patients found that although localized vulval pruritus (associated with candidiasis) was three times more common in diabetic than in non-diabetic women, the prevalence of generalized

753

Table 72.1. The skin and diabetes mellitus.

'Cutaneous markers' of diabetes
Necrobiosis lipoidica diabeticorum
Granuloma annulare
Diabetic dermopathy ('shin spots')
Diabetic thick skin (including diabetic hand syndrome)
Acanthosis nigricans
Diabetic bullae

Complications of diabetes
Neurovascular and ischaemic skin changes and foot
   ulceration
Digital gangrene (due to atherosclerosis)
Disordered sweating (with autonomic neuropathy)
Increased susceptibility to skin infections:
- bacterial (boils, erythrasma)
- yeasts (candidiasis — intertrigo, perineal infections,
  balanitis)
- fungal dermatoses

Complications of diabetic treatment
Sulphonylureas:
- maculopapular eruptions
- Stevens–Johnson syndrome
- purpura
- photosensitivity
- erythema nodosum
- porphyria cutanea tarda
- alcohol-induced flushing with chlorpropamide ('CPAF')
Insulin:
- localized allergy (late-phase, Arthus or delayed
  reactions)
- systemic allergy (urticaria, anaphylaxis)
- lipoatrophy
- lipohypertrophy
- idiosyncratic reactions (pigmentation, keloid formation)

Rare associations with endocrine and other syndromes
Glucagonoma (migratory necrolytic erythema)
Cushing's syndrome (skin atrophy, striae, hirsutes)
Acromegaly (thickened skin, increased sweating)
Partial and total lipodystrophy (variable loss of
  subcutaneous fat)
Ataxia telangiectasia

pruritis was the same (3%) in the diabetic as in the general population [3].

Cutaneous conditions considered markers of diabetes

Necrobiosis lipoidica diabeticorum (NLD)

This rare condition, first described by Oppenheim in 1929 [4] and named by Urbach in 1932 [5], has an incidence of 3 per 1000 diabetic patients per year. Three-quarters of cases are women, with an average age of onset of 34 years [6].

The appearance of the fully developed lesion is diagnostic: non-scaling plaques with atrophic yellow centres, surface telangiectasia and a violaceous or erythematous border (sometimes raised) are usually seen in the pretibial region (Fig. 72.1). The lesions vary in size, small papules often coalescing to form large irregular plaques, sometimes several centimetres in diameter. One-third of the lesions ulcerate. Multiple or bilateral lesions occur in most cases, and sites other than the pretibial are affected in 15% of patients.

The histological hallmark of the condition — 'necrobiosis' — refers to degeneration and thickening of collagen bundles in the dermis. The necrobiotic foci are acellular, associated with granular debris scattered throughout the dermis and surrounded by a mixed cellular infiltrate of lymphocytes, histiocytes, fibroblasts and epitheloid cells. Granulomata may form in some lesions. The epidermis is normal in early lesions, but later becomes thin and atrophic.

The pathogenesis of the disorder is not known [7] and the nature of the association between necrobiosis and diabetes is uncertain. The much-quoted statistic that 90% of people with NLD are diabetic, will develop diabetes or have a family history of the disease [6] derives from a retrospective review in 1966, in which the selection criteria are unknown and over 50% of the patients had not been seen for over 10 years. Moreover, 'impending diabetes' was presumed on the basis of glucose tolerance testing after prednisone treatment, a procedure since abandoned because it is non-specific and non-reproducible. Other studies of the time (when the diagnostic criteria for diabetes were less rigorous) found that about 60% of patients with necrobiosis had diabetes [8, 9]. A recent study showed normal HbA_1 levels in non-diabetic people with necrobiosis lipoidica, demonstrating that significant hyperglycaemia is not necessary for its development [10]. Overall, therefore, the association between NLD and diabetes seems weaker than previously assumed, and NLD may not be a specific marker for diabetes.

Evaluation of treatment of NLD, which must take into account the 20% spontaneous remission rate, has not yet been rigorously undertaken. Active red lesion margins may respond to steroids, either injected or applied locally, but topical steroids are contraindicated once atrophy is apparent; local emollients may then be used instead. Skin grafts of necrobiotic ulcers or lesions are often complicated by recurrence within or around the grafts.

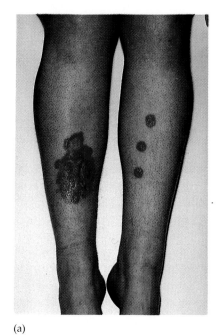 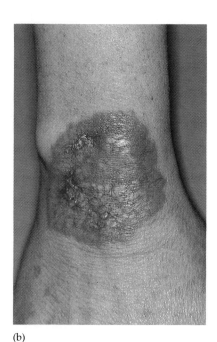

Fig. 72.1. Necrobiosis lipoidica diabeticorum. (a) A typical lesion on the front of the right shin, with three smaller areas on the left shin. (b) An area of necrobiosis with the typical yellow atrophic centre and telangiectases, on the unusual site of the dorsum of the wrist. (Courtesy of Dr Ian A. MacFarlane and Dr Geoffrey V. Gill.)

(a)   (b)

Granuloma annulare (GA)

Granuloma annulare was described by Fox in 1895 [11]. The most common form consists of one or more annular or arciform lesions with a raised, flesh-coloured papular border and a flat, often hyperpigmented centre (Fig. 72.2). In 63% of a large series, the dorsum of the hands and arms was affected; the feet, legs and trunk were less frequently involved [12]. An uncommon generalized form comprises numerous flesh-coloured papules which are distributed symmetrically, often on sun-exposed areas. Granuloma annulare differs histologically from NLD in that the epidermis is normal and the necrobiotic collagen is localized to the mid-dermis and associated with abundant mucin.

Clinically, it can be difficult to distinguish GA from NLD and this has led to attempts to establish an association between GA and diabetes, as reported for NLD. There are case reports of diabetic patients with GA [13, 14], particularly the disseminated form and an even rarer perforating type. However, both diabetes and GA are relatively common and chance associations are therefore likely. Several large studies [15, 16] have been unable to show a significant association between the two disorders, although a recent retrospective investigation reported a marginally higher than expected incidence of IDDM in patients with localized GA [17]. Patients with GA show no increased incidence of glucose intoler-

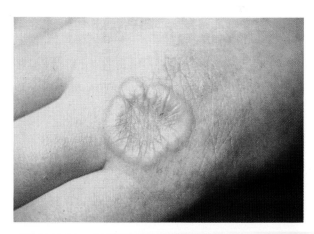

Fig. 72.2. Granuloma annulare. (Courtesy of Dr Geoffrey V. Gill.)

ance, or of the HLA phenotypes associated with IDDM [18, 19]. GA does not therefore seem to be definitely associated with diabetes.

Diabetic dermopathy (pigmented pretibial patches)

This condition, first described by Melin in 1964 [20] and subsequently named 'diabetic dermopathy' by Binkley [21], is also known as 'shin spots' or 'pigmented pretibial patches'. Despite its name, there is no strong evidence of an association with the chronic complications of diabetes and it is not pathognomic of the disease, having been reported in 1.5% of healthy medical students and in 20% of euglycaemic patients with various endocrine diseases [22].

Initially, lesions are round or oval, red or brownish papules which slowly evolve into discrete, sharply circumscribed, atrophic, hyperpigmented or scaly lesions (Fig. 72.3). Sometimes, only depressed areas of normal skin colour are seen. Ulceration is rare. Lesions are bilateral but not perfectly symmetrical. The anterior and lateral aspects of the shin are most commonly affected but other sites have been reported. Men are more often affected: dermopathy occurs in about 60% of male diabetic patients older than 50 years of age and in 29% of similarly aged female patients [20].

Histological features are not diagnostic and the underlying pathophysiology is not understood. Patients often associate the appearance of lesions with some preceding trauma but experimental skin damage has failed to reproduce the lesions [20]. Treatment is not required. Dermopathy may

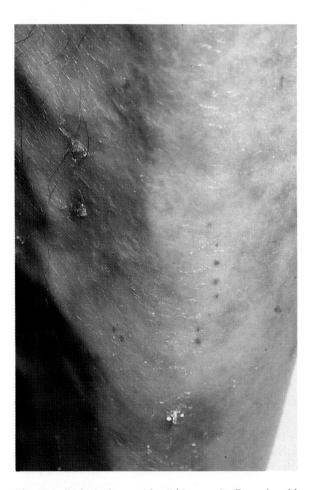

Fig. 72.3. Diabetic dermopathy ('shin spots'). (Reproduced by kind permission of Dr Julian Verbov, Royal Liverpool Hospital.)

regress spontaneously but new lesions continue to develop.

'Diabetic thick skin' (including scleroedema diabeticorum)

'Scleroedema' describes a rare condition with marked non-pitting induration and thickening of the skin. Two types have been described. The first is *scleroedema of Bushke*, which is not significantly associated with diabetes and may follow acute viral or streptococcal infection. The second type, *scleroedema diabeticorum*, which tends to be more persistent, is associated with IDDM. Both forms can involve the back of the neck and the upper part of the back, but that associated with diabetes frequently extends to involve the upper limbs and hands and can result in joint contractures [23].

More common 'diabetic thick skin' syndromes (see Chapter 73) may share a similar pathophysiological mechanism with scleroedema [24]. The diabetic thick skin syndrome includes fibroproliferative complications of the diabetic hand, namely Dupuytren's contractures (Fig. 72.4), sclerosing tenosynovitis of the palmar flexor tendons, Garrod's knuckle pads (Fig. 72.5) and carpal tunnel syndrome [25]. Various manifestations of diabetic thick skin syndrome are apparently common in IDDM, occurring in 22–40% of adult patients [23] and in 51% of diabetic children, many of whom have contractures and limited joint mobility of the fingers due to the condition [26]. The reported prevalence in NIDDM ranges from 4% to 70%.

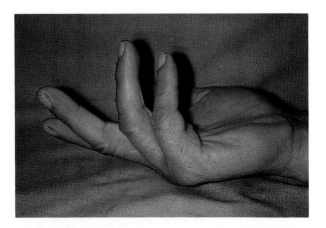

Fig. 72.4. Dupuytren's contracture in a diabetic patient with thickened skin and limited joint mobility. (Courtesy of Mr M.H. Matthewson, Addenbrooke's Hospital, Cambridge.)

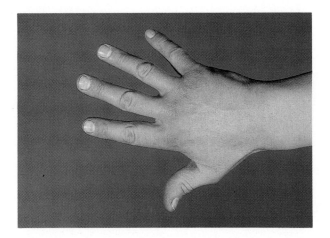

Fig. 72.5. Garrod's knuckle pads — thickening of the skin and superficial subcutaneous tissues — overlying the proximal interphalangeal joints in a patient with IDDM. (Courtesy of Mr M.H. Matthewson, Addenbrooke's Hospital, Cambridge.)

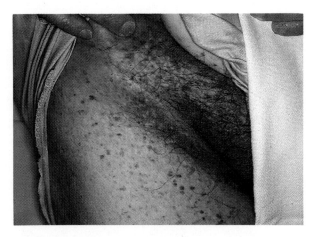

Fig. 72.6. Acanthosis nigricans in the groin. (Reproduced by kind permission of Dr Shevaun Mendelsohn, Royal Liverpool Hospital.)

The thickened skin of diabetic patients can be distinguished both histologically and ultrastructurally from other non-diabetic forms of thick skin such as progressive systemic sclerosis. Diabetic thick skin shows a normal epidermis and thickening of the dermis with hyalinized, disorganized collagen which extends into subcutaneous fat. Small amounts of acid mucopolysaccharide are often deposited in the papillary dermis. On electron microscopy, diabetic thick skin has a predominance of densely packed, large (>60-nm-diameter) collagen fibres, distinct from the bimodal distribution in scleroderma. The accumulation of large collagen fibres in diabetic thick skin can be explained by the known effects of hyperglycaemia on collagen metabolism [25, 27].

Most diabetic patients with thickened skin are asymptomatic and require no treatment. Diabetic knuckle pads can be treated by the application of liquid nitrogen, and Dupuytren's contractures by surgery. It is not yet known whether strict diabetic control can prevent or reverse diabetic skin thickening.

Acanthosis nigricans

This uncommon condition is characterized by brown, velvety, hyperkeratotic plaques which most often affect the axillae, back of the neck and other flexural areas. The lesions range in severity from minimal discoloration which spares the skin creases to thicker, more extensive hyperkeratotic areas (Fig. 72.6).

Histologically, the epidermis is extensively folded, slightly thickened and has increased cell density. The dark colour is caused by an increased number of melanocytes [28] (Fig. 72.7).

In 1976, Kahn et al. drew attention to the frequent association of acanthosis nigricans with a large heterogeneous group of disorders with the common feature of insulin resistance, ranging from asymptomatic hyperinsulinaemia to overt diabetes [29]. Flier [28] has classified the acanthosis–insulin resistance syndromes into two main groups, type A (genetic defects in the insulin receptor or post-receptor mechanisms) and type B (acquired insulin resistance, due to autoantibodies directed against the insulin receptor). These syndromes and their variants are described fully in Chapter 29.

Endocrine-associated acanthosis nigricans appears to be a true cutaneous marker, if not of overt diabetes, then at least of abnormal carbohydrate metabolism. The mechanism responsible for the development of acanthosis nigricans is uncertain, although the high circulating insulin concentrations associated with insulin resistance could promote epidermal growth (see Chapter 29).

Acanthosis and insulin resistance can also be associated in obesity, where receptor and post-receptor defects have been shown to play a role in the insulin-resistant state, and in various endocrinopathies (recently reviewed by Ober [30]). Acanthosis nigricans can also occur without insulin resistance, as a paraneoplastic syndrome (usually associated with gastrointestinal malignancy), in which epidermal growth may be stimulated by tumour-derived growth factors.

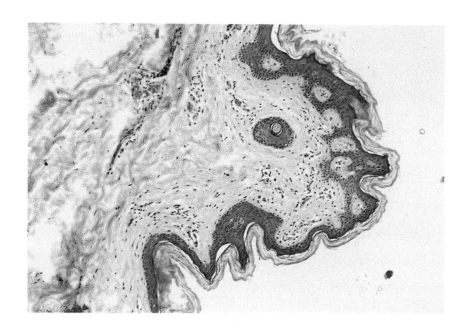

Fig. 72.7. Acanthosis nigricans, histological features (see text for explanation). Haematoxylin and eosin stain, ×350. (Reproduced by kind permission of Dr T.W. Stewart, Royal Liverpool Hospital.)

If necessary, the cosmetically disturbing appearance of acanthosis nigricans may be improved by applying mild peeling agents such as 5% salicyclic acid in a bland cream.

Bullosis diabeticorum (diabetic bullae)

This very rare condition, first described by Kramer [31], affects men more than women and has a predilection for patients with long-standing diabetes complicated by neuropathy [32]. One or more tense blisters on a non-inflammatory base appear suddenly, often overnight, with no preceding trauma, and heal during some weeks with or without scarring. The lesions are usually confined to the feet and lower legs but may involve the hands (see Fig. 72.8).

Recent electron-microscopical studies [32] have revealed a subepithelial blister with the split occurring at the level of the lamina lucida; the appearance of intra-epithelial splitting reported previously may have resulted from biopsies of older lesions in which the blister floor had re-epithelialized.

The condition can only be diagnosed in diabetic patients in whom other bullous disorders have been excluded by the absence of immunoglobulin deposition (demonstrated by direct immunofluorescence) in the skin. It is not clear how this entity differs from the localized variant of bullous pemphigoid, in which direct immunofluorescence of the basement membrane is frequently negative and the split is also in the lamina lucida.

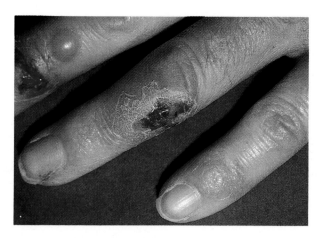

Fig. 72.8. Bullosis diabeticorum.

The aetiology is not understood, but a recent study showed a reduced threshold to suction-induced blister formation in diabetic patients [33].

Cutaneous complications of diabetic treatment

Complications of sulphonylureas

Various cutaneous reactions occur with first-generation sulphonylureas such as chlorpropamide and tolbutamide. These usually develop in the first two months of treatment and may be either toxic or allergic.

Two to three per cent of patients develop maculopapular eruptions [34]. Erythema multiforme major (Stevens–Johnson syndrome; see

Fig. 72.9), consisting predominantly of mucous membrane blistering, has been described with chlorpropamide [35]. Other rare skin manifestations include purpura (with or without thrombocytopenia), photosensitivity, erythema nodosum, and exacerbations of porphyria cutanea tarda. Generalized hypersensitivity reactions have also been reported. Alcohol-associated facial flushing (the 'chlorpropamide–alcohol flush', or CPAF) often develops with chlorpropamide [36].

Second-generation sulphonylureas are now widely prescribed, but seem to cause fewer cutaneous side effects: for example, skin reactions have been reported in only 0.21% of patients taking glyburide [37]. Alcohol-induced flushing does not occur commonly with second-generation sulphonylureas [36].

Complications of insulin treatment

Cutaneous reactions to insulin previously occurred in half of the patients treated, but have become much less frequent since purified pork and human insulins were introduced (see Chapter 40). The following reactions have been described.

INSULIN ALLERGY

This may be local or systemic and develops within 1–4 weeks of starting treatment (see also Chapter 40). *Local* allergy was extremely common in the 1960s with the use of 'impure' insulins [38], but the reported prevalence in patients receiving monocomponent porcine insulin was zero in one study [38] and 5% in another [39]. Local reactions are of three types. The commonest is the *late-phase reaction*, a biphasic IgE reaction characterized by immediate burning and pruritus with a wheal and flare at the injection site. It may resolve or become indurated, with pruritus continuing for hours to days. Two rarer forms are the *Arthus-type reaction*, producing a pruritic, painful nodule 6–8h after injection, and the *delayed hypersensitivity reaction*, which is similar but appears 12–24h after injection.

Systemic manifestations include generalized urticaria and, rarely, anaphylaxis. Urticarial allergic reactions to newer insulins are uncommon, with an incidence of 0.1–0.2% [40] and anaphylaxis is very rare. Even lower frequencies should be expected with the more widespread use of

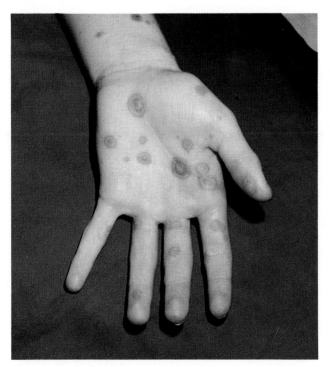

(a)

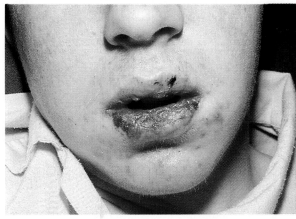

(b)

Fig. 72.9. Stevens–Johnson syndrome, showing typical 'target lesions' of erythema multiforme (a), and mouth ulceration (b). This is a rare complication of treatment with sulphonylureas. (Reproduced by kind permission of Dr Shevaun Mendelsohn, Royal Liverpool Hospital.)

human insulins, although patients sensitized to animal insulins may continue to suffer anaphylaxis even when changed to human insulin [41].

LIPODYSTROPHY

Lipoatrophy and insulin hypertrophy are complications of insulin injection. *Lipoatrophy* presents as circumscribed depressed areas of skin at the injection site and occasionally at distant sites as well (see Chapter 40). Before purified human insulins were available, lipoatrophy occurred in about 25% of insulin-treated patients [42]. Improvement or resolution of lesions has been noted in most patients after changing to purified porcine insulin [39]. Lipoatrophy may be due to a local immune response to injected insulin [43].

Insulin hypertrophy (*lipohypertrophy*) presents as a soft dermal nodule with normal surface epidermis at the injection site, which has often been used for many years (Fig. 72.10). This reaction may be due to the lipogenic action of insulin.

IDIOSYNCRATIC REACTIONS

Pigmentation can occur at the injection site, and rarely, keloids may form. Bilateral symmetrical plaques resembling acanthosis nigricans have also been reported at the site of repeated injections [44].

Glucagonoma syndrome (necrolytic migratory erythema)

This rare syndrome, due to a glucagon-secreting islet-cell neoplasm (Chapter 28), was first de-

scribed by Becker in 1942 [45]. Sixty to seventy per cent of glucagonoma patients develop a polymorphous, erythematous eruption with peripheral scaling which waxes and wanes in cycles of 7–14 days and may remit and relapse spontaneously. Superficial vesiculation can lead to erosions and necrosis. The eruption is usually worst around the mouth, in the groin and perineum and around the genitals. Associated features include painful glossitis, weight loss, relatively mild diabetes (in 80–90%), intermittent diarrhoea, mood changes and venous thrombosis (which commonly causes death). Other clinical features are described in detail in Chapter 28.

Similar rashes may occur without glucagonoma or elevated plasma glucagon levels and may also develop in zinc deficiency [46, 47]. The rash may respond to zinc supplementation and treatment with somatostatin or its analogues may be helpful, even when glucagon levels are not greatly suppressed [48]. The tumour and secondary deposits can be treated by chemotherapy (e.g. streptozotocin) or embolization.

SUSAN E. HILL

GARY R. SIBBALD

References

1 Braverman I. Cutaneous manifestations of diabetes mellitus. *Med Clin North Am* 1971; **55**: 1019–29.

2 Sibbald RG, Schachter RK. The skin and diabetes mellitus. *Int J Dermatol* 1984; **23**: 567–84.

3 Neilly JB, Martin A, Simpson N, MacCuish AG. Pruritus in diabetes mellitus. *Diabetes Care* 1986; **9**: 273–5.

4 Oppenheim M. *Eigentumliche disseminierte Degeneration des Bindegeswebes der Haut bei einem Diabetickes.* Vol 179. 1931: 1929–30.

5 Urbach E. Beiträge zu einer physiologischen und pathologischen Chemie der Haut; eine neue diabetische Stoffwechseldermatose: Nekrobiosis Lipoidica Diabeticorum. *Arch Dermatol Syphilol* 1932; **166**: 273–85.

6 Muller SA, Winkelman RK. Necrobiosis lipoidica diabeticorum. *Arch Dermatol* 1966; **93**: 272–81.

7 Jelinek JE. *The Skin in Diabetes.* Philadelphia: Lea & Febiger, 1986: 31–72.

8 Chernowsky ME. Current concepts of necrobiosis lipoidica. *South Med J* 1961; **54**: 25–9.

9 Heite HJ, Scharwenka HX. Erythema elevatum diutium, Granuloma annulare, Necrobiosis lipoidica und Granulomatosis disciformis Gottran-Miesches; eine vergleichende häufigkeitsanalytische Studie. *Arch Klin Exp Dermatol* 1959; **208**: 260–90.

10 Dandona P, Freedman D, Barter D, Majewski BB, Rhodes EL, Watson B. Glycosylated haemoglobin in patients with necrobiosis lipoidica and granuloma annulare. *Clin Exp Dermatol* 1981; **6**: 299–302.

11 Fox TC. Ringed eruption of the fingers. *Br J Dermatol* 1895; **7**: 91–5.

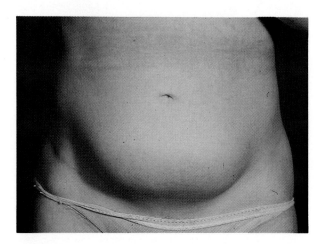

Fig. 72.10. Lipohypertrophy at site of habitual insulin injection.

12 Wells RS, Smith MA. The natural history of granuloma annulare. *Br J Dermatol* 1963; **75**: 199–205.

13 Romaine R, Rudner EJ, Altman J. Papular granuloma annulare and diabetes mellitus. *Arch Dermatol* 1968; **98**: 152–4.

14 Delaney TJ, Gold SC, Leppard B. Disseminated perforating granuloma annulare. *Br J Dermatol* 1973; **89**: 523–6.

15 Meier-Ewart H, Allenby CF. Granuloma annulare and diabetes mellitus. *Arch Dermatol Res* 1971; **241**: 194–8.

16 Mobacken H, Gisslen H, Johannison G. Granuloma annulare cortisone-glucose tolerance test in a non-diabetic group. *Acta Derm Veneneol* 1970; **50**: 440–4.

17 Muhlemann MF, Williams DRR. Localized granuloma annulare is associated with insulin dependent diabetes mellitus. *Br J Dermatol* 1984; **111**: 325–9.

18 Andersen BL, Verdich J. Granuloma annulare and diabetes mellitus. *Clin Exp Dermatol* 1979; **4**: 31–7.

19 Friedman-Birnbaum R, Haim S, Gideone O, Barzilai A. Histocompatibility antigens in granuloma annulare. *Br J Dermatol* 1978; **98**: 452–8.

20 Melin H. An atrophic circumscribed skin lesion in the lower extremities of diabetics. *Acta Med Scand* 1964; **176** (suppl 423): 1–75.

21 Binkley GW. Dermopathy in the diabetic syndrome. *Arch Dermatol* 1965; **92**: 625–34.

22 Danowski TS, Sabeh G, Sarver MF. Shin spots and diabetes mellitus. *Am J Med Sci* 1966; **251**: 570–5.

23 Editorial. Diabetic skin, joints and eyes. How are they related? *Lancet* 1987; ii: 313–4.

24 Hanna W, Friesen D, Bombardier C, Gladman D, Hanna A. Pathologic features of diabetic thick skin. *J Am Acad Dermatol* 1987; **16**: 546–53.

25 Seibold JR, Uitto J, Dorart BB, Prockop DJ. Collagen synthesis and collagenase activity in dermal fibroblasts from patients with diabetes and digital sclerosis. *J Lab Clin Med* 1985; **105**: 664–7.

26 Buckingham B, Perejda AJ, Sandborg C, Kershnar AK, Uitto J. Skin, joints, and pulmonary changes in type 1 diabetes mellitus. *Am J Dis Child* 1986; **140**: 420–3.

27 Ville DB, Powers ML. Effect of glucose and insulin on collagen secretion by human skin fibroblasts *in vitro. Nature* 1977; **268**: 156–8.

28 Flier JS. Metabolic importance of acanthosis nigricans. *Arch Dermatol* 1985; **121**: 193–4.

29 Kahn CR, Flier JS, Bar RS *et al.* The syndromes of insulin resistance and acanthosis nigricans. Insulin receptor disorders in man. *N Engl J Med* 1976; **294**: 739–45.

30 Ober KP. Acanthosis nigricans and insulin resistance associated with hypothyroidism. *Arch Dermatol* 1985; **121**: 229–31.

31 Kramer DW. Early warning signs of impending gangrene in diabetes. *Med J Rec* 1930; **132**: 338–42.

32 Toonstra, J. Bullosis diabeticorum: Report of a case with a review of the literature. *J Am Acad Dermatol* 1985; **13**: 799–805.

33 Bernstein JE, Levine LE, Medericn MM *et al.* Reduced threshold to suction-induced blister formation in insulin-dependent diabetes. *J Am Acad Dermatol* 1983; **8**: 790–1.

34 Stowers JM, Borthwick LJ. Oral hypoglycaemic drugs: clinical pharmacology and therapeutic use. *Drugs* 1977; **14**: 41–56.

35 Stewart RC, Piazza EU, Hyman J, Hurwitz D. Chlorpropamide therapy of diabetes. *N Engl J Med* 1959; **26**: 427–30.

36 Skillman TG, Feldman JM. The pharmacology of sulfonylureas. *Am J Med* 1981; **70**: 361–72.

37 BigBy M, Jick S, Jick H *et al.* Drug-induced cutaneous reactions: a report from the Boston Collaborative Drug Surveillance Program on 15,438 consecutive in-patients (1975–1982). *J Am Med Ass* 1986; **256**: 3358–63.

38 Arkins JA, Enghieing NH, Lennon EJ. *Allergy* 1926; **33**: 69.

39 Wright AD, Walsh CH, Fitzgerald MG, Malins JM. Very pure porcine insulin in clinical practice. *Br Med J* 1979; **1**: 25–7.

40 Anderson JA, Adkinson NF. Allergic reactions to drugs and biologic agents. *J Am Med Ass* 1987; **258**: 2891–9.

41 Fineberg SE, Galloway JA, Fineberg NS *et al.* Immunogenicity of recombinant DNA human insulin. *Diabetologia* 1983; **25**: 465–9.

42 Renold AE, Winegard AI, Martin DB. Diabète sucré et tissu adipeux. *Helv Med Acta* 1957; **24**: 322–7.

43 Reeves WG, Allen BR, Tattersall RB. Insulin-induced lipoatrophy: Evidence for an immune pathogenesis. *Br Med J* 1980; **280**: 1500–3.

44 Matthew G, Fleming MD, Stewart IS. Cutaneous insulin reaction resembling acanthosis nigricans. *Arch Dermatol* 1986; **122**: 1054–6.

45 Becker SW, Kahn D, Rothman S. Cutaneous manifestations of internal malignant tumours. *Arch Dermatol Syphilol* 1942; **45**: 1069.

46 Goodenberger DM, Lawley TJ, Strober W *et al.* Necrolytic migratory erythema without glucagonoma: Report of two cases. *Arch Dermatol* 1979; **115**: 1429–32.

47 Tucker SB, Schroeter AL, Brown PW *et al.* Acquired zinc deficiency: Cutaneous manifestations typical of acrodermatitis enteropathica. *J Am Med Ass* 1976; **235**: 2399–402.

48 Sohier J, Jeanmougin M, Lombrail P, Passa P. Rapid improvement of skin lesions in glucagonomas with intravenous somatostatin infusion. *Lancet* 1980; i: 40.

73 Connective Tissue and Joint Disease in Diabetes Mellitus

Summary

• Joint disease in diabetes is mainly due to either excessive collagen deposition or dysfunction of the autonomic nervous system.

• In the hand, there can be limited joint mobility (LJM), tenosynoviosclerosis (trigger finger), Dupuytren's disease and carpal tunnel syndrome.

• Diabetic collagenosis in the hand, particularly LJM, is associated with an increased prevalence of microvascular complications.

• Frozen shoulder (adhesive capsulitis) with painful restricted shoulder movement has a recurrent relapsing course with eventual recovery of some degree.

• Ankylosing hyperostosis of the spine (symptomless or causing back pain and stiffness) occurs mainly in NIDDM.

• Algodystrophy presents with pain, swelling, autonomic dysfunction and diffuse osteoporosis on X-ray; Charcot's joints and the shoulder—hand syndrome are examples of this disorder.

The first description of a neuropathic joint in diabetes was made in 1936 but it is only in the last two decades that the more subtle articular and periarticular features of diabetes have been clearly defined. The diabetic atherosclerotic plaque and capillary basement membrane thickening are both disorders of extracellular connective tissue and it is, therefore, not surprising that the interstitial connective tissues of bone, joints and periarticular structures are also affected (for reviews see [1-4]).

The disorders involving primarily skin and bone are described elsewhere (Chapters 72 and 74).

The diseases of joints and periarticular structures fall into two broad groups:

1 Diseases characterized by an excessive deposition of connective tissue (mainly collagen).

2 Diseases related to autonomic nervous system dysfunction.

Some disorders, for example shoulder—hand syndrome, may include both processes.

Articular and periarticular disease usually characterized by excessive collagen deposition

The hand

Lundbaeck described hand stiffness in young diabetic patients in 1957 and since then there has been increasing awareness of the link between many hand abnormalities and diabetes [5] (Table 73.1). One or more abnormalities may be present in the same patient: for example, limited joint mobility (LJM), tenosynoviosclerosis and carpal tunnel syndrome comprise a common triad in the adult diabetic hand. In many accounts, diagnosis of the specific abnormality has been imprecise and misleading and has led to unhelpful terms such as 'diabetic hand syndrome' and 'juvenile diabetic cheiro-arthropathy'. These are prejudicial as larger joints such as the elbow or knee may also be affected. In a severe case, the signs of thick, tight, waxy skin, joint restriction (with or without flexion contractures) and tenosynoviosclerosis are highly reminiscent of scleroderma ('pseudoscleroderma'). Occasionally, the dorsal dermal sclerosis can be seen proximal to the metacarpophalangeal (MCP) joints, thereby fulfilling the American Rheumatism Association criteria for frank scleroderma. In one study, 81% of diabetic children with dermal sclerosis of hands

Table 73.1. The diabetic hand (after Rosenbloom 1984 [5]).

Abnormality	Site	Comments
Thick, tight, waxy skin	Dorsal surface	Affects one-third of patients with limited joint mobility
Limited joint mobility (LJM)	MCP and PIP joints (often beginning at little finger) most commonly. Wrists, elbows knees, less commonly	Children and adults: painless
Stiff hand	All fingers	Adults; associated with skin thickening, calcified vessels and vascular insufficiency
Dupuytren's disease (DD)	MCP and PIP joints (especially middle and ring fingers)	Thickened palmar fascia; male:female ratio 6:1; 10−15% of patients with this abnormality are diabetic
Flexor tenosynoviosclerosis and tenosynovitis	Especially thumb, middle and ring fingers	Female preponderance; 'trigger finger'
Carpal tunnel syndrome	Median nerve distribution	5−16% of patients are diabetic; compression and neural factors
Reflex sympathetic dystrophy or algodystrophy	Contractures of finger joints	Usually part of 'shoulder−hand syndrome' with muscle atrophy and bone demineralization; painful

also had involvement of forefeet and toes [6]. Terminology emphasizing connective tissue disease of the diabetic hand should, therefore, be replaced by less committed terms such as 'diabetic collagenosis'.

LIMITED JOINT MOBILITY (LJM)

If the tips of fingers and palms of the normal hand are opposed, the MCP and proximal interphalangeal (PIP) joints can be fully extended. Inability to do this, the 'prayer sign' (Fig. 73.1), has proved a useful clinical screening test for LJM. It may also be positive in the presence of finger flexor tendon sheath disease, but it may be distinguished by the fingers involved (Table 73.1), a history of trigger finger or the palpation of a nodule in the tendon sheath. If the elbows are elevated, the degree of possible wrist extension can also be estimated (normally at least 90°).

The reported prevalence of LJM in young IDDM patients is between 8% and 42%. In the largest study, 30% of 309 patients aged 1−28 years had contractures and one-third of affected children had dermal sclerosis [7]. LJM is not apparently related to sex, insulin dosage or short-term metabolic control (as assessed by glycosylated haemoglobin). However, long-term quality of diabetic control may be relevant, as improvement has been reported if control is optimized. The development of LJM is linked to the duration of diabetes: two-thirds of affected young patients with diabetes for more than 5 years will have moderate or severe limitation of three or more joints and affected patients are 4 times more likely to fall below the 25th percentile for height [5]. LJM is not confined to children and young adults with IDDM, but is also a feature of adult-onset IDDM and of NIDDM, at similar prevalence rates [8, 9]. Although genetic factors have been suggested in the development of LJM, with an increased incidence in first-degree relatives, no HLA associations have been identified [10].

The significance of LJM is not the relatively mild disability which it imposes on some diabetic patients, but its possible role as a marker for more sinister diabetic complications. The relationship between LJM and retinopathy has been amply confirmed: 43% of those with LJM and more than 4 years' duration of diabetes had retinopathy, while only 15% of patients with matched disease duration without LJM had retinopathy [11]. Of 299 patients with retinopathy, 48% had LJM whereas only 24% of patients without retinopathy were affected [12]. The association between LJM and other microvascular compli-

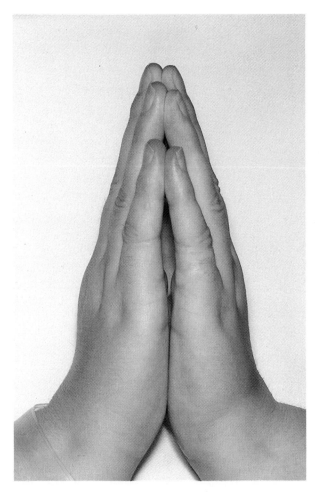

Fig. 73.1. The prayer sign. In normal subjects, finger tips and the palmar surfaces of fingers and palms can be perfectly apposed but in patients with LJM this is impossible. Flexion contractures at the metacarpo-phalangeal (MCP) and proximal interphalangeal (PIP) joints are demonstrated. Note the swelling of little-finger PIP joints and this patient's inability to extend her wrists fully.

cations, such as neuropathy and nephropathy, is less clear [9].

A defective microcirculation is likely to be the common denominator between diabetic patients with LJM, hypertensive subjects with LJM [13] and patients with scleroderma. The capillary loop abnormalities at finger nailfolds have been helpful in the assessment of scleroderma, but no abnormalities have been observed in diabetic patients with microvascular disease and LJM [14].

DUPUYTREN'S DISEASE (DD)

DD is diagnosed by observing or palpating thickened palmar fascia, a palmar or digital nodule (as opposed to a nodule in a tendon sheath), skin tethering and, in late cases, digital contracture.

The reported prevalence of DD in diabetes varies from 1.6–63% but is probably about 40% [2, 15]. About 10–15% of patients with DD are likely to have diabetes [5, 15]. The male:female ratio is about 6:1 [5]. It is linked to the duration of disease but may also be present in up to 16% of adult patients at the time of diagnosis of diabetes [2]. In non-diabetic DD, the lesions are mainly in the little and ring finger rays, but the middle and ring fingers are most affected in diabetes [15].

DD, like LJM, is a marker of microvascular disease [12, 13]. Thirty-six per cent of 299 patients with retinopathy had DD, as opposed to only 16% of diabetic subjects without retinopathy [12].

Increased amounts of type III collagen have been identified in the diseased palmar fascia and especially in the nodular tissue. The increased proportions of type III collagen and type I trimer are typical of embryonic collagen and increased amounts of sulphated glycosaminoglycans present in DD are characteristic of immature tendinous structures [16]. The active deposition of connective tissue in DD is by contractile 'myofibroblasts' and it is also worth noting that these cells have also been reported in the nodules of Ledderhose's disease of the plantar fascia and Peyronie's disease of the penis, both of which are more common in diabetes.

TENOSYNOVIOSCLEROSIS AND TENOSYNOVITIS

The deposition of excessive connective tissue in flexor tendon sheaths of the hand in diabetes can lead to 'trigger finger' [5, 6]. Palpation of the palm of the hand during passive movement of the fingers can sometimes demonstrate a nodule and finger contractures can occur in chronic involvement. The term 'tenosynoviosclerosis' may be preferred as inflammatory changes in the tendon sheaths are minimal or absent. The index and little fingers are relatively spared and there is a female preponderance [5]. Unlike LJM, trigger finger is often painful.

CARPAL TUNNEL SYNDROME (CTS)

In a series of 379 patients with CTS, 63 (16.6%) were found to be diabetic [17]. An association with LJM has been proposed, with the suggestion that the median nerve is compressed by excessive collagen deposition in the flexor retinaculum, but the pathogenesis of CTS in diabetes has been inadequately studied. It is certain that a true compression neuropathy can occur but the contribution of diffuse peripheral neuropathy is uncertain. There is some evidence that vitamin B6 (pyridoxine) deficiency may play a part but, although vitamin B6 deficiency has been reported in diabetes, anecdotal reports have failed to demonstrate improvement with vitamin B6 supplements in diabetic CTS; a formal study is awaited.

The shoulder

Adhesive capsulitis (or frozen shoulder) is characterized by painful restriction of all shoulder movements. Episodes of painful restriction of shoulders in diabetic patients are typically recurrent and multifocal. The thickened joint capsule is closely applied and adherent to the head of the humerus and arthrography demonstrates a marked reduction in volume of the glenohumeral joint. There may be increased periarticular uptake of bone-seeking isotopes followed by bone demineralization. A histological study of capsular tissue from a diabetic with frozen shoulder showed microvascular disease and the proliferation of fibroblasts and myofibroblasts as seen in DD. This contrasts with the more inflammatory histology of idiopathic capsulitis.

In one study of 800 diabetic patients, 10% had shoulder capsulitis compared with 2.5% of non-diabetic controls [18]; conversely, up to 28% of unselected patients with shoulder capsulitis have been found to have abnormal glucose tolerance.

By careful matching for age, sex and disease duration, Fisher et al. have demonstrated an increased incidence of shoulder capsulitis in diabetic patients who also have LJM of the hands [19]. However, it is unlikely that excessive connective tissue deposition in the shoulder capsule is the only factor in the development of the painful restricted shoulder, as the natural history is one of recurrent relapsing episodes with eventual partial or even complete recovery. Superadded inflammatory or autonomic neuropathic factors may contribute; formal comparison of the idiopathic with the diabetic frozen shoulder should provide further insight.

The spine

The main skeletal abnormality in diabetes, particularly in IDDM, is diabetic osteopenia (see Chapter 74). By contrast, some NIDDM patients display excessive bone deposition in certain sites, most commonly the spine. Ankylosing hyperostosis of the spine (Forestier's disease) occurs in 2–4% of the normal population aged over 40 years; the prevalence of 13% in diabetic patients (rising to 21% in the group aged 60–69 years) suggests that the association is genuine [20]. The condition is often asymptomatic or may cause back pain and stiffness. It is characterized by exuberant osteophytes which form anterior bridges between vertebrae and sclerosis of the underlying vertebral cortex. There is a predilection for the right side of the thoracic spine. The sparing of the posterior spinal joints may account for the preservation of relatively full spinal movements. Ankylosing spondylitis is easily distinguished by its younger age of onset, sacro-iliac joint involvement, its association with HLA B27 and the vertical syndesmophytes between vertebral bodies (rather than the curved, beak-like osteophytes of hyperostosis).

Lower limbs

It has been previously noted that patients with LJM of the hands may also have dermal sclerosis of the feet and lack full knee extension. Recently, an association between shoulder capsulitis and capsulitis of the hip in diabetes has been proposed. Of 61 diabetic patients with shoulder disease, 23 had hip restriction, especially of internal rotation, and in 18 this was bilateral [21].

Articular and periarticular disease related to autonomic dysfunction

Several syndromes of unknown pathogenesis variously described as 'Sudek's atrophy', 'reflex sympathetic dystrophy', 'transient osteoporosis', and 'migratory osteolysis' have been grouped convincingly under the single heading of algodystrophy [22] (Fig. 73.2). They present with pain (often severely disabling), sometimes swelling and invariably features of autonomic dysfunction. There may be a transient hyperaemic phase (which may persist in Charcot's neuroarthropathy) but, more commonly, patients present with a cold, cyanosed, shiny and tender limb. In established disease, X-rays may show a 'spotty' or diffuse osteoporosis. The condition usually resolves spontaneously, occasionally with fibrosis and contracture.

Trauma remains the commonest predisposing cause, but diabetic patients are also more prone. Of 108 consecutive cases, eight had diabetes: two had shoulder–hand syndrome, two had knee involvement and in four the foot was affected [23]. Few of these patients underwent glucose tolerance testing and the true prevalence may be higher.

SHOULDER–HAND SYNDROME

This may be considered a rarer, but exaggerated, form of adhesive capsulitis of the shoulder involving the whole upper limb with striking cold, vasomotor changes and distal oedema. Demineralization of the limb, especially the hand, often occurs. Early active mobilization of the limb is essential but regional intravenous guanethidine blockade or stellate ganglion blockade is often required.

TRANSIENT OSTEOPOROSIS OF THE HIP

In a study of 34 patients with algodystrophy of the hip, five had diabetes [22]. This may represent an advanced or more intense form of capsulitis of the hip.

NEUROARTHROPATHY OF THE LOWER LIMB (CHARCOT JOINTS)

This may involve, in order of decreasing frequency, the tarso-metatarsal joints, the metatarsophalangeal (MTP) joints, the ankle and the knee. It now seems clear that the initiating event is an increase in blood flow through the lower leg secondary to sympathetic neuropathy. Clinically, the ankle and foot are hot and swollen, often with less pain than might be anticipated. X-rays demonstrate local osteoporosis which may progress to frank osteolysis and fragmentation of bone and cartilage [3, 23] (Figs 73.3 and 73.4). It may progress through a 'coalescence' stage when the bone ends become sclerotic and then a 'reconstitution' stage, when a new joint space appears, but the evolution of a neuropathic joint may be arrested at any stage (see Chapter 70).

Since the decline of neurosyphilis, diabetes is now the commonest cause of neuropathic joints outside lepromatous regions. If there is any doubt about the diagnosis, however, it is essential to exclude septic arthritis, to which diabetic patients are also prone, by aspiration of a hot joint.

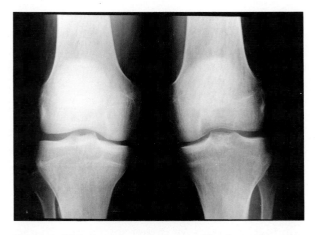

Fig. 73.2. Diabetic male aged 26 years. Algodystrophy: minor injury to left knee and increasing pain plus 10° fixed flexion deformity. Left knee was palpably cooler than the right. Normal arthroscopy. The X-ray shows normal right knee. There is demineralization of left femur and tibia. The intercondylar subcortical bone loss of the distal femur is very characteristic. Definite bone loss is seen extending above the patellar level and in the proximal tibia.

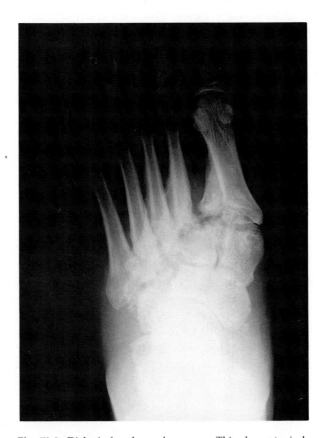

Fig. 73.3. Diabetic female aged 24 years. This shows typical Charcot-like changes in tarso-metatarsal joints with bone destruction and formation in a thoroughly disorganized fashion. (See also Figs 70.8–70.11.)

FOREFOOT OSTEOLYSIS

The pathogenesis of forefoot osteolysis is probably shared with Charcot's neuroarthropathy, but it seems to arise directly from the metatarsals themselves rather than the adjacent joints. The metatarsal heads can dissolve, producing a 'sharpened pencil' or 'sucked candy' appearance [3, 23]. Sclerosis of bone cortex and reformation of the metatarsal heads often occurs.

Other joint diseases which may be associated with diabetes

Osteoarthritis (OA)

It is obviously difficult to establish a relationship between such common diseases as OA and diabetes, but a positive correlation has been proposed by controlled studies [24]. The prevalence of OA was higher in young and middle-aged diabetic subjects, and joint damage started at an earlier age and was more severe than in controls. Clinical evidence is scanty but the evidence from studies *in vitro* is impressive (for reviews, see references [2, 3]). Cartilage growth is depressed in diabetes and there is reduced synthesis of sulphated proteoglycans, with a reduction in the size of high molecular-weight aggregates. Articular chondrocytes from diabetic hamsters undergo morphological changes and release more collagen-degrading enzymes. Insulin has been shown to stimulate cartilage growth activity and proteoglycan synthesis.

However, osteoarthritis is more than a simple depletion of proteoglycan from cartilage, also being characterized by bone osteophyte formation and periarticular osteosclerosis. The increased prevalence of ankylosing hyperostosis, a proliferative form of osteoarthritis affecting the spine (see above), suggests that diabetic patients are at increased risk of generalized osteoarthritis.

Rheumatoid arthritis (RA)

Thirty-nine out of 295 patients (13%) with RA had a first- or second-degree relative with IDDM [25] and Rudolf *et al.* described seven IDDM children with juvenile RA [26]. As both diseases are associated with HLA DR4, this is not surprising. However, a specific DQβ genotypic marker associated with DR4 has been identified, which is highly associated with diabetes but not with juvenile RA [27]. Payami *et al.* have proposed that IDDM is predisposed to by two HLA-linked alleles, one of which also confers susceptibility to RA [28].

Crystal arthropathy (gout and pyrophosphate arthropathy)

The triad of hyperglycaemia, hyperlipidaemia and hyperuricaemia is well recognized, but obesity is likely to be the linking factor. Although there have been reports of an increased prevalence of diabetes in gouty subjects, a study of glucose tolerance in weight-matched gouty and non-gouty subjects failed to demonstrate any difference [29]. Chronic glucose loading actually promotes uric acid excretion, and the onset of diabetes in patients with established gout is accompanied by a fall in serum urate levels and in the frequency and severity of attacks. However, diabetic ketoacidosis may be complicated by hyperuricaemia, as ketone bodies inhibit renal tubular secretion of uric acid (for review, see reference [2]). The critical role of renal function in the handling of uric acid in the presence of diabetes was emphasized in a recent study. The lowest uric acid levels were found in male diabetics but the strongest predictor of blood uric acid was plasma creatinine [30]. In conclusion, non-obese diabetics with normal renal function are less likely to develop gout than normal subjects and it is probable that non-obese gouty patients do not have an increased risk of diabetes.

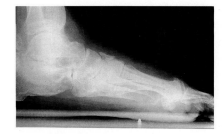 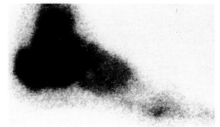

Fig. 73.4. Same patient as in Fig. 73.3. Very painful ankle. Bone destruction/osteolysis of talus and calcaneum with greatly increased uptake on bone scan (right). This is evolving into a Charcot arthropathy.

Early descriptions of pyrophosphate arthropathy — characterized by the radiographic appearance of chondrocalcinosis and the clinical syndrome of acute pseudogout — reported an apparent association with diabetes, which has not been confirmed in a large controlled study [31]. However, diabetes and chondrocalcinosis are both associated with haemochromatosis (see Chapter 27).

Pathophysiology of connective tissue changes in diabetes

Insulin deficiency is probably responsible for two processes highly dependent on insulin as a tissue growth factor: the reduced bone mass of the young diabetic at diagnosis of the disease and the depletion of cartilage proteoglycan in premature osteoarthritis (see above). With these exceptions, the hallmark of diabetic connective tissue is the excessive deposition of collagen at many periarticular sites and in the skin. It is possible that the increased permeability of diabetic capillaries may trigger proliferation of vessel wall and extravascular connective tissue. The excessive new bone formation found in ankylosing hyperostosis, hyperostosis frontalis interna and osteitis condensans ilii (all more common in diabetes) may be attributable to overactivity of bone growth factors, either through increased tissue concentrations (for example, of insulin-like growth factors [32]) or changes in receptor function. Such growth factors may also stimulate excess collagen deposition in the soft tissues of skin and periarticular structures.

The molecular basis of diabetic collagen deposition remains unclear, but could result from increased synthesis or reduced degradation of collagen. There is little evidence to support increased synthesis *in vivo*, although skin fibroblasts from IDDM patients may synthesize increased amounts of collagen *in vitro* [33]. Resistance of collagen to breakdown may be more important, and could result from biochemical modifications, such as non-enzymatic glycosylation of collagen and increased collagen cross-linking mediated by lysyl oxidase.

Hyperglycaemia *per se* increases non-enzymatic glycosylation of collagen, keratin and haemoglobin A, and the decreased solubility of glycosylated collagen in acetic acid suggests intermolecular cross-linking [34]. However, it now seems less likely that collagen glycosylation is the critical factor. Guitton *et al.* claimed that glycosylation actually *inhibits* cross-linking and maturation of collagen fibres [35]. Moreover, studies of forearm skin biopsies have confirmed increased tissue glycosylation in diabetic as compared with normal subjects, but found no differences in glycosylation between diabetic subjects with LJM and those without [36].

Chang *et al.* [37] concluded that the reduced solubility of collagen in diabetic rats was attributable to an increase in lysine-derived cross-links, as it could be inhibited by β-aminopropionitrile, an inhibitor of lysyl oxidase. Increased lysyl oxidase activity has been reported in diabetes [38] and may be crucial to the excess collagen deposition of LJM, tenosynoviosclerosis, carpal tunnel syndrome, DD, adhesive capsulitis of the shoulder and dermal sclerosis.

Treatment

General treatment

Tight control of blood glucose may ultimately reduce skin thickness and improve joint mobility [39, 40] and must obviously underpin all treatment.

Anecdotal reports, yet to be confirmed, have suggested that sorbinil, an aldose reductase inhibitor (Chapter 104), may improve the range of movement in patients with painful LJM and some peripheral nerve abnormalities [41]. It is unlikely to have a beneficial effect on painless LJM as defined by Rosenbloom [5]. Cyclo-oxygenase inhibitors prevent an increase in the thermal rupture time of rat-tail collagen (a measure of collagen stability) and may be useful in diabetic collagenosis [42] but no clinical evidence is available.

Specific treatment

Simple active and passive stretching exercises may help to limit joint contractures, and an active daily programme of shoulder exercises is mandatory in patients with adhesive capsulitis. Glucocorticoids are commonly injected locally into tendon sheaths, the carpal tunnel and the capsulitic shoulder, but seem to be less effective in diabetes than in traumatic or idiopathic cases. This is compatible with the minor, if any, inflammatory component in diabetic patients. Surgical decompression of tendon sheaths and the carpal tunnel, or arthrolysis of the shoulder, may be necessary. Excision of palmar fascia in DD is not worthwhile but surgery may be indicated if severe finger contractures develop.

Treatment of the autonomic disorders is very difficult. Early active mobilization of the capsulitic shoulder will help to prevent the development of shoulder−hand syndrome but if this does occur, regional intravenous guanethidine or stellate ganglion block is necessary. Calcitonin may be helpful in some cases of algodystrophy. The management of the neuropathic ankle and foot depends on providing appropriate protective footwear and on a strict non-weight-bearing policy during periods of active osteolysis (Chapter 70).

Finally, the hot swollen joint (which may not always be painful in diabetic patients) must always be assumed to be infected until this has been actively excluded by aspiration and culture.

ADRIAN J. CRISP

References

1 Gray RG, Gottlieb NL. Rheumatic disorders associated with diabetes mellitus. *Sem Arthr Rheum* 1976; **6**: 19−34.
2 Crisp AJ, Heathcote JG. Connective tissue abnormalities in diabetes mellitus. *J R Coll Physicians Lond* 1984; **18**: 132−41.
3 Johanson NA. Endocrine arthropathies. *Clin Rheum Dis* 1985; **11**: 297−323.
4 Crisp AJ. Diabetes mellitus and the rheumatologist. *Br J Rheum* 1986; **25**: 135−7.
5 Rosenbloom AL. Skeletal and joint manifestations of childhood diabetes. *Pediatr Clin North Am* 1984; **31**: 569−89.
6 Seibold JR. Digital sclerosis in children with insulin-dependent diabetes mellitus. *Arthr Rheum* 1982; **25**: 1357−61.
7 Rosenbloom AL, Silverstein JH, Lesotte DC, Richardson K, McCallum M. Limited joint mobility of childhood diabetes mellitus indicates increased risk for microvascular disease. *N Engl J Med* 1981; **305**: 191−4.
8 Fitzcharles MA, Duby S, Waddell RW, Banks E, Karsch J. Limitation of joint mobility in adult non-insulin dependent diabetic patients. *Ann Rheum Dis* 1984; **43**: 251−7.
9 Starkman HS, Gleason RE, Rand LI, Miller DE, Soeldner JS. Limited joint mobility of the hand in patients with diabetes mellitus: relation to chronic complications. *Ann Rheum Dis* 1986; **45**: 130−5.
10 Beacom R, Gillespie EL, Middleton D, Sawhney B, Kennedy L. Limited joint mobility in insulin-dependent diabetics: relationship to nephropathy, peripheral nerve function and HLA status. *Q J Med* 1985; **219**: 337−44.
11 Rosenbloom AL, Malone JI, Yucha J, Van Cader TC. Limited joint mobility and diabetic retinopathy demonstrated by fluorescein angiography. *Eur J Paediatr* 1984; **141**: 163−4.
12 Lawson PM, Maneschi F, Kohner EM. The relationship of hand abnormalities to diabetes and diabetic retinopathy. *Diabetes Care* 1983; **6**: 140−3.
13 Larkin JG, Frier BM. Limited joint mobility and

14 Trapp RG, Soler NG, Spencer-Green G. Nailfold capillaroscopy in type I diabetics with vasculopathy and limited joint mobility. *J Rheum* 1986; **13**: 917−20.
15 Noble J, Heathcote JG, Cohen H. Diabetes mellitus in the aetiology of Dupuytren's disease. *J Bone Jt Surg* 1984; **66B**: 322−5.
16 Brickley-Parsons D, Glimcher MJ, Smith RJ, Albin R, Adams JP. Biochemical changes in the collagen of the palmar fascia in patients with Dupuytren's disease. *J Bone Jt Surg* 1981; **63A**: 787−97.
17 Phalen GS. Reflections on 21 years' experience with the carpal tunnel syndrome. *J Am Med Ass* 1970; **212**: 1365−7.
18 Bridgeman JF. Periarthritis of the shoulder and diabetes mellitus. *Ann Rheum Dis* 1972; **31**: 69−71.
19 Fisher L, Kurtz A, Shipley M. Association between cheiroarthropathy and frozen shoulder in patients with insulin-dependent diabetes. *Br J Rheum* 1986; **25**: 141−6.
20 Julkunen H, Heinonen OP, Knekt P, Maatela J. The epidemiology of hyperostosis of the spine together with its symptoms and related mortality in a general population. *Scand J Rheum* 1975; **4**: 23−7.
21 Moren-Hybinette I, Moritz U, Schersten B. The clinical picture of the painful diabetic shoulder − natural history, social consequences and analysis of concomitant hand syndrome. *Acta Med Scand* 1987; **221**: 73−82.
22 Doury P, Dirheimer Y, Pattin S. *Algodystrophy*. Berlin: Springer-Verlag, 1981.
23 Brooks AP. The neuropathic foot in diabetes: Part II Charcot's neuroarthropathy. *Diabetic Med* 1986; **3**: 116−18.
24 Waine H, Nevinny D, Rosenthal J, Jaffe IB. Association of osteoarthritis and diabetes mellitus. *Tufts Fol Med* 1961; **7**: 13−19.
25 Thomas DJB, Young A, Gorsuch AN, Bottazzo GF, Cudworth AG. Evidence for an association between rheumatoid arthritis and autoimmune endocrine disease. *Ann Rheum Dis* 1983; **42**: 297−300.
26 Rudolf MCJ, Genel M, Tamborlane WV, Dwyer JM. Juvenile rheumatoid arthritis in children with diabetes mellitus. *J Pediatr* 1981; **99**: 519−24.
27 Nepom BS, Palmer J, Kim SJ, Hansen JA, Holbeck SL, Nepom GT. Specific genomic markers for the HLA-DQ subregion discriminate between DR4+ insulin-dependent diabetes mellitus and DR4+ seropositive juvenile rheumatoid arthritis. *J Exp Med* 1986; **164**: 345−50.
28 Payami H, Khan MH, Grennan DM, Sanders PA, Dyer PA, Thomson G. Analysis of genetic inter-relationship among HLA associated diseases. *Am J Hum Genet* 1987; **41**: 331−49.
29 Boyle JA, McKiddie M, Buchanan KD, Jasani MK, Gray HW, Jackson IMD, Buchanan WW. Diabetes mellitus and gout. *Ann Rheum Dis* 1969; **28**: 374−8.
30 Tuomilehto J, Zimmet P, Wolf E, Taylor R, Ram P, King H. Plasma uric acid level and its association with diabetes mellitus and some biologic parameters in a biracial population of Fiji. *Am J Epidemiol* 1988; **127**: 321−36.
31 Alexander GM, Dieppe PA, Doherty M, Scott DGI. Pyrophosphate arthropathy: a study of metabolic associations and laboratory data. *Ann Rheum Dis* 1982; **41**: 377−81.
32 Press M, Tamborlane WV, Sherwin RS. Importance of raised growth hormone levels in mediating the metabolic derangements of diabetes. *N Engl J Med* 1984; **310**: 810−5.
33 Smith BD, Silbert CK. Fibronectin and collagen of cultured skin fibroblasts in diabetes mellitus. *Biochem Biophys Res Commun* 1981; **100**: 275−82.
34 Buckingham BA, Uitto J, Sandborg C, Keens T, Kaufman F,

Landing B. Scleroderma-like syndrome and non-enzymatic glycosylation of collagen in children with poorly controlled insulin-dependent diabetes mellitus. *Pediatr Res* 1981; **15**: 626.

35 Guitton JD, LePape A, Sizaret PY, Muh JP. Effects of *in vitro* N-glucosylation on type I collagen fibrillogenesis. *Biosci Repts* 1981; **1**: 945–54.

36 Lyons TJ, Kennedy L. Non-enzymatic glycosylation of skin collagen in patients with Type I (insulin-dependent) diabetes mellitus and limited joint mobility. *Diabetologia* 1985; **28**: 2–5.

37 Chang K, Uitto J, Rowold EA, Grant GA, Kilo C, Williamson JR. Increased collagen cross-linkages in experimental diabetes: reversal by β-aminopropionitrile and D-penicillamine. *Diabetes* 1980; **29**: 778–81.

38 Madia AM, Rozovski SJ, Kagan HM. Changes in lung lysyl oxidase activity in streptozotocin-diabetes and in starvation. *Biochim Biophys Acta* 1979; **585**: 481–7.

39 Sherry DD, Rothstein RRL, Petty RE. Joint contractures preceding insulin-dependent diabetes mellitus. *Arthr Rheum* 1982; **11**: 1362–4.

40 Lister DM, Graham-Brown RAC, Burden AC. Resolution of diabetic cheiroarthropathy. *Br Med J* 1986; **293**: 1537.

41 Eaton RP, Sibbitt WL, Harsh A. The effect of an aldose reductase inhibiting agent on limited joint mobility in diabetic patients. *J Am Med Ass* 1985; **253**: 1437–40.

42 Yue DK, McLennan S, Handelsman DJ, Delbridge L, Reeve T, Turtle JR. The effects of cyclo-oxygenase and lipo-oxygenase inhibitors on the collagen abnormalities of diabetic rats. *Diabetes* 1985; **34**: 74–8.

74 Bone and Mineral Metabolism in Diabetes

Summary

• Diabetic osteopenia (reduced bone density) affects many IDDM patients and probably increases their susceptibility to fractures. NIDDM patients may be less affected.

• Bone loss is rapid in the first 2 years after diagnosis, declining to a steady value by 5 years.

• Diabetic osteopenia is a low turnover state, with reduced bone formation and continuing resorption.

• Diabetes has little effect on the mineral content of bone, or on serum calcium levels, although ketoacidosis and hyperglycaemia may cause magnesium and phosphate depletion.

• Hypercalciuria (due to predominant bone resorption) is common in diabetes and is reduced by improving metabolic control.

Diabetes has been associated both with localized changes in bone density (such as those affecting the diabetic foot: see Chapters 70 and 73) and with generalized disturbances of bone and mineral metabolism. The latter, particularly the diffuse reduction in bone density termed 'diabetic osteopenia', will be discussed here.

Diabetic osteopenia

Reports of the prevalence, extent and natural history of diabetic osteopenia vary widely, probably because of the different methods and study populations employed. Many clinical studies have measured bone density at a single site (commonly the forearm), either with non-invasive methods such as X-ray or photon absorptiometry or by histological examination of bone biopsies. Recently, non-invasive absorptiometric techniques and computerized tomography have been applied to investigate bone density in the axial skeleton, which includes the clinically relevant sites of the spine (Fig. 74.1) and proximal femur where significant osteoporosis leading to fractures is most likely to occur.

Prevalence

In IDDM, it is generally agreed that bone density (measured in the forearm in most studies) is significantly reduced below age-adjusted control values, over 50% of IDDM patients showing a reduction of >10% [1–3]. Significant bone loss may be present at the time of diagnosis (perhaps related to the preceding decline in insulin secretion) and is relatively rapid in the following 2 years, declining gradually thereafter to a steady-state value at about 5 years [3]. Poorly controlled IDDM patients probably suffer proportionately greater bone loss than those enjoying good metabolic control.

The situation in NIDDM is less clear-cut, possibly because of confounding variables such as age, race, obesity, menopausal status and the unknown duration of the disease before diagnosis. One study has reported a reduction in density of around 10% in as many as 60% of NIDDM patients [1], whereas others have found a decrease of this magnitude in only 20% [4]. The available data do not allow the time-course of these changes to be defined. One study has described a subgroup of NIDDM patients who show an *increase* in bone density [4]. This curious and unexpected finding is not apparently explicable by obesity but could be related to hyperinsulinaemia, which

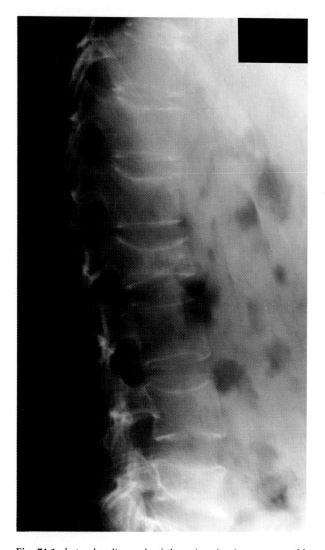

Fig. 74.1. Lateral radiograph of thoracic spine in a 23-year-old woman with IDDM, showing reduced bone density and collapse of vertebral bodies due to diabetic osteopenia. (Reproduced by kind permission of Dr Ian MacFarlane, Walton Hospital, Liverpool.)

has been associated with elevated insulin-like growth factor 1 (IGF-1) levels and as such could exert an anabolic effect on bone (see below; [5]).

Mechanisms of bone loss

Bone mass is normally maintained by close matching of bone resorption (osteoclastic activity) to bone formation (osteoblastic activity). Bone density can be reduced when these two opposing influences are uncoupled. Diabetic osteopenia appears to be a 'low turnover' state, with reduced bone formation rather than a primary increase in resorption [6] (Fig. 74.2). Bone formation is slowed in diabetes, the osteons taking 2–8 times longer to develop than in non-diabetic subjects [7]. His-

tomorphometric analyses of iliac crest biopsies have demonstrated increased surface areas, but normal volumes of trabecular and osteoid elements, indicating that resorption of bone is proportionately greater than its formation [8]. Levels of osteocalcin (a protein synthesized by osteoblasts) are reduced, consistent with decreased osteoblastic activity. The fact that the increase in bone resorption is relative and not absolute is confirmed by the urinary excretion of hydroxyproline (an indirect measure of total bone resorption), which is not increased in diabetes.

The factors mediating this uncoupling are unknown, but might involve the effects of insulin deficiency on the cytokines which are increasingly implicated in the local regulation of bone metabolism. In particular, insulin-like growth factors, IGF-1 [9] and probably IGF-2 [10] can stimulate osteoblastic precursors to replicate and differentiate into osteoblasts. In poorly controlled diabetes, growth hormone secretion is increased but circulating levels of IGF may be reduced [5], which could impede bone formation.

The calcium and phosphorus contents of bone are not significantly altered in diabetes; a minor reduction of magnesium levels in IDDM patients [12] does not seem to have any important effect on the degree of bone mineralization.

Bone loss does not appear to be related to other chronic diabetic complications, in that its time-course and prevalence do not match those of retinopathy or other microvascular complications [12].

Clinical implications

The tendency to reduced bone density in diabetes might be expected to increase diabetic patients' susceptibility to fracture. This is probably true, although the additional risk may not be great: a review of six studies showed the relative risk of fractures to vary between 1.16 and 2.86 times that of the non-diabetic population [12], although another study has found no excess risk. The risk may be higher in specific subgroups of subjects such as poorly controlled IDDM patients or those with additional risk factors for osteoporosis, notably perimenopausal women. The increasing availability of sensitive, non-invasive measurements of bone density will not only help to clarify the natural history of the condition, but should also allow at-risk patients to be screened. At present, the only rational measures to protect the skeleton in diabetic patients are probably the

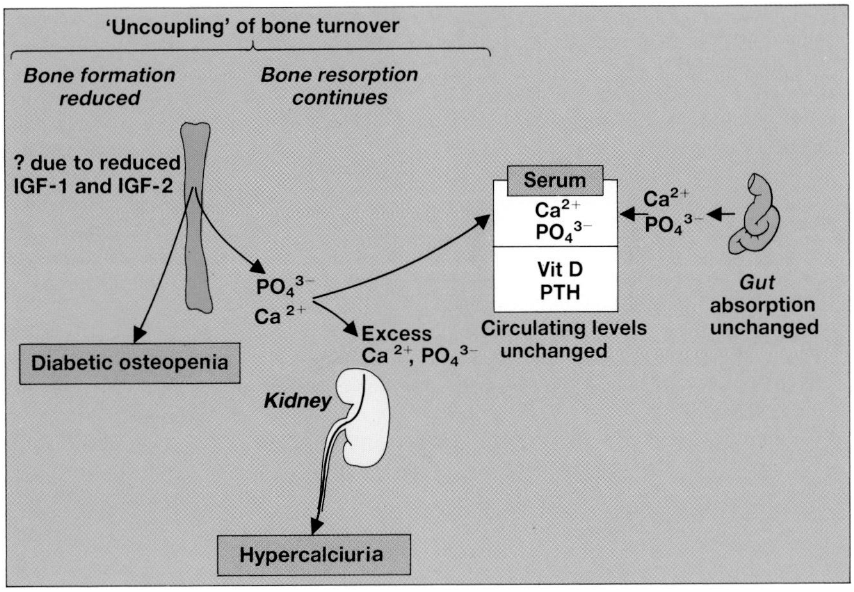

Fig. 74.2. Bone and mineral metabolism in diabetes. Bone formation is reduced while resorption continues at its normal pace; this 'uncoupling' liberates calcium from the skeleton (which is eliminated through the kidneys) and leads ultimately to diabetic osteopenia. Gut absorption of calcium and phosphate is normal. Serum levels of calcium and phosphate, and of parathyroid hormone (PTH) and 1, 25-dihydroxycholecalciferol (vitamin D) are unchanged in most diabetic patients. IGF-1, 2 = insulin-like growth factors 1 and 2.

maintenance of as good metabolic control as possible, and the possible use of hormonal replacement in postmenopausal women.

Effects of diabetes on calcium, phosphate and magnesium balance

Insulin is thought to have several effects on the turnover of calcium, magnesium and phosphate. It has complex actions on proximal and distal renal tubular handling of electrocytes, including enhanced phosphate reabsorption [16]. Insulin may also have a permissive effect on the 1-α-hydroxylase in the kidney which converts 25-hydroxycholecalciferol to its active metabolite, 1,25-dihydroxycholecalciferol [16].

The major disturbance in diabetes is hypercalciuria, which tends to fall but is not completely abolished by improved metabolic control [17]. Although the cause of hypercalciuria is unknown, the kidneys seem effectively to act to eliminate any excess calcium mobilized by the relatively increased bone resorption, and serum calcium concentrations generally remain within the normal range. Circulating levels of parathyroid hormone and of 1,25-dihydroxycholecalciferol are also unchanged, although other vitamin D metabolites may show alterations in diabetes [18, 19].

IDDM patients with ketoacidosis and hyperglycaemia may show variable total body depletion of both magnesium and phosphate, although serum levels only rarely fall to the point where clinical problems occur or treatment becomes necessary [21, 22].

RAYMOND BRUCE
JOHN C. STEVENSON

References

1 Levin ME, Boisseau VC, Avioli LV. Effects of diabetes mellitus on bone mass in juvenile and adult-onset diabetes. *N Engl J Med* 1976; **294**: 241–5.

2 Hui SL, Epstein S, Johnston CC. A prospective study of bone mass in patients with type 1 diabetes. *J Clin Endocrinol Metab* 1985; **60**: 74–80.

3 McNair P, Madsbad S, Christensen MS, Christiansen C, Faber OK, Binder C, Transbol I. Bone mineral loss in insulin treated diabetes mellitus: studies on pathogenesis. *Acta Endocrinol* 1979; **90**: 463–72.

4 De Leeuw I, Abs R. Bone mass and bone density in maturity-type diabetics measured by the ^{125}I photon absorption technique. *Diabetes* 1977; **26**: 1130–5.

5 Holly JMP, Amiel SA, Sandhu RR, Rees LH, Wass JAH. The role of growth hormone in diabetes mellitus. *J Endocrinol* 1988; **118**: 353–64.

6 Silberberg R. The skeleton in diabetes mellitus: a review of the literature. *Diabetes Res* 1986; **3**: 329–38.

7 Takahashi H, Frost HM. The kinetics of the resorption process in osteonal remodeling of diabetic rib. *Henry Ford Med Bull* 1964; **12**: 537–45.

8 De Leeuw I, Mulkens N, Vertommen J, Abs R. A histomorphometric study of the trabecular bone of diabetic subjects. *Diabetologia* 1976; **12**: 385–6.

9 Canalis E. Bone related growth factors. *Triangle* 1988; **27**: 11–19.

10 Strong DD, Beacher AL, Mohan S, Wegerdal JE, Linkhart TA, Baylink DJ. Multiple major skeletal growth factor (SGF) mRNA transcripts expressed in human bone cells. *J Bone Min Res* 1988; **3** (suppl 1): 294.

11 De Leeuw I, Vertommen J, Abs R. The mineral content of the trabecular bone of diabetic subjects (abstract). *Diabetologia* 1976; **12**: 386.

12 McNair P, Christensen MS, Christiansen C, Madsbad S, Transbol I. Is diabetic osteoporosis due to microangiopathy? (letter) *Lancet* 1981; i: 1271.

13 Selby PL. Osteopenia and diabetes. *Diabetic Med* 1988; **5**: 423–8.

14 Heath H, Melton LJ, Chu C-P. Diabetes mellitus and risk of skeletal fracture. *N Engl J Med* 1980; **303**: 567–70.

15 DeFronzo RA, Goldberg M, Agus ZS. The effects of glucose and insulin on renal electrolyte transport. *J Clin Invest* 1976; **58**: 83–90.

16 Henry HL. Insulin permits parathormone stimulation of 1, 25 dihydroxy Vit D3 in cultured kidney cells. *Endocrinology* 1981; **108**: 733–5.

17 Gertner JM, Tamborlane WV, Horst RL, Sherwin RS, Felig P, Genel M. Mineral metabolism in diabetes mellitus: changes accompanying treatment with a portable subcutaneous insulin infusion system. *J Clin Endocrinol Metab* 1980; **50**: 862–6.

18 Frazer TE, White NH, Hough S, Santiago JV, McGee BR, Bryce G, Mallon J, Avioli LV. Alterations in circulating vitamin D metabolites in the young insulin-dependent diabetic. *J Clin Endocrinol Metab* 1981; **53**: 1154–9.

19 Ishida H, Seino Y, Matsukura S, Ikeda M, Yawata M, Yamashita G, Ishizuka S, Imura H. Diabetic osteopenia and circulating levels of Vitamin D metabolites in type 2 (non-insulin dependent) diabetes. *Metabolism* 1985; **34**: 797–801.

20 Martin HE, Smith K, Wilson ML. The fluid and electrolyte therapy of severe diabetic acidosis and ketosis. *Am J Med* 1958; **24**: 376–89.

21 Guest GM. Organic phosphates of the blood and mineral metabolism in diabetic acidosis. *Am J Dis Child* 1942; **64**: 401–12.

75   Sexual Function in Diabetic Women

Summary

- Some diabetic women enter menarche later and have less regular cycles than non-diabetic women. Insulin requirements change (usually with an increase) in about 40% of diabetic women around the time of menstruation; the mechanism is unknown.
- Psychosexual development may be delayed in diabetic women, especially when diabetes presents at a young age.
- Fertility is essentially normal in most well-controlled diabetic women, unless serious complications (e.g. nephropathy) are present; contraception is therefore essential if pregnancy is not desired.
- Genito-urinary infections — especially candidiasis and perhaps genital herpes — are relatively common in diabetic women and often interfere with sexual intercourse. Good glycaemic control and specific anti-microbial treatment (e.g. fluconazole for candidiasis) are essential.
- Sexual responsiveness does not seem to be impaired in diabetic women, even though severe autonomic neuropathy might interfere with vaginal lubrication and other genital arousal responses.
- Diabetes in women does not appear to damage their relationship with their partner.

Most studies on sexuality in diabetes have concentrated on men. This section will review the limited work relating to sexuality in diabetic women.

Menstruation in diabetic women

Compared with their non-diabetic counterparts, diabetic women show a slight delay in physical maturation. They tend to reach the menarche a little later and to have less regular cycles [1, 2].

About 40% of diabetic women show some change in insulin requirements around the time of menstruation. Patterns vary from one individual to another, the commonest (occurring in about 20% of patients) being a modest increase in insulin requirement for the first two days of menstruation [3–5]. This can be covered by raising the insulin dose by a few units, although occasional patients need much greater increases. The older literature contains several reports of ketoacidosis recurring at the time of menstruation [6, 7]. This is unusual and probably has no true physiological basis; it seems more likely that the young girls with this problem are behaving in a manipulative way, perhaps omitting their insulin during episodes of premenstrual tension (see Chapter 88). About 10% of diabetic women experience a decrease in insulin requirement just before menstruation and this can be difficult to manage, particularly if cycles are irregular. Other less common patterns also occur.

These changes are not usually due to variation in diet or exercise and are likely to have a hormonal basis. Some diabetic women feel nauseated and eat less premenstrually, whereas others have cravings for carbohydrate, sometimes including sweet foods, at that time. Although major endocrine changes occur during the menstrual cycle, measurements of hormone levels have not so far shown any difference between those patients who show changes in their insulin requirements and those who do not. An interesting study by Walsh [8] demonstrated that glucose tolerance in *non-diabetic* women was impaired at the time of menstruation in some cases, but there was considerable individual variation [8]. On the other hand, Scott has shown that insulin sensitivity as measured by the artificial pancreas is unaffected by the phase of the menstrual cycle [9].

Psychosexual development

A high incidence of delay in psychosexual development has been described in insulin-dependent diabetic women. The younger the patient at diagnosis, the greater is the reported delay and it has been suggested that this phenomenon could be a factor in some cases of the adolescent turmoil so frequently noted in juvenile diabetic girls [10] (see Chapter 88).

Genito-urinary infections

Pruritus vulvae is a well-known presenting symptom of diabetes. Vaginal infections, particularly candidiasis, continue to be common, especially in poorly controlled diabetic patients as the yeasts thrive in glucose-containing media. Severe infections can be very irritating and painful, and may interfere with sexual intercourse. Treatment should aim to improve diabetic control in order to minimize the glycosuria, and the usual antifungal creams and pessaries should be used. In resistant cases, a single dose of the antifungal drug fluconazole may be very effective against candida. Vaginal warts may also be particularly common in diabetic women. Vaginal herpes also appears to be common and the accompanying systemic upset can lead to ketoacidosis. We do not yet know if HIV infection is more common or severe in diabetic patients.

Urinary tract infections are frequent in patients with poorly controlled diabetes and in those with autonomic neuropathy and bladder distension. These infections should be treated in the usual way, together with optimization of diabetic control [11].

Fertility

In the early days of insulin therapy, many women with IDDM were poorly controlled and suffered amenorrhoea and subfertility as a consequence of debility and general ill-health. Fortunately, most diabetic patients nowadays are very fit, and yet the belief persists in some quarters that diabetic women are infertile. One might expect that diabetic women would be slightly less fertile than the general population because of the high incidence of irregular cycles and perhaps an increased risk of pelvic infection. There is some evidence that this may be the case [12, 13]. Those with renal failure also have generally reduced fertility, but even some of these patients can and do conceive.

In practical terms, however, fertility is not significantly less than that of non-diabetics. It is important to explain this to diabetic girls and women because they often worry that they may be unable to conceive. Conversely, there can be unfortunate consequences for patients who think they do not need to use contraception because they have heard that diabetic women are infertile.

Sexual responsiveness

The problems of pregnancy in diabetes (Chapter 83) are well appreciated and documented but, unlike men, women rarely complain of sexual problems [14]. In 1971, Kolodny [15] reported a reduction in orgasm in diabetic women but the patients they studied were all in hospital. Ellenberg [16] found no difference in diabetic women with and without clinical evidence of autonomic neuropathy. Jensen [17] described very minor differences between diabetic and non-diabetic women, which were rather more marked in those with peripheral neuropathy.

The most comprehensive study is that of Tyrer [18], who examined 82 insulin-dependent diabetic women who had been married or cohabiting with their partners for at least a year. Fourteen had symptomatic autonomic neuropathy, 16 had abnormal autonomic function tests but no symptoms and 50 had normal autonomic function. They were compared with a control group of 47 healthy women attending a family planning clinic. During an interview with a psychologist, spontaneous sexual interest, the frequency and speed of vaginal lubrication, non-genital arousal, orgasm and vaginismus were rated on a 4–6 point scale. The only one of these ratings in which the diabetic group differed significantly from the controls was vaginal lubrication, the diabetic group having more individuals at the two extremes, i.e. 'inadequate lubrication' or 'always adequate'. The female psycho-physiological change most directly comparable to penile erection is vasocongestion of the vulva and vagina with associated vaginal lubrication. Abnormalities of lubrication might therefore be expected in diabetic women, particularly in those with autonomic neuropathy. However, this was not demonstrated. Two of the most severely affected patients, who died a few months after the study from sudden cardiorespiratory arrest (presumably due to autonomic neuropathy) appeared to lubricate normally. One had no sexual problems, although the other was troubled with diarrhoea during intercourse.

As might be anticipated from the disturbance of cardiovascular reflexes, patients with autonomic neuropathy reported slightly less non-genital arousal during sexual activity than the non-neuropathic diabetic and non-diabetic controls. In a further assessment, each woman rated the concepts of 'myself' and 'my partner' on a series of seven-point scales to give ratings of sexual attractiveness, sexual arousability, lovingness, calmness, potency and a general evaluation. The only finding of note was that diabetic women rated their partners significantly less potent than did the control group. A marriage-relationship questionnaire showed no difference between diabetic and control groups but, on direct questioning about the effect of diabetes on their marital relationship, 9% felt diabetes had a detrimental effect whereas 21% thought it had a beneficial effect because their husbands were more concerned.

Most studies have looked at IDDM women. Schreiner-Engel [19] studied 35 IDDM subjects and found no difference between them and a control group but also studied 23 NIDDM subjects and found reduced sexual desire, orgasmic capacity, lubrication and sexual activity. She also found a poorer relationship with the sexual partner as compared with a control group but surprisingly, the problems were not correlated with duration of diabetes. It is difficult to find an explanation for these interesting findings. The group studied was small and comprised volunteers; they were heavier, had more vaginitis and more of them were postmenopausal than the controls. The authors suggest that the neurovascular processes which regulate genital vasoconstriction may be important, but if this were the case, we should expect it to be commoner in long-standing diabetes. Autonomic nerve function was not evaluated in this study. The authors also suggest that NIDDM subjects have a poor sexual body image. This could be due to obesity, although details of weight are not given. This area merits further investigation in a larger number of patients.

Thus, there seem to be only minor disturbances in sexual function in diabetic women in contrast to the major problems seen in men. There may be sex-related differences in the way the autonomic nervous system controls genital responses. Another likely factor is that erection in the male is an all-or-nothing phenomenon; any impairment may therefore generate anxiety which can further inhibit the erectile mechanisms, whereas women focus on the subjective quality of their sexual relationship. At any sexual problem clinic, men tend to complain of difficulties with erection or ejaculation, whereas most women complain of inadequate enjoyment and only very few describe inadequate lubrication or orgasmic difficulties.

There is a tendency to become excessively preoccupied with the physiology of sexuality and to forget that, in human terms, a sexual encounter is a much more complicated phenomenon than mere spinal reflex activity. The central nervous system exerts its control, facilitating and inhibiting responses while adding its own special ingredients of fantasy, expectations, memories and emotions. Nocturnal sex dreams in men develop spontaneously in the teens, but in women only with a degree of conditioning based upon exposure and experience. Tenderness and security provided by the feeling of being loved are necessary requirements for the woman's response [20]. It seems likely that a more caring relationship in diabetic marriages can counteract any modest physiological deficit.

JUDITH M. STEEL

References

1 Bergquist N. The gonadal function in female diabetics. *Acta Endocrinol Suppl* (Copenhagen) 1954; **19**: 3–20.
2 Djursing H, Nyholm HC, Hagen C, Carstensen L, Pedersen LM. Clinical and hormonal characteristics in women with anovulation and insulin-treated diabetes mellitus. *Am J Obstet Gynecol* 1982; **143**: 876–82.
3 Steel JM. Sexual function in diabetic women. *Practical Diabetes* 1985; **2**: 10–11.
4 Walsh CM, Malins JM. Menstruation and control of diabetes. *Br Med J* 1977; **2**: 177–9.
5 Steel JM, Duncan LJP. The effects of oral contraceptives on insulin requirements in diabetics. *Br J Fam Plan* 1978; **3**: 77–8.
6 Hubble D. Insulin resistance. *Br Med J* 1954; **2**: 1022–4.
7 Sandstrom R. Diabetes mellitus and menstruation. *Nordic Med* 1969; **81**: 727–8.
8 Walsh CH, O'Sullivan DJ. Carbohydrate tolerance during the menstrual cycle in diabetics. *Lancet* 1973; ii: 413–15.
9 Scott AR, McDonald IA, Savage M, Bowman C, Jeffcoate WJ. Insulin sensitivity is unaffected by phase of menstrual cycle in women with insulin dependent diabetes. *Diabetic Med* 1987; **4**: 572A.

10 Surridge DHC, Erdahl DL, Lawson JS, Donald MW, Monga TN, Bird CE, Letemendia FJ. Psychiatric aspects of diabetes mellitus. *Br J Psychiatr* 1984; **145**: 169−76.

11 Sawers JS, Todd WA, Kellet HA, Mills RS, Allan PL, Ewing DJ, Clarke BF. Bacteriura and autonomic nerve function in diabetic women. *Diabetes Care* 1986; **9**: 460−3.

12 Steel JM, Johnstone FD, Smith AF, Duncan LJP. The pre-pregnancy clinic approach. In: Sutherland HW, Stowers JM, eds. *Carbohydrate Metabolism in Pregnancy and the Newborn*. Edinburgh: Churchill Livingstone, 1984: 75−86.

13 Randall J. Fertility and conception. In: Stowers JM, ed. *Carbohydrate Metabolism in Pregnancy and the Newborn*. Berlin: Springer Verlag 1989; 31−40.

14 Jensen SB. Emotional aspects of diabetes mellitus. A study of somatopsychological reactions in 51 couples in which one partner has insulin-treated diabetes. *J Psychosomat Res* 1985; **29**: 353−9.

15 Kolodny RC. Sexual dysfunction in diabetic females. *Diabetes* 1971; **20**: 557−9.

16 Ellenberg M. Sexual aspects of the female diabetic. *Mt Sinai J Med* 1977; **44**: 495−500.

17 Jensen SB. Diabetic sexual dysfunction, a comparative study of 160 insulin treated diabetic men and women and an age matched control group. *Arch Sexual Behav* 1981; **10**: 493−504.

18 Tyrer G, Steel JM, Clarke BF, Ewing DJ, Bancroft J. Sexual responsiveness in diabetic women. *Diabetologia* 1983; **24**: 166−71.

19 Schreiner-Engel P, Schiavi RC, Vietovisz D, Smith H. The differential impact of diabetes type on female sexuality. *J Psychosomat Res* 1987; **31**: 22−33.

20 Kant F. Factors in female sexuality. *Med Aspects Human Sexual* 1973; **7**: 31.

76   Sexual Function in Diabetic Men

Summary

• Impotence affects about one-third of diabetic men.

• Psychogenic causes, often associated with anxiety and/or depression, are common; nocturnal erections are maintained and patients may respond to expert counselling.

• Autonomic neuropathy may interrupt the parasympathetic outflow which normally produces vasodilatation and engorgement of the penile corpora.

• Vascular causes of impotence include both reduced arterial inflow (through obstruction of iliac or internal pudendal arteries) and venous leakage from the corpora.

• Impotence may also be due to alcohol or cannabis abuse, to antihypertensive or psychotropic drugs, or to hypogonadism.

• Treatments available for 'organic' causes of impotence include suction devices causing passive erection, intracorporeal injection of vasodilators, and surgical implantation of rigid or inflatable prostheses.

Impotence is the inability to achieve or sustain an erection satisfactory for sexual intercourse. It is one of the saddest complications of diabetes and is relatively common in diabetic men. However, in the UK at least, it is probably the least discussed problem related to the disease. Even though the ultimate prognosis in many cases is poor, patients will often appreciate the opportunity to discuss this once-taboo subject with their physician.

The prevalence of impotence in diabetic men is high — up to 35%, according to McCullough [1]. Associated factors at presentation in this study were increasing age and the presence of retinopathy and peripheral and autonomic neuropathy. There was no apparent relationship with the duration of the disease, but poor glycaemic control and excessive alcohol intake at presentation seemed to be important. In a follow-up study of the same population 5 years later, 28% of those originally potent had developed impotence and 9% of the impotent had become potent [2].

It is important to differentiate 'impotence in diabetic men' from 'diabetic impotence', as the latter term implies organic disease which is essentially irreversible and untreatable. The possible causes of impotence must therefore be carefully considered in each individual case.

Physiology of normal erection and ejaculation

The physiological complexity of the male sexual response (Fig. 76.1) underlines the many ways in which various organic and psychological factors may cause impotence.

Erection is a parasympathetic response to psychic, visual and other stimuli acting on higher cortical centres and to reflex tactile stimulation of the genitalia [3]. The sacral parasympathetic outflow (carried via the pudendal nerves) causes dilatation of the corporeal arteries (end-branches of the internal pudendal artery), leading to engorgement of the corpora cavernosa and corpus spongiosum. Sustained erection depends not only on increased arterial inflow but also on restriction of venous outflow from the corpora.

Ejaculation is a sympathetic response, mediated by the presacral nerves arising from the lower part of the thoraco-lumbar sympathetic outflow, which causes contraction of the vas deferens and seminal vesicles.

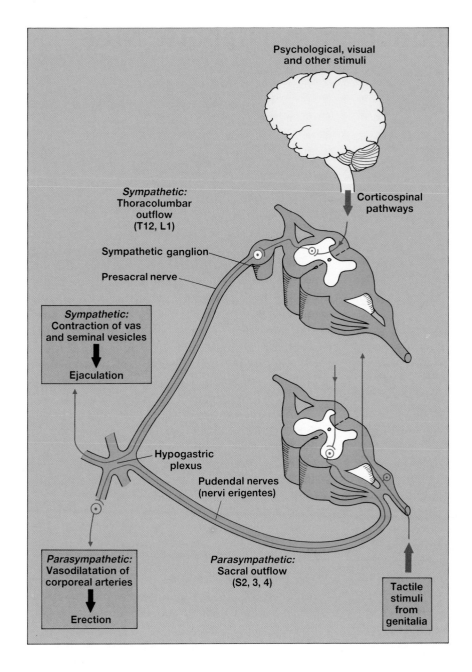

Fig. 76.1. Physiological basis of erection and ejaculation.

Causes of impotence in diabetes

These are summarized in Table 76.1, which shows the level at which various factors can interfere with the male sexual response to produce impotence and/or failure of ejaculation. Although a proportion of diabetic men will have irreversible organic impotence, other potentially treatable causes must be excluded. The development of impotence in any man will depend on many interrelated influences, including his marital relationship; basic personality and upbringing; cultural and personal attitudes to life and sex;

tendency to anxiety or depression; presence of and response to pressure at work or at home; and the use of drugs and alcohol. The particular pathophysiological complications and psychosocial pressures of diabetes itself will be superimposed upon and will interact with this complex and delicate background.

Psychological factors must also be considered in cases of impotence in diabetic men, as in the population at large [4]. Anxiety and depression are common in diabetic patients (see Chapter 77) and may be fuelled by the very knowledge that diabetes itself can cause impotence.

Table 76.1. Factors necessary for erection, and causes of impotence.

Component	Interfering factors causing impotence
Psychological arousal	Depression, anxiety (including that about diabetes) Psychotropic drugs Alcohol, cannabis
Tactile input from genitalia	Peripheral neuropathy
Parasympathetic outflow	Autonomic neuropathy Various antihypertensive and other drugs
Increased arterial inflow to corpora	Atheroma of iliac or pudendal arteries
Reduced venous outflow from corpora	Venous leakage
Adequate testosterone levels	Hypogonadism

Advanced autonomic neuropathy is almost invariably accompanied by impotence but the relationship of the latter to abnormal electrophysiological tests (see Chapter 63) is not so clear. Invasive research techniques have demonstrated a reduced conduction velocity in the dorsal nerve of the penis in patients with autonomic neuropathy, which was generally correlated with the presence of impotence [5].

Vascular problems, either by impeding arterial inflow or allowing excessive venous drainage, may also cause impotence. Atheroma in the common iliac arteries or more distally in the internal pudendal artery may reduce inflow. Arterial disease is difficult to assess non-invasively; in the latter case, the femoral pulses are frequently preserved. Doppler ultrasound may be used to assess penile blood flow: one study has found impaired blood flow in 65% of impotent patients as opposed to only 26% of potent patients with abnormal electrophysiological tests [6]. Abnormal leakage from the corpora into their draining veins can be demonstrated in some impotent patients by selective arteriography and infusion cavernosography [7] and probably contributes to detumescence.

Endocrine abnormalities remain a controversial cause of impotence in diabetic men (see Chapter 28). Although prolactin levels tend to be elevated in diabetes, there is no firm association with impotence [8]. However, serum free testosterone levels are apparently reduced in some impotent diabetic men [9].

Drugs, particularly antihypertensive and psychotropic agents (see Chapter 79), *alcohol* and *cannabis* are also associated with impotence.

From the above, it is obvious that many neurological, vascular and endocrine factors may potentially be involved and may be aggravated by coexisting psychogenic problems.

Investigation of the diabetic man with impotence

This is outlined in Table 76.2. The first step is to elicit an adequate history, concentrating on the above factors, during a free and open discussion with the patient and, ideally, with his partner. The subject is rarely mentioned spontaneously, but it is wrong for the clinician to assume that if it is not brought up, then it is not a problem. The patient should therefore be questioned directly, but it must be stressed that adequate assessment of an impotent man is a skilled task requiring

Table 76.2. Assessment of the diabetic man with impotence.

History and examination for evidence of:
Anxiety, depression
Impact of impotence
Drug and alcohol use
Autonomic neuropathy (especially involving bladder)
Peripheral neuropathy
Peripheral vascular disease (NB: poor correlation of
   femoral pulses with pudendal artery patency)
Hypogonadism

Further investigations
Formal psychological assessment of patient (and partner)
Autonomic function tests
Assessment of nocturnal erections (snap-gauge)

Specialist-centre investigations
Penile blood flow
Electrophysiological tests

special consideration and training, and is not a topic for a brief chat in a busy clinic.

The patient will also need a full physical examination, particularly to seek evidence of autonomic and peripheral neuropathy, peripheral vascular disease (with the above reservation regarding atheroma restricted to small distal arteries), hypogonadism and alcohol abuse.

The most important need is perhaps to identify the presence of psychogenic factors. Premature ejaculation, as distinct from failure of erection, is almost always psychogenic rather than organic in origin and the presence of nocturnal or early morning erection or emissions (even if erection cannot be maintained during full intercourse) again points to a psychogenic cause. The presence of nocturnal erections may be confirmed by measuring penile tumescence using a strain gauge [4] or maximal penile diameter using a snap-gauge fastener [10]. Although nocturnal erections are generally regarded as proof of organic normality, the erection may still not be rigid enough for satisfactory intercourse. The prevalence of psychogenic problems may be indicated by the finding by Hosking [11] of totally absent nocturnal tumescence in only six out of 30 impotent diabetic men. Other methods for detecting psychogenic problems include formal psychological assessments: the Minnesota multiphasic personality inventory has apparently been able to differentiate those more likely to have psychogenic impotence [12]. The viewing of erotic films to assess psychological state and induce erection does not completely separate organic from psychogenic causes, although responses were undoubtedly blunted in diabetic patients with autonomic dysfunction [13].

In routine clinic practice, basic tests of neurological and autonomic function can be performed and nocturnal penile tumescence assessed with a commercially available disposable snap-gauge. If serious organic disease is present, the possibility of psychological factors being reversible is greatly reduced. On the other hand, it should not be assumed that the presence of relatively minor physical abnormalities precludes a psychogenic component.

Management plan for the impotent diabetic man

Ideally, there should be close collaboration between the diabetologist, psychologist or psychiatrist, and urologist; all diabetic clinics should have a working relationship with expert marital and sexual therapists [14]. Much help and support can be provided, even if only to reassure the patient that he is not strangely abnormal.

General measures include exclusion of alcohol, withdrawal or substitution of any drugs which may be responsible, and improvement in metabolic control (which alone may help in some cases). Thereafter, the following scheme is suggested:
1 Establish whether there is a major problem causing personal or marital disharmony, and also whether his spouse or partner is willing to discuss the matter with the appropriate professionals. Many men or their partners will prefer to leave matters at this stage, but if possible, at least two interviews should be allowed intially so that thought and discussion can take place between the partners.
2 If there is a serious problem causing concern, the offer should be made of detailed assessment of the couple's sexual and psychological condition by a trained therapist or psychologist. The diabetologist should explain the likely treatment plan without giving too much graphic and possibly daunting detail about invasive procedures.
3 If an important psychogenic element appears likely, sexual counselling should be offered and may have a successful result.
4 If the problem is organic, then the patient should be offered the choice of the treatments listed below. No order of priority should be suggested, as the subject will no doubt wish to consider possible treatments and discuss them with his partner.

The treatments currently available are:
1 A non-invasive condom device (Erecaid®, Fig. 76.2) applies suction to the penis to cause blood to flow into the erectile tissue where it is trapped by a constricting band placed around the base of the penis [15]. Satisfactory erection can be maintained for intercourse. The device is popular with those who have taken part in clinical studies of this device [15], but it is very expensive.
2 Intracavernous injections of vasodilators, such as α_1-blockers (phentolamine, phenoxybenzamine) or smooth muscle relaxants such as papaverine (5–30 mg). Athough apparently an alarming procedure, patients readily learn to inject themselves and many report successful erection and intercourse [16]. Erections may last for 2 h, and priapism is a rare complication. Where available, this treatment should probably precede more

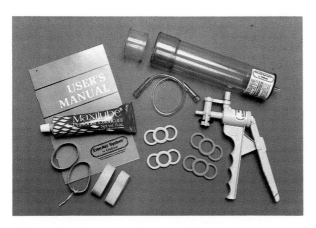

Fig. 76.2. The Erecaid Suction Tumescence System. Engorgement is induced by a simple suction device and the erection-like state is maintained using a constriction band. (Reproduced with permission from Wiles 1988 [15].) For further information contact Cory Bros. Co. Ltd. (Hospital Contracts), 4 Dollis Park, London N3 1HG, UK.

invasive surgical procedures.

3 Surgical implantation of permanently rigid or 'inflatable' prostheses into the corpora cavernosa is a well-established technique. Some sophisticated devices are inflated by a pump which is activated by pressing a button placed subcutaneously in the perineum. These devices are in use by only a relatively small number of diabetic subjects around the world, probably reflecting the attitudes of diabetologists and their patients. This approach may well not appeal to many people, but most treated patients are satisfied with its results [17].

Unfortunately, hormone treatment or vascular surgery seems to be of no benefit.

JOHN D. WARD

References

1 McCulloch DK, Campbell IW, Wu FC, Prescott RJ, Clarke BF. The prevalence of diabetic impotence. *Diabetologia* 1980; **18**: 279–83.

2 McCulloch DK, Young RJ, Prescott RJ, Clarke BF. The natural history of impotence in diabetic men. *Diabetologia* 1984; **26**: 437–40.

3 de Groat WC, Booth AM. Physiology of male sexual function. *Ann Intern Med* 1980; **92**: 329–31.

4 El-Bayoumi M, El Sherbini O, Mosrafa M. Impotence in diabetics: organic versus psychogenic factors. *Urology* 1984; **24**: 459–63.

5 Lin JT, Bradley WE. Penile neuropathy in insulin dependent diabetes mellitus. *J Urol* 1985; **133**: 213–19.

6 Jevitch MJ, Edson M, Jarman WD, Herrera HH. Vascular factors in erectile failure among diabetics. *Urology* 1982; **19**: 163–8.

7 Wagner G, Green R. *Impotence*. New York: Plenum Press, 1981.

8 Jensen SB, Hagen C, Froland A, Pederson PB. Sexual function and the pituitary axis in insulin treated diabetic men. *Acta Med Scand* 1979; **624** (suppl): 65–8.

9 Murray FT, Wyss HU, Thomas RG, Spevack M, Glaros AG. Gonadal dysfunction in diabetic men with organic impotence. *J Clin Endocrinol Metab* 1987; **65**: 127–31.

10 Bradley WE, Lin JT. Assessment of diabetic sexual dysfunction and cystopathy. *Diabetic Neuropath* 1987; **15**: 146–54.

11 Hosking DJ, Bennet T, Hampton JR, Evans DF, Clark AJ, Robertson G. Diabetic impotence: studies of nocturnal erection during REM sleep. *Br Med J* 1979; **2**: 1394–6.

12 Buvat J, Lemaire A, Buvat-Herbaut M *et al.* Comparative investigations in 26 impotent and 26 non-impotent diabetic patients. *J Urol* 1985; **133**: 34–40.

13 Bancroft J, Bell C. Simultaneous recording of penile diameter and penile arterial pulse during laboratory based erotic stimulation in normal subjects. *J Psychosom Res* 1985; **29**: 303.

14 McCulloch DK, Hosking DJ, Tobart A. A pragmatic approach to sexual dysfunction in diabetic men: psychosexual counselling. *Diabetic Med* 1986; **3**: 485–9.

15 Wiles PG. Successful non-invasive management of erectile impotence in diabetic men. *Br Med J* 1988; **296**: 161–2.

16 Brindley GS. Pilot experiments on the actions of drugs injected into the human corpus cavernosum penis. *Br J Pharmacol* 1986; **87**: 495–500.

17 Pfeifer M, Reenan A, Berger R, Best J. Penile prosthesis and quality of life. *Diabetes* 1983; **32**: 77A.

Summary

• Psychological disturbances and psychiatric disorders, mostly mild, are common in diabetic patients but are often missed in the routine diabetic clinic.

• All diabetic care teams should have easy and immediate access to a psychiatrist and/or a clinical psychologist who should have specialist knowledge of diabetes and its management.

• Patients learn to cope with the psychological stress induced by diabetes through a process of adaptation which may be complicated by reactions of denial, anger or depression. Failure to cope, or 'maladaptation', is manifested by emotional, physical and behavioural signs of psychological stress. Management is by 'self-help' measures and relaxation exercises as well as through social support and medical advice.

• A few animal studies and anecdotal case reports in man suggest that psychological stress may directly precipitate diabetes or aggravate diabetic control but there is no firm evidence that such a mechanism operates in human diabetes. Poor diabetic control in patients under psychosocial stress may be due to poor compliance or other factors.

• The commonest psychiatric disorder in diabetic patients is depression with or without anxiety, usually with sleep disturbance. Patients with visual impairment or other complications are particularly at risk.

• Depression frequently responds to general measures such as sympathetic discussion and advice to improve sleep. Moderate or severe depression requires antidepressants, of which tricyclic agents are the first choice. Patients at risk of suicide or antisocial behaviour need urgent psychiatric referral and possibly hospital admission.

• Other psychiatric problems encountered in diabetic patients include anorexia nervosa and other appetite disturbances, injection and needle phobias, obsessional disorders and factitious hyper- or hypoglycaemia.

Strictly defined, *psychology* is the study of normal and abnormal mental functioning and behaviour, and *psychiatry* the diagnosis and treatment of mental disorders. The purpose of this chapter is to discuss the psychological and psychiatric disorders occurring in diabetic patients, their possible causes and impact on diabetes, and their diagnosis, treatment and prognosis. Most of these observations apply equally to IDDM and NIDDM.

Psychological problems: stress, adaptation and coping

In common with other illnesses and traumatic life-events, diabetes and its sequelae impose a considerable burden of psychological stress. The term 'stress' is in many respects unsatisfactory, mainly because 'stress' cannot be readily defined or measured, but is convenient in that it is widely understood and is acceptable to patients. Moreover, the identification of those factors which cause 'stress' can suggest practical educational and behavioural tactics which may help to overcome them.

Patients attempt to come to terms with diabetes and its attendant psychological stress through a process of *adaptation*, which comprises two phases: first, the realization that certain attitudes and behaviours will have to change and secondly, the exploration of new ways of coping until satisfactory solutions are found. During adaptation, some patients may experience disagreeable emotional reactions, superficially resembling grief, over their potential loss of health and lifestyle. These reactions are usually transient and may include the following:

Disbelief and denial of the diagnosis, its implications or even the need for treatment may follow the initial shock of being diagnosed diabetic. These reactions are often accentuated by lack of knowledge and imperfect 'first-aid' education.

Anger is another common response, often directed at the illness but sometimes at the patient himself, his parents or the medical or nursing staff; the latter, if inexperienced, may unfortunately tend to neglect the angry patient, to the detriment of his diabetic care.

Depression often follows the realization that diabetes and the need for treatment and self-monitoring are in most cases lifelong, or that the disease carries the risk of long-term complications. Self-blame and withdrawal may be prominent and frequently accompany feelings of worthlessness and hopelessness. As discussed below, depression with or without anxiety may persist in the long term and represents the commonest psychiatric disorder in diabetic patients.

These reactions are usually short-lived but may be protracted and affect the patient's ability to cope with diabetes and life in general. It is not clear why some individuals cope with diabetes whereas others do not; possible determinants have been investigated in several studies (e.g. Koski [1]) but the tests used to measure 'coping ability' may have little relevance to the diabetic patient's struggle to regain control over his life [2]. *Maladaptation*, where the process of learning to cope is incomplete or prolonged, may be commoner in young patients or those with complications and is often signalled by 'warning signs' indicating psychological stress. These include emotional, physical and social or behavioural reactions (Tables 77.1–3), which must be actively sought and recognized early so that specialist advice and help can be provided if necessary. The commonest *emotional reactions* are increases in tension, irritability and moodiness which signify mounting depression and/or anxiety (Table 77.1). *Physical reactions* result from autonomic or endocrine responses to psychological stress and may need to be carefully distinguished from the symptoms

Table 77.1. Maladaptation: emotional reactions signifying depression and/or anxiety.

Feeling under pressure, threatened or frightened
Restlessness, inability to relax
Irritability, aggression, conflict with others
Inability to concentrate, make decisions or complete tasks quickly
Feeling tired or mentally drained
Feeling moody, pessimistic or a failure
Inability to feel pleasure
Tearfulness

Table 77.2. Maladaptation: physical reactions suggesting depression and/or anxiety.

Altered appetite or nausea
Indigestion or altered bowel habit
Insomnia, tiredness
Palpitations, breathlessness or chest pain
Frequent urge to pass urine
Paraesthesiae in fingers or toes or around the mouth
Sweating
Headache

Table 77.3. Maladaptation: social and behavioural reactions suggesting depression and/or anxiety.

Constant seeking of company, social support or reassurance
Avoidance of company, withdrawal and indifference to others
Capriciousness and unpredictability
Unreasonable expectations
Indecision in social matters
Altered sexual behaviour

of diabetes, its complications or treatment (Table 77.2). *Social and behavioural reactions* of people under stress may be striking, although more subtle features may be difficult to recognize (Table 77.3).

Management of maladaptation

Coping and adaptation will be greatly helped by a sympathetic and understanding approach to the patient, combined with effective education and ready availability of advice about diabetes and its management whenever the patient needs this; ways of providing this service are discussed in Chapter 97.

All members of the diabetes team must be alert to the features suggesting maladaptation (Tables

77.1–3) and should be able to discuss their significance with the patient and to suggest referral to a psychiatrist or psychologist if necessary. Regular supportive discussions and practical advice and reassurance about specific anxieties may be enough to help the patient to cope better. If not, a 'self-help' approach is often beneficial. The patient should be asked to keep a diary of the nature, severity and duration of his own 'warning signs' of stress and to try to identify their possible causes and anything which could help to alleviate them. Any practical solutions which suggest themselves should be tried and their success or failure evaluated; at the same time, the patient should be urged to try to stop worrying about any problems which are completely insoluble. The patient should review his diary and progress at regular intervals, either alone or with a diabetic team member, until he has reduced as many causes of stress as possible and has begun to feel in control again. Relaxation exercises can be very useful when patients experience acute tension or worry; instructional tapes (which should be played through and practised with a team member before the patient tries the procedure alone) can be obtained from most clinical psychology departments.

Adaptation may be particularly difficult in patients suffering diabetic complications such as loss of sight, amputation, sexual dysfunction, infertility or complications of pregnancy, renal failure or repeated hospital admissions with poor metabolic control. The basic psychological approach should be as above but individual advice and information will be needed. Some practical points are discussed in the relevant chapters of this book, and the series of *Coping with ...* booklets published by the British Diabetic Association provide valuable advice about specific problems. Local specialists or agencies may also be able to provide particular aspects of support and care, such as facilities for the blind and partially sighted (described in Chapter 60).

Metabolic effects of psychological stress in diabetic patients

The 'fight or flight' reaction provoked by acute physiological or psychological stress triggers the secretion of counter-regulatory hormones which antagonize the effect of insulin and tend to cause hyperglycaemia [3–5]. These observations have probably fuelled the popular and long-standing belief that psychological or psychosocial stress

may aggravate metabolic control in diabetic patients or even precipitate the disease.

There have been many anecdotal reports of diabetes (especially IDDM) developing suddenly after a traumatic life-event [6]. However, both diabetes and personal catastrophes are relatively common and will occasionally be associated by chance alone; this association may appear to gain strength when viewed retrospectively, which is a major flaw in the design of all such studies. Theoretical consideration of the central and metabolic effects of opioid peptides and other neurotransmitters (see Chapter 23) has led to speculation that chronic stress could act on the autonomic nervous system to induce a metabolic syndrome similar to NIDDM [7]. Recent animal studies have provided more direct and highly intriguing evidence that psychosocial stress (e.g. overcrowding and noise) may accelerate the development of diabetes in rats, either destined to develop an autoimmune IDDM-like condition [8] or treated with repeated subdiabetogenic doses of the B-cell toxin, streptozotocin [9]. It is not clear whether the diabetogenic effect of stress in these models is due to the counter-regulatory effects of the 'stress' hormones, their possible immunomodulatory actions, or some other factor. The relevance of these observations to man is unknown; at present, there are no convincing epidemiological or other data to suggest that psychological stress can precipitate either IDDM or NIDDM in humans.

The possible detrimental effects of psychological stress on metabolic control in people with established diabetes have also been debated for many years. A number of case reports, again anecdotal and retrospective, have claimed that psychological stress can aggravate metabolic control and even precipitate ketoacidosis in IDDM patients [10]. Several uncontrolled studies, often quoted but never repeated, have reported various metabolic disturbances in diabetic patients subjected to acute psychological stress, such as the (invented) threat of having a leg amputated. The metabolic responses described included diuresis and natriuresis and rises in circulating free fatty acid and ketone body levels; curiously, in view of the hyperglycaemic effects of the 'stress' hormones, the blood glucose level generally remained stable or fell slightly and rose only in occasional subjects [11–14]. As mentioned previously, 'stress' is impossible to quantify or administer in standardized 'doses'; currently used stressors — such as mental arithmetic, television games or simulated public speaking — may be ethically more acceptable than inducing the fear of amputation but may be just as remote from the patient's own sources of tension. Various psychological stressors can cause physiological changes which could affect metabolic control in diabetic patients, such as disturbing intestinal motility [15] and therefore perhaps food absorption, or subcutaneous blood flow [16] and therefore possibly insulin absorption. However, recent carefully controlled studies in IDDM patients with various levels of hyperglycaemia have demonstrated that psychological stress sufficient to produce significant physiological responses such as tachycardia, hypertension and increased plasma catecholamine levels had no effect on blood glucose, free fatty acid or ketone body levels [17].

Firm evidence that psychological stress may significantly worsen diabetic control is therefore lacking. Nonetheless, it is obvious that psychological stress and poor metabolic control frequently coexist, as exemplified by patients with 'brittle' diabetes (see Chapter 88). Numerous workers have reported that poor glycaemic control is associated with increased anxiety [18], mood disturbance [19] and stress scores [20], but may have fallen into the trap of confusing correlation with causation. Some patients under stress may fail to comply with diet or insulin treatment, whereas others may suffer stress through their inability to achieve adequate control. The picture is further clouded by the possibility that hyperglycaemia itself may be the cause rather than the effect of certain features of anxiety [21]. It is obvious that the precise interaction between psychological stress and metabolic control will only be elucidated when improved ways of delivering and measuring 'stress' relevant to the patient have been developed and rigid criteria for monitoring metabolic control applied [15, 22, 23].

Psychiatric disorders in diabetic patients

Prevalence

There have been no comprehensive epidemiological surveys of psychiatric disorder in the diabetic population. Wilkinson *et al*. [24], using a two-stage screening procedure, found the overall prevalence of psychiatric disorder in IDDM outpatients in Dundee to be 18% in men and 24% in women. These estimates corresponded closely to those in the local general community, as ascertained from general practitioners' records, and are at the lower end of the prevalences reported from hospital-based populations using the same technique. In specific groups of patients, such as those with unsatisfactory glycaemic control or diabetic complications, frank psychiatric illness may be more common. For example, depression and/or anxiety may affect up to 50% of poorly controlled youngsters with IDDM [25, 26] and a few have severe self-destructive tendencies which may end in suicide [27, 28]. The special problems of depression in blind or partially sighted diabetic patients are discussed in Chapter 60.

It must be emphasized that the Dundee prevalence data were derived from a study using strictly applied research criteria with the specific aim of identifying psychiatric disease; significant psychiatric disease will be detected much less frequently in the routine diabetic clinic. The diagnosis of psychiatric disorder depends on recognizing a pattern of mental and behavioural symptoms, which is intrinsically a subjective and uncertain process. It has been estimated that over one-half of cases of psychiatric disorder, diagnosable by research criteria, affecting general medical patients will be missed by their physicians [29]. In the case of diabetes, Wilkinson *et al*. [30] found that diabetologists in one large clinic detected only 28% of the psychiatric disorders identified by psychiatrists using a standardized psychiatric interview in a sample of out-patients. However, the diabetologists were correct in 94% of cases where they diagnosed psychiatric disorder, and were able to identify most of the cases with major psychiatric disorder requiring treatment.

The presence of specific diabetic complications may engender depression or anxiety in individual cases. However, in the general diabetic population overall, there does not seem to be any relationship between psychiatric disorder and the extent of complications, duration of diabetes, quality of glycaemic control (as measured by HbA_1) or method of treatment [26].

Nature of psychiatric disorder in diabetic patients

Most psychiatric disorder accompanying general medical conditions, including diabetes, comprises the single broad category of depression with or without anxiety. About one-half of these patients complain of sleep disturbance and various somatic symptoms which may be precipitated, exacerbated or maintained by psychological factors.

Other disorders, less commonly encountered in diabetic patients but usually readily recognized, include anorexia nervosa and other appetite disturbances (see Chapter 82); phobias about needles, injections and self-monitoring; obsessional disorders which may be fuelled by rigorous education and attention to detail in self-management [31]; alcohol and drug dependence which may masquerade as 'brittle' diabetes [32]; manic disorder; and schizophrenia. A problem which is probably underestimated is that of factitious hypo- or hyperglycaemia, which may be associated with significant psychiatric disorder; this difficult area is discussed in detail in Chapter 88. In many cases of mild psychiatric disorder, where true illness is difficult to distinguish from distress, a precise diagnosis may not be possible.

Diagnosis of psychiatric disorders in diabetic patients

As mentioned above, psychiatric disorders are commoner than generally suspected in diabetic patients. The busy diabetic clinic is clearly not the best place to elicit and discuss psychiatric symptoms. It is therefore essential for a psychiatrist and/or psychologist to be easily accessible for rapid referral of patients with suspected problems, and ideally part of the diabetic care team. It is best if these specialists have an interest in and a broad understanding of general medical diseases and diabetes in particular.

At the same time, physicians, nurses and other team members must remain alert to the possibility of psychiatric disorder in diabetic patients, particularly depression with or without anxiety, which may present in several ways (Table 77.4) and will frequently respond well to treatment. Some simple principles in interview technique have been suggested to make it easier for the

Table 77.4. Features of moderate and severe depression suggesting the need for antidepressant drugs.

Sleep disturbance, fatigue, loss of energy
Loss of appetite, loss of weight
Loss of interests, inactivity
Loss of libido
Inability to concentrate
Marked anxiety
Suicidal thoughts*

* Formal psychiatric referral is also indicated.

Table 77.5. Suggested interview style to improve detection of psychiatric disorders (from Goldberg & Huxley 1980 [33]).

Establish eye contact at the beginning of the consultation
Do not read notes while taking the history
Clarify the presenting complaint
Do not concentrate on the past history
Use direct questions for physical complaints
Use an empathic interview style
Be sensitive to non-verbal as well as verbal cues
Be able to deal with over-talkative patients

patient to volunteer and for the interviewer to detect the features of depression and/or anxiety [33] (see Table 77.5).

Treatment of psychiatric disorders

Many minor disorders will respond to simple supportive advice and the general measures outlined below but some will require medical treatment and specialist psychiatric referral. This section will deal with the commonest problem of depression with or without anxiety. The management of anorexia nervosa is discussed in Chapter 82 and the problems associated with 'brittle' diabetes in Chapter 88; other disorders will require specialist intervention and are beyond the scope of this chapter.

GENERAL MEASURES TO TREAT DEPRESSION

The diagnosis and the relationship of depression to the patient's symptoms should initially be explained. Specific causes of depression or anxiety (e.g. fear of blindness, renal failure, infertility, impotence) should be sought and discussed sympathetically but realistically. Practical advice for improving diabetic control and any other medical problems should be offered. The patient should be reassured that he can discuss the problem again if he so wishes and must be given a follow-up appointment.

Sleep disorder is common but will often respond to simple advice, such as to take regular exercise and avoid naps during the day and to avoid large meals, tobacco, alcohol or caffeine-containing drinks in the late evening. Relaxation exercises such as those developed by Surwit and colleagues [34, 35] may improve daytime restlessness or tension and may also improve glycaemic control in both IDDM [36] and NIDDM [37]. Benzodiazepines are best avoided because of the severe problems of dependency. Depressed patients should be advised to continue work and social contacts, in order to maintain self-esteem and avoid loneliness. Mustering friends and statutory or voluntary helping agencies to provide company is often beneficial, especially in the elderly.

ANTIDEPRESSANT DRUGS

Patients failing to respond to general measures or who display features of moderate to severe depression (Table 77.4) should be given a trial of antidepressant drugs. The more pronounced these features are, the greater is the likelihood that they will respond to these drugs; however, the source of the patient's depression and/or anxiety should also be identified and corrected if possible.

First-choice antidepressant drugs are generally the tricyclic or related agents, especially amitryptiline and imipramine. Guidelines for their use are shown in Table 77.6; they may also be useful in the treatment of painful diabetic neuropathy, as described in Chapter 62. Tricyclic drugs generally relieve certain depressive symptoms, often improving sleep and having a calming effect within the first few days. This may persist with a relatively sedative agent such as amitryptiline, whereas most patients treated with imipramine will then become more alert and energetic. Patients must be told that the maximum benefits of antidepressant treatment may not be felt for 4–6 weeks.

Other antidepressant drugs (such as tetracyclics, e.g. mianserin; serotonin reuptake inhibitors, e.g. fluvoxamine; monoamine oxidase inhibitors; lithium salts) are indicated in patients with medical conditions (especially cardiac disease) which preclude the use of tricyclic agents, or when these latter are ineffective or have significant side-effects. In this event, drug treatment is best supervised by a psychiatrist. Initially, only limited supplies of antidepressant drugs should be prescribed, because patients may show suicidal tendencies when they become more active. Most depressive episodes remit within 3–12 months; antidepressant treatment is generally continued at full dosage until the patient has felt well for a month and is then gradually reduced in steps lasting 1–2 weeks. Drugs can be gradually withdrawn in asymptomatic patients, although some

Table 77.6. Tricyclic antidepressants.

Examples
- Amitryptiline — sedative; use in agitated or anxious patients
- Imipramine — useful in withdrawn or apathetic patients

Dosages
- Start at 75 mg/day, increase to 150 mg/day after 1 week
- Use lower dosages in elderly patients
- Higher dosages (300 mg/day) need specialist supervision

Therapeutic effects
- Improved sleep and calming effect within few days
- Maximal clinical benefit may take 4–6 weeks

Duration of treatment
- Maintain full dosage until symptom-free for 1 month
- Gradually reduce dosage; do not withdraw abruptly
- Some patients require prolonged maintenance treatment (half of full dosage)

Side-effects (with specific contraindications in parentheses)
- Dry mouth ⎫
- Blurred vision (glaucoma) ⎬ Anticholinergic effects
- Hesitancy or retention of urine (prostatism)
- Tachycardia (arrhythmia, heart block) ⎭

- Hypotension (autonomic neuropathy)
- Sweating
- Excessive sedation (with amitryptiline)
- Late effects (after 2 weeks):
  tremor
  weight gain
  sexual dysfunction

patients benefit from continued treatment at half-dosage for several months to prevent recurrence. Treatment must not be stopped abruptly, and patients should be supervised closely in case symptoms recur.

Side-effects of tricyclic drugs (Table 77.6) may be severe but often improve within a few days of starting treatment and are fully reversible on withdrawing the drugs. Older people are particularly sensitive to dizziness and fainting. These drugs have no adverse metabolic effects but their hypotensive action demands caution in patients with symptomatic autonomic neuropathy and their anticholinergic action may rarely precipitate closed-angle glaucoma in patients with rubeosis iridis.

PROGNOSIS AND OUTCOME OF TREATMENT

Mild depressive disorders and those precipitated by upsetting life-events frequently improve spontaneously and may remit within a few days of starting general measures or medical treatment. Patients who fail to respond or who do so only temporarily, and those who are seriously ill and at risk of suicide will require immediate referral to a psychiatrist. Many psychiatrists now have expertise in the care of patients with general medical conditions. Hospital admission, compulsory if necessary, should be considered if there is a risk of suicide, harm to others or antisocial behaviour, or if home circumstances are unsuitable for the effective treatment of either the psychiatric disorder or the diabetes.

The management of the various psychological and psychiatric problems associated with 'brittle' diabetes is complicated and carries a poor record of success; various strategies are discussed in Chapter 88.

Conclusions

Psychological and emotional factors can affect patients with diabetes in many ways but the psychological and psychiatric aspects of diabetic management have largely been overlooked [38–40]. From this perspective, Williams et al. have suggested that the time is right for a re-appraisal of the impact that psychological factors have on metabolic control [23]. More importantly, there is a need for convincing evidence that the application of psychological techniques to diabetic care actually improves the patient's metabolic state and quality of life. On the other hand, Bradley has argued that we can only understand the patient's preferences for treatment and the factors affecting his motivation and compliance if treatment is evaluated in relation to his individual characteristics [41]. It therefore becomes necessary to measure psychological as well as clinical and metabolic factors in such studies and to recognize that, even if psychological factors are not measured, these may nevertheless influence outcome.

It is now apparent that psychological problems and psychiatric disorders are relatively common in diabetic patients and that all members of the diabetic care team must appreciate their possible impact on diabetic patients' ability to manage their disease. The need to include a psychiatrist and/or psychologist in the diabetic management team has been increasingly recognized in North America but many diabetic clinics in Britain still have only limited and difficult access to these specialists. It is to be hoped that they will play a wider role in the care of diabetic patients in the future.

GREG WILKINSON

References

1 Koski M-L. The coping process in childhood diabetes. *Acta Paediatr Scand* 1969; **198** (suppl): 1–56.

2 Cohen F, Lazarus RF. Coping with the stresses of illness. In: Stone GC, Cohen F, Adler N, eds. *Health Psychology: a Handbook*. San Francisco: Jossey-Bass, 1979: 217–54.

3 Cannon WB, De la Paz D. Emotional stimulation of adrenal secretion. *Am J Physiol* 1911; **28**: 64–70.

4 Bliss EL, Migeon CJ, Branch CHH, Samuels LT. Reaction of the adrenal cortex to emotional stress. *Psychosom Med* 1956; **18**: 56–76.

5 Miyabo S, Hisada T, Asato T, Muzushima N, Ueno K. Growth hormone and cortisol responses to psychological stress: comparison of normal and neurotic subjects. *J Clin Endocrinol Metab* 1976; **42**: 1158–62.

6 Hinkle LE, Conger GB, Wolf S. Studies on diabetes mellitus: the relation of stressful life situations to the concentration of ketone bodies in the blood of diabetic and non-diabetic humans. *Diabetes* 1952; **1**: 383–92.

7 Surwit RS, Feinglos MN. Stress and the autonomic nervous system in type II diabetes. A hypothesis. *Diabetes Care* 1988; **11**: 83–5.

8 Carter WR, Herman J, Stokes K, Cox DJ. Promotion of diabetes onset by stress in the BB rat. *Diabetologia* 1987; **30**: 674–5.

9 Mazelis G, Albert D, Crisa C et al. Relationship of stressful housing conditions to the onset of diabetes mellitus induced by multiple, sub-diabetogenic doses of streptozotocin in mice. *Diabetes Res* 1987; **6**: 195–200.

10 MacGillivray MH, Bruck E, Voorhess ML. Acute diabetic ketoacidosis in children: role of the stress hormones. *Pediatr Res* 1981; **15**: 99–106.

11 Hinkle LE, Wolf S. A summary of experimental evidence relating life stress to diabetes mellitus. *J Mt Sinai Hosp* 1952; **19**: 537–46.

12 Hinkle LE, Edwards CJ, Wolf S. Studies in diabetes mellitus. II. The occurrence of a diuresis in diabetic persons exposed to stressful life situations with experimental observations on its relation to the concentration of glucose in blood and urine. *J Clin Invest* 1951; **30**: 818–26.

13 Vandenburgh RL, Sussman KE, Titus CC. Effects of hypnotically induced acute emotional stress on carbohydrate and lipid metabolism in patients with diabetes mellitus. *Psychosom Med* 1966; **28**: 382–90.

14 Lustman P, Carney R, Amado H. Acute stress and metabolism in diabetes. *Diabetes Care* 1981; **4**: 658–9.

15 Cann PA, Read NW, Cammack J et al. Psychological stress and the passage of a standard meal through the stomach and small intestine in man. *Gut* 1983; **24**: 236–40.

16 Hildebrandt P, Mehlsen J, Sestoft L, Nielsen SL. Mild mental stress in diabetes: changes in heart rate and subcutaneous blood flow. *Clin Physiol* 1985; **5**: 371–6.

17 Kemmer FW, Bisping R, Steingruber HJ et al. Psychological stress and metabolic control in patients with type 1 diabetes mellitus. *N Engl J Med* 1986; **314**: 1078–84.

18 Anderson BJ, Miller JP, Auslander WF, Santiago JV. Family characteristics of diabetic adolescents: relationship to metabolic control. *Diabetes Care* 1984; **4**: 586–94.

19 Mazze RS, Lucido D, Shamoon H. Psychological and social correlates of glycemic control. *Diabetes Care* 1984; **7**: 360−7.

20 Chase HP, Jackson GC. Stress and sugar control in children with insulin-dependent diabetes mellitus. *J Pediatr* 1981; **98**: 1011−13.

21 Lustman PJ, Skor DA, Carney RM, Santiago JV, Cryer PE. Stress and diabetic control. *Lancet* 1983; i: 588.

22 Hauser ST, Pollets D. Psychological aspects of diabetes mellitus: a critical review. *Diabetes Care* 1979; **2**: 227−32.

23 Williams G, Pickup J, Keen H. Psychological factors and metabolic control: time for reappraisal? *Diabetic Med* 1988; **5**: 211−15.

24 Wilkinson G, Borsey DQ, Leslie P, Newton RW, Lind C, Ballinger CB. Psychiatric morbidity and social problems in patients with insulin-dependent diabetes mellitus. *Br J Psychiatr* 1988; **153**: 38−43.

25 Tattersall R, Walford S. Brittle diabetes in response to life stress: 'cheating and manipulation'. In: Pickup JC, ed. *Brittle Diabetes*. Oxford: Blackwell Scientific Publications, 1985, 76−102.

26 Orr DP, Golden MP, Myers G, Marrero DG. Characteristics of adolescents with poorly-controlled diabetes referred to a tertiary care center. *Diabetes Care* 1983; **6**: 170−5.

27 Flexner CW, Weiner JP, Sandek CD, Dans PE. Repeated hospitalization for diabetic ketoacidosis. The game of Sartoris. *Am J Med* 1984; **76**: 691−5.

28 Stearns S. Self-destructive behaviour in young patients with diabetes mellitus. *Diabetes* 1959; **8**: 379−82.

29 Goldberg D. Identifying psychiatric illness among general medical patients. *Br Med J* 1985; **291**: 161−2.

30 Wilkinson G, Borsey DQ, Leslie P, Newton RW, Lind C, Ballinger CB. Psychiatric disorder in patients with insulin-dependent diabetes mellitus attending a general hospital clinic: (i) two-stage screening; and detection by physicians. *Psychol Med* 1987; **17**: 515−17.

31 Beer SF, Lawson C, Watkins PJ. Neurosis induced by home monitoring of blood glucose concentrations. *Br Med J* 1989; **298**: 362.

32 Schade DS, Drumm DA, Duckworth WC, Eaton RP. The etiology of incapacitating, brittle diabetes. *Diabetes Care* 1985; **8**: 12−20.

33 Goldberg D, Huxley P. *Mental Illness in the Community. The Pathway to Psychiatric Care*. London: Tavistock Publications, 1980.

34 Forgione GA, Surwit RS, Page D. *Fear: Learning to Cope*. New York: Van Nostrand Reinhold, 1978.

35 Surwit RS. *Progressive Relaxation*. Durham, North Carolina: Duke University Medical Center, 1977.

36 Fowler JE, Budzynski TH, Vanderbergh RL. Effects of an EMG biofeedback relaxation program on the control of diabetes. *Biofeedback Self Regul* 1976; **1**: 105−12.

37 Surwit RS, Feinglos MN. The effects of relaxation on glucose tolerance in non-insulin-dependent diabetes. *Diabetes Care* 1983; **6**: 176−9.

38 Wilkinson G. Psychiatric aspects of diabetes mellitus. *Br J Psychiatr* 1981; **138**: 1−9.

39 Tattersall R. Psychiatric aspects of diabetes — a physician's view. *Br J Psychiatr* 1981; **139**: 485−93.

40 Wilkinson G. The influence of psychiatric, psychological and social factors on the control of insulin-dependent diabetes mellitus. *J Psychosom Res* 1987; **31**: 277−86.

41 Bradley C. Clinical trials — time for a paradigm shift? *Diabetic Med* 1988; **5**: 107−9.

SECTION 14
DIABETES AND
INTERCURRENT EVENTS

78   Exercise and Diabetes Mellitus

Summary

• Energy for muscular work is derived initially from the breakdown of muscle glycogen and later from circulating glucose and non-esterified fatty acids; muscle uptake of glucose may increase 20-fold during exercise, due to increased blood flow and glucose delivery and to enhanced glucose transporter activity.

• Hepatic glucose production (mainly from glycogenolysis) normally rises to meet increased glucose demands but ultimately may be unable to match glucose consumption; normal people may become hypoglycaemic after 2–3 h of strenuous exercise without caloric intake.

• During prolonged exercise, a normal subject's insulin secretion declines and release of counter-regulatory hormones increases.

• In IDDM, glycaemic changes during exercise depend largely on blood insulin levels and therefore on insulin administration and absorption; absorption may be accelerated by exercising an injected limb. Hyperinsulinaemia causes hypoglycaemia, which may persist for many hours as muscle glycogen stores are replenished. Hypoinsulinaemia, combined with counter-regulatory hormone excesses, leads rapidly to hyperglycaemia.

• Insulin-treated IDDM patients can reduce the risks of hypoglycaemia during acute exercise by taking 20–40 g extra carbohydrate before and hourly during exercise and/or by reducing pre-exercise insulin dosages by 30–50%. Glycaemia should be monitored during and after exercise; post-exercise hypoglycaemia may be delayed until the following day.

• In NIDDM, exercise increases peripheral glucose uptake but also decreases endogenous insulin secretion; hypoglycaemia is therefore rare and extra carbohydrate is not required. However, sulphonylureas may cause hypoglycaemia during exercise.

• Diabetic patients can undertake most sports, but insulin treatment contraindicates those where hypoglycaemia would be dangerous, and patients with proliferative retinopathy or severe arterial disease should not take strenuous exercise.

• Long-term physical training in normal and diabetic people increases insulin sensitivity and in diabetic subjects may improve glycaemic and lipaemic profiles. Physical training in youth may also protect against the subsequent development of NIDDM.

Due to its hypoglycaemic effect, exercise has traditionally been recommended as an important component of diabetic treatment. In recent years, much new information has accumulated regarding the beneficial and possible adverse effects of exercise for diabetic patients. This section focuses on the effects of acute exercise and physical training in diabetes and outlines practical recommendations for exercise. As a background to its implications for diabetes, the metabolic and hormonal responses to exercise in the healthy individual are first reviewed.

Metabolic effects of exercise in the healthy individual

Acute exercise enhances fuel utilization, necessitating several metabolic changes in order to ensure adequate substrate availability to both the exercising muscle and the non-exercising tissues.

Regular exercise leads to further metabolic adaptations which may also influence the resting state.

Acute exercise

GLUCOSE METABOLISM

During the first 5−10 min of exercise, muscle glycogen is the main source of energy. As exercise continues, the blood-borne substrates, glucose and non-esterified fatty acids (NEFA), become increasingly important. Glucose uptake by the exercising leg increases progressively up to 20-fold above the resting levels during intensive exercise (Fig. 78.1) [1]. If exercise of moderate intensity continues for several hours, the contribution of glucose diminishes and NEFA become the major fuel (Fig. 78.2) [2].

During the first hour of exercise, blood glucose levels remain virtually unchanged, because hepatic glucose production rises to meet the needs of the exercising muscle; with strenous exercise, hepatic glucose production may even exceed the rate of glucose utilization, when blood glucose increases. About 75% of hepatic glucose output is derived from glycogenolysis, the rest being formed from gluconeogenesis. If exercise lasts for several

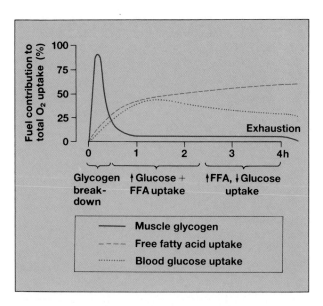

Fig. 78.2. The relative contributions of muscle glycogen breakdown and uptake of blood-borne glucose and non-esterified fatty acids to fuel utilization at various stages of prolonged exercise in normal man. The exercise intensity corresponds to 30% of maximal. (Adapted from Ahlborg et al. 1974 [2] with permission from the Journal of Clinical Investigation.)

hours, hepatic glucose production can no longer keep pace with increased utilization and glycaemia begins to decline. In normal man, hypoglycaemia may ensue after 2−3h of continuous exercise without caloric intake [3]. If exercise is preceded by a large sugar load causing hyperinsulinaemia when exercise begins, hypoglycaemia may develop within 30 min of exercise (Fig. 78.3) [4].

Exercise-induced stimulation of glucose uptake may involve several factors. First, increased blood flow enhances insulin delivery to muscle and opens up previously non-perfused capillaries, thus increasing both the effect of insulin and the surface area for glucose transport. Secondly, muscle contraction can stimulate glucose transport, possibly through translocation of glucose transporters from an intracellular pool into the cell membrane. Exercise and insulin have additive effects on muscular glucose transport, perhaps indicating two separate glucose transport systems, one insulin-dependent and the other contraction-dependent [5]. Thirdly, exercise increases insulin binding to blood cells [6], although not necessarily to muscle [7]. Thus, changes in insulin binding may not play a major role, since glucose uptake is augmented by exercise even in the absence of insulin [8].

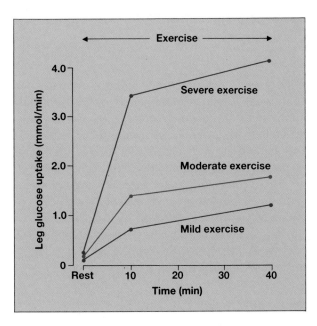

Fig. 78.1. Glucose uptake by the exercising leg during cycle ergometric exercise in a healthy man. Mild exercise corresponds to 65 W (about 25−30% of maximal capacity), moderate exercise to 130 W (50−60%) and severe exercise to 195 W (75−90%). (Adapted from Felig & Wahren 1975 [1] with permission of the New England Journal of Medicine.)

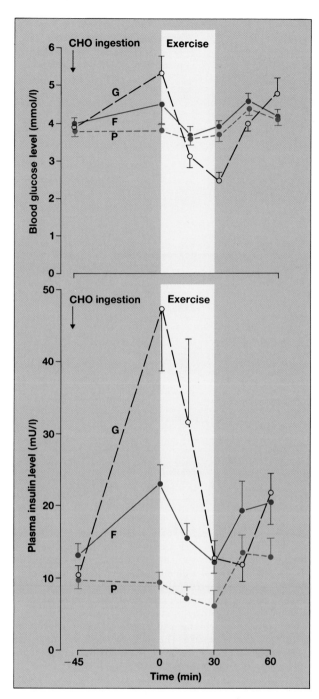

Fig. 78.3. Changes in blood glucose and plasma insulin concentrations in a healthy man during exercise performed 45 min after the ingestion of 75 g of glucose (G), fructose (F) or non-calorific placebo (P). In spite of elevated glucose levels at the beginning of exercise after glucose ingestion, the associated hyperinsulinaemia causes a rapid decline in blood glucose to hypoglycaemic levels during 30 min of exercise. The exercise intensity corresponds to 75% of maximal. (Redrawn with permission from the *Journal of Applied Physiology* [4].)

HORMONAL RESPONSES

Many endocrine changes occur during exercise (Table 78.1). These depend primarily on the

intensity and duration of muscular work [9] and serve to regulate fuel metabolism, cardiovascular changes and body temperature as well as fluid and electrolyte homeostasis.

Physical training

GLUCOSE METABOLISM

Aerobically trained athletes have low fasting plasma insulin levels and reduced insulin responses to a glucose challenge in the face of normal glucose tolerance, suggesting enhanced whole-body sensitivity to insulin. This has been confirmed directly, as insulin-mediated glucose disposal is increased [10]. In previously untrained subjects, muscle insulin sensitivity rises significantly after 4–6 weeks of intensive physical training, in proportion to the increase in maximal oxygen consumption. Physical training also increases hepatic insulin sensitivity [11]. Conversely, even a few days' immobilization can markedly impair glucose tolerance and insulin sensitivity [10].

LIPID METABOLISM

Physical training renders lipid and lipoprotein profiles less atherogenic: serum high-density lipoprotein (HDL) cholesterol levels increase, while total cholesterol levels remain unchanged or may decline [12]. The rise in HDL-cholesterol caused by physical training is related to increased lipoprotein lipase activity, which accelerates the conversion of very low density lipoprotein (VLDL) to HDL. Some studies also suggest that serum triglyceride levels decline after training.

Metabolic and hormonal effects of exercise in diabetes

Insulin-dependent diabetes

The metabolic and hormonal response to exercise in IDDM patients is determined by several factors, such as the intensity and duration of the exercise, the patient's level of metabolic control, the type and dose of insulin injected before the exercise, the site of insulin injection, and the timing of the previous insulin injection and meal relative to the exercise. Accordingly, blood glucose concentrations can decline (the commonest response), increase or remain unchanged (Table 78.2).

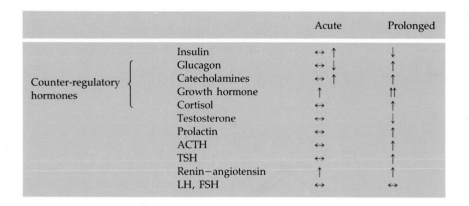

		Acute		Prolonged
Counter-regulatory hormones	Insulin	↔	↑	↓
	Glucagon	↔	↓	↑
	Catecholamines	↔	↑	↑
	Growth hormone	↑		↑↑
	Cortisol	↔		↑
	Testosterone	↔		↓
	Prolactin	↔		↑
	ACTH	↔		↑
	TSH	↔		↑
	Renin−angiotensin	↑		↑
	LH, FSH	↔		↔

Table 78.1. Hormonal response to acute and prolonged exercise. ↔ = no change; ↑, ↑↑ = moderate, marked increase; ↓ = decrease.

Table 78.2. Factors determining glycaemic response to acute exercise in IDDM patients.

Blood glucose decreases if:
- Hyperinsulinaemia exists during exercise
- Exercise is prolonged (>30−60 min) or intensive
- >3 h have elapsed since the preceding meal
- No extra snacks are taken before or during the exercise

Blood glucose remains unchanged if:
- Exercise is short
- Plasma insulin concentration is normal
- Appropriate snacks are taken before and during exercise

Blood glucose increases if:
- Hypoinsulinaemia exists during exercise
- Exercise is strenous
- Excessive carbohydrate is taken before or during exercise

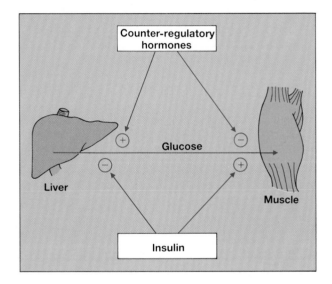

Fig. 78.4. Schematic representation of hormonal regulation of plasma glucose levels during exercise. Insulin diminishes hepatic glucose production and enhances glucose uptake by the muscle. In normal individuals, plasma insulin declines during prolonged exercise. Counter-regulatory hormones (glucagon, growth hormone, catecholamines, cortisol) stimulate hepatic glucose production and in high concentrations epinephrine and growth hormone reduce peripheral glucose uptake. The concentrations of counter-regulatory hormones increase during exercise in normal subjects; in diabetic patients this response is higher than normal.

The major determinant of the diabetic patient's glycaemic response to exercise is insulin availability. In normal subjects, insulin secretion declines during prolonged exercise. Exercise performed during *hyperinsulinaemia* will tend to cause hypoglycaemia. Insulin prevents the appropriate rise in hepatic glucose production and further accelerates the exercise-induced stimulation of glucose uptake into the contracting muscle (Fig. 78.4). Hyperinsulinaemia also prevents the normal increase in lipid mobilization during exercise, leading to reduced availability of NEFA as a fuel. Hyperinsulinaemia may occur for several reasons (Fig. 78.5). First, short-acting insulin injected a few hours previously may exert its peak action during exercise. This effect is exaggerated if the previously injected limb is exercised, as insulin absorption is accelerated by exercise [13]. Moreover, the use of long-acting insulin generally produces higher peripheral insulin levels than normal.

During *hypoinsulinaemia*, the inhibitory effect of insulin on hepatic glucose production and its stimulatory effect on glucose uptake are both reduced. In addition, the counter-regulatory response (catecholamines, glucagon, growth hormone, cortisol) to exercise is higher than normal during insulin deficiency [14]. The overall result is markedly increased hepatic glucose production and diminished glucose utilization by the exercising muscle, thus leading to hyperglycaemia. Extremely strenuous acute exercise may cause

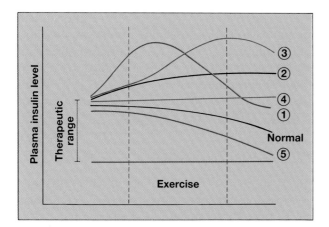

Fig. 78.5. Plasma insulin levels may vary widely during exercise in insulin-treated diabetic patients, whereas normal subjects show a steady decline during prolonged exercise. *Hyperinsulinaemia* and hypoglycaemia may occur when the peak action of short-acting (1) or intermediate-acting (2) insulin occurs during exercise or if exercise itself accelerates absorption from an injected leg (3). Steady insulin concentrations (4) may occur during CSII or after intermediate-acting insulin injection. Declining levels (5) and *hypoinsulinaemia* occur when the previous injections are exhausted.

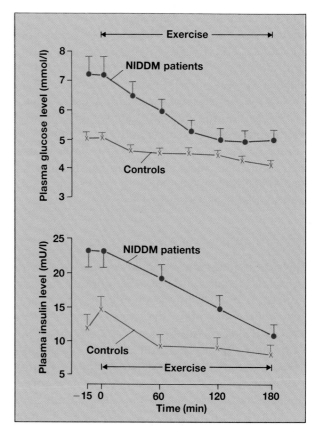

Fig. 78.6. Changes in plasma glucose and insulin concentrations during prolonged exercise in non-obese NIDDM patients. The exercise (30–35% of maximal) was performed after an overnight fast [20]. The fall in endogenous insulin secretion diminishes the risk of hypoglycaemia during exercise in NIDDM.

hyperglycaemia even without hypoinsulinaemia, because excessive counter-regulatory hormone action can stimulate glucose production beyond the limits of peripheral utilization [15]. Augmented lipid mobilization and ketogenesis in the liver increase blood ketone body concentrations: the hypoinsulinaemic patient may thus become hyper-ketonaemic and ketonuric after exercise.

Despite the complexities of glucoregulation, well-motivated IDDM patients can successfully undertake several hours of exhaustive exercise such as a marathon run [16] or competitive cross-country skiing [17], provided that both diet and insulin dose are adjusted appropriately before and during exercise. After prolonged exercise, patients may have hypoglycaemic symptoms for several hours or even on the following day. This can be explained by persistently enhanced glucose uptake by the exercised muscles to refill depleted gly-cogen stores [17].

Non-insulin-dependent diabetes

These patients are characterized by both hepatic and peripheral insulin resistance and hyperinsu-linaemia in the fasting state. During acute exer-cise, peripheral glucose uptake rises more than hepatic glucose production, and blood glucose concentration tends to decline [18]. At the same time, however, plasma insulin levels fall, and the risk of exercise-induced hypoglycaemia in NIDDM patients is small, even during prolonged exercise (Fig. 78.6) [19]. If NIDDM patients perform strenuous, glycogen-depleting exercise, both peri-pheral and hepatic insulin sensitivity are increased and remain so for 12–16 h after exercise [20]. Fast-ing glucose levels are lower on the morning after strenuous exercise due to decreased hepatic glucose production rather than increased glucose utilization.

Effects of physical training in diabetes

INSULIN-DEPENDENT DIABETES

Most IDDM patients are insulin-resistant. Physi-cal training in these patients improves whole-body insulin sensitivity as it does in healthy man, but will only improve metabolic control if the training programme is accompanied by blood glucose monitoring and appropriate changes in the diet and insulin in order to avoid hypoglycaemia and reactive hyperglycaemia during and after the acute bouts of exercise [21–4]. Like normal subjects, IDDM patients show a fall in serum total cholesterol level with a rise in HDL-cholesterol during physical training [21]. As well as these metabolic changes, physical training can confer psychological benefits, particularly in diabetic children, including improved feelings of well-being, better acceptance by peers and family and greater self-esteem [23].

NON-INSULIN-DEPENDENT DIABETES

Physical training also improves insulin sensitivity in subjects with NIDDM, the improvement in glucose disposal lasting for months after the training programme ends. Glycaemic control also improves, HbA$_1$ falling by 1.0–1.5% after 6 weeks of training, due to the cumulative effects of individual exercise bouts [25]. In addition, participation in the exercise programme may improve dietary compliance, which can also contribute to the improvement in control. Oral glucose tolerance may [25–7] or may not [19, 28, 29] improve after physical training; an improvement is more likely in patients with a high insulin secretory capacity in whom insulin resistance is the major cause of diabetes [27, 29].

Physical training in NIDDM patients has been reported to produce anti-atherogenic blood lipid changes and to reduce other risk factors for coronary heart disease (hypertension, obesity, coagulation abnormalities), in some but not in all studies [28, 30, 31]. The prophylactic value of physical exercise may be greater in younger individuals, who have neither established atherosclerosis nor musculo-skeletal or other problems which may prevent effective exercise. In elderly patients with relatively advanced atherosclerosis, physical training is less effective in retarding atherogenesis [30].

Exercise in the prevention of diabetes

There is no evidence that exercise can prevent the development of IDDM, but indirect data suggest that regular exercise may protect against NIDDM. In population studies, glucose tolerance is better in physically active than in inactive subjects [32]. In former college athletes, the prevalence of NIDDM was 2.7% as compared with 7.6% in the non-

athlete population [33]. These cross-sectional data do not exclude the possibility of natural selection, but insulin resistance — an important pathogenetic factor in NIDDM — is significantly less in older athletes than sedentary subjects [34], which may contribute to the lower prevalence of NIDDM among former athletes.

Recommendations for exercise in diabetes

Most sports can be recommended to diabetic patients. Guidelines are outlined in Tables 78.3–78.5. These guidelines should be tailored to the individual, taking into account his interests and fitness. Poor glycaemic control should be corrected primarily with diet and insulin or oral agents, and exercise used only as an adjunct to these other therapeutic modalities. In general, diabetic patients should be encouraged to exercise regularly. On the other hand, if the patient is interested in sports or even a professional athlete, diabetes should not interfere with his career and

Table 78.3. Cautions and advice regarding exercise in diabetes.

Contraindications
Insulin treatment: sports where hypoglycaemia would be dangerous (e.g. diving, climbing, single-handed sailing, motor racing)
Proliferative retinopathy: strenuous exercise (risk of possible haemorrhage)

Cautions
Cardiovascular disease (especially in NIDDM)
Peripheral neuropathy (risk of injury to feet)

General advice
Take exercise regularly, daily if possible
Strenuous exertion is not necessary; even regular walking has metabolic benefits
Tailor exercise schedules to the patient's individual needs and physical fitness

Table 78.4. Guidelines for exercise in IDDM.

- Monitor glycaemia before, during and after exercise
- Avoid hypoglycaemia during exercise by:
  – starting exercise 1–2 h after a meal
  – taking 20–40 g extra carbohydrate before and hourly during exercise
  – avoiding heavy exercise during peak insulin action
  – using non-exercising sites for insulin injection
  – reducing pre-injection insulin dosages by 30–50% if necessary
- After prolonged exercise, monitor glycaemia and take extra carbohydrate to avoid delayed hypoglycaemia

Table 78.5. Guidelines for exercise in NIDDM.

- Hypoglycaemia is unlikely during exercise and extra carbohydrate is therefore generally unnecessary
- Exercise used to reduce weight should be combined with dietary measures
- Exercise should be part of the daily schedule

treatment should be adjusted according to the demands of the physical activity.

ADJUSTMENT OF DIET AND INSULIN TREATMENT DURING EXERCISE

In IDDM patients, rapid glycaemic changes can be prevented by adjusting diet, insulin dose or both (Table 78.4). Adjustments must be tailored individually; even in the same patient, requirements can vary during different exercise periods. Blood glucose monitoring before, at the end and a few hours after exercise is helpful in guiding therapy. During short-term, occasional exercise, hypoglycaemia is most easily prevented by ingesting extra calories before and during the exercise. However, with long-term or regular exercise, or when hypoglycaemia ensues in spite of extra snacks, or if it is impractical to ingest enough calories, adjustment of the insulin dosage should be considered.

Diet. There are few controlled studies regarding the appropriate type and amount of calories to be taken with exercise. A clinical recommendation is to take approximately 20 g of carbohydrate before and at 60-min intervals during exercise. During strenuous exercise, at least part of this can be taken as a sucrose-containing soft drink. If exercise is performed postprandially, the need is less, whereas if some hours have elapsed since eating, larger snacks should be taken. During strenuous, long-term exercise, a carbohydrate intake of 40 g/h combined with a reduced insulin dosage (see below) can maintain near-normoglycaemia [17]. The breakfast before long-term exercise should contain about 20–30 g protein and approximately 40 g carbohydrate [17].

Insulin. In patients receiving multiple injections, short-acting insulin taken before exercise can be reduced by 30% to 50%, instead of dietary adjustment [35]. If exercise lasts for several hours, the insulin dose can be reduced by 40% and extra carbohydrate taken during exercise [17]. The insulin dose to be reduced is that which has its main action at the time of exercise.

If blood glucose increases during exercise and is not due to over-eating, the insulin dose should be slightly increased or the injection schedule changed in order to achieve higher plasma insulin concentrations during the exercise.

In NIDDM patients, exercise does not usually cause hypoglycaemia and, in obese patients, is a valuable tool in losing weight. For these reasons, no extra calories are needed with exercise (Table 78.5). If blood glucose declines rapidly during exercise, as may occur in patients taking oral hypoglycaemic agents, the dose of the drug should be reduced.

VEIKKO A. KOIVISTO

References

1 Felig P, Wahren J. Fuel homeostasis in exercise. *N Engl J Med* 1975; **293**: 1078–84.
2 Ahlborg G, Felig P, Hagenfeldt L, Hendler R, Wahren J. Substrate turnover during prolonged exercise in man: splanchnic and leg metabolism of glucose, free fatty acids and amino acids. *J Clin Invest* 1974; **53**: 1080–90.
3 Felig P, Cherif A, Minagawa A, Wahren J. Hypoglycemia during prolonged exercise in normal man. *N Engl J Med* 1982; **306**: 895–900.
4 Koivisto VA, Karonen S-L, Nikkilä EA. Carbohydrate ingestion before exercise: comparison of glucose, fructose and sweet placebo. *J Appl Physiol* 1981; **51**: 783–7.
5 Wallberg-Henriksson H. Repeated exercise regulates glucose transport capacity in skeletal muscle. *Acta Physiol Scand* 1986; **127**: 39–43.
6 Koivisto VA, Soman V, Conrad P, Hendler R, Nadel E, Felig P. Insulin binding to monocytes in trained athletes. *J Clin Invest* 1979; **64**: 1011–19.
7 Bonen A, Tan MH, Clune P, Kirby RL. Effects of exercise on insulin binding to human muscle. *Am J Physiol* 1985; **248**: E403–8.
8 Wallberg-Henriksson H, Holloszy JO. Contraction activity increases glucose uptake by muscle in severely diabetic rats. *J Appl Physiol* 1984; **57**: 1045–1049.
9 Galbo H. The hormonal response to exercise. *Diabetes Metab Rev* 1986; **1**: 385–408.
10 Koivisto VA, Yki-Järvinen H, DeFronzo R. Physical training and insulin sensitivity. *Diabetes Metab Rev* 1986; **1**: 445–81.
11 DeFronzo RA, Sherwin RS, Kraemer N. Effect of physical training on insulin action in obesity. *Diabetes* 1987; **36**: 1379–85.
12 Huttunen JK, Länsimies E, Voutilainen E, Ehnholm C, Hietanen E, Penttilä I, Siitonen O, Rauramaa E. Effect of moderate physical exercise on serum lipoproteins: a controlled clinical trial with special reference to serum high-density lipoproteins. *Circulation* 1979; **60**: 1220–9.
13 Koivisto VA, Felig P. Effects of leg exercise on insulin absorption in diabetic patients. *N Engl J Med* 1978; **298**: 77–83.
14 Berger M, Berchtold P, Cüppers HJ *et al.* Metabolic and

hormonal effects of muscular exercise in juvenile type diabetes. *Diabetologia* 1977; **13**: 355−65.

15 Mitchell TH, Schiffrin A, Marliss E. Hyperglycemia following intense exercise in type 1 diabetes. *Diabetes* 1986; **35** (suppl 1): 10A.

16 Meinders AE, Willekens FLA, Heere LP. Metabolic and hormonal changes in IDDM during long-distance run. *Diabetes Care* 1988; **11**: 1−7.

17 Sane T, Helve E, Pelkonen R, Koivisto VA. The adjustment of diet and insulin dose during long-term endurance exercise in Type 1 (insulin-dependent) diabetic men. *Diabetologia* 1988; **31**: 35−40.

18 Minuk HL, Vranic M, Marliss E, Hanna AK, Albisser AM, Zinman B. Glucoregulatory and metabolic response to exercise in obese non insulin-dependent diabetes. *Am J Physiol* 1981; **240**: E458−64.

19 Koivisto VA, DeFronzo RA. Exercise in the treatment of type II diabetes. *Acta Endocrinol* 1984; **262** (suppl): 107−11.

20 Devlin JT, Hirshman M, Horton ED, Horton ES. Enhanced peripheral and splanchnic insulin sensitivity in NIDDM men after single bout of exercise. *Diabetes* 1987; **36**: 434−9.

21 Wallberg-Henriksson H, Gunnarsson R, Henriksson J, DeFronzo R, Felig P, Östman J, Wahren J. Increased peripheral insulin sensitivity and muscle mitochondrial enzymes but unchanged blood glucose control in type 1 diabetics after physical training. *Diabetes* 1982; **31**: 1044−50.

22 Yki-Järvinen H, DeFronzo R, Koivisto VA. Normalization of insulin sensitivity in type 1 diabetic subjects by physical training during insulin pump therapy. *Diabetes Care* 1984; **7**: 520−7.

23 Rowland T, Swadba LA, Biggs DE, Burke EJ, Reiter EO. Glycemic control with physical training in insulin-dependent diabetes mellitus. *Sports Med* 1985; **139**: 307−10.

24 Wallberg-Henriksson H, Gunnarsson R, Rössner S, Wahren J. Long-term physical training in female Type 1 (insulin-dependent) diabetic patients: absence of significant effect on glycaemic control and lipoprotein levels. *Diabetologia* 1986; **29**: 53−7.

25 Schneider SH, Amorosa LF, Khachadurian AK, Ruderman NB. Studies on the mechanism of improved glucose control during regular exercise in Type 2 (non-insulin-dependent) diabetes. *Diabetologia* 1984; **26**: 355−60.

26 Saltin B, Lindegärde F, Houston M, Hörlin R, Nygaard E, Gad P. Physical training and glucose tolerance in middle-aged men with chemical diabetes. *Diabetes* 1979; **28** (suppl 1): 30−2.

27 Rönnemaa T, Mattila K, Lehtonen A, Kallio V. A controlled randomized study on the effect of long-term physical exercise on the metabolic control in type 2 diabetic patients. *Acta Med Scand* 1986; **220**: 219−24.

28 Ruderman NB, Ganda OP, Johansen K. The effect of physical training on glucose tolerance and plasma lipids in maturity-onset diabetes. *Diabetes* 1979; **28** (suppl 1): 89−92.

29 Holloszy JO, Schultz J, Kusnierkiewicz J, Hagberg JM, Ehsani AA. Effects of exercise on glucose tolerance and insulin resistance. *Acta Med Scand* 1986; **711** (suppl): 55−65.

30 Skarfors ET, Wegener TA, Lithell H, Selinus I. Physical training as treatment for Type 2 (non-insulin-dependent) diabetes in elderly men. A feasibility study over 2 years. *Diabetologia* 1987; **30**: 930−3.

31 Schneider SH, Vitug A, Ruderman N. Atherosclerosis and physical activity. *Diabetes Metab Rev* 1986; **1**: 513−53.

32 Cederholm J, Wibell L. Glucose tolerance and physical activity in a health survey of middle-aged subjects. *Acta Med Scand* 1985; **217**: 373−8.

33 Frisch RE, Wyshak G, Albright TE, Albright NL, Schiff I. Lower prevalence of diabetes in former college athletes compared with nonathletes. *Diabetes* 1986; **35**: 1101−5.

34 Seals DR, Hagberg JM, Allen WK, Hurley BF, Dalsky GP, Ehsani AA, Holloszy JO. Glucose tolerance in young and older athletes and sedentary men. *J Appl Physiol* 1984; **56**: 1521−5.

35 Schiffrin A, Parikh S. Accommodating planned exercise in type 1 diabetic patients on intensive treatment. *Diabetes Care* 1985; **8**: 337−42.

79   Drugs and Diabetes Mellitus

Summary

- Corticosteroids are the drugs with the greatest hyperglycaemic effect. Diabetic treatment must be adjusted before starting high-dose steroid therapy: most IDDM patients require a 50% increase in insulin dosage and many NIDDM patients treated with diet or oral agents will need insulin.
- Thiazide diuretics are diabetogenic in non-diabetic and NIDDM subjects (possibly by inhibiting insulin secretion) but have no hyperglycaemic effect in IDDM patients receiving insulin. Frusemide or other loop diuretics are not diabetogenic and are the diuretics of choice in NIDDM.
- Oral contraceptives containing low-dose oestrogen and progestogen or progestogen alone have no significant hyperglycaemic action and are acceptable in IDDM and probably in NIDDM and women with previous gestational diabetes. The progestogen, levonorgestrel may be diabetogenic.
- β_2-adrenergic agents (e.g. salbutamol, ritodrine) given as intravenous infusion stimulate gluconeogenesis and cause hyperglycaemia.
- β-blocking agents, both β_1-selective and non-selective, mask important hypoglycaemic symptoms and should be prescribed cautiously in patients taking insulin or sulphonylurea drugs.
- Many drugs either reduce or increase the hypoglycaemic action of the sulphonylureas; potential interactions must always be checked before starting other drugs in sulphonylurea-treated patients and blood glucose levels should be carefully monitored. The elderly and tightly controlled patients are at particular risk of hypoglycaemia.

Unlike many adverse reactions to drugs, effects on blood glucose control are often unrecognized by both patient and doctor. Exacerbation of hyperglycaemia in diabetes or impairment of glucose tolerance in previously normoglycaemic subjects may be caused by several groups of drugs which are used for long-term therapy. Conversely, hypoglycaemia is frequently caused or exacerbated by drugs which interact with sulphonylurea agents.

Drugs inducing hyperglycaemia

The mechanisms by which drugs may cause hyperglycaemia are illustrated in Fig. 79.1, and important examples are listed in Table 79.1 (see Appendix to Chapter 79).

Corticosteroids

Corticosteroids have by far the most powerful influence on glucose tolerance of any group of drugs. Steroids decrease hepatic and peripheral tissue sensitivity to insulin by acting at a post-receptor level, leading to an inappropriately raised hepatic glucose output and impaired uptake of glucose by muscle and fat [1]. Even inhaled or topically applied steriods may induce metabolic abnormalities if given in sufficient dosage [2]. Normal subjects given high-dose prednisolone (30 mg per day or more) rapidly develop significant increases in fasting blood glucose and serum insulin concentrations [3], and unselected subjects receiving chronic steroid therapy have an estimated prevalence of impaired glucose tolerance (IGT) or diabetes of between 14% and 28% [4, 5]. The incidence of abnormality does not appear to rise with increasing duration of treatment and the decrease in glucose tolerance appears to be

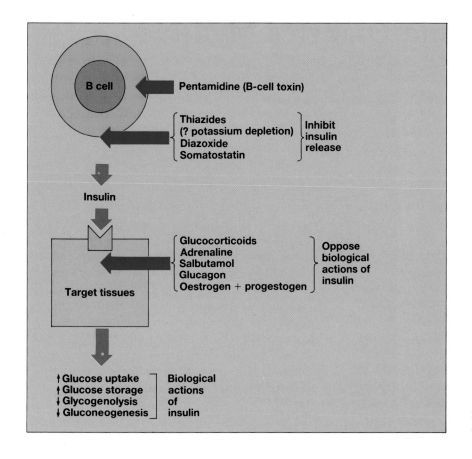

Fig. 79.1. Mechanisms by which drugs may induce hyperglycaemia.

strictly dose-related and has not been observed at doses of less than 7.5 mg/day of prednisolone [5].

In diabetic subjects, both IDDM and NIDDM, steroid therapy inevitably exacerbates hyperglycaemia. Administration of steroids to any diabetic subject requires prospective adjustment of hypoglycaemic therapy and close monitoring of glycaemic control, as outlined below and in Fig. 79.2.

Thiazide and other diuretics

Within a year of the introduction of the first benzothiadiazine diuretic, chlorothiazide, hyperglycaemia was reported as a side-effect [6]. The mechanism of the thiazides' effect on glucose tolerance is uncertain. It is widely believed that potassium depletion may be involved by impairing insulin release, although the reported relationship between hypokalaemia and reduced glucose tolerance is contentious. Normal and IDDM individuals may be affected, the degree depending on pre-existing glucose tolerance and genetically determined pancreatic reserve [7, 8]. Clinical observation suggests that thiazides cause deterioration in blood glucose control in all NIDDM

subjects, but with individual variability. At least in NIDDM patients, concurrent treatment with propranolol has an additional deleterious influence upon glucose tolerance. Thiazide-induced hyperglycaemia may appear rapidly [9, 10]. However, in insulin-treated IDDM patients, thiazides do not alter blood glucose control [11].

It has long been suggested that frusemide has an effect on glucose tolerance similar to that of the thiazide diuretics [12]. However, the handful of reported cases of loop diuretics worsening glycaemic control (including their possible role in hyperosmolar coma) may simply represent chance associations, as serious systemic illness requiring potent diuretic therapy may be expected to increase insulin resistance. Published evidence falls far short of proving a significant hyperglycaemic effect of frusemide, ethacrinic acid or bumetanide [13]. Indeed, frusemide, in a low dose, is the diuretic of choice in NIDDM.

Oral contraceptive agents

As oral contraceptive agents are taken by large numbers of young women for many years, any effect upon glucose tolerance could be of great importance. Early studies suggested that the prevalence of abnormal glucose tolerance in women taking the contraceptive pill was increased from approximately 4% to 35% [14], and in women who displayed glucose intolerance during pregnancy, subsequent oral contraceptive therapy made the development of diabetes more likely [15, 16]. However, conflicting results arose from subsequent studies with low-oestrogen preparations, largely as a result of the different doses of oestrogen and the different types and doses of progestogen employed. Decreased glucose tolerance appears to be related not only to oestrogen doses greater than 75 µg/day, but also to the type of progestogen, levonorgestrel having a greater deleterious effect [17–19]. Like glucocorticoids, sex steroids probably act at a postreceptor level.

For IDDM subjects, the combined low-dose contraceptive pill or the progesterone-only pill exert no significant effect on glycaemic control. For those with NIDDM, a strong family history of the same or a history of gestational diabetes, there is insufficient information upon which to base firm recommendations, but it seems reasonable to avoid those containing levonorgestrel, pending the results of further studies (see Chapter 85).

Other drugs causing hyperglycaemia

β_2-adrenergic agonists (e.g. salbutamol and ritodrine, used to treat asthma and premature labour) increase glycogenolysis in the liver and skeletal muscle, but also stimulate insulin secretion. Human studies have confirmed that intravenous salbutamol increases hepatic glucose output and stimulates insulin release [20], the net effect being hyperglycaemia. This effect is particularly pronounced in IDDM patients, especially when β-agonists are used in conjunction with dexamethasone for preterm labour (see Chapter 83); indeed, this combination may produce acute metabolic decompensation even in previously normoglycaemic patients. Acute administration of adrenaline may also cause large increases in blood glucose levels [21].

Asparaginase in therapeutic dosages, and phenytoin and salicylates in overdose, are well established as causing hyperglycaemia. Pentamidine is a pancreatic B-cell toxin, closely related to the experimental diabetogenic agent, alloxan. Pentamidine may also cause acute hypoglycaemia in as many as 14% of patients because of insulin

release from degenerating B cells [22]. The antihypertensive agent, diazoxide (a sulphonylurea derivative) inhibits insulin secretion and has a powerful diabetogenic effect which is occasionally exploited in the medical treatment of insulinoma. Somatostatin blocks insulin secretion but also inhibits the release of the counter-regulatory hormones, glucagon and growth hormone (see Chapters 33 and 104); because of these opposing actions, glucose tolerance is often unchanged during somatostatin treatment, although some acromegalic patients develop glucose intolerance or frank diabetes [23]. Certain synthetic steroids with androgenic properties (e.g. oxymetholone, danazol) interfere with insulin action at or beyond the receptor, stimulating compensatory hyperinsulinaemia and occasionally producing glucose intolerance [24]. Recently, atenolol and metoprolol have been shown to decrease insulin sensitivity [25]. Many other drugs have been implicated in causing hyperglycaemia, although evidence usually rests upon anecdotal reports.

There is no firm evidence to link decreased glucose tolerance with angiotensin converting enzyme (ACE) inhibitors, calcium channel blockers or other longer-established antihypertensive agents (see Chapter 69).

Treatment of drug-induced diabetes

As in all drug-induced disorders, the responsible agent should be withdrawn if possible. If thiazide-induced hyperglycaemia occurs, the indication for diuretic treatment should be reappraised and, if this is still required, a small dose of frusemide or bumetanide should be substituted.

Withdrawal of steroid therapy is often not immediately feasible and the diabetes must be controlled rapidly. Management depends entirely upon the degree of hyperglycaemia, as illustrated in Fig. 79.2. The random blood glucose level is shown as the basis for decision-making, as this is often the only information available in clinical practice, but the values quoted should be regarded only as approximate guides, and therapy must be continually assessed. In most situations requiring steroid therapy, resistance to infection is already decreased and added susceptibility as a consequence of hyperglycaemia should be avoided. Simple relief of symptoms alone is therefore inadequate. The target fasting blood glucose of less than 8 mmol/l applies only in the short term and if long-term steroid therapy is likely, then the usual criteria for good control apply (see Chapter 34).

In the face of significant hyperglycaemia caused by high-dose steroid therapy (prednisolone 40 mg/day or more), insulin therapy may be started, as indicated in Fig. 79.2, at 0.5 U/kg body weight/day divided between morning and evening doses of short- and intermediate-acting insulin. This dosage is unlikely to produce hypoglycaemia and indeed may need to be increased day by day, as dictated by blood glucose monitoring. If the patient presents as a hyperglycaemic emergency, then standard therapy (see Chapter 49) should be started, initially with an intravenous insulin infusion of 12 U/h.

For patients with known diabetes about to begin high-dose steroid therapy, prospective adjustment of their diabetic treatment is essential. NIDDM patients treated by diet alone whose fasting blood glucose concentration is 7–10 mmol/l will require addition of a sulphonylurea or insulin, and the need for insulin therapy may be anticipated for those patients poorly controlled by high dosages of oral agents. For patients already taking insulin, the dosage should be increased by 50% initially, starting on the same day as steroid therapy. Further adjustments will be based upon results of blood glucose monitoring.

Drug interactions with oral hypoglycaemic agents

Hypoglycaemia can be induced in various ways by a number of drugs, as illustrated in Table 79.2. In addition, many drugs may increase or decrease the effectiveness of sulphonylureas; Table 79.3 lists the important interactions. (See Appendix to Chapter 79 for Tables). The incidence of symptomatic hypoglycaemia produced as a result of drug interactions is unknown, not least because such events may not come to medical attention or may be misdiagnosed. A distinction should be made between mechanisms likely to cause hypoglycaemia at the onset of therapy (such as by acute interference with hepatic drug metabolism, or acute displacement of sulphonylurea from plasma protein binding sites) and those which predispose to hypoglycaemia during chronic therapy (such as by decreasing rates of drug clearance or by interfering with counter-regulatory homeostatic responses) [26].

The elderly and those achieving near-normal blood glucose control with sulphonylurea therapy are at greatest risk of iatrogenic hypoglycaemia. Frequent monitoring of control is required if these subjects are prescribed any drug able to increase the hypoglycaemic effect of sulphonylureas. If the pancreas is unable to respond adequately to maximal doses of sulphonylureas (i.e. if glycaemic control is poor), drug-induced hypoglycaemia is unlikely unless starvation ensues.

Clinically significant interactions with metformin have not been reported, although care should be taken in using drugs which may impair renal function (e.g. non-steroidal anti-inflammatory agents, or high-dose frusemide). Guar gum and α-glucosidase inhibitors may alter the intestinal absorption of other drugs, but their action in delaying glucose absorption is not known to be significantly affected by other drugs.

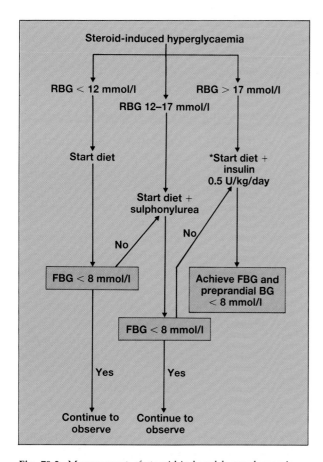

Fig. 79.2. Management of steroid-induced hyperglycaemia. RBG, random blood glucose; FBG, fasting blood glucose. * Intravenous insulin and fluids may be needed, depending upon clinical state. Plasma electrolytes must be checked.

Hypoglycaemia and β-blockers

All β-blocking drugs decrease awareness of hypoglycaemia, an effect which is clinically important in the context of therapy with either insulin or sulphonylureas. Certain early warning symptoms of adrenergic overactivity, especially tremor and tachycardia (but not sweating), are entirely suppressed by adequate β-blockade with either selective or non-selective agents [27]. Although it is theoretically possible that non-selective β-blockers might inhibit catecholamine-mediated glycogenolysis in liver and muscle (a β_2-adrenoceptor effect), there is no evidence to suggest that this is clinically important. Propranolol has occasionally been associated with hypoglycaemia in non-diabetic subjects who are malnourished [28], a condition in which gluconeogenesis is more important in maintenance of blood glucose. There is no evidence that this occurs with selective β_1-blockers.

The risk of masking hypoglycaemia, coupled with undesirable effects upon the peripheral circulation and plasma lipids, limits the use of β-blockers in both IDDM and NIDDM.

Other considerations

Certain drugs are relatively or absolutely contraindicated in the presence of certain diabetic complications. Important examples are shown in Table 79.4.

Although urine testing is now used less frequently it is still favoured by many elderly patients and it is important to remember that a number of drugs can interefere with measurements of urinary glucose [29].

ROY TAYLOR

References

1 Rizza RA, Mandarino LJ, Gerich JE. Cortisol-induced insulin resistance in man. Impaired suppression of glucose production and stimulation of glucose utilisation due to a postreceptor defect of insulin action. J Clin Endocrinol Metab 1982; **54**: 131–8.
2 Gomez EC, Frost P. Induction of glycosuria and hyperglycaemia by topical corticosteroid therapy. Arch Dermatol 1976; **112**: 1559–62.
3 Pagano G, Caballo-Perin P, Cassader M, Bruno A, Ozzello A, Masciola P, Dall'omo AM, Imbimbo B. An in vivo and in vitro study of the mechanism of prednisolone-induced insulin resistance in healthy subjects. J Clin Invest 1983; **72**: 1814–20.
4 Schubert GE, Schultz HD. Contribution to the clinical picture of steroid diabetes. Deutsch Med Wschr 1963; **8**: 1175–88.
5 Lieberman P, Patterson R, Kunske R. Complications of long-term steroid therapy for asthma. J Allergy Clin Immunol 1972; **49**: 329–36.
6 Wilkins RW. New drugs for the treatment of hypertension.

Ann Intern Med 1959; **50**: 1–10.
7 European Working Party on Hypertension in the Elderly. Glucose intolerance during diuretic therapy. Lancet 1978; i: 681–3.
8 Lewis PJ, Kohner EM, Petrie A, Dollery CT. Deterioration of glucose tolerance in hypertensive patients on prolonged diuretic treatment. Lancet 1976; i: 564–6.
9 Dornhorst A, Powell SH, Pensky J. Aggravation by propranolol of hyperglycaemic effect of hydrochlorothiazide in type II diabetics without alteration of insulin secretion. Lancet 1985; i: 123–6.
10 Nardoni DA, Bouma DJ. Hyperglycaemia and diabetic coma: possible relationship to diuretic propranolol therapy. South Med J 1979; **72**: 1604–6.
11 Schmitz O, Hermansen K, Hother Nielsen O, Christensen CK, Arnfred J, Hansen HE, Mogensen CE, Ørskov H, Beck-Nielsen H. Insulin action in insulin-dependent diabetics after short-term thiazide therapy. Diabetes Care 1986; **9**: 630–7.
12 Toivonen S, Mustala O. Diabetogenic actions of frusemide. Br Med J 1966; **1**: 920–1.
13 Taylor R. Drugs and glucose tolerance. Adv Drugs React Bull 1986; **121**: 452–5.
14 Spellacy WN. A review of carbohydrate metabolism and the oral contraceptives. Am J Obstet Gynecol 1969; **104**: 448–60.
15 Szabo AJ, Cole HS, Grimaldi RD. Glucose tolerance in gestational diabetic women during and after treatment with a combination type oral contraceptive. N Engl J Med 1970; **282**: 646–50.
16 Beck P, Wells SA. Comparison of the mechanisms underlying carbohydrate intolerance in subclinical diabetic women during pregnancy and during post-partum oral contraceptive steroid treatment. J Clin Endocrinol Metab 1969; **29**: 807–18.
17 Wynn V, Adams PW, Godsland I et al. Comparison of effects of different combined oral-contraceptive formulations on carbohydrate and lipid metabolism. Lancet 1979; i: 1045–9.
18 Perlman JA, Russell-Briefel R, Eggati T, Lieberknecht G. Oral glucose tolerance and the potency of contraceptive progestins. J Chron Dis 1985; **10**: 857–64.
19 Wynn V. Effect of low dose oral contraceptive administration on carbohydrate metabolism. Am J Obstet Gynecol 1982; **142**: 739–46.
20 Gundogdu AS, Brown PM, Juul S, Sachs L, Sönksen PH. Comparison of hormonal and metabolic effects of salbutamol infusion in normal subjects and insulin-requiring diabetics. Lancet 1979; ii: 1317–21.
21 Hamburg S, Hendler R, Sherwin RS. Influence of small increments of epinephrine on glucose tolerance in normal humans. Ann Intern Med 1980; **93**: 566–8.
22 Waskin H, Stehr-Green JK, Helmick CG, Sattler FR. Risk factors for hypoglycemia associated with pentamidine therapy for pneumocystis pneumonia. J Am Med Ass 1988; **260**: 345–7.
23 Verschoor L, Lamberts SWJ, Nitterlinden P, Del Pozo E. Glucose tolerance during long term treatment with a somatostatin analogue. Br Med J 1986; **293**: 1327–8.
24 Wynn V. Metabolic effects of danazol. J Int Med Res 1977; **5** (Suppl 3): 25–35.
25 Pollare T, Lithell H, Selinus I, Berne C. Sensitivity to insulin during treatment with atenolol and metoprolol: a randomised, double blind study of effects on carbohydrate and lipoprotein metabolism in hypertensive patients. Br Med J 1989; **298**: 1152–7.

26 Ferner RE. Oral hypoglycemic agents. *Med Clin N Am* 1988; **72**: 1323–35.

27 Deacon SP, Karunanayake A, Barnett D. Acebutolol, atenolol, and propranolol and metabolic reponses to acute hypoglycaemia in diabetics. *Br Med J* 1977; **2**: 1255–7.

28 Feller JM. Dangers of hypoglycaemia with use of propranolol. *Med J Austr* 1976; **2**: 92 (let).

29 Rotblatt MD, Koda-Kimble MA. Review of drug interference with urine glucose tests. *Diabetes Care* 1987; **10**: 103–10.

Appendix to Chapter 79

The help of Jackie Williams and Adrian Brown (South Sefton Drug Information Service, Fazakerley Hospital, Liverpool) in preparing the following tables is gratefully acknowledged.

Table 79.1. Drugs causing or exacerbating hyperglycaemia.

System indication	Drug class and examples	Mechanisms	Effects and comments
Cardiovascular drugs	β-adrenergic blockers	• Inhibit insulin secretion (β$_2$ action) and sensitivity	• May impair glucose tolerance in NIDDM or non-diabetic people • Rarely clinically significant
	Potassium-losing diuretics: Thiazides (e.g. bendrofluazide) Thiazide-related (e.g. chlorthalidone, metolazone)	• Cause potassium depletion which may impair insulin secretion	• May impair glucose tolerance in NIDDM or non-diabetic people • Thiazides combined with β-blockers more deleterious • No firm evidence that loop diuretics (e.g. frusemide) worsen glucose tolerance
	Vasodilator: Diazoxide	• Directly inhibits insulin secretion	• Hyperglycaemia may develop after a few injections
	Anti-arrhythmic drug: Encainide [*]	• Unknown	• Hyperglycaemia may develop after some weeks of treatment
Respiratory system drugs	*β$_2$-adrenergic stimulants*: Salbutamol, terbutaline	• Increase hepatic glucose output	• Acute hyperglycaemia only with high intravenous dosages • May precipitate ketoacidosis in IDDM patients
Anti-microbial agents	Pentamidine	• Causes B-cell destruction	• Often initial hypoglycaemia • Irreversible hyperglycaemia may occur during or even weeks after treatment
	Rifampicin [†]	• Enhances glucose absorption from gut	• Mild postprandial hyperglycaemia • Clinically unimportant
Obstetric drugs	*β$_2$-adrenergic stimulants*: Salbutamol, terbutaline, ritodrine	• Increase hepatic glucose output	• Acute hyperglycaemia only with high intravenous dosages • Exacerbated by dexamethasone given concurrently to accelerate fetal lung maturation

Table continued on p. 810.

Table 79.1. Cont'd

System indication	Drug class and examples	Mechanisms	Effects and comments
Endocrine drugs	*Glucocorticoids*: Cortisone, hydrocortisone, prednisolone, dexamethasone; also corticotrophin (ACTH)	• Postreceptor inhibition of insulin action; increase glycogenolysis and gluconeogenesis	• Dose-related hyperglycaemia • Only occurs with doses > 7.5 mg/day prednisolone or equivalent
	Oral contraceptives: Synthetic oestrogens and/or progestogens	• Postreceptor inhibition of insulin action	• Hyperglycaemia due mainly to oestrogens; some progestogens also implicated • On present evidence, sequential low-oestrogen or progestogen-only pills cause little metabolic disturbance
	Anabolic and related steroids: Oxymetholone, danazol, stanozolol	• Postreceptor inhibition of insulin action	• Impairment of glucose tolerance may result
	Growth hormone	• Postreceptor inhibition of insulin action	• Impairment of glucose tolerance may result
	Somatostatin analogues: Octreotide [‡]	• Inhibits insulin secretion; also inhibits glucagon and growth hormone secretion and glucose absorption from gut	• May worsen glucose tolerance in normal subjects; little change in NIDDM; improved in insulin-treated patients

Notes: General references may be found in the References for this chapter, and in: Young LY, Koda-Kimble MA, eds. *Applied Therapeutics: The Clinical Use of Drugs* (4th edn). Vancouver: Applied Therapeutics Inc., 1988, 1726–8. Specific references for this Table: [*] Salerno DM *et al., Am J Med* 1988; **84**: 39–44; [†] Takasu N *et al., Am Rev Respir Dis* 1982; **125**: 23–7; [‡] Davies RR *et al., Diabetic Med* 1989; **6**: 103–11.

Table 79.2. Drugs causing or exacerbating hypoglycaemia or its symptoms.

System indication	Drug class and examples	Mechanisms	Effects and comments
Cardiovascular drugs	*β-adrenergic blockers*	• Block catecholamine action	• Reduce some symptoms of hypoglycaemia (tremor, tachycardia) and possibly neuroglycopaenia • May delay recovery from hypoglycaemia
	Anti-arrhythmic drugs: Quinidine	• Stimulates insulin secretion	• May cause hypoglycaemia, especially in overdose and in fasting or severely ill patients
	Lipid-lowering drugs: Fibrates, e.g. bezafibrate, gemfibrozil	• Reduce free fatty acid levels, so stimulate peripheral glucose utilization	• Clinically not important
Analgesics and anti-inflammatory drugs	Salicylates	• Decrease hepatic glucose output	• In high therapeutic doses or overdosage • Especially in children; often fatal in this group
	Paracetamol	• Acute hepatic necrosis reduces hepatic glucose output	• In acute overdose; often fatal
Anti-microbial agents	Quinine	• Stimulates insulin secretion	• High risk in malaria, mainly cerebral in children and in pregnancy; exaggerated in renal failure; often fatal
	Sulphamethoxazole (in co-trimoxazole)	• Stimulates insulin secretion (sulphonylurea-like action)	• In elderly patients receiving high doses • Exaggerated in renal failure
	Pentamidine	• Causes insulin release due to B-cell damage	• Hypoglycaemia during first weeks of treatment • Irreversible hyperglycaemia may follow
Miscellaneous	Ethanol	• Inhibits gluconeogenesis • Effect exaggerated if hepatic glycogen is depleted	• Especially in malnutrition • Profound hypoglycaemia may follow 2–3 h after drinking alcohol with high-glucose food or drink

Table 79.3. Drugs interacting with oral hypoglycaemic agents.

Sulphonylureas Increased hypoglycaemic effect	Decreased hypoglycaemic effect
Hypoglycaemic agents (see Table 79.2)	*Hyperglycaemic agents (see Table 79.1)*
Decreased sulphonylurea clearance:	*Increased hepatic sulphonylurea clearance:*
• Azapropazone[§]	• Alcohol (chronic intake)
• Phenylbutazone[§], oxyphenbutazone[§]	• Rifampicin
• Sulphinpyrazone[§]	• Chlorpromazine
• Sulphonamides[§]	
• Salicylates[§]	
• Probenecid[§]	
• Monoamine oxidase inhibitors[§]	
• Chloramphenicol	
• Nicoumalone[§] (but not warfarin or phenindione)	

Metformin
Cimetidine reduces renal clearance of metformin, thus raising its plasma levels and increasing the risks of toxicity

§ indicates drugs which are strongly bound to plasma proteins; acute displacement of bound sulphonylureas may contribute to their hypoglycaemic actions.

Table 79.4. Drugs requiring caution in specific diabetic complications.

Complication and drug	Problem	Action to be taken
Nephropathy Sulphonylureas	• Accumulate in renal failure; increased risk of hypoglycaemia and toxicity	• Use insulin or a sulphonylurea not cleared through the kidneys (e.g. gliquidone, gliclazide)
Metformin	• Accumulates in renal failure; increased risk of lactic acidosis	• Avoid completely
Cardiovascular disease β-adrenergic blockers	• Accentuate hypoglycaemia • May cause modest VLDL elevation	• Consider alternative antihypertensive, anti-anginal or anti-arrhythmic drugs (e.g. ACE inhibitors, calcium channel blockers)
Thiazide diuretics	• Aggravate glycaemic control in NIDDM • Exacerbate hyperlipidaemia	• Use loop diuretic or alternative anti-hypertensive drugs
Retinopathy Mydriatics (eyedrops or systemic atropinic drugs)	• In patients with rubeosis or previous eye surgery, glaucoma may be precipitated	• Seek ophthalmological advice before dilating pupils
Anticoagulants and thrombolytic drugs	• May predispose to vitreous haemorrhage in patients with proliferative changes	• Avoid if possible
Autonomic neuropathy: *Postural hypotension* Ganglion-blocking agents and vasodilators	• Aggravate postural hypotension	• Avoid, especially in the elderly
Impotence Ganglion-blocking agents β-adrenergic blockers Clonidine α-methyldopa Thiazide diuretics (?)	• Aggravate erectile failure	• Use alternative antihypertensive drugs, e.g. ACE inhibitors, calcium channel blockers or prazosin

80　Infection and Diabetes Mellitus

Summary

• Infection impairs glycaemic control in diabetic patients and is one of the commoner identified precipitating factors for diabetic ketoacidosis.

• The presence of diabetes impairs several aspects of phagocyte function, including cell movement, phagocytosis and intracellular killing of microorganisms; hyperglycaemia reduces oxidative killing capacity because increased glucose metabolism through the polyol pathway consumes NADPH, which is necessary to generate superoxide radicals.

• Although diabetic patients are strikingly prone to unusual infections with rare organisms (e.g. mucormycosis, enterococcal meningitis, osteomyelitis), to tuberculosis and to complicated urinary tract infections, it is not clear whether their general susceptibility to infection is increased or not.

It is widely believed that patients with diabetes are more prone to infection than their non-diabetic peers. This assumption is often based on personal experience of a few patients with difficult and protracted episodes of infection. There is no doubt that diabetic patients have higher carriage rates of staphylococci on the skin and of candida on the oral and genital mucosae. Therefore, it is not surprising that when these surfaces are breached by surgery or instrumentation, there is a higher incidence of wound infections and genital or oral candidiasis. However, it is still unclear whether diabetic people have a general increase in the rate of infection. Indirect evidence from a study of American factory workers showed that 28% of the diabetic employees were absent for 10 days or more in one year due to infections as compared with 15% of the controls; however, this difference was not statistically significant [1].

Infection undoubtedly disturbs blood glucose control [2] and infection is one of the commonest precipitating causes of diabetic ketoacidosis [3] (see Chapter 49). Studies have shown a relationship between the level of blood glucose and carriage rates of staphylococci [4] and, further, the rates of infection [5]. The effect of glucose control is multifactorial and related to defects in the cellular and humoral immune systems.

Cellular defects

Abnormalities of all aspects of phagocyte function have been described in diabetes, namely adherence [6], cell movement [7], phagocytosis [8] and intracellular killing [9].

Cell movement

Cell movement (cytotaxis, chemotaxis or leucotaxis) is difficult to measure and its relevance to the clinical situation is dubious (except in the rare inherited disorder of Job's syndrome or the 'lazy leucocyte disorder' of poor cell movement). However, movement does appear to be generally depressed in diabetes, with no additive effects of poor glycaemic control. Poor cell movement may, in fact, be inherited, as defects have been reported in the first-degree relatives of patients with IDDM [7].

Phagocytosis

This is the process of ingestion of a target particle, and encompasses recognition, adherence and engulfment. The phagocyte (neutrophil or macrophage) must first recognize the target as foreign, which it does via receptors on the cell membrane for immunoglobulin (IgG), complement (C3b) and lectins (simple sugars). Immunoglobulin IgA and IgG levels in patients with diabetes may be reduced in those subjects bearing HLA B8/DR3 [10, 11]. However, the levels of antibodies against specific microorganisms (e.g. *Pneumococcus* [12]) have shown no differences between diabetic subjects and controls. Complement deficiency is common in IDDM, with 25% of subjects having low C4 levels [13]. The genes encoding C4 are in linkage disequilibrium with HLA B8/DR3 [14]. It is not clear what effect these abnormalities might have on recognition in general.

Various techniques have been employed to measure phagocytosis. Many of the methods are relatively imprecise and involve visual evaluation of target engulfment or plating techniques which measure phagocytosis by counting the remaining viable colonies of target bacteria. These differing techniques may partly explain the divergent reports relating to defects in phagocytosis. In the author's experience, phagocytosis is a very robust process, unaffected by hyperglycaemia of up to 50 mmol/l [15]. Subtle improvements in phagocytosis have been reported during improvements in diabetic control: treatment of patients with intravenous insulin to reduce the blood glucose concentration from 18 to 5 mmol/l resulted in enhanced phagocytosis [16].

Killing

Following ingestion of the target organism into the phagocyte, lysosomal granules are discharged into the phagocytic vacuole and killing proceeds by both oxidative and non-oxidative means. Oxidative killing occurs at an earlier stage than non-oxidative [17], and employs active oxygen products, e.g. superoxide, hydrogen peroxide and hypochlorite. The energy for this process is provided by the hexose monophosphate shunt (HMPS). Oxidative killing is initiated by a membrane oxidase which utilizes the electron donor, NADPH, and produces superoxide radicals. The neutrophil membrane is permeable to glucose, high intracellular levels of which greatly reduce the availability of NADPH. Under normal circumstances, glucose enters the HMPS and generates NADPH but in hyperglycaemia, high glucose levels swamp the HMPS and are metabolized by aldose reductase through the polyol pathway [18]. Aldose reductase is an NADPH-requiring enzyme and competes for this, thereby reducing the cell's ability to mount an oxidative attack and thereby inhibiting killing. Aldose reductase inhibitors have been shown to reverse these abnormalities, and these agents can restore both superoxide levels and impaired killing capacity to normal [18].

There are several methods for measuring organism-killing ability. Neutrophils can be simply incubated with test organisms and subsequently lysed, when viable bacteria are counted. More reliable and reproducible are the radiometric assays, based on the principle that only viable organisms can take up a radio-labelled marker [19]. Such assays, using specific test strains of *Candida albicans* (which should be obtained from a centre experienced in the technique), can be used for both research and clinical screening of neutrophil function.

Unusual infections

Patients with diabetes are prone to unusual infections with rare organisms, such as rhinocerebral mucormycosis, Gram-negative enterococcal meningitis, malignant external otitis and emphysematous cystitis or cholecystitis. It is important to recognize these infections, as prompt antimicrobial therapy — sometimes combined with surgery — greatly increases the chances of cure.

Rhinocerebral mucormycosis

This is a fungal infection, usually with *Mucor* (Figs 80.1 and 80.2) or *Rhizopus* spp., which may infect diabetic patients (whether well-controlled or in diabetic ketoacidosis), and especially those who abuse alcohol. It most commonly affects the lungs but may involve the paranasal air sinuses, and in diabetic or immunosuppressed subjects, may invade the skull, orbit or even brain (Fig. 80.3). Even with aggressive treatment, the established infection still carries a mortality of up to 50%. The clinical picture is often that of severe sinusitis with a bloody nasal discharge, but features such as proptosis, limitation of eye movements and failing vision (suggestive of orbital involvement) or of pain and discoloration of the tip of the nose should alert the physician, even in the UK [20]. The patient is also likely to have a severe, persistent acidaemia. Diagnosis is by his-

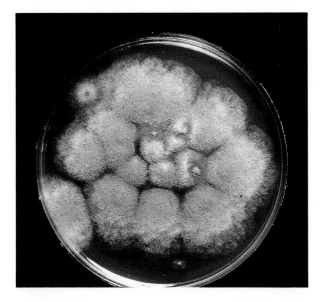

Fig. 80.1. Culture plate showing growth of *Mucor*. (Reproduced by kind permission of Dr R.C. Spencer, Royal Hallamshire Hospital, Sheffield.)

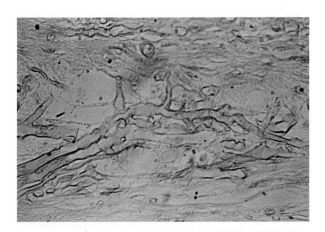

Fig. 80.2. Histological section of nasal submucosa, showing invasion by hyphae of *Mucor* (×400). (Reproduced by kind permission of Dr R.C. Spencer, Royal Hallamshire Hospital, Sheffield.)

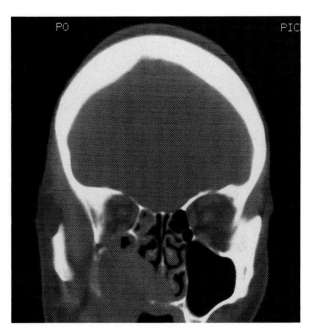

Fig. 80.3. CT scan showing rhinocerebral mucormycosis in a diabetic patient. The right maxillary sinus is filled and there is invasion of the floor of the orbit and the turbinates. (Reproduced by kind permission of Dr R. Nakielny, Royal Hallamshire Hospital, Sheffield.)

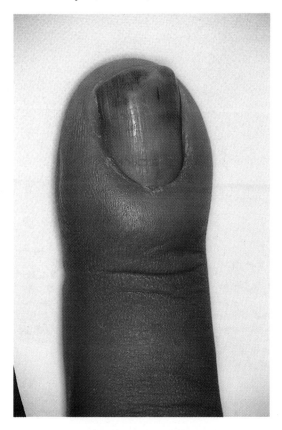

Fig. 80.4. Bolstering of the nail-fold due to chronic paronychia involving candida. (Reproduced by kind permission of Dr Ian MacFarlane, Walton Hospital, Liverpool.)

tology and culture of biopsies of affected mucosae (Figs 80.1 and 80.2). Intravenous amphotericin-B is the drug of choice, and extensive surgical debridement may be necessary.

Malignant external otitis

This infection can be extremely serious, hence its description as 'malignant'. It is almost always due to *Pseudomonas* spp. and may follow syringing of the external auditory canal. It should be suspected in a patient with otalgia and otorrhoea, and poor diabetic control. Standard antipseudomonal agents should be used and a surgical opinion sought.

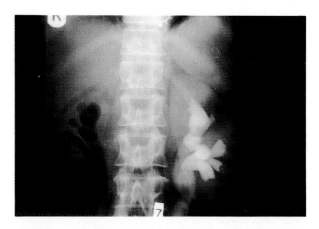

Fig. 80.5. Emphysematous pyelonephritis. Intravenous pyelogram showing gas filling the pelvicalyceal system of the right kidney. (Reproduced by kind permission of Dr Ian MacFarlane, Walton Hospital, Liverpool.)

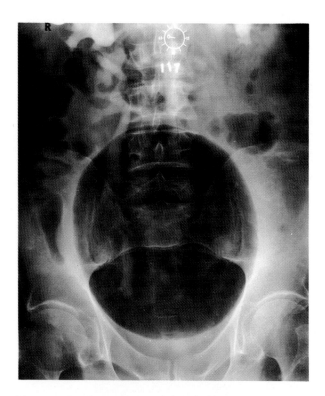

Fig. 80.6. Emphysematous cystitis. The bladder is grossly distended with gas. (Reproduced by kind permission of Dr Ian MacFarlane, Walton Hospital, Liverpool.)

Enterococcal meningitis

The classical physical signs of meningitis may be absent in this infection. The patient is likely to be ketoacidotic and the Gram-negative organisms should be obtainable from blood cultures.

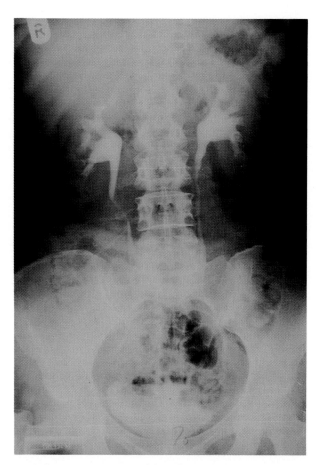

Fig. 80.7. Acute papillary necrosis, showing loss of a papilla and a calyceal ring shadow in the left kidney. (Reproduced by kind permission of Dr Ian MacFarlane, Walton Hospital, Liverpool.)

Infections of the skin and subcutaneous tissues

These seem to be common in newly presenting or poorly controlled diabetic patients, and may significantly worsen metabolic control. Acute and chronic paronychia, often involving candida (Fig. 80.4) may occur. *Necrotizing cellulitis* (progressive synergistic gangrene) is usually a combined infection involving streptococci and staphylococci or Gram-negative organisms; this often spreads rapidly under the skin, which can be of deceptively normal appearance. It is rare and tends to affect older and debilitated patients. It demands immediate treatment with high-dose intravenous antibiotics and often requires surgical debridement or even amputation. Mortality is high, as with *Fournier's gangrene* which involves the scrotum and perineum. Diabetic foot ulcers frequently have an infective component and are usually colonized by multiple organisms, aerobic or anaerobic and sometimes gas-forming, often

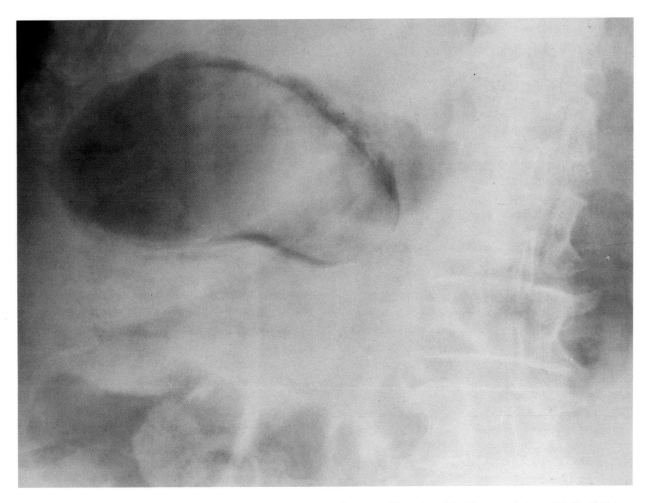

Fig. 80.8. Plain abdominal radiograph showing emphysematous cholecystitis. (Reproduced by kind permission of Dr R. Nakielny, Royal Hallamshire Hospital, Sheffield.)

acting synergistically [21]. Infection may spread into the surrounding soft tissues, fascial spaces and bones of the feet (see Figs 70.5 and 70.6). Because infection with several organisms is so common, both aerobic and anaerobic cultures should be set up from material taken from the deeper parts of the wound. Fastidious organisms (e.g. *Eikenella* spp.) should be sought on repeated culture in patients who fail to respond to initial antibiotic therapy.

Infections of the urinary tract

Cystitis is common in diabetic women and relatively often is complicated by ascending infection: renal scarring due to *pyelonephritis* is several times commoner in diabetic than in non-diabetic subjects. Renal infections may rarely be complicated by *emphysematous pyelonephritis*, in which Gram-negative rods or other organisms generate gas within the substance of the kidney [22]; the radiographic appearances may be diagnostic (Fig. 80.5). *Emphysematous cystitis* (Fig. 80.6) is another severe and fortunately rare sequel of lower urinary tract infection. Other complications include *perinephric abscess* and *papillary necrosis*, in which fragments of sloughed medullary tissue can be identified histologically in the urine and retrograde pyelography may demonstrate loss of papillae and 'ring shadows' lying in the calyces or pelvis (Fig. 80.7). It must be remembered that intravenous pyelography may precipitate acute renal failure in papillary necrosis and should not be performed if the diagnosis is suspected. All these conditions have a high mortality and must be treated rapidly and energetically.

Infections of the lung, gut and other sites

Tuberculosis was previously common in diabetic patients but now, as in the general population, is relatively rare. Asian and Afro-Caribbean diabetic

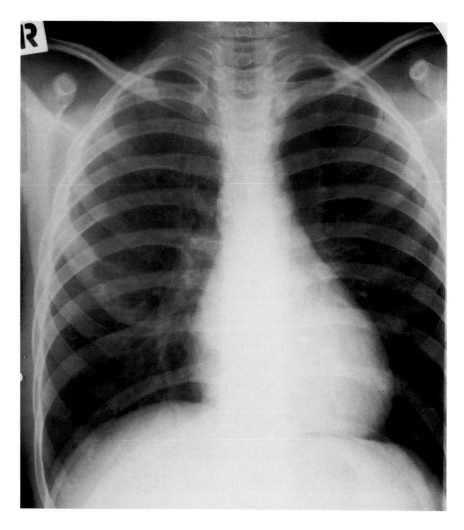

Fig. 80.9. Chest radiograph showing osteomyelitis in the left fourth rib of a diabetic child. (Reproduced by kind permission of Dr A. Barringdon, Royal Hallamshire Hospital, Sheffield.)

patients (in the UK) are still at increased risk of developing tuberculosis. Infection is usually due to reactivation of an old focus rather than through fresh contact.

Emphysematous cholecystitis (Fig. 80.8) is another rare infection, relatively commoner in diabetic patients, in which clostridia and other gas-forming organisms cause inflammation and often necrosis of the gall-bladder. *Ascending cholangitis*, with gas formation in the biliary system and liver, may ensue and mortality is very high. *Gingivitis* and *periodontal disease* are common in diabetic patients, particularly if poorly controlled.

Osteomyelitis in the diabetic foot (Fig. 70.6) is discussed fully in Chapter 70. *Vertebral osteomyelitis*, sometimes associated with epidural abscess formation, may present with backache. Other sites may occasionally be involved (Fig. 80.9). Diagnosis of osteomyelitis may be difficult, especially in the foot, where rarefaction of the bones and periosteal reactions (localized thickening of cor-

tical bone) and non-specific radiographic findings are common (see Chapter 73). Three-phase radionuclide bone scans may demonstrate abnormalities in early blood flow which are apparently more specific [23].

R. MALCOLM WILSON

References

1 Pell D, D'Alonzo CA. Sickness absenteeism in employed diabetics. *Am J Public Health* 1967; **57**: 253–60.
2 Colwell AR. Clinical use of insulin. In: Ellenberg M, Rifkin H, eds. *Diabetes Mellitus, Theory and Practice.* New York: McGraw-Hill, 1970: 624–37.
3 Nabarro JDN. Diabetic acidosis. In: Leibel BS, Wrenshall, eds. *Nature and Treatment of Diabetes.* New York: Excerpta Medica, 1965: 545–63.
4 Lipsky BA, Pecoraro BE, Chen MS, Koepsell MD. Factors affecting staphylococcal colonisation among NIDDM outpatients. *Diabetes Care* 1987; **10**: 483–6.
5 Rayfield EJ, Ault MJ, Kensch GT, Brothers MJ, Nechemias C, Smith H. Infection and diabetes: the case for glucose control. *Am J Med* 1982; **72**: 439–50.

6 Wilson RM, Galvin AM, Robins RA, Reeves WG. A flow cytometric method for the measurement of phagocytosis of candida by polymorphonuclear leucocytes. *J Immunol Methods* 1985; **76**: 247–53.

7 Molenaar DM, Palumbo PJ, Wilson WR, Rims RE. Leucocyte chemotaxis in diabetic patients and their non-diabetic first degree relatives. *Diabetes* 1976; **25** (Suppl 2): 880–3.

8 Bybee JD, Rogers DE. The phagocytic activity of polymorphonuclear leucocytes obtained from patients with diabetes mellitus. *J Lab Clin Med* 1964; **64**: 1–13.

9 Wilson RM, Reeves WG. Neutrophil function in diabetes. In: Nattrass M, ed. *Recent Advances in Diabetes*, Vol 2. Edinburgh: Churchill Livingstone, 1986: 127–39.

10 Smith WI, Rabin BS, Huellmontel A, Van Thiel DH, Drash A. Immunopathology of juvenile-onset diabetes mellitus. I. IgA deficiency and juvenile diabetes. *Diabetes* 1978; **27**: 1092–7.

11 Hoddinott S, Dornan J, Bear JC, Farid NR. Immunoglobulin levels, immunodeficiency and HLA in Type 1 (insulin-dependent) diabetes mellitus. *Diabetologia* 1982; **23**: 326–9.

12 Lederman MM, Rodman HM, Schacter BZ, Jones PK, Schiffman G. Antibody response to pneumonococcal polysaccharides in insulin-dependent diabetes mellitus. *Diabetes Care* 1982; **5**: 36–9.

13 Vergani D, Johnston C, B-Abdullah N, Barnett AH. Low serum C4 concentrations: an inherited predisposition to insulin dependent diabetes. *Br Med J* 1983; **286**: 923–8.

14 Charlesworth JA, Timmermans V, Golding J. The complement system in Type 1 (insulin-dependent) diabetes. *Diabetologia* 1987; **30**: 372–9.

15 Wilson RM, Reeves WG. Neutrophil phagocytosis and killing in insulin-dependent diabetes. *Clin Exp Immunol* 1986; **63**: 478–84.

16 Kjersem H, Hilsted J, Madsbad S, Wandall JH, Johansen KS, Borregaard N. Polymorphonuclear leucocyte dysfunction during short term metabolic changes from normo- to hyperglycaemia in Type 1 (insulin dependent) diabetic patients. *Infection* 1988; **16**: 215–21.

17 Nathan CF. Secretion of oxygen intermediates: Role in effector functions of activated macrophages. *Federation Proc* 1982; **41**: 2206–11.

18 Wilson RM, Tomlinson DR, Reeves WG. Neutrophil sorbitol production impairs oxidative killing in diabetes. *Diabetic Med* 1987; **4**: 37–40.

19 Bridges CG, Da Silva GL, Yamamura M, Valdimarsson H. A radiometric assay for the combined measurement of phagocytes and intracellular killing of *Candida albicans*. *Clin Exp Immunol* 1980; **42**: 226–33.

20 Larkin JG, Butcher IG, Frier BM, Brebner H. Fatal rhinocerebral mucormycosis in a newly-diagnosed diabetic. *Diabetic Med* 1986; **3**: 266–8.

21 Wheat LJ, Allen SD, Henry M *et al*. Diabetic foot infections. Bacteriologic analysis. *Arch Int Med* 1986; **146**: 1935–40.

22 Zabbo A, Montie JE, Popowniak KL, Weinstein AJ. Bilateral emphysematous pyelonephritis. *Urology* **1985**; 25: 293–6.

23 Seldin DW, Heikin JP, Feldman F, Alderson PO. Effect of soft-tissue pathology on detection of pedal osteomyelitis in diabetics. *J Nucl Med* 1985; **26**: 988–93.

Surgery and Diabetes Mellitus

Summary

- Surgical 'stress' suppresses insulin release and stimulates counter-regulatory hormone secretion, increasing catabolism overall; in insulin-deficient diabetic patients, hyperglycaemia and ketosis may result.
- Hypoglycaemia due to excessive insulin or sulphonylurea treatment in starved patients is the other major hazard of surgery.
- Successful management of surgery in diabetic patients requires a simple and safe procedure which is fully understood by all staff.
- Long-acting sulphonylureas or insulins should be changed for shorter-acting agents some days before surgery, to reduce the risk of hypoglycaemia.
- Well-controlled NIDDM patients undergoing minor surgery only require close glycaemic monitoring.
- Poorly controlled NIDDM patients, or those requiring major surgery, should be treated as for IDDM.
- IDDM patients require continuous administration of both insulin and glucose during surgery, ideally with potassium to prevent hypokalaemia. The standard 'cocktail' is 15 U short-acting insulin plus 10 mmol KCl in 500 ml of 10% dextrose, given intravenously at 100 ml/h. The insulin dosage should be changed in case of hyper- or hypoglycaemia.
- Open-heart surgery requires higher rates of insulin delivery because of glucose-rich solutions and inotropes used during bypass, and the metabolic effects of hypothermia.

The metabolic response to surgery

Trauma in general, and surgery in particular, in-duces a complex series of hormonal and metabolic changes [1]. Insulin secretion is suppressed, and the production of counter-regulatory or 'stress' hormones (particularly cortisol and catecholamines) is greatly increased. In general, the greater the degree of surgical trauma, the greater the endocrine upset.

The metabolic result of these changes is a strong catabolic flux, with increased hepatic glucose production and breakdown of protein and fat. Normally, these changes are of little clinical significance, but in the diabetic patient — compromised by absolute or relative insulin deficiency — catabolism is enhanced and dangerous glycaemic instability and ketosis may result. These problems may be compounded by the period of starvation which accompanies surgery.

Principles of management

Management principles are determined by the degree of surgical trauma, the period of starvation necessary, and the patient's insulin reserves. Insulin-treated patients (mostly IDDM) must be assumed to have no endogenous insulin, whereas non-insulin-treated subjects can be considered to have at least some residual B-cell function. Thus, for IDDM patients to undergo surgery safely, a system of exogenous insulin and carbohydrate supply is needed. NIDDM patients will need a similar system only for major surgery; otherwise, simple observation is generally sufficient. These principles are outlined in Table 81.1, and practical details are discussed below.

'Safety and simplicity' are the watchwords of surgical diabetic management. Safety should be ensured if the above basic principles are observed.

Table 81.1. Principles of diabetes management during surgery.

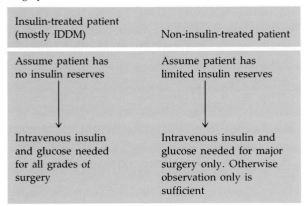

Insulin-treated patient (mostly IDDM)	Non-insulin-treated patient
Assume patient has no insulin reserves	Assume patient has limited insulin reserves
↓	↓
Intravenous insulin and glucose needed for all grades of surgery	Intravenous insulin and glucose needed for major surgery only. Otherwise observation only is sufficient

Simplicity is essential, as surgery is frequently required in the diabetic patient and its bedside management is usually undertaken by junior doctors with little or no special knowledge of diabetes. Protocols of management should *not* aim for normoglycaemia or even near-normoglycaemia, as this has been shown to be unnecessary: outcome is not improved and the risks of hypoglycaemia are considerably increased [2]. It is particularly important to avoid hypoglycaemia, as the surgical or postsurgical patient may be unaware of or unable to communicate this. Sensible glycaemic targets are outlined in Table 81.5. A further point is that it is not so much the treatment method itself, but rather the skill, care and enthusiasm with which it is performed, which determines the overall results. This is well shown in Table 81.2, which compares glycaemic control and complications in two nearby hospitals using quite different systems of diabetic surgical care. The results are good, and almost identical in both hospitals, despite the differences in management.

In general, wound healing and infection rates are now similar to those in non-diabetic people [2], although operations on ischaemic diabetic feet are an exception. Postoperative mortality and morbidity figures should also be at non-diabetic levels, and the length of stay in hospital little different from the norm.

Surgery and the patient with NIDDM

Preoperative assessment, for both IDDM and NIDDM patients, is outlined in Table 81.3. The essentials are to ensure reasonable glycaemic control and also to confirm fitness for anaesthesia. Close liaison with anaesthetic staff is essential. Chlorpropamide, if used, should be stopped at least 5 days before surgery, and if necessary a shorter-acting sulphonylurea (e.g. tolbutamide) substituted. This is because of the very long duration of action of chlorpropamide, and hence its potential hypoglycaemic hazards during starvation.

NIDDM patients undergoing major surgery which requires prolonged starvation are best managed with a system of continuous glucose and insulin delivery as for IDDM patients. Poorly

Table 81.2. Diabetic management during surgery — results of two different systems.

	Method 1	Method 2
	Glucose−potassium−insulin intravenous infusion	Subcutaneous insulin injections + intravenous glucose infusion
Number of patients	68	136
Mean preoperative blood glucose	8.6 mmol/l	7.6 mmol/l
Mean postoperative blood glucose	10.4 mmol/l	10.4 mmol/l
Hypoglycaemic episodes	1	0
Postoperative ketoacidosis	0	0

Note: The above results refer to IDDM patients managed during surgery at the Freeman Hospital (Method 1) and the Royal Victoria Infirmary (Method 2), Newcastle-upon-Tyne. Despite the different management methods, glycaemic control and occurrence of complications were not significantly different.

Table 81.3. Preoperative assessment of the diabetic patient requiring surgery.

- Assess glycaemic control
- Adjust diabetic treatment as necessary to optimize glycaemic control; substitute shorter-acting preparations for chlorpropamide or ultralente
- Arrange other investigations if needed, e.g. chest X-ray, electrocardiogram, renal function
- Arrange for surgery in morning if possible
- Liaise with anaesthetist

controlled NIDDM subjects should also be treated in this way, after initial stabilization on insulin (either in hospital or at home). Except in these situations, the remaining endogenous insulin reserves of the NIDDM patient will generally see them safely through surgery, and a system of simple observation only is needed [3].

Throughout the perioperative period, frequent glycaemic monitoring is required and glucose-containing infusion fluids must be avoided. Sulphonylurea drugs, if used, should be omitted until the first postoperative meal (Table 81.4).

Surgery and the patient with IDDM

Many management methods have been advocated in the past [4, 5], perhaps demonstrating previous imperfections in treatment. Simple omission of insulin was an early system, later giving way to a series of methods utilizing 'split normal doses' [6]. These involved giving various proportions of the patient's usual morning insulin dose (usually one-half or two-thirds), followed by glucose

Table 81.4. Management of NIDDM subjects during surgery.

Minor surgery, good glycaemic control
- Admit day before surgery
- Operate in morning if possible
- Omit breakfast and oral hypoglycaemic drugs on day of surgery
- Avoid glucose-containing intravenous infusions
- Monitor blood glucose with strips 2-hourly initially, reducing frequency later as necessary
- Restart oral hypoglycaemic drugs with the first postoperative meal

Major surgery, poor glycaemic control
- Admit 2–3 days before surgery
- Stabilize glycaemic control using short-acting insulin
- Treat as for IDDM on day of surgery

NB: Poor glycaemic control = fasting blood glucose level >8 mmol/l, other values >10 mmol/l.

infusions of various rates and concentrations. A more physiologically attractive version of these now-outdated methods is to give the *full* morning insulin dose, followed by a glucose infusion (usually 10%) at a rate to match the patient's usual dietary intake.

Nowadays, however, systems which continuously provide intravenous glucose and insulin are preferred. 'Mini-pump' methods [7] utilize low insulin doses (0.5–1.0 U/h) given by intravenous pump infusion; this is usually accompanied by a glucose drip, although for relatively brief operations this is sometimes omitted. Glycaemic control using the 'mini-pump' system is not always good, and with such low insulin delivery rates, there must be some risk of metabolic decompensation. Larger doses of both insulin (2–4 U/h) and glucose (5–10 g/h) are therefore preferable. These provide greater 'metabolic protection', and give more room for dose adjustments to achieve acceptable glycaemic control.

In practice, there are two methods by which insulin and glucose can be delivered in this way. The first is to use separate intravenous lines, one to deliver glucose (usually 100 ml 10% dextrose solution given per hour, preferably by electronic drip-counter pump), together with a 'piggy-backed' infusion of insulin given by a syringe-driver (usually at 2–4 U/h) [8] (Fig. 81.1). The second 'combined infusion' method is now the more popular, and comprises glucose and insulin mixed in a single infusion bag, usually with a small amount of potassium to prevent hypokalaemia. This is the so-called 'glucose–potassium–insulin' or 'GKI' system [4] (Fig. 81.2), which has gained widespread acceptance due to its simplicity and effectiveness [9].

The glucose–potassium–insulin ('GKI') system

The combined GKI infusion (Table 81.5) generally contains 500 ml 10% dextrose, 10 mmol potassium chloride (KCl), and 15 U short-acting insulin, infused over 5 h. It therefore delivers similar amounts of glucose and insulin to the 'separate line' system, but is considerably simpler and does not require electronic gadgetry. It also avoids one of the main problems of separate drips and pumps, i.e. failure of one of the lines (through the infusion running out, the infusion cannula becoming blocked or dislodged, pump malfunction, etc.) whilst the other continues, a situation which could lead to dangerous hypo- or hyperglycaemia.

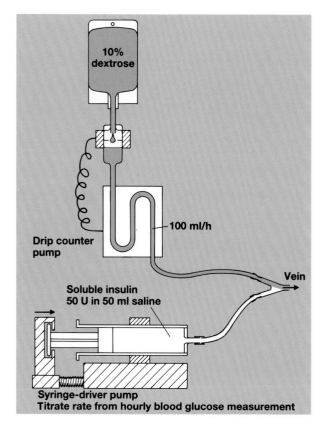

Fig. 81.1. The 'separate line' method of continuous intravenous glucose and insulin infusion. The glucose is delivered by drip-counter at a constant rate of 100 ml 10% dextrose (10 g glucose) hourly. The pump contains 50 U short-acting insulin in 50 ml 0.9% saline (1 U/ml), the rate being varied according to hourly bedside blood glucose testing.

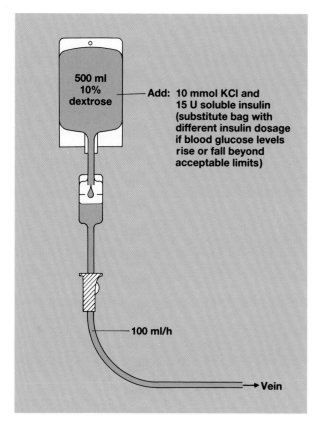

Fig. 81.2. The 'GKI' infusion system for continuous intravenous delivery of glucose and insulin. The single infusion bag contains 500 ml 10% dextrose with 15 U short-acting insulin and 10 mmol KCl. It is infused at 100 ml/h. The amount of insulin in the infusion is varied by substituting a new bag if bedside blood glucose tests are outside acceptable limits (see Table 81.5).

When adding insulin and potassium solutions to the bag, it is important to use a needle which is long enough to clear the self-sealing bung, to mix the bag well and to label it clearly with the additions. The insulin content of the infusion is altered by substituting a new bag according to frequent blood glucose monitoring (Table 81.5), and the potassium content is varied depending on the results of regular plasma electrolyte tests. Dilutional hyponatraemia may rarely occur when GKI infusion is prolonged. This should be treated by additional saline infusion, and if necessary slowing the GKI slightly. When volume overload is a problem, more concentrated dextrose infusions (e.g. 20%) are given in smaller volumes, with appropriate adjustments of insulin and potassium content.

GKI infusion can also be used for radiological and endoscopic investigations in IDDM patients which require starvation. It is also a useful and versatile maintenance infusion when vomiting or anorexia prevents eating.

Postoperative management

As soon as the patient is able to eat normally again, the usual treatment regimen can be restarted. Frequent glycaemic monitoring is essential because of the variable effects of surgical trauma and other factors such as inactivity, postoperative infection and changes in other medication.

Practicalities of management

Some teaching hospitals operate a 'diabetes team' for the care of diabetic patients undergoing surgery. The average district general hospital is not so luxuriously staffed, but this in no way precludes the operation of a successful service. A simple, brief and concise protocol of management should be agreed upon by the diabetes specialist, surgeons and anaesthetists. Copies of this protocol can then be widely distributed (Fig. 81.3), and the system put into operation by junior surgical and anaes-

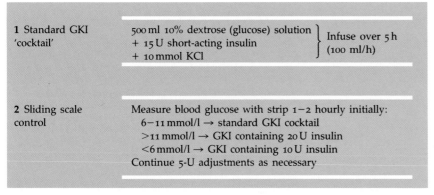

1 Standard GKI 'cocktail'	500 ml 10% dextrose (glucose) solution + 15 U short-acting insulin + 10 mmol KCl	Infuse over 5 h (100 ml/h)
2 Sliding scale control	Measure blood glucose with strip 1–2 hourly initially: 6–11 mmol/l → standard GKI cocktail >11 mmol/l → GKI containing 20 U insulin <6 mmol/l → GKI containing 10 U insulin Continue 5-U adjustments as necessary	

Table 81.5. The glucose–potassium–insulin or 'GKI' infusion system.

Notes: (1) Any short-acting insulin can be used, e.g. Humulin S, or, Actrapid. (2) The frequency of monitoring can usually be reduced later. (3) In practice, alterations in the standard GKI infusion are not often needed; if so, the current infusion bag should be taken down and a new bag (containing the altered insulin dosage) substituted.

1 **Ensure satisfactory preoperative control. Operate in morning if possible**

2 **Liaise with anaesthetist**

3 **Omit breakfast, and insulin or oral hypoglycaemic drug, on morning of surgery**

4 **Non-insulin treated diabetic patients, having non-major surgery, need observation only. Chart 2-hourly glucose reagent strips on day of surgery. Patients taking oral hypoglycaemic drugs can restart those with next meal**

5 **Glucose-potassium-insulin ('GKI') is used in all other cases, i.e.**
(a) all insulin-treated diabetics; and
(b) major surgery in non-insulin treated diabetics

(i) At 8–9 a.m. on morning of surgery, start GKI infusion:

500 ml 10% dextrose
+15 U short-acting insulin   Infuse 5-hourly
+10 mmol KCl   (100 ml/h)

(ii) Check blood glucose 2-hourly initially and aim for 6–11 mmol/l.
If > 11 mmol/l, change to GKI with 20 U insulin
If < 6 mmol/l, change to GKI with 10 U insulin
Continue to adjust as necessary
(iii) Continue GKI until patients eat, then revert to usual treatment. If GKI is prolonged (> 24 h), check electrolytes daily for possible Na$^+$ or K$^+$ abnormalities

Fig. 81.3. A simple protocol for diabetes management during surgery.

thetic staff, leaving the diabetologist to supervise difficult cases.

A vital aspect of care is adequate blood glucose monitoring. This is generally done by nursing staff at the bedside, using glucose–oxidase reagent strips, read either visually or by meter. Measurements should be made 2-hourly on the day of surgery, extending the interval later as necessary. Accuracy with these monitoring methods may be poor [10], and an occasional laboratory measurement may be advisable. Nowadays, all hospitals using reagent strips for diabetic monitoring should have some form of quality-control system to ensure

reasonable accuracy, and all relevant staff should be carefully trained in their use.

Special surgical situations

Emergency surgery

Diabetic patients needing urgent rather than elective surgery must first be fully assessed clinically and biochemically. Not infrequently, the problem necessitating surgery may have led to metabolic decompensation, which should first be corrected, unless the need for surgery is immediate. The general management methods are as described above, although in insulin-treated patients, the time of their last injection must be noted. Insulin injected relatively recently will continue to be absorbed during and after surgery, and this will need to be remembered when prescribing intravenous fluids. Careful monitoring is needed, and sometimes a separate-line system is advisable.

Open-heart surgery

Cardiac surgery with cardiopulmonary bypass requires considerably greater amounts of insulin than other operations [11]. This is mainly because glucose-containing fluids are used to prime the bypass pump [11, 12], although even without such solutions, insulin requirements are still relatively high and also erratic [13]. These difficulties are probably due to the unusual degree of surgical trauma, the effect of induced hypothermia in impairing insulin action and the liberal use of inotropic drugs which also have counter-regulatory actions. Under these circumstances, GKI solutions are not effective [11], and a separate-line system with very frequent blood glucose monitoring is advisable [13, 14]. During the procedure, glucose must be infused slowly (if at all), but should be restarted at conventional rates immediately after surgery. Careful use of this system can achieve results which compare well with the artificial pancreas [13].

Caesarean section

For induced labour in insulin-treated diabetic women, a separate-line system of control is preferred; if caesarean section becomes necessary, this can simply be continued throughout the procedure. For elective caesarean section, however, the GKI system is simplest. Patients in late pregnancy are usually taking relatively high doses of insulin (see Chapter 83), and an infusion containing 20 U soluble insulin in 500 ml 10% dextrose may be best tried initially, with an appropriate adjustment to the 'sliding scale' used (Table 81.5). Use of the β-adrenergic agonist, ritodrine (to delay labour) or of glucocorticoids (to encourage fetal lung maturation) will increase insulin requirements. Insulin requirements drop dramatically at the time of delivery of the placenta, and the GKI should be stopped at this point. It can be restarted in the recovery room or ward, with a GKI solution containing less insulin (usually one-

half or two-thirds of the dosage used during labour). Subcutaneous insulin injections can be resumed — usually at close to the prepregnancy dosage — when the patient is able to eat again.

Surgery and ultralente regimens

A growing number of IDDM patients are being treated with multiple injections of short-acting insulin, usually by a pen-device injector, together with an evening injection of long-acting insulin [15] (see Chapter 39). The latter is often an ultralente preparation [16], which may have a particularly long duration of action and demands the same considerations as chlorpropamide in the NIDDM diabetic patient (see above). Ideally, a lente or isophane insulin should be substituted several days before surgery. If not, then less insulin will be needed in the GKI infusion used, and closer monitoring required.

GEOFFREY V. GILL

References

1 Elliott MJ, Alberti KGMM. Carbohydrate metabolism — effects of pre-operative starvation and trauma. *Clin Anaesthesiol* 1983; **1**: 527–50.

2 Hjortrup A, Sørensen, C, Dyremose E, Hjortso N-C, Kehlet H. Influence of diabetes mellitus on operative risk. *Br J Surg* 1985; **72**: 783–5.

3 Thompson J, Husband DJ, Thai AC, Alberti KGMM. Metabolic changes in the non-insulin dependent diabetic undergoing minor surgery: effect of glucose—insulin—potassium infusion. *Br J Surg* 1986; **73**: 301–4.

4 Alberti KGMM, Thomas DJB. The management of diabetes during surgery. *Br J Anaesthesiol* 1979; **51**: 693–710.

5 Alberti KGMM, Gill GV, Elliott MJ. Insulin delivery during surgery in the diabetic patient. *Diabetes Care* 1982; **5**: 65–77.

6 Shuman CR, Podolsky S. Surgery in the diabetic patient. In: Podolsky S, ed. *Clinical Diabetes: Modern Management*. New York: Appleton—Century—Crofts, 1980: 509–35.

7 Goldberg NJ, Wingert TD, Levin SR, Wilson SE, Viljoen JF. Insulin therapy in the diabetic surgical patient: metabolic and hormone response to low dose insulin infusion. *Diabetes Care* 1981; **4**: 279–84.

8 Podolsky S. Management of diabetes in the surgical diabetic patient. *Med Clin North Am* 1982; **66**: 1361–72.

9 Husband DJ, Thai AC, Alberti KGMM. Management of diabetes during surgery with glucose—insulin—potassium infusion. *Diabetic Med* 1986; **3**: 69–74.

10 Hutchison AS, Shenkin A. BM strips: how accurate are they in general wards? *Diabetic Med* 1984; **1**: 225–6.

11 Gill GV, Sherif IH, Alberti KGMM. Management of diabetes during open heart surgery. *Br J Surg* 1981; **68**: 171–2.

12 Crock PA, Ley CJ, Martin IK, Alford FP, Best JD. Hormonal and metabolic changes during hypothermic coronary artery bypass surgery in diabetic and non-diabetic subjects. *Diabetic Med* 1988; **5**: 47–52.

13 Elliot MJ, Gill GV, Home PD, Noy GA, Holden MP, Alberti

KGMM. A comparison of two regimens for the management of diabetes during open heart surgery. *Anaesthesiology* 1984; **60**: 364–8.

14 Watson BG, Elliott MJ, Pay DA, Williamson M. Diabetes mellitus and open heart surgery. A simple, practical closed loop insulin infusion system for blood glucose control. *Anaesthesia* 1986; **41**: 250–7.

15 Jefferson IG, Marteau TM, Smith MA, Baum JD. A multiple injection regimen using an insulin injection pen and pre-filled cartridged soluble human insulin in adolescents with diabetes. *Diabetic Med* 1985; **2**: 493–7.

16 Holman RR, Steemson J, Darling P, Reeves WG, Turner RC. Human ultralente insulin. *Br Med J* 1984; **288**: 665–8.

82   Eating Disorders and Diabetes Mellitus

Summary

• Eating disorders — anorexia and bulimia (food bingeing) — are apparently commoner in diabetic patients (particularly young women) than in the general population.

• Inflexible education about 'ideal' diet and weight may be partly responsible; fear of hypoglycaemia may encourage overeating.

• Diabetic patients may also lose weight by deliberately reducing or omitting insulin treatment.

• Life-threatening electrolyte disturbances and acute renal failure may result from induced diarrhoea or vomiting.

• Abnormal eating attitudes can be identified by standard questionnaires ('EAT' and 'EDI'), but diabetes-biased questions should be avoided.

• Eating disorders are frequently accompanied by poor diabetic control and may precipitate or aggravate acute painful neuropathy and other microvascular complications.

• Eating disorders are difficult to treat in diabetic patients, but may respond to psychotherapy or behavioural therapy; expert psychiatric help is needed.

Sir William Gull described anorexia nervosa in 1874 [1]. His patients, predominantly young girls, felt a compulsion to be thin and insisted they were too fat even when cachectic. They avoided fattening foods and many had bizarre and often secretive eating habits; some also abused laxatives, induced vomiting or exercised strenuously to reduce weight.

The diagnostic criteria for anorexia nervosa [2, 3] stipulate weight loss (exceeding 25% of pre-

morbid weight according to some authorities [3]) due to abnormal eating behaviour, amenorrhoea and a morbid fear of becoming fat.

Bulimia ('the hunger of an ox') described formally by Russell in 1979 [4] also mostly affects young women. Patients have binges when they eat large quantities of high-calorie foods (often several thousand calories at a time), followed by vomiting or use of laxatives or severe dietary restriction. They are frightened that they cannot stop eating voluntarily and have feelings of depression and self-depreciation after a binge. This condition is much more difficult to recognize than anorexia nervosa as patients may be obese, of normal weight or thin. Clinical examination is usually normal, although some will have erosion of the front teeth as a result of repeated vomiting.

Severely affected patients with these eating disorders may develop major electrolyte disturbances, especially profound hypokalaemia and acute renal failure due to vomiting and/or laxative-induced diarrhoea, and can die as a result of their illness.

Eating disorders have become increasingly recognized over the last 20 years, probably in part through enhanced media publicity, although there is also evidence that anorexia and bulimia are becoming commoner [5–7]. In parts of the world where many people do not have enough to eat, obesity is encouraged as a sign of prosperity. In the Western world, it used to be considered beautiful for women to be plump but in recent years it has become increasingly fashionable to be thin, as is witnessed by the diminishing vital statistics of beauty queens and photographic models. There is therefore a great deal of pressure — particularly from women's magazines — on all women of today to be thin, and this may contribute to the increased prevalence of eating disorders.

Psychiatric hospital units with a special interest in eating disorders have found that while initially they saw many patients with anorexia nervosa, more recently they have seen increasing numbers of patients with bulimia and now patients with 'multiple impulsive bulimia' — bulimia associated with other self-damaging forms of behaviour, e.g. multiple overdoses, repeated self-mutilation, drug abuse, sexual disinhibition and stealing.

The association with diabetes

Eating disorders were first associated with diabetes in 1980 by Fairburn and Steel, who reported three cases [8]. There followed several series of case reports suggesting that the association was commoner than would be expected by chance [9–11]. In a survey of 208 female IDDM patients aged 16–25 years, Steel et al. found that 7% had a clinically apparent eating disorder [12]. Even this high prevalence was probably an underestimate, particularly of bulimia, as only known cases were included; patients were not specifically questioned.

In order to try to assess more accurately the size of the problem and attitudes to eating in more detail, several workers have carried out surveys using standard questionnaires such as the EAT (Eating Attitude Test) and EDI (Eating Disorder Inventory) designed by Garner [13]. The EAT has been widely used to screen for cases of anorexia nervosa in groups at high risk for this disorder, for example among college students [14], and the EDI to assess psychological characteristics relevant to anorexia nervosa and bulimia [15]. Results of the original questionnaires may be difficult to interpret, as answers to some questions (e.g. 'Do you avoid foods with sugar in them?') are likely to be affected by diabetes per se [16]. Wing and colleagues found higher scores in diabetic patients using the unmodified EAT and Rodin et al. [17], applying the original EAT and EDI to 46 female diabetic patients, found an incidence of 19% for clinically significant disorders of eating and weight. Rosmark removed diabetes-related questions and found that 41 female diabetic patients had higher mean EAT scores than either female non-diabetic controls or male diabetic subjects [18]. Steel et al. [19] compared cohorts of 152 young IDDM women and 139 young IDDM men with age- and sex-matched controls, using the EAT and EDI. After diabetes-related questions were excluded, female diabetic patients scored significantly higher than their controls, whereas there was no difference between male diabetic and non-diabetic subjects. These studies add to the mounting evidence that clinical and subclinical eating disorders are particularly common in young female diabetic patients.

The clinical problem

It has become clear from clinical experience that, in addition to the usual artifices used by patients with anorexia nervosa and bulimia, diabetic patients commonly choose to omit insulin injections or reduce the dose of insulin to control their weight [9–11, 19–22]. The relationship between eating disorders and diabetic control is complex (Fig. 82.1). Many patients with diabetes and eating disorders described in the literature have been poorly controlled [20–24] (see Table 82.1) and those with pathologically high EAT and EDI scores tend to have a high HbA_1 [18]. Psychiatrists seeing patients referred to them by physicians because of an eating disorder stress that eating disorders cause poor control [24]. There are undoubtedly cases, particularly those with bulimia, where this appears to be the case. On the other hand, diabetologists seeing patients in the context of life-long diabetes suggest that eating disorders tend to occur more frequently in patients who are already poorly controlled [11], and that the emergence of an eating disorder in such patients appears to be another facet of long-standing behavioural disturbance. Indeed, eating disorders are a feature of 'brittle' diabetes (Chapter 88).

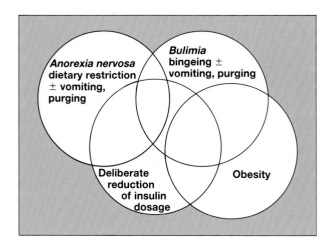

Fig. 82.1. The relationship between eating disorders and diabetic control.

Table 82.1. Metabolic and microvascular complications in 15 patients with clinically apparent eating disorders, identified from a randomly selected population of 208 female IDDM patients aged 16–25 years. (Adapted from Steel *et al.* 1987 [12].)

Complication	Number of patients affected
Persistent hyperglycaemia	11
Ketoacidosis	5
Hypoglycaemia	3
Retinopathy	11
(proliferative retinopathy)	(6)
Peripheral neuropathy	6
Nephropathy	6

There are, however, small numbers of patients who manage to control their diabetes well despite suffering from an eating disorder. Some with anorexia nervosa manage to reduce their carbohydrate intake and insulin dose in parallel without developing either ketoacidosis or hypoglycaemia. Some with bulimia increase their insulin in an attempt to compensate for a large binge and some try hard to control their eating disorder for fear of upsetting their diabetic control.

In addition to those who fulfil the formal criteria for an eating disorder, there is a large number of diabetic patients who possess the psychological characteristics of an eating disorder and who, as well as the usual tactics used by patients with anorexia nervosa and bulimia, commonly choose to reduce or omit their insulin injections to cause weight loss through diuresis and catabolism [9–11, 19–22]. Many of these patients are overweight, although their weight can be normal or low. This syndrome has been provisionally labelled 'MIDMED' ('Manipulation of Insulin Dose as a Manifestation of an Eating Disorder') [25]. These different clinical situations are summarized in Fig. 82.1.

Relationship to diabetic complications

There appears to be a high incidence of early-onset microvascular complications — retinopathy, nephropathy, autonomic neuropathy and peripheral neuropathy — in diabetic patients with eating disorders [8, 10, 20] (see Table 82.1). Patients have also been described with acute painful neuropathy coinciding with the development of an eating disorder, becoming very severe at the time of maximum weight loss and remitting as weight was regained [12] (see Fig. 61.7). Poor metabolic control is likely to be of major importance in

the aetiology of these microvascular complications but nutritional factors may also contribute.

Why does diabetes predispose to eating disorders?

The most obvious explanation for the high prevalence of abnormal eating attitudes in diabetic women is that they are constantly educated to focus on diet and food in order to control their diabetes. They are discouraged from eating sweet foods, which they may particularly enjoy, and made to feel guilty if they 'cheat'.

They are also encouraged to control their weight. Many diabetic people rightly associate insulin with weight gain, which often follows the start of treatment through a combination of rehydration and the anabolic effect of insulin, and there may be a marked increase during the first year after diagnosis. Even though many patients do not become overweight according to standard height–weight tables, they may find the rapid change in their body image frightening. Diabetic women tend to score highly on the 'drive for thinness' and 'body dissatisfaction' subscales of the EDI. Insulin-treated diabetic patients tend to be slightly heavier than their peers, probably partly because insulin delivered systemically rather than into the portal circulation over-stimulates adipose tissue formation. Another undoubted factor is that many patients find it easy to eat more than their dietary allowance but difficult to eat less, because of the risk of developing hypoglycaemia; occasionally patients overeat frequently because of a fear of hypoglycaemia.

Diabetes presents a challenge to an adolescent's self-esteem. Young diabetic patients often have low self-esteem and feel ineffective, psychological characteristics which predispose to the development of eating disorders.

It has also been suggested that the conflict between dependence and independence, which is an integral part of adolescent development, is greatly intensified in the diabetic adolescent who is dependent on treatment for survival but who is forced to assume a major role in regulating therapy. Such conflict may also be important in the development of eating disorders [10].

Treatment of eating disorders in diabetes

Treatment of these conditions is difficult. Patients should be referred for psychiatric help, preferably to a unit specifically interested in eating disorders. These units use behavioural, cognitive and psychotherapy often in combination with family therapy and group therapy. The emphasis may vary depending on the centre. Well-equipped units also have facilities for art and drama therapy, relaxation training, body image work, and may run anxiety management programmes.

Those unwilling to see a psychiatrist may be helped by an experienced, understanding physician preferably working closely with an interested psychiatrist. Patients with bulimia can be helped by discussing their problems and explaining that many others have similar difficulties. Diabetic patients usually already keep a diary in which they record insulin dose, blood glucose levels, hypoglycaemia, etc. and they should be encouraged also to record everything they eat and drink and particularly binges, vomiting and the use of laxatives. They should also be asked to record their feelings at the time of a binge. The diaries should then be discussed and patients encouraged to understand why they binge, to develop strategies to avoid it and to eat regularly (not avoiding meals after a binge), explaining that they may expect to gain weight initially. It is usually necessary to see patients fairly frequently for several months and it is important to involve members of the family.

Antidepressants have a place for those who are depressed and are also helpful in controlling bulimia in some who are not depressed.

Some patients refuse all help because their overwhelming desire to be thin blinds them to the need for a change in their behaviour. In severe cases, in-patient treatment is required and very occasionally it may be necessary to detain a patient compulsorily in a psychiatric unit if his or her life is in danger.

Conclusions

Eating disorders are particularly disabling in diabetic patients and present special management difficulties. These patients tend to be poorly controlled and often develop serious complications of diabetes. The first step towards more effective treatment is an increased awareness of the problem. Early recognition, sympathetic discussion of the patient's attitude to body weight and to eating and the avoidance of rapid weight gain in the first few months after diagnosis should all help to forestall the more serious manifestations of eating disorders in a substantial proportion of susceptible patients.

JUDITH M. STEEL

References

1 Gull WW. Anorexia nervosa (Apepsia hysterica, Anorexia hysterica). *Trans Clin Soc Lond* 1874; **7**: 22.
2 Russell GFM. Anorexia nervosa: its identity as an illness and its treatment. In: Price JH, ed. *Modern Trends in Psychological Medicine*, vol 2. London: Butterworths, 131–64.
3 *Diagnostic and Statistical Manual of Mental Disorders*, 3rd edn. Washington DC: American Psychiatric Association, 1980: 69.
4 Russell GFM. Bulimia nervosa, an ominous variant of anorexia nervosa. *Psychol Med* 1979; **6**: 429–48.
5 Kendell RE, Hall DJ, Hailey A, Babigian HM. Epidemiology of anorexia nervosa. *Psychol Med* 1976; **3**: 200–3.
6 Crisp AH, Palmer RL, Kalvey RS. How common is anorexia nervosa? A prevalence study. *Br J Psychiatr* 1976; **128**: 549–54.
7 Cooper PJ, Fairburn CG. Binge eating and self-induced vomiting in the community. A preliminary study. *Br J Psychiatr* 1983; **142**: 139–44.
8 Fairburn CG, Steel JM. Anorexia nervosa in diabetes mellitus. *Br Med J* 1980; **280**: 1167–8.
9 Roland OM, Bhanji S. Anorexia nervosa occurring in patients with diabetes mellitus. *Postgrad Med J* 1982; **58**: 354–6.
10 Powers PS, Malone JE, Duncan J. Anorexia nervosa and diabetes mellitus. *J Clin Psychiatr* 1983; **44**: 133–5.
11 Szmukler GI. Anorexia and bulimia in diabetics. *J Psychosomat Res* 1984; **28**: 365–9.
12 Steel JM, Young RJ, Lloyd GG, Clarke BF. Clinically apparent eating disorders in young diabetic women associated with painful neuropathy and other complications. *Br Med J* 1987; **294**: 859–62.
13 Garner DM, Garfinkel PE. The eating attitudes test: an index of the symptoms of anorexia nervosa. *Psychol Med* 1979; **9**: 273–9.
14 Garner DM, Garfinkel PE. Socio-cultural factors in the development of anorexia nervosa. *Psychol Med* 1980; **10**: 647–56.
15 Garner DM, Olmsted MP, Polivy J. Development and validation of a multidimensional eating disorder inventory for anorexia nervosa and bulimia. *Int J Eating Disord* 1983; **2**: 15–34.
16 Wing RA, Nowalk MP, Marcus MD, Koeske R, Finegold D. Subclinical eating disorders and glycemic control in adolescents with type I diabetes. *Diabetes Care* 1986; **9**: 162–7.
17 Rodin GM, Daneman D, Johnson LE, Kenshole A, Garfinkel PE. Anorexia nervosa and bulimia in female adolescents with insulin dependent diabetes mellitus, a systematic study. *J Psychiatr Res* 1985; **19**: 381–4.
18 Rosmark B, Berne C, Holmgren L, Lago C, Renholm G, Schilberg S. Eating disorders in patients with insulin dependent diabetes mellitus. *J Clin Psychiatr* 1986; **47**: 547–50.
19 Steel JM, Young RJ, Lloyd GG, Macintyre CCA. Abnormal eating attitudes in young insulin dependent diabetics *Br J Psychiatr* 1989; **155**: 515–21.

20 Garner S. Anorexia nervosa in diabetes mellitus. *Br Med J* 1980; **281**: 1144.

21 Hudson MS, Wentworth SM, Hudson J. Bulimia and diabetes. *N Engl J Med* 1983; **309**: 431−2.

22 Szmukler GI, Russell GFM. Diabetes mellitus, anorexia nervosa and bulimia. *Br J Psychiatr* 1983; **142**: 305−8.

23 Hudson JI, Hudson MS, Wentworth SM. Self-induced glycosuria. A novel method of purging in bulimia. *J Am Med Ass* 1983; **249**: 2501.

24 Hillard JR, Hillard PJA. Bulimia, anorexia nervosa and diabetes. Deadly combinations. *Psychiatr Clin North Am* 1984; **7**: 367−79.

25 Steel JM. Eating disorders and diabetes. *Practical Diabetes* 1987; **4**: 256.

SECTION 15
DIABETES IN SPECIAL GROUPS

83   Pregnancy and Diabetes Mellitus

Summary

• In the absence of increased insulin administration, glycaemic control worsens during pregnancy; possible causes include metabolic effects of the pregnancy hormones, tissue resistance to insulin and impaired insulin secretion.

• Mortality of the diabetic mother is now minimal; although there are no precise figures, it is probably slightly higher than in the general population.

• Retinopathy may worsen during pregnancy, perhaps because of the sudden improvement in metabolic control. This complication should be assessed and treated, preferably before pregnancy. Nephropathy also worsens during pregnancy and the nephrotic syndrome may develop.

• Perinatal mortality for diabetic pregnancies has improved vastly in the last 50 years but varies widely from country to country, with the standard of living and general (non-diabetic) perinatal mortality. In the UK in 1980, the general perinatal mortality was 14 per 1000 births and that for diabetic pregnancies 56 per 1000 births.

• The major causes of perinatal mortality are stillbirths (about half the cases), congenital malformations (3 times higher than in the general population) and the respiratory distress syndrome (RDS), especially in babies born prematurely.

• Malformations are possibly caused by maternal hyperglycaemia and the associated metabolic perturbations in the first trimester, at the time of organogenesis — emphasizing the need for strict glycaemic control in the first 10 weeks of pregnancy.

• Babies of diabetic mothers are heavier and longer (macrosomia) than those of non-diabetic mothers, a response to increased nutrient supply to the fetus and hypersecretion of insulin by the fetal islets. Macrosomia may lead to dystocia.

• Neonatal problems include increased proneness to RDS and jaundice (diseases of prematurity), hypoglycaemia (continued hypersecretion of insulin from the B cell), polycythaemia (due to relative fetal hypoxia) and hypocalcaemia (hyposecretion of parathyroid hormone).

• The management of a diabetic pregnancy requires a team approach and starts with pre-pregnancy counselling to offer contraceptive advice, explain the risks and relative contra-indications of pregnancy, treat complications and above all help the woman to achieve better glycaemic control.

• Antenatal visits at weekly or up to monthly intervals should include assessment and management of glycaemic control, diabetic complications including hypertension, and potential obstetric complications, especially pre-eclampsia, hydramnios and urinary tract infections.

• Control may be optimized by dietary and insulin adjustments, the latter based on home glucose monitoring data. HbA_1 will provide a check on glycaemic control. Continuous adjustments of insulin dose will need to be made and more than two insulin injections per day may be required.

• Delivery should be after at least 38 weeks in the absence of obstetric problems. Normoglycaemia is advisable, particularly in prolonged labour, and can be provided by intravenous insulin and dextrose infusions. Vaginal delivery is preferable; the indications for caesarean section are pelvic disproportion, an abnormal

uterus, placenta praevia, marked macrosomia and presentations other than cephalic.
• Gestational diabetes mellitus (GDM) is diabetes which presents in pregnancy, commonly in the middle of the second trimester. The frequency is between 1 and 2% of pregnancies, with an increased risk in the obese and those with a family history of diabetes.
• GDM is rarely symptomatic and can only be detected by screening. Though there is no consensus, screening at 28 weeks detects the majority of GDM. A random blood glucose of >6.0 mmol/l, or a value >8.0 mmol/l 1 h after a 75-g oral glucose tolerance test, is suggestive of GDM. A full oral glucose tolerance test should then be performed to confirm the diagnosis.
• Management of GDM includes assessment of diet and appropriate adjustments to reduce obesity. Adequate glycaemia is not achieved in about one-third of the women; insulin must then be added and postpregnancy follow-up is desirable to ensure that diabetes has resolved.

Historical perspective

The outlook for pregnancy in diabetic women has improved greatly during the last few decades. Before the discovery of insulin, it was rare for diabetic women to become pregnant and the prognosis was gloomy for those who did, with a maternal mortality rate approaching 50% and only a slender chance of the baby surviving [1]. Nowadays, the mortality rate in pregnant diabetic women is minimal [2, 3] and the perinatal mortality has fallen to around 5% [4–7]. There are many reasons for this improvement. The first and most dramatic change was due to the introduction of insulin. In the preinsulin era, the only treatment available was the 'starvation' diet (see Chapter 1) with which survival was barely possible; the increased insulin demands of pregnancy commonly precipitated ketoacidosis which often led to the death of both fetus and mother. The second change, less impressive but nonetheless important, has been the recognition of the need for very strict glycaemic control during pregnancy, assisted by the introduction of home blood glucose monitoring about a decade ago [8]. It is probable that the previously favoured regimen of a single daily injection of short-acting plus protamine–zinc insulin, coupled with hopelessly

inadequate self-monitoring methods based on glycosuria, helped to maintain the high perinatal mortality [9] and to encourage the development of serious and sometimes life-threatening microvascular complications [10]. In developed countries, pregnant diabetic women are now routinely treated with intensified insulin schedules, usually based on multiple daily injections, in conjunction with home blood glucose monitoring which is essential for their effective use [11].

From the mother's viewpoint, diabetic pregnancy has become safe; only very serious micro- or macrovascular complications are now regarded as relative contraindications to pregnancy (see below). The prospects for the fetus have also greatly improved. Our eventual aim — not yet realized — must be for pregnancy in diabetic women to be no more hazardous to either mother or fetus than pregnancy in the non-diabetic population.

The object of this chapter is to discuss the interactions between diabetes and pregnancy, and to suggest logical guidelines for the management of the diabetic pregnancy.

Effect of pregnancy on glucose tolerance

Pregnancy tends to alter carbohydrate tolerance, although the effect in normal women is subtle. Fasting plasma glucose falls slightly whereas postprandial values rise. Insulin secretion is increased and plasma levels are higher. Glycaemic control worsens in pregnant women with established diabetes if increases in insulin administration are not made. Diabetes may appear for the first time during pregnancy and most of these cases will have 'gestational' diabetes (see below), although some of these patients (perhaps as many as 50% [12]) may subsequently go on to develop permanent diabetes. There is also evidence that the incidence of true IDDM may increase during pregnancy [13].

The diabetogenic effect of pregnancy has been attributed to many different causes, ranging from accelerated breakdown of insulin by the placenta (no longer thought important) to the metabolic effects of sex steroids and other hormones whose secretion increases in pregnancy. Recent work has documented resistance to the biological actions of insulin during the second half of pregnancy (from mid-second trimester onwards) in both non-diabetic and diabetic animals and in man. Probably because of methodological problems, the precise level of the defect remains controversial, with insulin receptor numbers being reported variously as normal or reduced [14]. A separate postreceptor abnormality (manifested by reduced ability of insulin to promote the uptake and metabolism of glucose by its target tissues) has been attributed to the action of several hormones (including progesterone, cortisol, prolactin and placental lactogen) which rise in pregnancy [15]. Insulin secretion may also be relatively impaired [14] and so unable to generate the hyperinsulinaemia necessary to overcome the block to its action.

Effects of diabetes on pregnancy

Uncontrolled diabetes threatens both mother and fetus. The risks to each will be considered in turn; the subject of the teratogenic effect of diabetes is discussed fully in Chapter 84.

Risks of diabetes to the mother

MORTALITY

The general maternal mortality rate in the UK is currently two deaths per 10000 pregnancies. Although the precise figures are not known, the rate is probably higher in diabetic women. Of the 773 women registered in the 1980 UK Diabetic Pregnancy Survey [7], two died (one of keto-acidosis and the other of heart failure), and a North American study [2] has also reported an increased death rate. Most of the deaths notified to the American study were potentially avoidable as they were associated with ketoacidosis, hypoglycaemia or haemorrhage after the traumatic delivery of a macrosomic baby [2]. A few women aged 30–40 years have died from cardiac failure associated with major macrovascular disease (which could be regarded as a contraindication to pregnancy).

MORBIDITY

Women with IDDM develop microvascular complications, whose prevalence is closely related to the duration of the disease (Chapter 52). In the UK Diabetic Pregnancy Survey [7], the mean duration of diabetes was just under 10 years; 12% were reported to have retinopathy, 4% hypertension and 3% had evidence of nephropathy at their first antenatal visit.

Retinopathy tends to worsen during pregnancy [16] but usually does not lead to long-term loss of vision [17]. This deterioration may be associated with the sudden improvement in metabolic control achieved during pregnancy rather than the pregnant state itself [18]. Women with retinopathy should, therefore, undergo careful ophthalmological assessment and be treated if necessary before pregnancy can be advised. If glycaemic control is poor, it should be gradually improved before pregnancy is attempted. Stable, photocoagulated retinopathy appears to present no extra risk to patients whose glycaemic control is already good and is maintained [19].

Nephropathy can pose a more serious threat to the mother. Renal function tends to deteriorate in pregnancy and proteinuria may sometimes reach nephrotic proportions. If there is some degree of renal failure and/or hypertension, the baby may also be at risk: unlike diabetes in general, the fetus grows poorly, and the incidences of intrauterine growth retardation, prematurity and respiratory distress syndrome (RDS) are high [20]. The perinatal mortality is also increased.

Neuropathy per se is unlikely to influence the outcome of diabetic pregnancy but established symptomatic autonomic neuropathy may cause specific problems. In particular, women suffering from gastric stasis and intermittent vomiting (which is often associated with diarrhoea) tend to vomit throughout pregnancy and can therefore be very difficult to manage.

Risks of diabetes to the fetus

MORTALITY

As mentioned above, the outlook for the baby has also improved considerably. Perinatal mortality figures vary widely from country to country and tend to reflect the standard of living [5, 21, 22]. In 1938, the general perinatal mortality rate in England and Wales was 60 per 1000 births, but was almost 400 per 1000 births for children of diabetic mothers [9]. Since then, perinatal mortality has declined steadily throughout Europe; the rates during 1974–8 ranged from 12 per 1000 births (in Denmark) to 23 per 1000 births (in Italy) [23]. Of the European countries, only Norway has gathered comprehensive data relating specifically to established diabetic women: for the period 1967–76, the overall perinatal mortality was 18 per 1000 births compared with 60 per 1000 births for the babies of diabetic women [5]. A limited study carried out in the UK in 1979–80 found a perinatal mortality rate of 56 per 1000 births following 773 registered pregnancies in women with established diabetes, compared with a general rate of 14 per 1000 births [7]. The excess mortality in babies of diabetic mothers has therefore fallen considerably in the developing countries as a whole (Fig. 83.1), although centres with experienced and committed teams have achieved consistently better results than others [6, 9, 24, 25].

About half of the perinatal mortality in diabetic pregnancies is attributable to stillbirth, which is often associated with very poor glycaemic control throughout pregnancy [26]. Hyperglycaemia, like pregnancy-induced hypertension, reduces placental blood flow [27]; this could impair oxygen delivery to the fetus, favouring anaerobic metabolism and causing fetal death through lactic acid production and acidaemia. This hypothesis is supported by data from the few cord centeses which have been performed in diabetic pregnancies.

Another important cause of fetal and neonatal death is major congenital malformations which currently account for about one-third of the perinatal mortality [26].

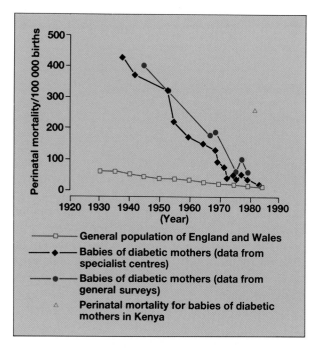

Fig. 83.1. Comparison of perinatal mortality figures for the general population of England and Wales and for babies of diabetic mothers. Note declining perinatal mortality which is lower in specialist centres and markedly higher in Kenya than England and Wales.

FETAL MALFORMATIONS

Disappointingly, the fall in perinatal mortality in diabetic pregnancies has not been matched by a fall in the frequency of severe (fatal or non-fatal) congenital malformations in the children of diabetic mothers [28].

The incidence of congenital malformations in diabetes depends on the frequency of birth defects in the background population as well as on the definition of malformation. In the UK [26], USA [29], Denmark [6] and Norway [5], the incidence in diabetic pregnancy is about 7%, about 3 times higher than in the respective general populations. Various defects are associated with maternal diabetes, particularly major cardiac abnormalities, microcephaly and skeletal malformations (notably sacral agenesis) (Figs 83.2, 83.3 and 84.1). Multiple defects are approximately 5 times commoner than in non-diabetic pregnancies. Table 83.1 illustrates the incidence of major abnormalities reported in the UK survey [7] and the USA study of diabetes in early pregnancy [30].

The pathogenic processes which may mediate the teratogenic effect of diabetes are discussed in detail in Chapter 84 (see also [31–33]). Of the various biochemical factors which could be responsible, glucose has attracted the most attention. During normal pregnancy, despite the tendency to insulin resistance, glycaemic homeostasis remains tight and blood glucose concentrations range between about 3 and 7 mmol/l. Hyperglycaemia during the first trimester (when organogenesis is taking place most rapidly) may be particularly teratogenic. Several studies have reported that diabetic women with elevated HbA_1 concentrations during the first trimester give birth to significantly more malformed babies than those with more normal HbA_1 levels [34–36]. This finding was not confirmed by the Diabetes in Early Pregnancy Study Group (DEPSG) in the USA [30], but this may be because only 5% of the women in this latter report achieved optimal glycaemic control. Moreover, both the DEPSG and the 1980 UK Diabetic Pregnancy Survey (Table 83.2) found that the malformation rate was halved in diabetic women whose glycaemic control had been monitored during the first trimester, and factors other than improved glycaemic control (such as advice about diet and smoking) could obviously have been important. The possible role of *hypoglycaemia* in causing fetal malformation has been much debated and is highly relevant to

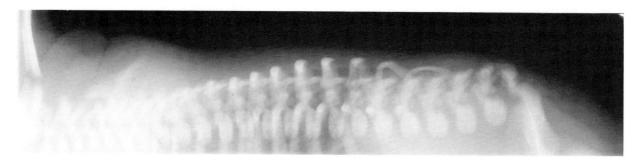

Fig. 83.2. X-ray showing sacral agenesis (right).

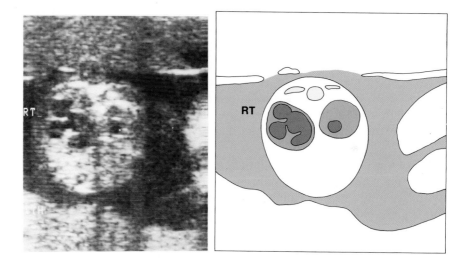

Fig. 83.3. Ultrasound scan of fetal abdomen showing a major abnormality — hydronephrosis of the right kidney.

Table 83.1. Incidence of congenital malformations.

	UK survey*	USA survey†
Number of diabetic women observed	773	626
Number of babies with malformations	55	43
% Malformations	7.1	6.8

* Lowy *et al.* 1986 [7].
† Mills *et al.* 1988 [30].

the generally accepted policy to intensify insulin treatment as far as possible. Although profound glucose deprivation has been associated with malformations in animal fetuses, both *in vitro* [37] and *in vivo* [38], there is not yet any convincing evidence for such an effect in man.

Other metabolites, particularly ketone bodies, can impede somite formation in rodents and under certain conditions can simulate some of the skeletal abnormalities seen in human diabetic

Table 83.2. Malformations categorized by early or late first-trimester attendance.

	Number of women observed	% Babies malformed
UK survey: blood glucose reported in first trimester	460	5.0
UK survey: no blood glucose reported in first trimester	313	10.2
USA survey: women seen before 21 days after conception	347	4.8
USA survey: women first seen 21 days after conception	279	9.3

pregnancy [39]. The precise role of ketone bodies in human teratogenesis remains uncertain, partly because of confusion between two quite different situations in which ketonuria may develop in pregnant diabetic women. Ketonuria is often seen in obese patients with gestational diabetes whose calorie intake is over-restricted. These patients have virtually normal insulin secretion and only minimal disturbances of glucose, free fatty acid and amino acid levels. By contrast, ketonuria in women with true IDDM is likely to be associated with significant hyperglycaemia and markedly increased free fatty acid levels. The possible divergent effects on the fetus of hyperketonaemia superimposed on these two different metabolic backgrounds need to be explored further. Another possible contributory factor is smoking, which may act with diabetes as a coteratogen [40].

The time-course of teratogenesis in diabetes is crucial to the management of the diabetic pregnancy. Gross malformations are due to disorders of organogenesis, which is largely completed within the first trimester: by day 50 after fertilization, the fetus has a beating heart and most of the organs have formed by day 70. During the second and third trimesters, the fetus grows and matures, but the structure of the organs is already determined. Assuming that fetal malformations are due to some disturbance of the maternal metabolic *milieu*, it is clearly vitally important to achieve optimal glycaemic control during the first 10 weeks of pregnancy. As the woman may not suspect that she has become pregnant for 2–3 weeks or even longer, there is an obvious need to plan ahead and to optimize diabetic control before pregnancy is attempted.

MACROSOMIA

Babies born to diabetic mothers tend to be heavier and longer — so-called 'macrosomia'. Although the increased birth weight is most obvious, excessive growth involves much of the body which, as in overfed children, has a disproportionately high fat content [41] (Fig. 83.4). Macrosomia is due mainly to disordered growth during the second and third trimesters, but is also dependent on events which occurred during the first trimester. This may be one reason why babies of established diabetic mothers are only slightly larger than those born to women developing gestational diabetes, which causes lesser

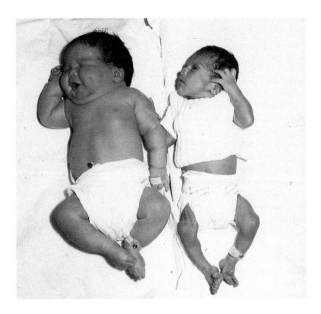

Fig. 83.4. Left: a macrosomic baby born to a diabetic mother. Right: a normal baby born to a non-diabetic mother.

hyperglycaemia, and generally only in the latter half of pregnancy.

Fetal growth depends on delivery of nutrients (glucose, amino acids and free fatty acids [42]) and oxygen, which are governed by placental blood flow and their respective concentration gradients across the placenta. In diabetic women, blood concentrations of all three classes of nutrient are raised and their delivery to the fetus increased. Moderately elevated glucose and amino acid levels stimulate the fetal B cells, which hypersecrete insulin and become hypertrophied [43, 44]. The combination of increased nutrient availability and excessive insulin secretion appears to promote fetal growth. The importance of insulin in fetal growth has been emphasized by the observation that growth-retarded fetuses in severely hyperglycaemic pregnant rats with insulin-deficient diabetes are themselves hyperglycaemic but hypoinsulinaemic [45]. Moreover, Rhesus monkey fetuses infused with insulin *in utero* become grossly macrosomic with no change in maternal blood glucose concentration [46] as has also been observed for babies in whom nesidioblastosis or insulinoma is diagnosed in the neonatal period [47]. A parallel situation may apply to the macrosomic babies born to mildly diabetic women who were treated with sulphonylurea drugs during pregnancy [48]: although maternal glycaemic control may be satisfactory, these agents cross the placenta and stimulate fetal insulin secretion.

Sustained high glucose concentrations (>20 mmol/l) may paradoxically inhibit insulin secretion, at least in animals. This mechanism could theoretically reduce fetal growth in severely hyperglycaemic women, and could partly explain the rather weak correlation found between birth weight and maternal glycaemic control during the third trimester [49, 50].

The most important consequence of macrosomia is dystocia; vaginal delivery may be impossible for grossly macrosomic babies. As described below, serial ultrasound examinations can help to identify macrosomia, although not with absolute certainty.

NEONATAL PROBLEMS

The respiratory distress syndrome (RDS) is, after stillbirth, the second most important cause of perinatal death. RDS is a disease of prematurity which affects about 6% of babies born at 36.5–38.5 weeks' gestation to healthy mothers, but about 19% of those of similar gestational age born to diabetic women [51]. Hyperglycaemia is apparently an important determinant of RDS, as babies born at term to mothers with normal HbA$_1$ levels were not affected [52]. There is increasing experimental evidence that excessive levels of both glucose and insulin may retard the maturation of lung surfactant, although in a subtle way. The lecithin:sphingomyelin ratio in amniotic fluid, generally taken to indicate fetal lung maturity, tends to be spuriously high in diabetic pregnancies and may therefore be misleading [53]. Measurements of the amniotic fluid concentrations of individual surfactant phospholipids (e.g. reduced phosphatidylcholine or phosphatidylglycerol levels) may be a more reliable predictor of the risks of the fetus developing RDS [54].

Hypoglycaemia, usually mild and transient, affects about 20% of newborn babies of diabetic mothers, especially if macrosomic. The cause is continuing hypersecretion of insulin from the neonate's hypertrophied B cells, which can be further stimulated by maternal hyperglycaemia during labour. It is therefore essential to maintain the mother's blood glucose concentration close to normal throughout labour and to check the baby's blood glucose concentration at regular intervals for at least 6 h after birth. Most babies will need to be fed early; persistent hypoglycaemia will require intragastric or intravenous dextrose. The degree of hypoglycaemia at which intervention is required is not universally agreed but in a multicentre study of premature babies whose mothers were not diabetic, plasma glucose values between 1.5–2.5 mmol/l were associated with significant reduction in the Mental Development Index [55].

Babies of diabetic mothers are also prone to develop jaundice, probably largely because of prematurity, and polycythaemia, which may be due to increased erythropoietin production following minor hypoxia *in utero* [41]. Polycythaemia and increased blood viscosity may occasionally cause thrombosis of placental or fetal blood vessels. Transient hypocalcaemia is another recognized complication of the first 2–3 days of life of babies of diabetic pregnancies, especially if premature or suffering from RDS; temporary and reversible hyposecretion of parathormone is apparently responsible.

LATER DEVELOPMENT

Several studies have suggested that diabetic pregnancy, especially if maternal metabolic control is poor, may cause more subtle effects on the child which possibly extend far beyond the neonatal period. Of a group of children born to diabetic mothers, those whose crown–rump length during the first trimester was significantly reduced were subsequently found to be late in reaching their developmental milestones as toddlers [56]. Maternal ketonuria during pregnancy has also been reported to impair the child's intellectual status at 5 years of age [57]. Another study, while failing to demonstrate any such long-term effects, found an increased incidence of IDDM in the children of diabetic mothers, with a calculated prevalence of 1.5% at 25 years of age [58].

Management of pregnancy in diabetic women

Successful management of pregnancy in women with established diabetes demands careful planning, close links between the patient and a co-ordinated medical team, and intensive monitoring of the diabetes and the pregnancy. Management should begin before conception and be maintained continuously until the neonatal period.

Care is best administered by a dedicated, combined diabetic and obstetric antenatal clinic. Many reports over the last 40 years have confirmed that perinatal mortality is lower in these specialized units than in general [9, 59]. The combined clinic team should consist of a diabetes specialist nurse, diabetologist and obstetrician and later in pregnancy should also include a neonatologist. Those general practitioners who organize diabetic mini-clinics may also wish to become involved in antenatal management (Chapter 99); in this case, details of prepregnancy counselling should be conveyed to the general practitioner so that he can reinforce the advice and help to ensure prompt referral when pregnancy occurs.

However, as only 2−4 per 1000 pregnant women have diabetes, the establishment of a formal combined clinic may not represent an effective use of resources. A possible compromise is for all diabetic clinics caring for women of fertile age to organize prepregnancy counselling clinics to educate diabetic women to achieve near-normoglycaemia when pregnancy is first contemplated. This should protect the embryo during organogenesis and the patient can then be transferred to a combined clinic further afield when pregnancy is confirmed.

Prepregnancy counselling

As diabetes exerts many of its harmful effects on the fetus early in gestation — perhaps before pregnancy is confirmed or even suspected — it is essential for pregnancy to be well planned in advance and, ideally, for the patient and the diabetes care team to have rehearsed the management plan for pregnancy. Good glycaemic control should already have been obtained before conception and any other threats to health which may be aggravated by pregnancy (e.g. proliferative retinopathy) should be identified and treated.

Safe and satisfactory contraception is the first requisite of pregnancy counselling, without which it is impossible to achieve planned parenthood. Appropriate methods are discussed in Chapter 85.

Although modern management has greatly reduced the risks of diabetic pregnancy, the prospective parents should be informed of the potential hazards to both mother and child and a specific time should be set aside to counsel both partners. Pregnancy can now be considered in all but a few diabetic women; the relative contra-indications and major issues to be discussed are shown in Table 83.3. The commonest contra-indication — fortunately remediable in most cases — is poor maternal metabolic control. With better understanding of diet and careful attention to insulin treatment and self-monitoring, almost all diabetic women can achieve nearly normal

Table 83.3. Key facts for prepregnancy counselling.

Do the prospective parents understand the risks?
- To the mother:
  - Diabetes increases the risk of death slightly compared with the general population
  - Active retinopathy, nephropathy, and heart disease may get worse
  - Caesarean section is more likely

- To the baby:
  - Diabetes increases the risk of death about threefold
  - Malformations are 3 times commoner and more often multiple
  - Serious neonatal complications are commoner
  - Long-term risk of developing diabetes is slightly increased

Note: these risks are based on survey data and should be substantially reduced if sensible advice is given and heeded

Does the mother understand what a diabetic pregnancy involves?
- Close supervision with frequent antenatal visits
- Home blood glucose monitoring several times per day
- Two or more insulin injections per day
- Careful attention to diet
- Stopping smoking and drinking alcohol

Does the father understand that mother and baby will need much attention?

Do the prospective parents need:
- Contraceptive advice? (Chapter 85)
- Genetic counselling? (Chapter 86)

glycaemic control, as judged by HbA_1 measurements. The prospective mother should be told that the risks to the fetus and herself will be decreased if she can obtain satisfactory blood glucose profiles [60]; fortunately, most diabetic women are highly motivated and are receptive to this advice.

The choice of whether to start a family rests ultimately with the parents. There is no absolute contraindication to pregnancy in diabetic women; babies have been born to women receiving peritoneal dialysis and to others who have undergone renal transplantation [61], although such cases are very much the exception.

Routine antenatal assessments

When pregnancy is confirmed, diabetic women should be advised to attend the combined clinic at weekly to monthly intervals. Provided that pregnancy proceeds uneventfully, hospital admission should not be necessary until delivery.

At the first visit, it is advisable to make a full obstetric and diabetic assessment (Table 83.4). Glycaemic control should be carefully evaluated and, if necessary, improved further. The patient's understanding of her treatment and its adjustment on the basis of home blood glucose monitoring should be checked. Patients are encouraged to bring self-monitored results to the clinic and these should be discussed so that suggestions can be made for changes in diet, insulin dose and frequency of injections. The presence of diabetic complications should already have been documented. Visual acuity should be checked and the fundi carefully examined through dilated pupils, with referral to an ophthalmologist if preproliferative or proliferative changes are seen or suspected.

Urine should be tested for proteinuria and the plasma urea, creatinine and electrolyte concentrations measured. Any symptoms of autonomic neuropathy, especially vomiting, should be noted. The blood pressure should be checked and evidence of significant cardiac failure or vascular disease sought.

At subsequent visits (Table 83.5), glycaemic control will need to be carefully evaluated and the diet and insulin schedule adjusted if necessary. Evidence of progression of micro- or macrovascular complications must be sought. Patients with retinopathy will require regular fundoscopy and measurements of visual acuity throughout pregnancy. Possible obstetric complications, particularly pre-eclampsia, hydramnios and urinary tract infection, should be monitored. Fetal development should be followed with serial ultrasound measurements of biparietal diameter or head circumference, abdominal girth and femur length. Head size and abdominal girth should be

Table 83.5. Subsequent evaluation of the pregnant diabetic woman in the combined diabetic obstetric clinic.

Optimize glycaemic control (as above)

Assess diabetic complications

Check for obstetric complications
Pre-eclampsia
Hydramnios
Urinary tract infections

Assess fetal growth by ultrasound examination
Crown–rump measurement in first trimester
  (confirm dates)
17 weeks: detailed survey for major malformations
19–20 weeks: detailed examination of fetal heart
Regular head and abdominal girth measurements to
  assess growth progress and to detect macrosomia

Table 83.4. Initial evaluation of the pregnant diabetic woman.

Optimize glycaemic control
Self-monitoring and education
Adjust insulin regimen if necessary
Check diet
Check HbA_1

Targets
Preprandial BG 3–5 mmol/l
Postprandial BG <10 mmol/l
HbA_1 in non-diabetic range (4–8%)

Assess diabetic complications
Retinopathy (visual acuity, fundoscopy)
Nephropathy (proteinuria, blood urea, creatinine)
Vascular disease (hypertension, ischaemic heart and peripheral vascular disease)
Autonomic neuropathy (vomiting)

Discourage smoking and drinking alcohol

Obstetric assessment

plotted and compared at regular intevals; progressive mismatching of the two values, with a disproportionately large abdominal girth, indicates the development of macrosomia (Fig. 83.5). At 17 weeks, a detailed scan should be performed to identify possible major malformations and the fetal heart should be examined at 19 weeks; as cardiac lesions are amongst the commonest serious defects and the most difficult to detect on ultrasound.

Hospital admission is only indicated for obstetric complications such as pre-eclampsia or, rarely, for very poor metabolic control. The latter is almost always due to erratic and inappropriate eating patterns or a difficult home environment.

Occasionally, the question of whether to terminate the pregnancy will be raised by the detection of a severe fetal malformation or a threat to the mother's life through metabolic or other complications of diabetes. In our opinion, the decision to terminate must be made by the parents and should only be recommended by the medical team if the fetus has a malformation incompatible with a satisfactory life.

Optimizing glycaemic control in pregnancy

DIET IN DIABETIC PREGNANCY

Women with established diabetes should already have received some dietary advice. In pregnancy, some 50% of the caloric intake should be provided by carbohydrate and the diet should include adequate fibre, calcium and vitamins (especially vitamin D). Standard iron and folate supplements should be given to diabetic women unless they cause nausea and vomiting. The adequacy of total calorie intake can be assessed from the rate of weight gain: on average, non-diabetic and well-controlled diabetic women gain about 11 kg during pregnancy. Most women will require 30–35 kcal/kg body weight, although obese women will need less.

Appetite may be distorted in pregnancy, and vague anorexia or hunger are not uncommon. The former can present problems in slender women but can usually be overcome by frequent and small meals, accompanied by more rest. Increased appetite can cause very erratic glycaemic control which may require hospital admission for supervision of food intake.

INSULIN TREATMENT IN DIABETIC PREGNANCY

Concomitant with increasing insulin resistance, insulin requirements rise as pregnancy advances, sometimes to as much as 3 times the prepregnancy dosage. In the final few weeks of gestation, however, fasting blood glucose concentration and total daily insulin dosage may fall slightly, probably because of the fetus's growing glucose consumption (about 1 mmol/min). After delivery, there is usually an immediate and rapid fall in insulin requirements.

Most women can be managed with mixtures of short- and intermediate-acting insulins, given 2–4 times daily. Overnight glycaemic control may be difficult; the troublesome combination of early morning hypoglycaemia and fasting hyperglycaemia may be overcome by 'splitting' the

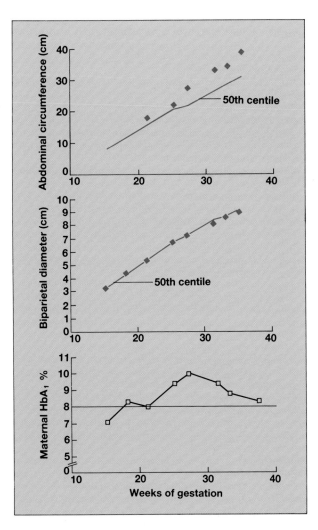

Fig. 83.5. Graphs showing ultrasound-measured abdominal circumference of a fetus outstripping biparietal diameter, and thus indicating macrosomia.

evening dose, giving the short-acting insulin before the evening meal and the intermediate-acting injection with a snack before retiring to bed (see Chapter 51).

In the first trimester, morning nausea and vomiting are common and may restrict food intake at breakfast-time. To avoid hypoglycaemia, affected patients may prefer to eat a little first and then inject an appropriate dose of insulin some time afterwards. As insulin requirements increase through pregnancy, particularly in its latter half, it may become impossible to reduce hyperglycaemia before the evening meal simply by increasing the morning dose of intermediate-acting insulin; an additional injection at midday may be effective. From 36 weeks onwards, the tendency for the fasting blood glucose concentration to fall may require reduction or even omission of the evening injection of intermediate insulin.

In most cases, intermittent insulin injections will achieve satisfactory metabolic control, although continuous subcutaneous insulin infusion (CSII) (see Chapter 42) may produce better results in some cases. CSII should only be attempted by units familiar with the technique and where there is constant access to experienced staff. The possible hazards of pump failure, including both hyperglycaemia and hypoglycaemia, must not be forgotten.

MONITORING METABOLIC CONTROL IN DIABETIC PREGNANCY

The mean diurnal blood glucose concentration in non-diabetic pregnant women is around 5 mmol/l at 30 weeks' gestation [62]. Diabetic women should aim at this level of control, attempting to obtain fasting and preprandial values of between 3 and 5 mmol/l and postprandial values of less than 10 mmol/l. This target can only be reached by frequent and accurate home blood glucose monitoring combined with good understanding of the action and duration of different insulin preparations and of dietary schedules.

Women should measure their blood glucose concentrations 2–6 times/day at home, so that they can recognize glycaemic patterns. Initially, dosages can be adjusted by the medical team, but the aim should be for the woman to do this herself, if necessary following advice by a member of the team (one of whom should be constantly available by telephone for consultation). Calculation of the mean and range of home blood glucose values at each clinic visit provides an overview of performance, which should be carefully discussed with the patient.

HbA$_1$ levels should also be measured regularly as this provides an objective assessment of glycaemic control. HbA$_1$ values tend to fall slightly in pregnancy: in our unit, the mean value in mid-pregnancy in non-diabetic women is 6%, and this should be the target for diabetic patients. Ideally, the current result should be available to compare with the recorded glycaemic profiles. Any discrepancy between the HbA$_1$ value and the self-recorded glucose profiles must raise the suspicion of poor monitoring technique (which should be checked) or of deliberate falsification of results (which may be quite common [63]), although other possible confounding factors such as haemoglobinopathy must first be excluded (see Chapter 34).

Attempts to achieve this level of control will inevitably make hypoglycaemia commoner. Many patients fear hypoglycaemia, and this may be a bar to compliance in some cases. The home treatment of hypoglycaemia should be reviewed in the clinic with the patient and other family members or friends. Many patients either over- or undertreat hypoglycaemia. Three or four dextrose tablets, half a glass of a carbonated glucose drink or a small chocolate bar are suitable for minor attacks. Carbohydrate in a convenient form must always be to hand. If severe hypoglycaemia occurs, prompt treatment is essential. If the patient cannot take glucose orally, jam or glucose gel can be smeared around the inside of the mouth in the first instance and, if the episode is prolonged, glucagon should be injected subcutaneously or intramuscularly; the husband or other family members should be shown how to do this.

Management of labour and delivery

Timing of delivery

The aim is to deliver the mother of a normal-sized, full-term baby, but this goal cannot always be achieved. Provided that there are no obstetric complications and that fetal growth is satisfactory, pregnancy should continue to at least 38 weeks; diabetic women are commonly delivered at 37 weeks in the hope of avoiding stillbirth, but most fetal deaths in fact occur earlier in gestation. The sick fetus which will require earlier delivery may be identified from serial home records of fetal movements and monitoring of fetal heart rate and reactivity, or Doppler measurements of cord blood flow. As mentioned above, estimation of the lecithin:sphingomyelin ratio or of specific phospholipid concentrations in amniotic fluid may be difficult to interpret as a guide to fetal lung maturity, and is only useful if the timing of delivery can be influenced by the result obtained.

Metabolic control during labour

Maternal blood glucose concentrations must be maintained as close to normal as possible throughout labour, as hyperglycaemia will cause fetal hyperinsulinaemia and increase the risk of neonatal hypoglycaemia. Intermittent insulin injections may continue to provide adequate control, but for prolonged labour, a combined intravenous infusion of glucose with insulin may be needed (see p. 822). Whatever the mode of insulin delivery, blood glucose levels must be measured at least hourly. Insulin may not be required during the first stage of labour. Various drugs sometimes given during labour may significantly affect glycaemic control, notably synthetic glucocorticoids (given to promote fetal lung maturation) and β-agonists such as ritodrine (used to delay or retard delivery), both of which cause hyperglycaemia. The sudden drop in insulin requirements following delivery of the placenta should also be anticipated.

Mode of delivery

Vaginal delivery is undoubtedly safest and preferable, unless specific indications for caesarean section are present. These are:
1 pelvic disproportion, an abnormal uterus, or placenta praevia;
2 marked macrosomia;
3 presentations other than cephalic.

It remains difficult to define fetal size in relation to the birth canal. As mentioned above, serial ultrasonographic measurements of fetal head and abdominal size may indicate macrosomia and computerized tomographic estimation of shoulder width may be used to identify babies whose birth weight will exceed 4 kg [64]. Although these methods generally indicate fetal size, their diagnostic accuracy for serious shoulder dystocia is still poor. As a result, many obstetricians prefer to perform a caesarean section rather than subject the fetus to the hazards of birth asphyxia or brachial plexus lesions. Elective caesarean sections are generally performed under epidural anaesthesia, as the baby is not exposed to the anaesthetic and the mother can both experience the birth and recover more quickly from the operation.

The puerperium

After delivery, the insulin resistance of pregnancy rapidly disappears, and insulin dosages should immediately be reduced to those which were appropriate before pregnancy; women who were started on insulin treatment during pregnancy can safely have their insulin discontinued after delivery. Failure to reduce the insulin dosage may cause profound hypoglycaemia, which previously has caused several maternal deaths.

A neonatologist should be present at birth and should immediately examine the baby and check its blood glucose concentration. Macrosomic, small-for-dates or premature babies should be nursed initially in a specialized neonatal unit because of the risks of hypoglycaemia and RDS. Some 15–20% of all babies born to diabetic mothers experience a transient fall in blood glucose level to below 2.0 mmol/l, so that frequent measurements are mandatory. Hypoglycaemia generally responds to early feeding but occasionally intravenous glucose infusion may be needed, although usually for only a few hours.

Diabetic mothers do not usually need to stay in hospital after delivery for longer than their non-diabetic counterparts.

Gestational diabetes

Gestational diabetes mellitus (GDM) is best defined as glucose intolerance which presents in pregnancy. As discussed above, there is evidence that impaired insulin secretion and defects at or beyond the insulin receptor might be responsible [14]. The reported incidence of GDM varies enormously between populations, with figures ranging from 0.15% (UK) to 12.3% (USA) [65]. The overall incidence in the UK and most of Europe is about 1–2%. GDM may develop at any time during pregnancy, but most commonly appears after the middle of the second trimester. Risk factors for GDM include obesity (>90 kg) and a strong family history (in first-degree relatives) of diabetes.

The impact of GDM on the pregnancy is similar

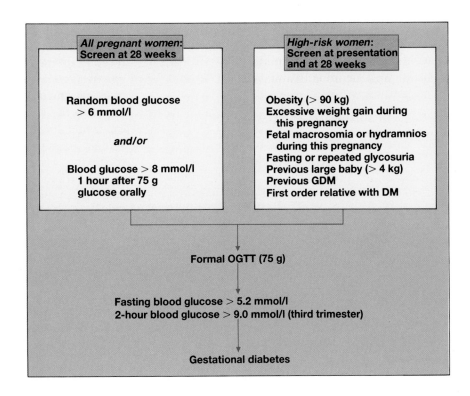

Fig. 83.6. Screening and diagnosis of gestational diabetes.

to that of established diabetes, although its complications are generally fewer and less severe; nonetheless, the condition must be identified and treated effectively before the start of the third trimester in order to reduce the hazards to both mother and fetus. Women with GDM are seldom symptomatic and patients therefore have to be screened for the disease. Guidelines for screening, diagnosis and treatment are outlined below (Fig. 83.6).

Effects of GDM on the fetus

As during pregnancy in women with established diabetes, GDM promotes fetal growth and causes macrosomia and obesity. Approximately 30% of neonates born following GDM pregnancy exceed the 90th centile for weight. The risks of dystocia and birth trauma are therefore increased. There is also a slightly increased stillbirth rate, which is largely unexplained. As GDM is usually a disease of late pregnancy and appears after organogenesis is completed, fetal abnormalities are much rarer than in established diabetic mothers.

Effects on the neonate

RDS, hypoglycaemia and the other problems affecting babies of women with established diabetes can occur, but their incidence and severity are generally lower and are also influenced to some extent by the efficacy of treatment during pregnancy.

Long-term effects of GDM on mother and child

GDM often recurs in subsequent pregnancies. Recent long-term follow-up studies have suggested that as many as 50% of women with GDM will subsequently develop permanent diabetes, either NIDDM or IDDM [12]. Continuing obesity has been identified as a risk factor for future susceptibility to NIDDM, but even about half of the women of ideal weight have been shown to have some blood glucose and insulin secretory abnormalities following a glucose challenge [66]. By contrast, relatively few insulin-treated GDM patients develop true IDDM. It is therefore important to identify women with GDM and obesity, as prophylactic dietary advice may be able to reduce their chances of developing NIDDM, or at least retard its onset.

Maternal GDM may also have surprisingly long-term sequelae for the offspring. Both experimentally induced diabetes in animals and longitudinal studies in the Pima Indians suggest that fetuses exposed to GDM are at increased risk of developing diabetes themselves in adult life [67]. These observations emphasize the importance of early detection and vigorous treatment of GDM.

Screening and diagnosis of GDM

GDM can only be diagnosed by demonstrating abnormal hyperglycaemia. As blood glucose concentrations in pregnancy are not distributed bimodally, an arbitrary cut-off level has to be selected. At present, there is no consensus as to which test is best, when testing should be performed, or which patients should be tested.

A suggested scheme for screening and diagnosis is shown in Fig. 83.6. As mentioned previously, most women with GDM are asymptomatic and the use of clinical screening criteria alone probably misses one-third of cases [68]. The fall in renal threshold during pregnancy greatly limits the usefulness of routine testing for glycosuria, although women with fasting or recurrent glycosuria require further evaluation and an oral glucose tolerance test. Measurements of HbA_1 are convenient but, because of frequent false-positive and false-negative results, do not reliably indicate the presence or absence of GDM. Because of these uncertainties, many clinics have adopted a comprehensive screening programme in which all pregnant women have their blood glucose concentration measured, either in a random sample or at a set interval after an oral glucose load given in the fasting state. Diagnostic levels are not universally agreed, but a random concentration exceeding 6 mmol/l or a value which exceeds 8.0 mmol/l 1 h after ingesting 75 g glucose are strongly suggestive of GDM and indicate the need for a formal oral glucose tolerance test.

GDM may develop at any time during pregnancy but shows a predilection for its second half. Twenty-eight weeks is therefore generally considered to be the optimal time to screen for GDM and also allows enough time for effective intervention. Women at high risk of GDM will obviously be examined in detail before 28 weeks, as appropriate. In view of the wide geographical variation in incidence of GDM, the effort and time devoted to screening for GDM will be determined by its local frequency and the availability of health resources.

As with the screening tests, several different diagnostic tests and criteria are in use throughout the world. The European Association for the Study of Diabetes (through a multicentre study organized by its Diabetic Pregnancy Study Group) have recently defined the 95th centile for fasting blood glucose as 5.2 mmol/l and for the 2-h value after 75 g oral glucose as 9.0 mmol/l [69]. These values apply to the third trimester; women with values exceeding these values should therefore be considered to have GDM and should be treated accordingly. However, there are two important considerations concerning testing, namely the stage of pregnancy and the geographical population examined. Glucose tolerance may improve slightly during the first half of pregnancy; the 97.5% limits for the 2-h blood glucose concentration in a UK study have been found to be 7.5 mmol/l during the second trimester and 9.6 mmol/l for the third [70]. There may also be significant racial differences in carbohydrate metabolism during pregnancy. These variations and other topics have recently been reviewed [71].

Treatment of GDM

Most women with GDM are obese, and their hyperglycaemia may respond to dietary restriction alone. A full dietary assessment should be carried out when GDM is diagnosed and total energy intake reduced to about 1500–1800 kcal/day. Unrefined carbohydrate should constitute at least 50% of the energy intake but *refined* carbohydrates (such as the fizzy glucose drinks widely promoted for pregnant women) should be avoided.

At least one-third of women with GDM cannot achieve satisfactory glycaemic control (as defined above for pregnancy in women with established diabetes) by diet alone. Indeed, it has been argued that current dietary allowances are too generous and that even greater restriction is necessary for moderately or severely obese women (body mass index >27 kg/m² [72]). The proposal has even been made that women who, according to currently accepted glycaemic criteria, are adequately controlled by dietary restriction alone should be treated by 'prophylactic' insulin, as this seems essential to prevent macrosomia and its attendant hazards of birth trauma and the need for caesarean section [73].

Because of the risks of fetal hyperinsulinaemia and macrosomia, there is no place for the use of sulphonylurea drugs in GDM. Insulin is best given as injections of intermediate-acting insulin (e.g. isophane), with or without short-acting insulin, two or more times daily. The precise schedule used will be individual and determined by the patient's glycaemic profile and HbA$_1$ values (as discussed above). Daily insulin requirements vary greatly, from as little as 15 U up to 300 U, but in a given patient, will tend to rise to a plateau between 30 and 36 weeks gestation.

Labour and the puerperium are managed as for established diabetes. Women who have had GDM should be followed up by blood glucose series and an oral glucose tolerance test if necessary to ensure that diabetes has disappeared, and will require careful supervision during subsequent pregnancies.

CLARA LOWY

References

1 Whitridge A, Williams J. The clinical significance of glycosuria in pregnant women. *Am J Med Sci* 1909; **137**: 1−26.

2 Gabbe SG, Mestman JH, Hibbard LT. Maternal mortality in diabetes mellitus. *Obstet Gynecol* 1976; **48**: 549−51.

3 Cousins L. Pregnancy complications among diabetic women: review 1965−1985. *Obstet Gynecol Surv* 1987; **42**: 140−9.

4 Drury MI, Greene AT, Stronge JM. Pregnancy complicated by clinical diabetes mellitus. A study of 600 pregnancies. *Obstet Gynecol* 1977; **49**: 519−22.

5 Jervell J, Bjerkedal T, Moe N. Outcome of pregnancies in diabetic mothers in Norway 1967−1976. *Diabetologia* 1980; **18**: 131−4.

6 Molsted-Pedersen L. Pregnancy and diabetes: a survey. *Acta Endocrinol* 1980; **238** (suppl): 13−19.

7 Lowy C, Beard RW, Goldschmidt J. The UK diabetic pregnancy survey. *Acta Endocrinol* 1986; **277** (suppl): 86−9.

8 Sönksen PH, Judd SL, Lowy C. Home monitoring of blood glucose. *Lancet* 1978; i: 729−32.

9 Peel J, Oakley W. The management of pregnancy in diabetes. *Obstet Gynaecol* 1949; 161−83.

10 Hare JW, White P. Pregnancy in diabetes complicated by vascular disease. *Diabetes* 1977; **26**: 953−5.

11 Blumenthal SA, Abdul-Karim RW. Diagnosis, classification and metabolic management of diabetes in pregnancy: therapeutic impact of self-monitoring of blood glucose and of newer methods of insulin delivery. *Obstet Gynecol Surv* 1987; **42**: 593−604.

12 O'Sullivan JB. Subsequent morbidity among gestational diabetic women. In: Sutherland HW, Stowers JM, eds. *Carbohydrate Metabolism in Pregnancy and the Newborn.* Edinburgh: Churchill Livingstone, 1984: 174−80.

13 Bushard K, Buch I, Molsted-Pederson L, Hougaard P, Kühl C. Increased incidence of true type 1 diabetes acquired during pregnancy. *Br Med J* 1987; **294**: 275−9.

14 Kuhl C, Honnes PJ, Andersen O. Etiology and pathophysiology of gestational diabetes mellitus. *Diabetes* 1985; **34** (suppl 2): 66−70.

15 Ryan EA, Enns L. Role of gestational hormones in the induction of insulin resistance. *J Clin Endocrinol Metab* 1988; **67**: 341−7.

16 Molony JBM, Drury IM. The effect of pregnancy on the natural course of diabetic retinopathy. *Am J Ophthalmol* 1982; **93**: 745−56.

17 Horvat M, Maclean H, Goldberg L, Crock GW. Diabetic retinopathy in pregnancy: a 12 year prospective survey. *Br J Ophthalmol* 1980; **64**: 398−403.

18 Phelps RL, Sakol P, Metzger BE, Jampol LM, Freinkal N. Changes in diabetic retinopathy during pregnancy. *Arch Ophthalmol* 1986; **104**: 1806−10.

19 Jovanovic R, Jovanovic L. Obstetric management when normoglycemia is maintained in diabetic pregnant women with vascular compromise. *Am J Obstet Gynecol* 1984; **149**: 617−23.

20 Kitzmiller JL, Brown ER, Phillippe M, Stark AR, Acker D, Kaldany A, Singh S, Hare JW. Diabetic nephropathy and perinatal outcome. *Am J Obstet Gynecol* 1981; **141**: 741−51.

21 Wheeler FC, Gollmar CW, Deeb LD. Diabetes in South Carolina. Prevalence, perinatal mortality and neonatal mortality in 1978. *Diabetes Care* 1982; **5**: 561−5.

22 Fraser RB. The fate of the pregnant diabetic in a developing country: Kenya. *Diabetologia* 1982; **22**: 22−4.

23 Holland WW. In: *European Community Atlas of Avoidable Death.* Oxford: Oxford University Press, 1988: 276.

24 White P. Diabetes mellitus in pregnancy. *Clin Perinatol* 1974; **1**: 331−47.

25 Jovanovic L, Druzin M, Peterson CM. Effect of euglycemia on the outcome of pregnancy in insulin-dependent diabetic women as compared with normal control subjects. *Am J Med* 1981; **71**: 921−7.

26 Lowy C, Beard RW, Goldschmidt J. Congenital malformations in babies of diabetic mothers. *Diabetic Med* 1986; **3**: 458−62.

27 Lunell NO. Obstetric complications in diabetic pregnancy. *Acta Endocrinol* 1986; suppl **277**: 117−21.

28 Ballard JL, Holroyde J, Tsang RC, Chan G, Sutherland JM, Knowles HC. High malformation rates and decreased mortality in infants of diabetic mothers managed after the first trimester of pregnancy. 1956−1978. *Am J Obstet Gynecol* 1984; **148**: 1111−18.

29 Mills J. Malformations in infants of diabetic mothers. *Teratology* 1982; **25**: 385−94.

30 Mills JL, Knopp RH, Simpson JL et al. Diabetes in early pregnancy study group. Lack of relation of increased malformation rates of diabetic mothers to glycemic control during organogenesis. *N Engl J Med* 1988; **318**: 671−6.

31 Mills JL, Baker L, Goldman AL. Malformations in infants of diabetic mothers occur before the seventh gestational week. *Diabetes* 1979; **28**: 292−3.

32 Eriksson U. Congenital malformations in animal models. *Diabetes Res* 1984; **1**: 57−66.

33 Sadler TW, Horton WE, Hunter ES. Mechanisms of diabetes-induced congenital malformations as studied in mammalian embryo culture. In: Jovanovic L, Peterson CM, Fuhrmann K, eds. *Diabetes and Pregnancy: Teratology, Toxicity and Treatment.* New York: Paiger, 1986; 51−71.

34 Leslie RDG, Pyke DA, John PN, White JM. Haemoglobin A1 in diabetic pregnancy. *Lancet* 1978; ii: 958−9.

35 Miller E, Hare JW, Cloherty JP. Elevated maternal hemoglobin A$_1$ in early pregnancy and major congenital anomalies in infants of diabetic mothers. *N Engl J Med* 1981; **304**: 1331−4.

36 Ylinen K, Aula P, Stenman UH, Kesaniemi-Kuokkanen T, Teramo K. Risk of minor and major fetal malformations in diabetics with high HbA1c values in early pregnancy. *Br Med J* 1984; **289**: 345−6.

37 Ellington SKL. Development of rat embryo cultured in glucose deficient media. *Diabetes* 1987; **36**: 1372−8.

38 Buchanan TA, Schemmer JK, Freinkel, N. Embryotoxic effects of brief maternal insulin hypoglycemia during organogenesis in the rat. *J Clin Invest* 1986; **78**: 643−9.

39 Eriksson UJ, Dahlström E, Hellerström C. Diabetes in pregnancy. Skeletal malformations in the offspring of diabetic rats after intermittent withdrawal of insulin in early gestation. *Diabetes* 1983; **32**: 1141–5.

40 Brooke OL, Anderson HR, Bland JM, Peacock JL, Stewart CM. Effect on birth weight of smoking, alcohol, caffeine, socioeconomic factors, and psychosocial stress. *Br Med J* 1989; **296**: 795–801.

41 Pedersen J. *The Pregnant Diabetic and her Newborn*, 2nd edn. Copenhagen: Munksgaard, 1977: Ch 10, 123–91.

42 Knopp RH, Warth MR, Carles D, Childs M, Li JR, Mabuchi H, VanAllen M. Lipoprotein metabolism in pregnancy, fat transport to the fetus and the effects of diabetes. *Biol Neonate* 1966; **50**: 297–317.

43 Grasso G, Palumbo G, Fallucca F, Lanzafame S, Indelicato B, Sanfilippo S. The development and function of the endocrine pancreas of fetuses and infants born to normal and diabetic mothers. *Acta Endocrinol* 1986; suppl 277: 130–5.

44 Reiher H, Fuhrmann K, Noack S, Woltanski K, Jutzi E, Dorsche HH, Hahn HJ. Age-dependent insulin secretion of the endocrine pancreas *in vitro* from fetuses of diabetic and nondiabetic patients. *Diabetes Care* 1983; **6**: 446–51.

45 Eriksson U, Andersson A, Efendic S, Elde R, Hellerström C. Diabetes in pregnancy: effects on the foetal and newborn rat with particular regard to body weight, serum insulin concentration and pancreatic contents of insulin, glucagon and somatostatin. *Acta Endocrinol* 1980; **94**: 354–64.

46 Susa JB, Schwartz R. Effects of hyperinsulinemia in the primate fetus. *Diabetes* 1985; **34** (suppl 2): 36–41.

47 Soltesz G, Jenkins PA, Aynsley Green A. Hyperinsulinaemic hypoglycaemia in infancy and childhood: a practical approach to diagnosis and medical treatment based on experience of 18 cases. *Acta Paediatr Hung* 1984; **25**: 319–32.

48 Kemball ML, McIver C, Milner RD, Nourse CH, Schiff D, Tiernan JR. Neonatal hypoglycaemia in infants of diabetic mothers given sulphonylurea drugs in pregnancy. *Arch Dis Child* 1970; **45**: 693–701.

49 Visse GHA, Van Ballegooie E, Sluiter WJ. Macrosomy despite well controlled diabetic pregnancy. *Lancet* 1984; i: 284–5.

50 Small M, Cameron A, Lunan B, MacCuish AC. Macrosomia in pregnancy complicated by insulin-dependent diabetes mellitus. *Diabetes Care* 1987; **10**: 594–9.

51 Minouni F, Miodovnik M, Whitsett JA, Holroyde JC, Siddiqi T, Tsang R. Respiratory distress syndrome in infants of diabetic mothers in the 1980s: no direct adverse effect of maternal diabetes with modern management. *Obstet Gynecol* 1987; **69**: 191–5.

52 Ylinen K. High maternal levels of haemoglobin A1c associated with delayed lung maturation in insulin dependent diabetic pregnancies. *Acta Obstet Gynecol Scan* 1987; **66**: 263–6.

53 James DK, Chiswick ML, Harkes A, Williams M, Tindall VR. Maternal diabetes and neonatal respiratory distress. 1 Maturation of fetal surfactant. *Br J Obstet Gynaecol* 1984; **91**: 316–24.

54 James DK, Chiswick ML, Harkes A, Williams M, Tindall VR. Maternal diabetes and neonatal respiratory distress. 11 Prediction of fetal lung maturity. *Br J Obstet Gynecol* 1984; **91**: 325–9.

55 Lucas A, Morley R, Cole TJ. Adverse neurodevelopmental outcome of moderate neonatal hypoglycaemia. *Br Med J* 1988; **297**: 1304–8.

56 Bloch-Petersen M, Pedersen SA, Greisen G, Fog-Pedersen J, Molsted-Pedersen L. Early growth delay in diabetic pregnancy: relation to psychomotor development at age 4. *Br Med J* 1988; **296**: 598–600.

57 Stehbens JA, Baker GL, Kitchell M. Outcome at ages 1, 3 and 5 years of children born to diabetic women. *Am J Obstet Gynecol* 1977; **127**: 408–13.

58 Perrson B. Long term morbidity in infants of diabetic mothers. *Acta Endocrinol* 1986; **277**: 156–8.

59 Traub AI, Harley JMG, Cooper TK, Maguiness S, Hadden DR. Is centralized hospital care necessary for all insulin-dependent pregnant diabetics? *Br J Obstet Gynaecol* 1987; **94**: 957–62.

60 Fuhrmann K, Reicher H, Semmler K, Fischer F, Fischer M, Glockner E. Prevention of congenital malformations in infants of insulin dependent diabetic mothers. *Diabetes Care* 1983; **6**: 219–23.

61 Grenfell A, Bewick M, Brudenell JM, Carr JV, Parsons V, Snowden S, Watkins PJ. Diabetic pregnancy following renal transplantation *Diabetic Med* 1986; **3**: 177–9.

62 Gillmer MDG, Beard RW, Brooke FM, Oakley NW. Carbohydrate metabolism in pregnancy. Part 1. Diurnal plasma glucose profile in normal and diabetic women. *Br Med J* 1975; **2**: 399–402.

63 Williams CD, Scobie IN, Crane R, Lowy C, Sönksen PH. Use of memory meters to measure reliability of self blood glucose monitoring. *Diabetic Med* 1988; **5**: 459–62.

64 Kitzmiller J, Mall JC, Gin GD, Hendricks SK, Newman RB, Scheerer L. Measurement of fetal shoulder width with computed tomography in diabetic women. *Obstet Gynecol* 1987; **70**: 941–5.

65 Hadden DR. Geographic, ethnic and racial variation in the incidence of gestational diabetes mellitus. *Diabetes* 1985; **34** (suppl 2): 8–12.

66 Efendic S, Hanson U, Persson B, Wajngot A, Luft R. Glucose tolerance, insulin release, and insulin sensitivity in normal-weight women with previous gestational diabetes mellitus. *Diabetes* 1987; **36**: 413–19.

67 Pettitt DJ, Bennett PH, Knowler WC, Baird HR, Alick KA. Gestational diabetes mellitus and impaired glucose tolerance during pregnancy. *Diabetes* 1985; **34** (suppl 2): 119–22.

68 Jovanovic L, Peterson CM. Screening for gestational diabetes. *Diabetes* 1985; **34** (suppl 2): 21–3.

69 Lind T. *The WHO Recommend OGTT*. 4th International Colloquium on Carbohydrate Metabolism in Pregnancy and the Newborn. Berlin: Springer Verlag (in press).

70 Hatem M, Anthony F, Hogston P, Rowe DJF, Dennis KJ. Reference values for 75 g oral glucose tolerance test in pregnancy. *Br Med J* 1988; **296**: 676–8.

71 Okonofua FE, Amole FA, Ayangade SO, Nimalaraj T. Criteria for oral glucose tolerance test in pregnant and non-pregnant Nigerian women. *Int J Gynecol Obstet* 1988; **27**: 85–9.

72 Algert S, Shragg P, Hollingworth DR. Moderate calorie restriction in obese women with gestational diabetes. *Obstet Gynecol* 1985; **65**: 485–91.

73 Coustan DR, Imarah J. Prophylactic insulin treatment of gestational diabetes reduces the incidence of macrosomia, operative delivery and birth trauma. *Am J Obstet Gynecol* 1984; **150**: 836–42.

84   Mechanisms of Teratogenesis in Diabetes Mellitus

Summary

• The common abnormalities caused by diabetes during embryogenesis are cardiac malformations, neural tube defects, impaired ossification (especially caudal regression) and malformations of the gut and urogenital system.
• The identity of the teratogen(s) in diabetes has not been proven.
• In experimental animals, hyperglycaemia has a dose-related effect in inducing malformations but hypoglycaemia may also be teratogenic; the precise dependence of malformations on glycaemic control in man is unknown.
• Hyperglycaemia and hyperketonaemia may impair the activities of important cellular enzymes through glycosylation and alterations in osmolarity and pH.
• Insulin deficiency may reduce availability of cations (zinc, magnesium, calcium); this could interfere with the function of certain enzymes and with ossification.
• Reduced placental blood flow in diabetes may compromise yolk-sac perfusion and metabolism, and so lead to both growth retardation and malformations.
• Later effects of diabetes on the fetus include macrosomia (due to fetal hyperinsulinaemia, stimulated by maternal hyperglycaemia), delayed lung maturation and neonatal hypoglycaemia and hypocalcaemia.

It is hardly surprising that maternal diabetes can have serious consequences for the infant, as a major aspect of pregnancy is to ensure adequate fetal nutrition, and as the levels of all major nutrients and several minerals are often disturbed in diabetes. Until recently, the most common abnormality in the infants of diabetic mothers was macrosomia, but careful observation has now demonstrated a range of anomalies including growth retardation and malformations (for review see Chapter 83 and [1, 2]). Many of these have been reproduced experimentally in animals with chemically induced or genetically inbred diabetes, or *in vitro* (for review see [3]). In the search for a unifying mechanism for the teratogenic effects of diabetes, several separate but physiologically related putative teratogens need to be considered.

Pre-embryonic and placental development

The first 18 days of human gestation (5−6 days in the rat) can be regarded as the pre-embryonic period. Diabetes may impair the earlier processes of ovulation, fertilization, movement along the oviduct and implantation [3] but these effects are not strictly considered as teratogenesis.

The fertilized egg in the oviduct is virtually independent of maternal physiology, deriving metabolic energy from cytoplasmic stores of pyruvate and lactate. By 7 days, the morula has become a hollow blastocyst and has begun to implant in the uterus. Yolk-sac development may be disrupted by diabetes, and impaired vessel formation and reduced numbers of mitochondria [4] may inhibit cellular metabolism, especially glycolysis. As anaerobic glycolysis is the major source of metabolic energy during early development, this may partly explain the association between fetal growth retardation and congenital malformations in general [5] and in infants of diabetic mothers in particular [1−3].

In diabetic pregnancy, there is often an increase in placental weight despite a reduction in blood flow [6]. The increased weight reflects excess stores of glycogen and lipid, together with deposits of fibrin and mucopolysaccharides [7]. An increase in villous surface area has been observed in some, but not all, studies [8]. Recently, Thomas *et al.* [9] found that, despite an elevated maternal–fetal glucose gradient, net glucose transfer to the fetus was reduced. However, Herrera *et al.* [10] found a linear relationship between maternal glucose and placental glucose transfer. Thus, the effect of glycaemia on facilitated glucose transport remains to be clarified.

Embryogenesis

Teratogenesis strictly refers to disruptions during organ formation, i.e. the period spanning 2.5 to 8 weeks in human gestation or days 6–11 in rats. The wide variety of abnormalities observed in infants of diabetic mothers suggests that the mechanism(s) of teratogenesis must operate across a range of systems. The common problems include neural tube defects, impaired ossification, gut and urogenital malformation and congenital heart disease.

Between days 18–25 in humans (8.5 to 10.5 days in rodents), the neural plate folds and closes to form the neural tube. This critical stage is susceptible to various teratogens [11] and the malformation rate is increased at least tenfold in infants of diabetic mothers [3]. Exencephaly, anencephaly (Fig. 84.1), and hydrocephaly all occur both in humans [1, 2], and experimentally in rats *in vivo* [12] and *in vitro* [13].

Hyperglycaemia *per se* has a dose-dependent effect and improved glycaemic control consistently improves malformation rates in experimental animals [3, 12, 13]. High glucose concentrations apparently induce cytoarchitectural changes in the neuroepithelium, including a reduction in cell mitosis and premature differentiation [13]. On the other hand, Sadler and Hunter [11] recently demonstrated a failure of neural development in mouse embryos as a result of *low* glucose levels in the culture medium for as little as 12 h. Growth retardation only accompanied the malformation if the glucose deprivation was more severe or prolonged. A common mechanism by which hypo- and hyperglycaemia give rise to the same malformation has not been described, but pH and osmolarity may be implicated, as acid conditions contribute to neural tube defects [14] and as glucose is weakly ionized under physiological conditions. The caudal regression syndrome (causing sacral agenesis in man) is almost exclusive to infants of diabetic mothers [15] and comparable rat models [12, 16] and arises early in embryogenesis [16]. The defect is probably in the mid-posterior axis of the mesoderm but the mechanism has not been clarified (Fig. 84.2).

Ossification may be delayed or defective in infants of diabetic mothers and in various animal models, giving rise to micrognathia, cleft palate, malformed ribs and femoral hypoplasia [12, 16–18]. Disturbed enzyme function may be involved. Renal β-glucuronidase shows severely reduced activity, in parallel with delayed ossification [17]. This enzyme may be involved in breakdown of cartilage during ossification, or it may merely reflect a group of enzymes specifically affected by hyperglycaemia or some other disturbance of diabetes. The fact that β-glucuronidase is a glycoprotein and therefore liable to excessive glycosylation may be relevant to its susceptibility to inhibition by maternal diabetes.

In a study of diabetic rats by Eriksson [19], in which micrognathia was the most common abnormality, a significant decrease in total fetal body zinc was observed. This was accompanied by excessive accumulation of zinc, copper and manganese in maternal liver; dietary zinc supplements to the diabetic mothers did not increase fetal zinc levels. Since zinc deficiency *per se* is teratogenic and may inhibit DNA synthesis via decreased activity of zinc-dependent enzymes [20], this may be an important mechanism for some teratogenic effects of diabetes, especially as many other zinc-dependent enzymes have important roles in cellular function. It is also possible

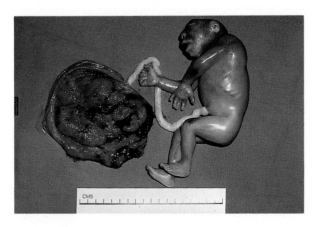

Fig. 84.1. Anencephaly in the stillborn child of a diabetic mother. (Reproduced with permission from Mr R.B. Fraser, University of Sheffield).

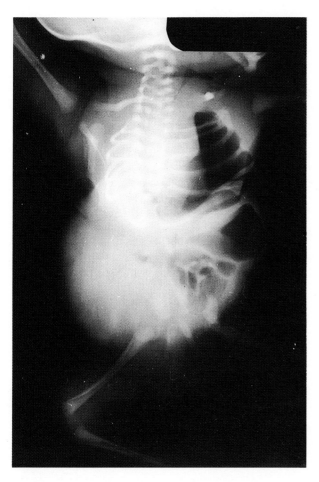

Fig. 84.2. Radiograph of the fetus of a diabetic mother, showing sacral agenesis (the 'caudal regression syndrome'). (Reproduced by kind permission of Dr Ian MacFarlane, Walton Hospital, Liverpool.)

Identity of the teratogen in diabetes

As hyperglycaemia is the most obvious metabolic derangement in diabetes, it has been considered the most likely teratogen in infants of diabetic mothers, and many studies, especially those *in vitro*, support this conclusion. Nonetheless, Mills et al. have recently observed a lack of correlation between maternal glycaemia during weeks 5–12 and malformation rate in infants of diabetic mothers [23]. Experiments with other sugars have demonstrated, however, that some of the effects attributable to glucose may be due to changes in osmolarity [24] and/or pH [14].

In very poorly controlled diabetes, ketone bodies are present in the maternal circulation and freely cross the placenta. High levels of 3-hydroxybutyrate *in vitro* caused growth retardation and malformations, and synergism has been demonstrated between subteratogenic doses of 3-hydroxybutyrate and glucose in rat embryos [25]. It has also been suggested that hyperketonaemia during pregnancy may lower intellectual capacity in the offspring, although this is disputed [2] (see Chapter 83).

There has been concern that hypoglycaemia, which is common during the tight control recommended during pregnancy, may also be teratogenic. Whereas Sadler and Hunter [11] found that hypoglycaemia impaired neural development, another study [26] which induced severe hypoglycaemic shock in pregnant rats found no evidence of abnormalities. The excess placental glycogen laid down during the diabetic pregnancy may protect the fetus against maternal hypoglycaemia by releasing glucose into the fetal circulation.

The possible role of insulin — which promotes growth — as a teratogen is unresolved, although it can cause malformations in chick embryos [27]. The human placenta is not permeable to insulin, so periods of maternal hyperinsulinaemia probably do not affect the embryo, although abnormal nutrient levels and particularly hyperglycaemia are likely to influence fetal insulin production. Insulin and primitive B cells have been detected in fetuses from day 14 in rats or week 9 in humans; insulin secretion may be raised in the fetus of the diabetic mother, and probably contributes to macrosomia (see Chapter 83).

Figure 84.3 summarizes the possible mechanisms of diabetic teratogenesis. The major maternal disruptions are hypoinsulinaemia leading to

that bone mineral constituents are reduced; hypocalcaemia is observed in up to 50% of infants of diabetic mothers within 72 h of birth [21] but embryonic levels have not been determined. Serum levels of magnesium, a mainly intracellular cation whose metabolism is partly linked with calcium and is partly insulin-dependent, are lower than normal in both diabetic mothers [22] and neonatal infants of diabetic mothers [21], but again embryonic data are not available.

During weeks 5–8 in humans, the gut, urogenital system, cardiovascular system and limbs develop and abnormalities may appear. Anomalies particularly associated with maternal diabetes include gastroschisis, renal agenesis, duodenal and anorectal atresia, and, most commonly, congenital heart disease, especially transposition of the great vessels [2, 12]; many of these are fatal *in utero* or in the neonatal period.

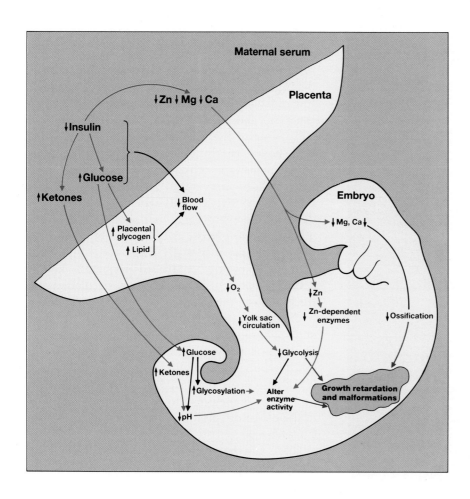

Fig. 84.3. Possible mechanisms for teratogenic effects of maternal diabetes during embryogenesis. Red arrows represent observed effects; black arrows represent speculative or unconfirmed mechanisms; blue arrows indicate that these processes may influence outcomes but mechanisms are not clarified.

hyperglycaemia and disturbed intermediary metabolite levels, which lead to alterations in pH and osmolarity in the embryo and impaired metabolism. Altered cation and mineral availability may impair ossification. The activity of a wide variety of enzymes is probably altered. These defects, and others as yet unknown, may lead to the specific malformations associated with diabetes.

Further disturbances of development occur during fetal development due to altered nutrient and hormone levels, as described in the following section.

Fetal development

From week 8 onwards, the human conceptus has recognizable limbs, digits, face and internal organs and is described as a fetus. Subsequent development involves an increase in size from 30 to 500 mm, the appearance and maturation of endocrine and neural systems, and preparation for breathing and feeding. Maternal diabetes may have serious effects on various aspects of this maturation, particularly on total growth, adipose stores, pulmonary maturation and pancreatic development [1, 2]. A combination of abnormal nutrient levels, insulin, insulin-like growth factors (IGF), placental lactogen and IGF inhibitors interact to disrupt normal development. Insulin is certainly required for fetal survival and growth, and fetal hyperinsulinaemia (stimulated by maternal hyperglycaemia) may be responsible for overgrowth of adipose tissue, leading to macrosomia, as postulated by Pedersen [28].

Alterations at this stage can be serious, but do not result in malformations. For further details of effects of diabetes on fetal development see [29, 30] and Chapter 83.

CAROLINE J. CRACE

References

1 Freinkel N. Of pregnancy and progeny. Banting Lecture 1980. *Diabetes* 1980; **29**: 1023–35.
2 Reece EA, Hobbins JC. Diabetic embryopathy: pathogenesis, prenatal diagnosis and prevention. *Obstet Gynecol Surv* 1986; **41**: 325–35.

3 Eriksson U. Congenital malformations in diabetic animal models: a review. *Diabetes Res* 1984; **1**: 57−66.

4 Pinter E, Reece EA, Leranth C. Yolk sac failure in embryopathy due to hyperglycaemia. Ultrastructural analysis of yolk sac differentiation in rat conceptuses under hyperglycaemic culture conditions. *Teratology* 1986; **33**: 363−8.

5 Van den Berg BJ, Yerushalmy J. The relationship of the rate of intrauterine growth of infants of low birthweight to mortality, morbidity and congenital abnormalities. *J Pediatr* 1966; **69**: 531−45.

6 Eriksson U, Janssen L. Diabetes in pregnancy: decreased placental blood flow and disturbed fetal development in the rat. *Pediatr Res* 1984; **18**: 735−8.

7 Diamant YZ, Metzger BE, Freinkel N, Shafrir E. Placental lipid and glycogen content in human and experimental diabetes mellitus. *Am J Obstet Gynecol* 1982; **144**: 5−11.

8 Boyd PA, Scott A, Keeling JW. Quantitative structural studies on placentas from pregnancies complicated by diabetes mellitus. *Br J Obstet Gynaecol* 1986; **93**: 31−5.

9 Thomas CR, Eriksson GL, Kihlstrom I, Eriksson UJ. The effects of diabetes on placental glucose metabolism and transport in the rat. (Abstract) *Diabetologia* 1987; **30**: 588A.

10 Herrera E, Palacin M, Martin A, Lasuncion A. Relationship between maternal and fetal fuels and placental glucose transfer in rats with maternal diabetes of varying severity. *Diabetes* 1985; **34** (suppl 2): 42−6.

11 Sadler TW, Hunter ES. Hypoglycemia: how little is too much for the embryo? *Am J Obstet Gynecol* 1987; **157**: 190−3.

12 Brownscheidle CM, Wootten V, Mathieu MH, Davis DL, Hofmann IA. The effects of maternal diabetes on fetal maturation and neonatal health. *Metabolism* 1983; **32** (suppl 1): 148−55.

13 Reece EA, Pinter E, Leranth CZ *et al*. Ultrastructural analysis of malformation of the embryonic neural axis by *in vitro* hyperglycaemia. *Teratology* 1985; **32**: 363−73.

14 Nau H, Scott WJ. Weak acids may act as teratogens by accumulating in the basic milieu of the early mammalian embryo. *Nature* 1986; **323**: 276−8.

15 Mills JL, Baker L, Goldman AS. Malformations in infants of diabetic mothers occur before the seventh gestational week: implications for treatment. *Diabetes* 1979: **28**: 292−3.

16 Eriksson UJ, Styrud J. Congenital malformations in diabetic pregnancy: the clinical relevance of experimental animal studies. *Acta Paediatr Scand Suppl* 1985; **320**: 72−8.

17 Wilson GN, Howe M, Stover JM. Delayed developmental sequences in rodent diabetic embryopathy. *Pediatr Res* 1985; **19**: 1337−40.

18 Johnson JP, Carey JC, Gooch WM, Petersen JP, Beattie JF. Femoral hypoplasia−unusual facies syndrome in infants of diabetic mothers. *J Pediatr* 1983; **102**: 866−72.

19 Eriksson UJ. Diabetes in pregnancy: retarded fetal growth, congenital malformations and feto-maternal concentrations of Zn, Cu, Mn in the rat. *J Nutr* 1984; **114**: 477−84.

20 Duncan JR, Hurley LS. Thymidine kinase and DNA polymerase activity in normal and zinc deficient developing rat embryos. *Proc Soc Exp Biol Med* 1978; **159**: 39−43.

21 Mimouni F, Tsang RC, Hertzberg VS, Miodovnik M. Polycythemia, hypomagnesemia, and hypocalcemia in infants of diabetic mothers. *Am J Dis Child* 1986; **140**: 798−800.

22 Wibell L, Gebbre-Medhin M, Lindmark G. Magnesium and zinc in diabetic pregnancy. *Acta Paediatr Scand Suppl* 1985; **320**: 100−6.

23 Mills JL, Knopp RH, Simpson JL *et al*. Lack of relation of increased malformation rates in infants of diabetic mothers to glycemic control during organogenesis. *N Engl J Med* 1988; **318**: 671−6.

24 Cockroft DL, Coppola DT. Teratogenic effects of excess glucose on head-fold rat embryos in culture. *Teratology* 1977; **16**: 141−6.

25 Lewis NJ, Akazawa S, Freinkel N. Teratogenesis from B-hydroxybutyrate during organogenesis in rat embryo organ culture and enhancement by subteratogenic glucose. (Abstract) *Diabetes* 1983; **32** (suppl 1): 11A.

26 Ream JR, Weingarten PL, Pappas AM. Evaluation of the prenatal effects of massive doses of insulin in rats. *Teratology* 1970; **3**: 29−32.

27 Landauer W. Rumplessness of chicken embryos produced by the injection of insulin and other chemicals. *J Exp Zool* 1945; **98**: 65.

28 Pedersen JF, Bojsen-Moller B, Poulsen H. Blood sugar in newborn infants of diabetic mothers. *Acta Endocrinol* 1954; **15**: 33−52.

29 Hill DJ, Milner RDG. The role of peptide growth factors and hormones in the control of fetal growth. In: Chiswick ML, ed. *Recent Advances in Perinatal Medicine*, vol 2. Edinburgh: Churchill Livingstone, 1985; 79−102.

30 Crace CJ, Hill DJ, Milner RDG. Mitogenic actions of insulin on fetal and neonatal rat cells *in vitro*. *J Endocrinol* 1985; **104**: 61−8.

85   Contraception for Diabetic Women

Summary

• Most diabetic women can safely have children, but pregnancy is contraindicated by advanced nephropathy, ischaemic heart disease, severe symptomatic autonomic neuropathy and untreated proliferative retinopathy. Sterilization may be indicated in some cases.

• Contraceptive advice must be carefully tailored to the couple's needs.

• Combined oral contraceptive pills containing high-dose oestrogens aggravate glycaemic and lipaemic profiles, and are not recommended in diabetic women. Newer, low oestrogen-dose pills have very high success rates and few metabolic side-effects, and are suitable in young patients with no diabetic complications or risk factors for vascular disease.

• Progestogen-only pills have no adverse metabolic effects and are effective if used regularly. They may cause menstrual disturbance, including amenorrhoea.

• Intra-uterine devices have no metabolic side-effects but have a generally higher failure rate and may carry an increased risk of infection in diabetic women.

• Mechanical methods (condom or diaphragm) have high failure rates unless used carefully and are not recommended if pregnancy is contraindicated.

Planning of pregnancies, in the fullest sense of the term, is particularly important for diabetic women for many reasons. The majority of diabetic women can safely have children, although those with severe complications may be best advised against pregnancy. The outcome of pregnancy is improving, but hazards to the fetus remain (Chapter 83). The main considerations are the importance of periconceptional diabetic control [1, 2], the constraints imposed by diabetes in pregnancy, the specific problems of patients with diabetic complications and the reduced life expectancy of women with IDDM. Good contraceptive advice is therefore essential.

Contraindications to pregnancy (see also Chapter 83)

These are shown in Table 85.1. The commonest contraindication is advanced nephropathy (creatinine clearance <40 ml/min), in which pregnancy usually has a poor outcome and the mother's life expectancy may be very limited [3, 4]. Pregnancies in those with less advanced nephropathy and adequate renal function are usually successful [4]. The outcome is related to the level of creatinine clearance, the degree of proteinuria and the severity of associated hypertension [5], which should be assessed at the prepregnancy clinic. In patients with either good or extremely poor renal function, a decision is easy to make but in borderline cases this can be quite difficult. Nevertheless, successful pregnancies have been reported in a few very high-risk patients [6] and in others who have received renal transplantation [7].

Severe ischaemic heart disease is an accepted contraindication to pregnancy, although no large series of patients with this complication have been published. In 1977, Hare reported that three out of four high-risk patients died during pregnancy [8]. Since then, there have been a few other reports and Silfen has recommended that, because of the extremely high maternal mortality, sterilization should be considered in such women [9]. Each case requires

Table 85.1. Contraindications to pregnancy in diabetic women.

- Advanced nephropathy
  - creatinine clearance <40 ml/min
  - heavy proteinuria or nephrotic syndrome
  - associated severe hypertension
- Significant coronary heart disease
- Proliferative retinopathy, if left untreated
- Autonomic neuropathy with severe hyperemesis

careful investigation and should be discussed with a cardiologist. An exercise electrocardiogram should be carried out at the prepregnancy clinic.

Severe autonomic neuropathy in pregnancy is rare but can be extremely difficult to manage. Such patients usually have other complications and therefore a limited life expectancy, and severe autonomic neuropathy *per se* may occasionally be a contraindication to pregnancy because of the intractable vomiting which tends to accompany it.

There is some argument about the effect of pregnancy on retinopathy but most authorities agree that rapid deterioration can occur and until the mid-1970s, proliferative retinopathy was generally considered a contraindication to pregnancy [10–12]. However, it is now clear that proliferative retinopathy successfully treated with photocoagulation or vitrectomy only rarely deteriorates during pregnancy [13, 14]. Retinopathy is thus no longer a contraindication, but it must be effectively treated before pregnancy [15, 16].

Methods of contraception

All forms of contraception carry some risks. Every couple and their relative risks must be considered individually in order to find the method most

suitable for them. The reliability and other features of the methods are shown in Tables 85.2 and 85.3.

Oral contraceptives

THE COMBINED ORAL CONTRACEPTIVE PILL

Certain contraceptive steroids have adverse metabolic effects, including hyperglycaemia and hyperlipidaemia. In the past, high-dose oestrogen pills caused an increase in insulin requirements in a small proportion of women with IDDM. The dosage increase was usually small and did not present a clinical problem [17]. The newer, low-dose preparations rarely cause any change in insulin requirements.

In the case of women with IDDM at increased risk of vascular disease, there is obviously concern about the further increase in risk of vascular disease associated with the combined pill, although this is largely based on anecdotal evidence [18]. Adverse changes in blood lipids and coagulation factors caused by the combined pill are similar to those associated with diabetes itself and are related to the amount of oestrogen and the amount and androgenic potency of the progestogen. In recent years, the dose of oestrogen in combined pills has been reduced and the type and dose of progestogen have changed; the triphasic preparations have a low total dose and the most recent combined pills contain even less. There is a reduced risk of thromboembolic disease with the lower-dose pills and it seems likely that the risk of arterial disease will also be diminished, although this has not yet been established. Skouby [19] studied 27 women with IDDM and compared the metabolic effects of four oral contraceptives, a monophasic combination of a non-alkylated oestrogen with 500 µg

Table 85.2. The chances of pregnancy with various contraceptive methods: the number of women who will become pregnant for each 100 couples who use the method for 1 year is indicated. If no method is used, 80/100 women will become pregnant per year.

Method	If method is used correctly	General experience of method
Withdrawal	20	40
Rhythm method	10	25
Spermicides	10	20
Diaphragm	5	10
Condom	5	10
IUCD	4	4
Contraceptive pill	<1	2
Vasectomy	<1	<1
Tubal sterilization	<1	<1

Table 85.3. Main contraceptive methods available for diabetic women.

Methods	Adverse effects on: Glycaemia	Lipidaemia	Thrombo-embolic risk	Other comments
Oral contraceptive pill:				
Combined {high-dose E + P	+	+	+	Avoid combined pills if other risk factors for coronary disease are present: smoking, hypertension, hyperlipidaemia, positive family history
low-dose E + P	−	±	±	
low-dose E + P, triphasic	−	±	±	
Progestogen only ('mini-pill')	−	−	−	Menstrual irregularity; use other contraceptive method if more than one pill missed (e.g. by omission, vomiting or diarrhoea)
Intra-uterine contraceptive device	−	−	−	Possibly increased risk of pelvic infection; relatively high failure rate
Barrier methods (± spermicide)	−	−	−	High failure rate; avoid if pregnancy absolutely contra-indicated

Notes: E, oestrogen; high dose ⩾50 μg of ethinyl oestradiol or equivalent; low dose ⩽30 μg.

norethisterone; a monophasic, low-dose oestrogen (35 μg ethinyl oestradiol) with 500 μg norethisterone); a progestogen-only pill (300 μg norethisterone); and a low-dose, triphasic preparation. No differences were found in fasting plasma glucose level, insulin requirements, HbA_1, non-esterified fatty acids, or low-density to high-density lipoprotein cholesterol (LDL:HDL) ratios between the treatment groups. However, the low-dose combined pill produced significant increases in plasma triglyceride and very low density lipoprotein cholesterol levels [19]. Interestingly, diabetic and non-diabetic subjects may react differently to the same preparation. It is reassuring that Radberg, using a preparation of ethinyl oestradiol 50 μg and lynestrol 2.5 mg, found much less deleterious effects on lipids in IDDM than in non-diabetic women [20].

It seems reasonable to restrict the use of the combined pill to young patients without serious diabetic complications or additional risk factors (smoking, hypertension or a strong family history of ischaemic heart disease), and to use it for a limited period, regularly checking blood pressure and fundi. The available data favour a triphasic preparation or the newest low-dose preparations.

THE COMBINED PILL IN PATIENTS WITH PREVIOUS GESTATIONAL DIABETES

Early metabolic studies with 50-μg oestrogen preparations demonstrated decreased glucose tolerance, and it was suggested that oral contraceptives should not be prescribed to women with a previously abnormal glucose tolerance test [21]. It has now been shown that the low-dose combined pill and the triphasic pill produce no change in glucose tolerance in patients with previous gestational diabetes, although a slight rise in plasma insulin levels suggests decreased insulin sensitivity. Most authorities now feel that it is reasonable to use low-dose preparations in women with previous gestational diabetes [22].

THE PROGESTOGEN-ONLY PILL

For most patients electing to take an oral contraceptive, the progestogen-only pill ('mini-pill') has many advantages. There is no epidemiological evidence to associate the progestogen-only pill with vascular disease. Some progestogens in association with oestrogens cause an increase in LDL and a decrease in HDL-cholesterol levels. However, the norethisterone dose in progestogen-only preparations (300–350 μg) is less than that in any combined preparations and causes no change in blood lipids or clotting factors in either diabetic or non-diabetic subjects [20]. The progestogen-only pill has very few side-effects.

The progestogen-only pill is usually criticized on two accounts. First, it is said to be less reliable than the combined pill, although its performance in diabetic women has been very satisfactory [23]. The reported high failure rates are apparently due to patient failure; for once, the rigid schedule of the diabetic patient may confer the advantage of reminding her to take the pill, with her evening insulin, at the recommended time of about 18.00. A second problem is menstrual irregularity. Intermenstrual bleeding usually responds to changing the preparation or doubling the dose for a few cycles. Amenorrhoea may also occur. It is difficult to understand why doctors change contraception when this happens. Most patients are satisfied when reassured that the absence of bleeding is harmless. It is, of course, important to arrange a pregnancy test in a woman who develops amenorrhoea; if this is negative, the preparation is inhibiting ovulation in addition to its basic action on cervical mucus and is therefore particularly effective as a contraceptive.

Injectable progestogens

The injectable progestogen preparations have a place in a few patients when compliance with other methods is likely to be poor and when the risks of an unwanted pregnancy may greatly outweigh any theoretical risks due to changes in blood lipids. Prolonged irregular bleeding can be a problem. An implantable progestogen-containing capsule which can be removed at any time is being developed and may overcome this problem.

The intra-uterine contraceptive device (IUCD)

The IUCD has the advantages of not causing detrimental metabolic effects and not depending on patient compliance. The main concern (and the reason that it is now rarely used in the United States) is the risk of infection, which might theoretically be increased in diabetic patients who are particularly susceptible to various forms of bacterial infection. Moreover, high failure rates of IUCDs in IDDM women have been reported [24, 25] and attributed to differences in the endo-metrial reaction in diabetic women [26–28]. However, some centres (notably Copenhagen) have used large numbers of IUCDs with very few problems and no increased failure rate [29]. These differences in failure rate between various centres may be related to the type of device and the degree of diabetic control.

Whether or not it is increased in diabetic women, the failure rate of an IUCD is rather high (Table 85.2), particularly in the first year of use. This fact, together with the risks of menorrhagia and infection, often rules out the IUCD as the method of first choice, although it may be the best option for a particular patient.

Mechanical (barrier) methods

Barrier methods (condoms, cervical diaphragms) are considered unaesthetic and unreliable and have become generally unfashionable, although with the spread of AIDS, the sheath is making a comeback. The high failure rate is usually because they are not used correctly or not used at all; they are not recommended if pregnancy is absolutely contraindicated. They have no metabolic consequences and are usually free from local side-effects, although a slightly raised incidence of urinary tract infections has been reported in women using a diaphragm [30]. The recently described vaginal shield may be more satisfactory. Highly motivated couples taught to use the diaphragm and sheath correctly may find this an effective and acceptable form of contraception, especially if combined with the use of a spermicidal cream or gel.

Other methods

The 'natural' family planning method of Billings [31] has obvious religious and aesthetic attractions for some patients, but requires much motivation and long periods of abstinence. There is no information regarding its reliability for diabetic women.

There are numerous possibilities for the future. Vaginal rings may be used to deliver steroids more evenly. Immunization against the zona pellucida or against human chorionic gonado-trophin, various potential male contraceptive agents, and antigestogens to be used as postcoital or postconceptional compounds are all under investigation. The induction of electric fields to 'stun' sperm before they enter the cervical canal is another new and interesting approach.

Sterilization

Unfortunately, it may be necessary to advise sterilization in a few patients with serious diabetic complications, as discussed at the beginning of this chapter. Many diabetic mothers request sterilization when they have completed their families, and this is often the contraceptive method of choice at this stage. For some couples, vasectomy may be appropriate; however, because this procedure is often irreversible, the reduced life expectancy of a woman with long-standing IDDM must be borne in mind when considering this option.

JUDITH M. STEEL

References

1 Steel JM, Parbosingh J, Cole RA, Duncan LJP. Pre-pregnancy counselling, a logical prelude to the management of the pregnant diabetic. *Diabetes Care* 1980; **3**: 371−3.

2 Steel JM, Johnstone FD, Smith AF, Duncan LJP. Five years' experience of a pre-pregnancy clinic for insulin-dependent diabetics. *Br Med J* 1982; **285**: 353−6.

3 Bear RA. Pregnancy in patients with renal disease. *Obstet Gynecol* 1976; **48**: 13−18.

4 Grenfell PJ. Pregnancy in diabetic women who have proteinuria. *Q J Med* 1986; **228**: 379−86.

5 Main EK, Main DM, Gabbe SG. Factors predicting perinatal outcome in pregnancies complicated by diabetic nephropathy. *Diabetes* 1984; **33** (suppl 1): 201A.

6 Kitzmiller JL, Brown ER, Phillippe M, Stark AR, Acker D, Kaldany A, Singh S, Hare JN. Diabetic nephropathy and perinatal outcome. *J Obstet Gynaecol* 1981; **141**: 741−51.

7 Nesler CL, Sinclair SH, Schwartz SS, Gabbe SG. Diabetic nephropathy in pregnancy. *Clin Obstet Gynaecol* 1985; **28**: 528−35.

8 Hare JW. Pregnancy in diabetes complicated by vascular disease. *Diabetes* 1977; **26**: 953−5.

9 Silfen SL, Wapner RL, Gabbe SG. Maternal outcome in class H diabetes mellitus. *Obstet Gynecol* 1980; **55**: 749−51.

10 Beetham WP. Diabetic retinopathy in pregnancy. *Trans Am Ophthalmol Soc* 1950; **48**: 205−19.

11 Maloney JM, Drury MI. The effect of pregnancy on the natural course of diabetic nephropathy. *Am J Ophthalmol* 1982; **93**: 745−56.

12 White P. In: Marble A, White P, Bradley R, Krall L, eds. *Joslin's Diabetes Mellitus.* Philadelphia: Lea and Febiger, 1971: 595−7.

13 Dibble CM, Kochenour NK, Worley RJ, Tyler FH, Swartz M. Effect of pregnancy on diabetic retinopathy. *Obstet Gynecol* 1982; **59**: 699−702.

14 Young LB, Steel JM, West CP, Chawla H. Pregnancy after vitrectomy for proliferative diabetic retinopathy. *Diabetic Med* 1987; **4**: 77−8.

15 Steel JM. Pre-pregnancy counselling and contraception in the insulin-dependent diabetic patient. *Clin Obstet Gynaecol* 1985; **28**: 553−66.

16 Steel JM, Johnstone FD, Smith AF. Pre-pregnancy preparation. In: Sutherland HW, Stowers JM, eds. *Carbohydrate Metabolism in Pregnancy and the Newborn.* Fourth International Colloquium. Berlin: Springer Verlag 1989; 129−39.

17 Steel JM, Duncan LJP. The effect of oral contraceptives on insulin requirement in diabetics. *Br J Fam Plan* 1978; **3**: 77−8.

18 Steel JM, Duncan LJP. Serious complications of oral contraception in insulin dependent diabetics. *Contraception* 1978; **17**: 291−5.

19 Skouby SO, Molsted-Pedersen L, Kühl C, Bennet P. Oral contraceptives in diabetic women: metabolic effects of four compounds with different oestrogen/progestogen profiles. *Fertil Steril* 1986; **46**: 858−64.

20 Radberg T, Gustafson A, Skryten A, Karlsson K. Oral contraception in diabetic women, diabetes control, serum and high density lipoprotein lipids during low-dose progestogen, combined oestrogen/progestogen and non-hormonal contraception. *Acta Endocrinol* 1981; **98**: 246−51.

21 Mishell DR. Current status of oral contraceptive steroids. *Clin Obstet Gynaecol* 1976; **19**: 744−64.

22 Skouby SO, Molsted-Pedersen L, Kühl C. Low dosage oral contraception in women with previous gestational diabetes. *Obstet Gynecol* 1982; **59**: 325−8.

23 Steel JM, Duncan LJP. The progestogen only contraceptive pill in insulin-dependent diabetes. *Br J Fam Plan* 1981; **6**: 108−10.

24 Steel JM, Duncan LJP. Contraception for the insulin dependent diabetic. *Diabetes Care* 1980; **3**: 557−60.

25 Wiese J. Contraception in diabetic patients. *Acta Endocrinol* 1974; **182** (suppl): 87−94.

26 Larsson B. Fibrinolytic activity of the endometrium in diabetic women using copper IUCDs. *Contraception* 1977; **28**: 422−5.

27 Gosden C, Steel J, Ross A, Springbett A. Intrauterine contraceptive devices in diabetic women. *Lancet* 1982; i: 530−5.

28 Craig GM. Diabetes, intrauterine devices and fibrinolysis. *Br Med J* 1981; **283**: 1184.

29 Molsted-Pedersen L, Skouby SO. Contraception in diabetic women. In: Sutherland HW, Stowers J, eds. *Carbohydrate Metabolism in Pregnancy and the Newborn.* Third International Colloquium. Edinburgh: Churchill Livingstone, 1984; **119−30**.

30 Vessey MP. Urinary tract infection and the diaphragm. *Br J Fam Plan* 1988; **13**: 41−3.

31 Billings EL, Billings JJ. The idea of the ovulation method. *Australian Family Physician* 1973; **2**: 81−5.

86   Genetic Counselling in Diabetes Mellitus

Summary

• The vast majority of diabetic patients need *not* be advised against having children.

• The risks of a child developing IDDM are about 6% if the father has IDDM, 1% if the mother is affected and 30% if both parents have the disease.

• The overall risk of the sibling of an IDDM patient developing the disease is about 8%; The risks are increased considerably if the sibling is HLA-identical with the patient (16%) or has islet-cell antibodies (up to 76%), and are greatly reduced (about 1%) if the sibling either is HLA-non-identical with the patient or lacks islet-cell antibodies.

• About 10% of *non-identical* twins, and about 35% of *identical* twins, of co-twins with IDDM will ultimately develop the disease. The exact risk depends on age at diagnosis of diabetes, HLA-type and islet-cell antibody status.

• The risks of a child developing NIDDM are about 15% if one parent has the disease and probably about 75% if both are affected.

• The overall risk of NIDDM developing in the sibling of a patient with NIDDM is about 10%.

• The chances of the *non-identical* twin of a patient with NIDDM developing the disease are about 10%, and virtually 100% for an *identical twin*.

• Some varieties of NIDDM (particularly MODY) are apparently transmitted as an autosomal dominant gene; the chances of a child or a sibling of an affected person developing the disease are each 50%.

Genetic counselling about any familial disease has two aspects: firstly, advice about the risk of a given individual developing the disorder, and secondly, humane but realistic discussion about morbidity, mortality and quality of life should this occur.

In the case of diabetes mellitus, accurate genetic counselling presents some problems. The susceptibility of certain families to diabetes was noted by Rondolet in 1574 and by Morton in 1696 and, indeed, the ancient Hindus believed that the disease ran in families. However, it is now obvious that 'diabetes' is a group of conditions of various aetiologies to which hereditary factors make quite different contributions. The first step in genetic counselling is therefore to consider the patient's personal and family history, clinical features and biochemical and other markers, in order to determine whether he has IDDM, NIDDM or one of the minor types of diabetes. Genetic counselling for each of these categories will be considered below in the context of what is known about their inherited predisposition and general outcome. The key statistics are summarized in Tables 86.1 and 86.2.

In most cases, the prognosis of diabetes in both patients and their offspring is sufficiently good that prospective diabetic parents need not be advised against having children [1]. The single exception to this rule is when the patient's life expectancy is so poor (e.g. with advanced diabetic nephropathy) that he or she is unlikely to survive to bring up the child. In this case, it is the risk to the patient rather than the child which determines the suitable course.

Counselling in insulin-dependent diabetes

Epidemiological and aetiological background

IDDM is predominantly a disease of childhood

	IDDM	NIDDM	MODY
One parent diabetic	2% overall (6% if father, 1% if mother)	15% (?)	50%
Both parents diabetic	30% (?)	75% (?)	100%

(?) — Indicates inexact data due to lack of rigorous longitudinal studies.

Table 86.1. Chances of the child of diabetic parent(s) developing diabetes.

	IDDM		NIDDM	MODY
Overall frequency	8%		10%	50%
Subdivided according to:				
HLA-identity with patient				
HLA-identical	16%	after 25 years	HLA-type does not predict risk	—
HLA-haploidentical	9%	after 25 years		
HLA-non-identical	1%	after 25 years		
Islet-cell antibody (ICA) status				
ICA positive	42%		ICA status does not predict risk	—
(complement-fixing ICA-positive	76%)			
ICA negative	1%			
(complement-fixing ICA-negative	3%)			

Note: Risks to twins of diabetic patients are considerably increased, especially with NIDDM (see text).

Table 86.2. Chances of the sibling of a diabetic patient developing diabetes.

with a peak age incidence of 10–15 years [2, 3] (see Chapter 7). The exact prevalence in older people is unknown, although those with organ-specific autoimmune disorders such as Addison's disease and hypothyroidism are at increased risk of the disease [4] (see Chapter 28). The prevalence of IDDM also varies with race and latitude, increasing with distance from the equator and being some 15 times higher in Scandinavia than in Japan [5] (see Chapter 7).

The genetic basis of IDDM has become clearer in recent years. Genes in the class II region of the HLA system on chromosome 6 are associated with IDDM, most notably HLA-DR3 and HLA-DR4 and the HLA-DQ genes linked to these DR genes [6] (see Chapter 14). The presence of an amino acid residue other than aspartate at position 57 of the DQβ chain confers the greatest disease risk. When such substitutions occur in both HLA-DQ β chains, the chance of developing IDDM is 107 times greater than without these genetic changes [7]. However, these genes are not specific for IDDM: up to 20% of the 'normal' population possess them, and only a minority of these subjects will develop the disease.

Other possible indices of risk may be derived from the cellular and humoral immune changes which accompany and indeed precede the clinical onset of IDDM [8] (see Chapter 15). In particular, islet-cell antibodies may have a powerful predictive value, although the family studies performed to date may not be applicable to the general population.

Risks to the children of IDDM parents

The overall risk that a parent with IDDM will have a similarly affected child is small (about 2%). The possibility is greater if the father has IDDM (about 6%) rather than the mother (about 1%), an intriguing observation not attributable to the increased miscarriage rate in diabetic women [9]. When both parents have IDDM, the risk is apparently greater and may reach 30%, though accurate data are not available.

An independent risk to the fetus of a diabetic mother is that of malformation (see Chapter 84); severe malformations (especially sacral agenesis and cardiac abnormalities) affect about 4% of fetuses, about 4 times the risk in the general population. However, there is no evidence that the risk of fetal malformation is genetically determined, and poor diabetic control at around the time of conception and in the first trimester appears to be critical [10] (see Chapter 83). Careful and detailed discussion about the need for impeccable glycaemic control during pregnancy must therefore be part of the counselling offered to diabetic women contemplating pregnancy.

Risks to the siblings of IDDM patients

The siblings of a patient with IDDM are at increased risk of developing the disease. Overall, this amounts to about 8% [11], although the risk is not equal amongst siblings but depends crucially on the number of HLA haplotypes shared with the diabetic index sibling (proband). The cumulative risk of a sibling developing IDDM by the age of 25 years is about 16% when two HLA haplotypes are shared with the proband, 9% when only one haplotype is shared and about 1% for those with none in common [11]. The relative risk compared with the overall risk for siblings of a diabetic proband is about 3.0 for HLA-identical siblings, 1.1 for those who are HLA-haploidentical and 0.05 for non-identical siblings.

Siblings with islet-cell antibodies also have an increased risk of developing IDDM, which amounts to about 42% after 8 years, as compared with 1% for those without islet-cell antibodies [11]. Of those siblings with complement-fixing islet-cell antibodies, 76% developed IDDM within 8 years as compared with only 3% of those without these antibodies [11]. Islet-cell antibodies are therefore a better predictor of the subsequent development of IDDM than HLA status.

Risks to the twins of IDDM patients

The chances of a non-diabetic twin developing IDDM when his co-twin has the disease depend on whether the twins are non-identical or identical.

Probably about 10% of the *non-identical* co-twins of a twin with IDDM develop the disease themselves; the precise figure is not known, as an actuarial analysis of such twins has not yet been performed.

For *identical* co-twins of a twin with IDDM, the risk (estimated by actuarial analysis) is considerably higher at 35% [12], although much lower than in NIDDM (see below). The risk for identical twins apparently depends on the age at diagnosis of the index twin, the time from diagnosis of the index twin, HLA status and the presence of islet-cell antibodies. Identical co-twins of IDDM patients diagnosed before the age of 15 years have a 51% risk of developing IDDM themselves, as compared with 22% of co-twins whose diabetic twin was diagnosed after this age [12]. The risk of developing diabetes falls sharply with time from the diagnosis of the index twin, being about 10% after 4 years and less than 2% after 12 years [12]. Approximately 50% of twins with both HLA-DR3 and DR4 develop IDDM, as compared with about 20% of twins who do not possess both these HLA types [12]. The chance that an identical twin with islet-cell antibodies will develop IDDM is 77%, and 100% for those with persistent complement-fixing islet-cell antibodies [13].

Counselling in non-insulin-dependent diabetes

Epidemiological and aetiological background

NIDDM is the commonest variety of diabetes, affecting about 1% of the British population and up to 50% of adults in certain well-circumscribed groups such as the Pima Indians and Nauruans (see Chapter 7). NIDDM is rare in young people and is mainly a disease of middle and old age; impaired glucose tolerance (IGT) affects up to 15% of people aged over 70 years.

The aetiology of the disease is undoubtedly heterogeneous, comprising a variable combination of a relative impairment of insulin secretion (distinct from the absolute insulin deficiency of IDDM) and decreased tissue sensitivity to insulin (see Chapters 21 and 22). NIDDM is commoner in fat than in lean people and NIDDM patients are, on average, overweight. However, most obese subjects are not diabetic and as many as 60% of patients with NIDDM are not obese. Thus, the role of obesity in the pathogenesis of NIDDM remains unclear (see Chapter 20).

Unlike IDDM, NIDDM is not associated with genes in the HLA region. However, the available evidence suggests that NIDDM is at least in part an inherited condition, although the nature of the genetic defects and their mode of inheritance remain elusive (see Chapter 19). The lack of a genetic marker of the disease means that assessments of disease risk must depend on the family history of the disease, a notoriously unreliable source of information.

Risks to the children of NIDDM parents

In most cases, the inheritance of NIDDM is apparently polygenic. The risk that a parent with NIDDM will have a similarly affected child is not accurately known, as adequate longitudinal studies have not been performed. However, about one-third of children have IGT, of whom perhaps one-half can be expected to develop diabetes, giving an overall risk of about 15% [14, 15]. When both parents have NIDDM, the risk to the offspring is substantial, possibly as high as 75%.

Some variants of NIDDM are inherited in a pattern consistent with a single autosomal dominant gene. The most notable example is maturity-onset diabetes of the young (MODY; see Chapter 25) [16] but similar transmission also occurs in Nauruans and in families with hyperproinsulin-aemia [17, 18] (see Chapter 30).

Patients with NIDDM of early onset (25 to 40 years of age) without a family history consistent with an autosomal dominant mode of inheritance have a very high prevalence of diabetes and glucose intolerance in parents (92%) and in siblings (69%); they may have inherited diabetes genes from both parents [19].

Risks to the siblings of NIDDM patients

About 10% of patients with NIDDM have a similarly affected sibling. In patients with MODY, 50% of siblings are affected and in patients with early-onset NIDDM which is not MODY, 69% of the siblings have diabetes [16, 19].

Risks to the twins of NIDDM patients

In contrast to IDDM, virtually all *identical* twins of patients with NIDDM ultimately develop the disease themselves, usually within 10–15 years of the first twin becoming diabetic [20, 21].

Non-identical twins of patients with NIDDM probably have about a 10% chance of becoming diabetic, although large-scale prospective studies have not been performed. The striking concordance rate in identical twin pairs and the difference between identical and non-identical twins emphasizes the importance of genetic factors in causing NIDDM.

Conclusions

The immediate aim of genetic counselling is to provide accurate estimates of disease risk. Once a disease can be predicted, intervention studies to prevent the phenotypic expression of its inherited basis can be contemplated. The last decade has witnessed major advances in the ability to predict the risks of developing diabetes, particularly IDDM. Given progress in the understanding of the causes of the disease, the ultimate aim — to prevent diabetes — becomes an exciting and realistic prospect.

DAVID LESLIE

References

1 Deckert T, Poulsen JE, Larsen M. Prognosis of diabetics with diabetes onset before the age of thirty-one. *Diabetologia* 1978; **14**: 363–70.

2 Christau B, Kromann H, Christy M, Ortved-Anderson O, Nerup J. Incidence of insulin-dependent diabetes mellitus (0–29 years at onset) in Denmark. *Acta Med Scand* 1979; **642**: 54–60.

3 Crossley JR, Upsdell M. The incidence of juvenile diabetes mellitus in New Zealand. *Diabetologia* 1980; **18**: 29–30.

4 MacLaren NK, Riley WJ. Thyroid, gastric and adrenal auto-immunities associated with insulin-dependent diabetes mellitus. *Diabetes Care* 1985; **8**: 34–8.

5 Taha TH, Moussa MAA, Rashid AR, Fenech FF. Diabetes mellitus in Kuwait: incidence in the first 29 years of life. *Diabetologia* 1983; **25**: 306–8.

6 Michelson B, Lernmark A. Molecular cloning of a polymorphic DNA endonuclease fragment associates insulin-dependent diabetes with HLA-DQ. *J Clin Invest* 1987; **75**: 1144–52.

7 Todd JA, Bell JI, McDevitt HO. HLA DQ beta gene contributes to susceptibility and resistance to insulin-dependent diabetes mellitus. *Nature* 1987; **329**: 599–604.

8 Leslie RDG, Lazarus NR, Vergani D. Events leading to insulin-dependent diabetes. *Clin Sci* 1989; **76**: 119–24.

9 Warram JH, Krolewski AS, Gottlieb MS *et al.* Differences in risk of insulin-dependent diabetes in offspring of diabetic mothers and diabetic fathers. *N Engl J Med* 1984; **311**: 149–52.

10 Leslie RDG, Pyke DA, John PN, White JM. Haemoglobin A1 in diabetic pregnancy. *Lancet* 1978; ii: 958–9.

11 Tarn AC, Thomas JM, Dean BM, Ingram D, Schwartz G, Bottazzo GF, Gale EAM. Predicting insulin dependent diabetes. *Lancet* 1988; i: 845–50.

12 Olmos P, A'Hern R, Heaton DA, Millward BA, Risley D, Pyke DA, Leslie RDG. The significance of the concordance rate for Type 1 (insulin-dependent) diabetes in identical twins. *Diabetologia* 1988; **31**: 747–50.

13 Johnston C, Hoskins P, Millward BA, Leslie RDG, Bottazzo GF, Pyke DA. Islet cell antibodies as predictors of the later development of Type 1 (insulin-dependent) diabetes: a study in identical twins. *Diabetologia* 1989; **32**: 382–6.

14 Leslie RDG, Volkmann HP, Poncher M, Hanning I, Ørskov H, Alberti KGMM. Metabolic abnormalities in children of non-insulin-dependent diabetics. *Br Med J* 1986; **293**: 840–2.

15 Keen H, Jarrett RJ, McCartney M. The ten-year follow-up of the Bedford survey (1962–1972): glucose tolerance and diabetes. *Diabetologia* 1982; **22**: 73–00.

16 Fajans SS, Cloutier MC, Crowther RL. Clinical and

etiological heterogeneity of idiopathic diabetes mellitus. *Diabetes* 1978; **27**, 1112–25.

17 Zimmet P. Type 2 (non-insulin-dependent) diabetes — an epidemiological review. *Diabetologia* 1982; **22**: 399–411.

18 Robbins DC, Shoelson SE, Rubinstein AH, Tager HS. Familial hyperproinsulinemia: two cohorts secreting indistinguishable Type II intermediates of proinsulin conversion. *J Clin Invest* 1984; **73**: 714–19.

19 O'Rahilly S, Spivey RS, Holman RR, Nugent Z, Clark A, Turner RC. Type II diabetes of early onset: a distinct clinical and genetic syndrome? *Br Med J* 1987; **294**: 923–8.

20 Barnett AH, Eff C, Leslie RDG, Pyke DA. Diabetes in identical twins: a study of 200 pairs. *Diabetologia* 1981; **20**: 87–93.

21 Newman B, Selby JV, King M-C, Slemenda C, Fabsitz R, Friedman GD. Concordance for Type 2 (non-insulin-dependent) diabetes mellitus in male twins. *Diabetologia* 1987; **30**: 763–8.

87 Diabetes Mellitus in Childhood and Adolescence

Summary

• Over 95% of cases of diabetes in childhood are due to IDDM, which has a peak age of onset of 12 years.

• IDDM presents in children with classical symptoms, including polyuria and nocturia (often with enuresis), polydipsia, weight loss and malaise. Non-specific presentations include growth failure and abdominal pain. Symptoms are usually present for a few days and occasionally up to several weeks.

• Diabetes should be diagnosed by confirming significant hyperglycaemia (fasting blood glucose concentration > 7.7 mmol/l or random level >11 mmol/l) on two occasions. Hyperglycaemia not due to diabetes is extremely rare in childhood.

• With the support of home visits by the diabetes specialist nurse, newly presenting diabetic children who are not ketotic need only a short hospital admission to begin insulin treatment and learn 'first aid' knowledge of diabetes. Full education and dietary instruction can be given gradually over the following weeks and months.

• Initial insulin dosages average 0.5 U/kg/day but are very variable. Many children show a temporary fall in insulin requirements during the first few months of treatment. This 'honey-moon period', due to transient recovery of B-cell function following reduction of hyperglycaemia, generally lasts a few months.

• Most children eventually need twice-daily insulin injections as their daytime activities become prolonged. Two-thirds of the total daily dosage may be given before breakfast and one-third before the evening meal. Biphasic, pre-mixed insulin preparations may be useful in some cases. 'Pen' devices may help compliance with multiple injection regimens.

• Insulin injection sites should be rotated. The child should gradually be encouraged to inject himself, with no age set for the child to become independent.

• Insulin dosages should be adjusted according to glycaemic control, using self-monitored blood glucose values and HbA_1, and in the longer term, by growth rate and pubertal development. Diet and exercise are also important in improving glycaemic control. Physiological and behavioural changes at puberty often disturb diabetic control.

• Dietary recommendations for children with IDDM are as for adults. Foods rich in complex carbohydrate and fibre should be encouraged, whereas fat and simple sugars should be avoided.

• Exercise-induced hypoglycaemia can often be prevented by planned reductions in insulin dosage before exercise, together with extra 'long-acting' carbohydrate (biscuits, chocolate) taken if blood glucose is less than 4 mmol/l before exercise. As for all children, sport and exercise should be encouraged.

• Intercurrent illnesses frequently cause hyperglycaemia and occasionally hypoglycaemia. Insulin must *never* be stopped and often needs to be increased. Blood glucose levels must be monitored frequently; hypoglycaemia may be controlled by sugar-rich fluids. Medical assistance is needed if symptoms last more than 12 hours, blood glucose persistently exceeds 22 mmol/l, ketonuria appears, or vomiting or diarrhoea develop.

• Adequately treated diabetes generally has little effect on growth, development, school attendance, academic performance or sporting

and other activities.
- Many diabetic children do not comply fully with their management. Compliance will often be improved by providing flexible and considerate advice and is often damaged by criticism from parents or the diabetic care team.
- Diabetic ketoacidosis still carries a high morbidity and mortality in childhood. Presentation includes both classical and non-specific symptoms. Important cases include intercurrent infection, omission of insulin and poor diabetic education.
- In treating ketoacidosis, frequent monitoring of blood glucose, urea and electrolytes and arterial blood pH and blood gases is essential. ECG monitoring may be needed for patients with cardiac arrhythmias or blood potassium disturbances.
- Accurate and controlled intravenous fluid replacement is essential in managing ketoacidosis. The volumes needed should be calculated from the estimated fluid deficit, plus the daily maintenance intake, plus any further fluid losses during treatment. Isotonic saline is given initially and changed to 5% dextrose or dextrose-saline when blood glucose has fallen to 10 mmol/l. Plasma expanders are occasionally needed to treat severe hypotension. Potassium must be replaced carefully according to need.
- Intravenous bicarbonate may paradoxically aggravate intracellular acidosis and may predispose to cerebral oedema. Small amounts of bicarbonate (e.g. 500 ml of isotonic (1.4%) solution) may be given if arterial blood pH is less than 7.0.
- Insulin is best given as a continuous intravenous infusion of insulin diluted in isotonic saline, delivered by a syringe-driver pump. A suitable starting dose is 0.1 U/kg/h but must be adjusted on the basis of frequent glycaemic monitoring. The aim is to reduce blood glucose levels to 10 mmol/l in 6 hours or so; faster rates of fall may precipitate cerebral oedema.
- Cerebral oedema remains a significant cause of death from ketoacidosis in childhood. It is unexplained, but acute changes in osmolality — perhaps due to over-rapid delivery of fluid (hypotonic saline and bicarbonate have been implicated), insulin and a sudden glycaemic fall may contribute. Clinically significant cerebral oedema causes headache and a deterioration in conscious level due to

brain herniation, sometimes with papilloedema. CT scanning confirms the diagnosis. Intravenous mannitol or dexamethasone, given within 10 minutes of brain herniation, may sometimes reduce intracranial pressure.
- Hypoglycaemic symptoms vary considerably but may include faintness, hunger, sweating, abdominal pain and irritability or aggression. Profound and prolonged neuroglycopenia may cause fitting and unconsciousness and occasionally death. There is no firm evidence that repeated mild or moderate hypoglycaemia causes permanent brain damage.
- Hypoglycaemia should be treated immediately with oral carbohydrate or, if consciousness is impaired, with glucose-containing gels smeared inside the cheeks or glucagon injected intramuscularly or deep subcutaneously. Severe hypoglycaemia may require intravenous glucose and glycaemic monitoring for several hours.
- Children with diabetes for several years may develop features of microvascular disease. These are normally subclinical, although 'malignant microangiopathy' with rapidly-deteriorating retinopathy may appear in late adolescence following long-standing diabetes.
- At least 70% of diabetic children will escape significant complications and will live long and relatively healthy lives.
- Care of diabetic children and adolescents is best delivered by a specific children's diabetic care team, comprising medical and nursing staff, a diabetes specialist nurse, dietitian, social worker and paediatric psychiatrist or psychologist.
- Children with diabetes of several years' standing should be reviewed annually, with checks of blood pressure, fundi and albuminuria.
- Diabetic camps and activity holidays are greatly enjoyed by diabetic children and often help to reinforce practical and theoretical aspects of diabetic education. However, glycaemic control and ability to cope with diabetes are not apparently improved in the long term.

Diabetes affecting children is a relatively common problem. The peak age of onset of IDDM — which accounts for virtually all cases of childhood diabetes — is around 12 years [1, 2] and the average district general hospital in Britain will encounter some 12–16 new cases among children and teenagers each year. The basic disease process is identical to that in adults but the treatment of diabetes in childhood is greatly influenced by the physiological processes of growth and maturation during childhood and puberty, together with changes in the child's capacity for self-management and the interplay between family life and emotional and social development.

Prevalence and geographical variation

There is marked geographical variation both between and within countries in the frequency of diabetes in young people [1] (see Fig. 87.1 and Chapter 7). The average annual incidence of diabetes in children under 15 years of age ranges from 1.7/100000 in Japan to 29.5/100000 in Finland and generally rises steadily with increasing distance from the equator. Within the UK, annual incidence varies from 8 to 21/100000 of the population under 16 years of age, being highest in North-East Scotland. Rural areas may have higher incidence rates than urban [3, 4].

These variations, together with the tendency to clustering of cases in the late autumn and spring [2], suggest that environmental agents, perhaps viral infections of childhood, may contribute to the development of IDDM (Chapter 16). Other evidence in favour of an environmental influence includes the increase in incidence of IDDM during the last three decades in Britain [5, 6], a trend also seen in other European countries, notably Finland and Poland. Diabetes in children less than 5 years of age also appears to be increasing [7].

Aetiology of diabetes in childhood

Over 95% of cases of childhood diabetes are due to IDDM but a number of genetic syndromes, either associated with chromosomal abnormalities or single-gene defects, are well recognized. The major syndromes are shown in Table 87.1 and discussed in detail in Chapter 31. Secondary diabetes is occasionally seen in chronic childhood diseases which cause pancreatic damage, such as cystic fibrosis, thalassaemia and cystinosis. The diabetes in these cases is nearly always non-ketotic and clinically similar to NIDDM. Diabetes follows total pancreatectomy, which in infancy is usually performed for intractable hypoglycaemia caused by nesidioblastosis (generalized B-cell hyperplasia) [8]; the resulting diabetes is insulin-dependent but, perhaps because of the loss of pancreatic glucagon, is relatively mild, with low insulin requirements and little tendency to keto-acidosis [9]. Maturity-onset diabetes of the young (MODY) may present in teenagers and is diagnosed by a positive family history and the other features described in Chapter 25.

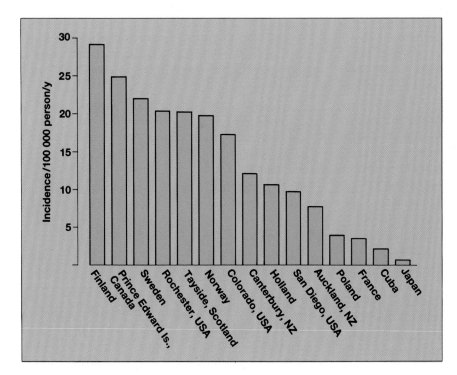

Fig. 87.1. Age-adjusted (world standard) incidence of IDDM in children aged under 15 years in 1980. (Data from Diabetes Epidemiology Research International Group [1].)

Table 87.1. Principal causes of diabetes mellitus in childhood.

Insulin-dependent diabetes mellitus (IDDM) — over 95% of cases

Maturity-onset diabetes of the young (MODY)

Secondary diabetes:
- Chromosomal abnormalities: Down's syndrome
  Turner's syndrome
  Klinefelter's syndrome

- Inherited disorders: Prader−Willi syndrome
  Laurence−Moon−Biedl syndrome
  DIDMOAD syndrome

  Leprechaunism
  Lipodystrophy   ⎫
  Ataxia-telangiectasia   ⎬ with insulin resistance
  (Rabson) Mendenhall syndrome ⎭
  Cystic fibrosis ⎫
  Cystinosis   ⎬ with pancreatic damage
  Thalassaemia   ⎭

- Postpancreatectomy

MODY is described in detail in Chapter 25 and genetic disorders associated with diabetes in Chapter 31.

Presentation and diagnosis

The presentation of diabetes in childhood and adolescence is extremely variable (Table 87.2). Symptoms range from mild to severe and may be present for only a few days or several weeks (which is often realized only in retrospect). Common symptoms include polyuria, especially the sudden onset of nocturia and unexpected night-time incontinence in previously toilet-trained children; polydipsia, which may be difficult to assess in young children whose daytime fluid input is often high; weight loss and growth failure; and abdominal pains, vomiting and general malaise. Other presenting complaints include infections, especially of the urinary tract or skin (abscesses, balanitis, perineal candidiasis), visual disturbance (due to reversible osmotic changes in the lens) and behavioural disturbance. Any child who is unwell should be screened for diabetes by urine or capillary blood glucose testing.

Diagnostic criteria and tests

Hyperglycaemia not due to diabetes is extremely uncommon in childhood but may occasionally develop during an acute illness (e.g. acute appendicitis) or following trauma, when it usually lasts less than 24 hours and is not accompanied by persistent ketosis. These children have no symptoms or evidence of pre-existing diabetes such as growth failure or marked weight loss. Most children found to have transient glycosuria or an isolated raised blood glucose measurement, require no follow-up or counselling after the return to normal has been confirmed.

Virtually all children presenting with diabetes will be symptomatic and in these cases, confirmation of hyperglycaemia (fasting blood glucose concentration >7.7 mmol/l or random concentration >11.0 mmol/l, measured by a laboratory method) on two occasions is diagnostic. Most cases will also have at least some degree of

Table 87.2. Presenting symptoms of IDDM in childhood.

- Polyuria, including nocturia and incontinence
- Thirst and polydipsia
- Weight loss
- Growth failure (falling below height and weight centiles)
- Increased appetite, especially for carbohydrate-rich foods
- Abdominal pains and vomiting
- Blurred vision
- Muscle cramps
- Infections: (a) boils, urinary tract infections
  (b) genital or perineal candidiasis
- Behavioural disturbance, poor school performance
- Inability to concentrate
- Tiredness, lack of energy
- Ketoacidosis: (a) acidotic (Kussmaul) breathing
  (b) protracted vomiting
  (c) dehydration and postural hypotension
  (d) disturbance of consciousness
  (e) coma

ketonuria, which may occasionally occur in the absence of diabetes in children who have been vomiting and anorexic for some days. Formal oral glucose tolerance testing is generally unnecessary. If further investigation is indicated in an asymptomatic child (e.g. because of a family history of diabetes or parental anxiety), the fasting blood glucose level, height and weight can be checked intermittently.

Management of childhood diabetes

Management immediately after diagnosis

Children presenting with diabetic ketoacidosis and dehydration must be treated urgently with intravenous fluids and insulin (see below). Those without ketoacidosis, however, do not usually require emergency treatment [10]. Symptoms have usually been present for several days or weeks and, provided that the child is not ketoacidotic, insulin can be delayed until before the evening meal or even the following morning. If polyuria and polydipsia are present with marked hyperglycaemia (>22 mmol/l), a small dose (0.3–0.5 U/kg) of a soluble insulin may be required.

Most families suffer no harm from the child being admitted for a short stay (up to 48 h) in a modern paediatric ward; prolonged admission to achieve 'good control' and teach the child everything about diabetes is unnecessary and may cause anxiety. Deliberate induction of hypoglycaemia is unnecessary and unlikely to mimic the initial hypoglycaemic episodes. These are usually mild and frequently do not occur for several months, by which time the growing child will have forgotten about his 'artificial' attack in hospital. Nothing will alleviate the parents' anxiety which is provoked by the first hypoglycaemic episode at home. The newly presenting diabetic child can be managed at home if the diabetes team can provide close supervision and instruction (e.g. help with the prebreakfast insulin injections) until confidence has been gained. The child should be instructed to avoid sweets and to change to 'diet-style' soft drinks; other formal dietary advice should be delayed until a home visit by the dietitian.

The results of this less intensive approach, recently adopted at the Children's Diabetic Clinic in Dundee, are illustrated in Fig. 87.2. Children in group 1 were admitted to hospital for only a short stay or not at all (0–1 day), to begin insulin treat-

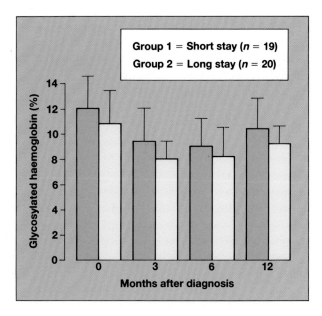

Fig. 87.2. Mean glycosylated haemoglobin levels in newly presenting IDDM children. Group 1 (pink) were admitted for a short (0–1 day) hospital stay, with detailed education and dietary advice delayed for some weeks after diagnosis. Group 2 (yellow) had a conventional longer stay in hospital (7–14 days) with intensive education. Error bars are SD. There are no significant differences between the two groups at any time up to 12 months after diagnosis.

ment and to receive 'first aid' education. Those in group 2 were admitted for a conventional longer stay, with intensive education. All were closely supervised after discharge by the diabetes liaison nurse, who adjusted the insulin regimens as necessary. There were no significant differences in the glycaemic control achieved by the two groups during the first year after diagnosis (Fig. 87.2). Increasing numbers of newly diagnosed diabetic children are now not admitted to hospital at all, but begin treatment at home under the guidance of the diabetes liaison nurse.

INITIAL DIABETES EDUCATION

The diagnosis of diabetes in children and teenagers produces considerable anxiety in the patients and their parents. The diagnosis should be given by a senior doctor, preferably the paediatrician taking charge of the child's diabetic management, who should be optimistic about the future and give any negative information as simply as possible. Initial education is vitally important. Basic information about diabetes, insulin and its action and blood glucose monitoring should be given, together with 'first aid' advice about what to do if hypoglycaemia, hyperglycaemia or vomiting develop. The family should be told how to contact the diabetic care team in an emergency. More detailed discussion about the causes and consequences of diabetes can then take place over the next few months, ideally during home visits by the medical or nursing staff. All children and their families will initially need to have a basic knowledge of diabetes and its management, but additional information (e.g. the causes of diabetes, specific complications, intensified insulin regimens) should be adapted to individual needs. The child's understanding of diabetes and his practical skills will need to be regularly checked, corrected and updated; it must be emphasized that diabetes education is a life-long process (see Chapter 97).

Parents often ask about the inheritance of diabetes and the risks of their other children developing the disease. The genetics of IDDM are discussed in Chapter 14 and genetic counselling in Chapter 86. Other common questions concern a possible 'cure' for diabetes. They should be told that this is an active area of research but that any advances are unlikely to be applied clinically for the foreseeable future. Immunosuppressive treatment with steroids [11], plasmapheresis [12], or cyclosporin therapy [13, 14] in childhood diabetes seems generally disappointing and can only be considered in the context of well-coordinated research studies [15] (see Chapter 103). Pancreatic transplantation (see Chapter 106) is showing promise but also remains experimental. Nonetheless, the child and his parents must be told that diabetes can be controlled if not cured and that its prognosis is increasingly hopeful.

Insulin therapy in childhood diabetes

The daily insulin requirement of the newly diagnosed diabetic child varies considerably. An average initial dose is 0.5 U/kg/day, but this will be adjusted according to the glycaemic response and, in the longer term, the child's general health and growth. Many children show a significant 'honeymoon period', with a marked fall in the daily insulin dose to less than 0.3 U/kg/day during the first 6 months or so after diagnosis. This is due to transient recovery of B-cell function and rarely lasts more than 12 months [16]. The daily insulin dose will need to be increased as the child grows, often to around 0.8–1.0 U/kg/day by the end of the first year. Children frequently require alterations of their daily dose and redistribution of insulin because of changes in their lifestyle and poorly understood factors such as seasonal variation, viral infections and physical and emotional development.

ONE DAILY INJECTION OR TWO?

A single daily injection of an intermediate-acting insulin preparation (0.3–0.5 U/kg/day) is currently thought to be satisfactory for children up to around 6 years of age but is inadequate for most children as they grow older. This should be carefully explained to children and their families who will then usually accept eventual transfer to a conventional twice-daily regimen. Some children manage well with a single injection; there is no reason to change as long as growth is maintained, hypoglycaemia is minimal and the HbA_1 concentration is satisfactory, although the situation must be reviewed regularly.

Twice-daily schedules do not necessarily achieve better glycaemic control than single daily injections; indeed, studies comparing the two regimens under various conditions have shown no significant differences between them [17–19]. In most children, however, prolongation of daytime activities requires a twice-daily regimen, as increasing a single morning dose will produce significant afternoon hypoglycaemia while failing to reduce the evening hyperglycaemia. The frequency of insulin injections must be determined individually for each child; their differing needs may be due to variables such as persisting basal residual insulin secretion, regularity of meal-times and levels of exercise.

When insulin is given twice daily, the same total daily dosage can be divided into two-thirds given before breakfast and one-third before the main evening meal. For simplicity, and given the difficulties of drawing up small doses of insulin, premixed insulins have a useful place in the treatment of children and may well become more acceptable with the wider use of preloaded 'pen' devices (see Chapter 39).

INSULIN INJECTIONS

Basic injection technique is similar to that in the adult. Accuracy in drawing up the insulin should be checked. The current recommendation is for the needle to be inserted perpendicularly to the skin, although there is a possibility that some insulin may be injected intramuscularly. There is no need to swab the skin with spirit beforehand. Injection sites should be rotated. Most children and their parents rapidly become confident with injections and settle into a routine. For the very young child, the injection has to be given by the parents, which requires both confidence and time, particularly in the mornings. Both parents should be instructed and should give injections. The child should gradually be encouraged to inject himself, with no specific target age set for him to become independent. Some children and their families find the trauma of injections hard to overcome. Simple advice about technique, best given at home by the liaison nurse or at a children's camp, is often enough to solve the problem.

INTENSIFIED INSULIN REGIMENS

The hectic lifestyle of the adolescent, with irregular eating times and erratic night-day cycles and exercise routines, suggests that they should be ideal candidates for more flexible, multiple-injection regimens [20, 21]. Many teenagers find that 'pen' devices provide greater personal freedom and more individual control over their diabetes (see Chapter 39). However, no significant glycaemic improvement has been reported during long-term use of multiple-injection regimens. This fact should not deter use of the 'pens', in view of their popularity with youngsters.

Continuous subcutaneous insulin infusion (CSII: see Chapter 42) has also been used by children and teenagers but for the immediate future seems likely to remain a research tool [22, 23].

CHANGES IN INSULIN TREATMENT AROUND PUBERTY

Insulin secretion and sensitivity are reported to change during puberty in non-diabetic children and many diabetic children require more insulin at this stage [24]. In an attempt to improve control, the insulin dosage is often increased to 1.0–2.0 U/kg/day; paradoxically, however, higher dosages generally fail to improve diabetic control and, particularly in girls, may lead to obesity [25]. Insulin dosages should therefore be increased in response to changes in the overall clinical situation, rather than on the basis of glycaemic criteria alone. Other management strategies (diet, exercise) should also be employed to improve blood glucose control.

Diet

Dietary advice for children with IDDM is basically similar to that given to adults [26] (Chapter 41). Specific dietary therapy may be difficult for the young child, but the family should continually be encouraged to adopt general dietary guidelines which nowadays are increasingly seen as appropriate for everyone. About half the energy intake should derive from starchy carbohydrate; simple sugars should be avoided, and a high dietary fibre and reduced fat intake should be encouraged. For diabetic children, regular timing of meals and snacks is important.

The dietary advice should be tailored to the family's understanding and capabilities. Some children may rebel (for example, by eating sweets) if the general dietary rules are too severe. Dietary advice should be reinforced regularly and re-assessed to ensure that the caloric intake is sufficient to sustain growth. A paediatric dietitian is a key member of the team managing diabetic children.

Assessment of diabetic control

The basic methods of monitoring can all be used by children. Urine glucose testing (nowadays using disposable strips) is probably favoured by most young children, although many parents prefer the greater accuracy of blood glucose monitoring. Blood glucose testing is well established in most paediatric clinics and becomes the main technique of monitoring in the teenager [27]. Children should not be overburdened with too many requests for tests and their parents should not be converted into zealots in blood glucose monitoring. One test per day at varying times is perfectly acceptable for the child or adolescent in good health [28].

Very young children tolerate blood glucose testing surprisingly well. Test-sites should include both fingers and toes, in rotation. A night-time test is often reassuring for parents with diabetic infants or toddlers, particularly in view of their relatively long sleeping hours. Urine and blood testing must not be duplicated and blood testing should be encouraged as the main form of monitoring after the age of 10 years or so.

HbA$_1$ or fructosamine estimations, used and interpreted as for adults (Chapter 34), are valuable and for many families are the only acceptable form of 'invasive' routine monitoring. The results, their implications and any discrepancies with self-recorded measurements must be fully discussed with the child and the parents.

Glycaemic control is generally good in the young schoolchild with short-duration diabetes [25], but often worsens in adolescence [25, 29, 30], presumably because of both physiological and behavioural changes. Despite their abnormally elevated HbA$_1$ levels around puberty, sometimes accompanied by delayed growth and puberty, most diabetic children finally achieve a normal adult height [31, 32].

Glycaemic control is influenced by residual insulin secretion, as reflected by C-peptide secretion. Many children and adolescents will retain substantial B-cell reserve, which appears from most studies to relate to the duration of diabetes [16]; severe or absolute C-peptide deficiency may produce marked instability of the diabetes [33].

OTHER MEASURES OF CONTROL

The overall quality of control can be assessed by comparing the child's growth, particularly his height, with the expected population centile charts. Height must be measured at least twice per year. Severe growth failure secondary to chronic poor blood glucose control is nowadays a rare phenomenon. The 'Mauriac syndrome', comprising short stature, poor glycaemic control and hepatomegaly associated with high insulin dosages (Fig. 87.3), was probably iatrogenic, produced by inappropriate insulin regimens, and is now rarely seen [34, 35]. If growth failure occurs, other causes — especially those associated with diabetes, such as coeliac disease, hypothyroidism, and polyendocrine deficiency syndrome — should be sought.

Exercise

The metabolic effects of exercise in normal and diabetic people are discussed in Chapter 78. Hypoglycaemia due to abnormally elevated plasma insulin levels during acute intensive random exercise is the most frequent clinical problem in childhood diabetes (Fig. 87.4). Most children respond readily to oral glucose given at the time; routine 'preloading' with extra glucose is probably unnecessary for most children and is often a method by which otherwise-forbidden sweets are obtained.

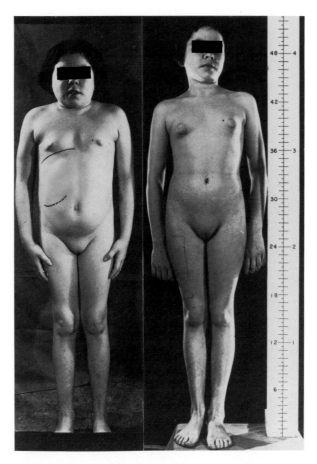

Fig. 87.3. 'Mauriac syndrome' in a 13½ year old girl, with typical obesity, short stature, hepatomegaly (outlined), growth failure and pubertal delay (left). One year later, after a two-thirds reduction in insulin dosage, growth and sexual development have resumed and obesity and hepatomegaly have begun to improve. (Reproduced from Lasalle R, Chicoine L, *Union Méd Canad* 1962; **91**: 963–8, with kind permission of the Editor.)

Exercise patterns and daily energy expenditure are fairly constant for most children [36] and must be carefully considered when planning the schedules of insulin injections and meals. For the older child, specific sports events are best covered either with a planned reduction in insulin (adjusted on an individual basis) or extra carbohydrate at meal times, with carbohydrate readily available in case hypoglycaemia develops during exercise. The blood glucose concentration can be checked before exercise and some 'long-acting' carbohydrate (e.g. biscuits or a small chocolate bar) taken if pre-exercise levels are already low (<4 mmol/l). Although most hypoglycaemic episodes occur during or soon after exercise, some episodes are delayed by up to several hours or even until the next day (see Chapter 78) and

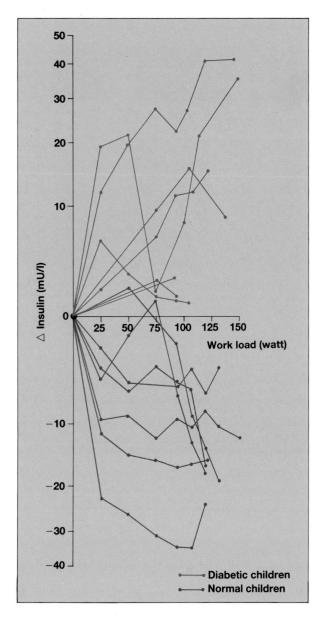

Fig. 87.4. Changes in plasma free insulin levels during acute exercise increasing stepwise to maximum work capacity in seven diabetic and seven non-diabetic children. The opposite changes in insulin concentration — a rise in the diabetic, a fall in the non-diabetic children — account for hypoglycaemia during exercise in diabetic children. In non-diabetic children, blood glucose levels remain constant even during severe exercise.

patients should be warned of this possibility. Some children need less insulin during school holidays, whereas others become noticeably less energetic when not at school.

Education of the children, parents, friends and school staff is essential if hypoglycaemia is to be contained and restricted to mild, short-lived events. Above all, diabetes must not be regarded as a bar to exercise, which indeed should be encouraged.

Intercurrent illness and surgery

Acute viral illnesses, particular upper respiratory tract infections and gastroenteritis, are a frequent cause of unstable metabolic control in children. Hyperglycaemia generally results but hypoglycaemia may occasionally occur. Blood glucose monitoring should be increased during periods of illness and medical advice sought if symptoms persist for over 12 hours; if severe vomiting or diarrhoea develop; if the blood concentration exceeds 22 mmol/l for more than a few hours and fails to fall after insulin injection; or if significant ketonuria (++ or +++) appears. Ketonuria is a particularly serious warning sign, and urine should be tested to check for this during intercurrent illness or periods of hyperglycaemia.

Insulin must *never* be stopped, even if the child cannot eat, and often needs to be increased during acute pyrexial illnesses. Hypoglycaemia may be avoided in anorexic children by changing carbohydrate intake to small but frequent amounts of glucose-rich liquids (e.g. yoghurt, fruit juice or squash, sugar-containing fizzy drinks).

Parents must understand these 'first aid' rules (Table 87.3) and be encouraged to contact the diabetes care team (who should provide a 24-hour advice service) as soon as problems appear. Severe symptoms and marked loss of control will often require intravenous insulin and fluid therapy in hospital.

Living with diabetes

Diabetic control in children is affected by many different complex influences (Fig. 87.5), but

Table 87.3. Instruction during intercurrent illness.

- *Never* stop insulin (you will often need more)

- *Always* check your blood glucose level at least 4-hourly (take food or glucose drinks to prevent hypoglycaemia if necessary)

- *Contact* the diabetes care team or general practitioner if:
  (a) symptoms last more than 12 hours
  (b) vomiting or diarrhoea develop
  (c) blood glucose exceeds 22 mmol/l for more than 4 hours or does not fall with insulin
  (d) ketonuria ++ or +++ develops

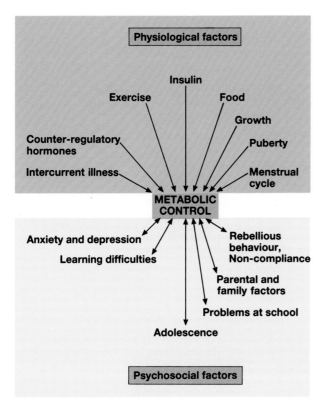

Fig. 87.5. Some factors suggested to influence blood glucose control in children with diabetes mellitus.

fortunately most families generally cope well with the practical management of the disease. The growth, development, school attendance and success in higher education of diabetic children are generally as expected in non-diabetic children [37].

Although a few forms of employment and sport are unsuitable for adolescents with diabetes (see Chapter 92), most teenagers have the same hopes and aspirations as their non-diabetic peers. It should be stressed that many diabetic youngsters go on to achieve considerable success in their chosen careers and pastimes.

All families have overt difficulties at some stage with the management of their diabetes and in coping with the 'hidden anxieties' of the disease [38–40]. Many problems are minor and will be solved by practical help, common-sense advice and understanding. In other cases, however, such problems may come to dominate the lives and irrevocably alter the lifestyle of the child and other family members. Psychological upsets and psychiatric illnesses are common in adults with diabetes (see Chapter 77) and do not spare children. Formal psychiatric and family therapy support

may be needed in some cases, and psychiatric support as well as advice about the physical aspects of diabetes should be readily available from the diabetic care team. Ideally, the team should include a child psychiatrist and/or counsellor; the general lack of these invaluable specialists is a major deficiency of diabetic care teams in the UK.

Compliance with treatment over a long period of time presents many difficulties for children, teenagers and their families. Indeed, lack of compliance in dietary advice, monitoring and clinic attendance is so common, particularly in adolescence, that it could almost be regarded as normal behaviour [41–43]. Many children will not adhere to rigid constraints which they dislike, even after many years of diabetes. Advice must be offered with this in mind and should be flexible and considerate and, wherever possible, presented in a novel way. Realistic goals for each child and his parents should be worked out on an individual basis and praise must be given whenever these aims are achieved. Conversely, criticism by the medical team will discourage the child and almost certainly damage compliance. The major task for diabetic families is to keep the child out of hospital, at school and growing up, and most deserve congratulation for achieving this.

Complications of childhood diabetes

Diabetic ketoacidosis

This is an extremely serious condition in children and, despite significant refinements in management, still carries a significant morbidity and mortality and remains the commonest cause of death in British diabetic patients under the age of 20 years [44]. It is a prolonged medical emergency which requires close medical and nursing supervision.

Children present with a range of symptoms and signs: polyuria, polydipsia, abdominal pains, vomiting, dehydration, acidotic breathing, disturbed consciousness, and ultimately circulatory failure and coma (Table 87.4). Usually the symptoms develop over a few hours, although in some cases ketoacidosis may have been present for several days; in such children, protein loss may be more prominent than dehydration and fluid therapy should be altered appropriately. The biochemical disturbances of ketoacidosis and its diagnostic criteria are described in Chapter 49.

Table 87.4. Features of diabetic ketoacidosis in children.

- Polyuria, nocturia, incontinence
- Thirst, polydipsia
- Abdominal pain
- Vomiting
- Acidotic (Kussmaul) breathing, smell of ketones on breath
- Dehydration, hypotension, collapse
- Disturbed consciousness
- Coma

MANAGEMENT

As in adults, treatment must restore fluid and electrolyte balance (the most immediate threat to life), correct insulin deficiency and restore the supply of glucose and other nutrients to the tissues.

All cases require urgent admission to hospital. Paediatric units should have a preplanned schedule to treat ketoacidosis, such as that outlined in Table 87.5, which will be modified as necessary according to frequent clinical and biochemical assessments. On admission, the child should be weighed if possible or his weight calculated from growth charts; this is essential for controlled fluid replacement. Venous access must be secured immediately, if necessary with a 'cut-down' or central venous cannula. Continuous electrocardiographic monitoring may be needed in case of cardiac arrhythmias or to indicate plasma potassium levels. In comatose children, the need for intubation and assisted ventilation must be constantly reviewed. A nasogastric tube should be passed if the child is unconscious or vomiting or shows clinical or radiological signs of gastric dilatation. The bladder should be catheterized if the child is unconscious, has a palpable bladder or has not passed urine within 3–4 hours of starting fluid replacement.

BIOCHEMICAL MONITORING

On admission, venous plasma glucose, sodium, potassium and bicarbonate concentrations and arterial blood pH and base excess are measured. Electrolyte levels should be re-checked 3-hourly until stable and blood glucose concentrations measured every hour in finger-prick samples; a reflectance meter is adequate if used correctly by trained staff.

Table 87.5. Management of diabetic ketoacidosis in children.

Urgent hospital admission

Fluid replacement:
- Volumes (see Fig. 87.6)
- Isotonic saline; dextrose-saline when blood glucose <10 mmol/l
- Consider bicarbonate if arterial blood pH <7.0
- Consider plasma or plasma expander (25 ml/kg) initially if severe hypotension and coma

Potassium replacement:
- Generally 20 mmol per litre intravenous fluid
- Adjust according to plasma potassium (or ECG)

Insulin replacement:
- Continuous intravenous infusion, initially 0.1 U/kg/h
- Adjust by blood glucose monitoring

Other measures:
- Blood glucose monitoring, hourly until stable
- Fluid balance monitoring
- Plasma urea and electrolytes monitoring, 3-hourly until stable
- Arterial blood gases and pH monitoring if acidotic or hypoxaemic
- Consider oxygen; review need for intubation and ventilation
- ECG monitoring, if arrhythmias or electrolyte disturbances develop
- Nasogastric intubation, if persistent vomiting or gastric stasis occurs
- Urinary catheterization, if retention or apparent oliguria develops
- If cerebral oedema suspected:
  (a) avoid fluid overload and use of hypotonic solutions
  (b) consider intravenous mannitol or dexamethasone

FLUID BALANCE

Fluid replacement in young children must be undertaken with great care, as even small volumes may represent a significant proportion of the body's water content. Constant monitoring of fluid input and output will avoid the need to give large volumes intermittently. A scheme such as that in Fig. 87.6 should therefore be followed in every case. The child's immediate fluid requirements are the sum of his calculated fluid deficit (the product of body weight and estimated percentage dehydration) and normal daily fluid intake, estimated from his age and weight. Twenty percent of this volume should generally be given in the first 2 hours, 20% over the next 4 hours and the remaining 60% during the following 20 hours. Every few hours, fluid losses (in urine, gastric aspirate and diarrhoea) should be calculated and added to the volume to be given during the next few hours. This schedule will obviously need to be altered in circumstances such as circulatory collapse or fluid overload.

The composition of the fluid replacement is also important. Isotonic saline should be given initially and until the blood glucose level has fallen to around 10 mmol/l, when 5% dextrose or isotonic dextrose-saline should be substituted. True hyperosmolar coma (see Chapter 49) is rare in children; even if plasma osmolality is significantly raised, many authorities now advise against giving hypotonic (0.45%) saline, as this may increase the risks of cerebral oedema (see below).

Unless hyperkalaemia is present (plasma potassium concentration >5 mmol/l), potassium should be added to the intravenous fluid at 20 mmol per litre of fluid (or 40 mmol/l if the plasma potassium level is less than 3.5 mmol/l).

The place of bicarbonate administration in treating diabetic ketoacidosis is now controversial because of the possible hazards of paradoxically aggravating intracellular acidosis (see Chapter 49) and cerebral oedema and of precipitating hypokalaemia. Many paediatricians give small amounts of bicarbonate (50–100 ml of hypertonic 8.4% solution or 500 ml of isotonic 1.4% solution over 30 minutes) to children with an arterial blood pH of less than 7.0. If bicarbonate is to be given, the isotonic preparation may be safer as the hypertonic solution causes thrombosis of peripheral veins and extensive local tissue necrosis if extravasated.

Plasma or plasma expanders are sometimes indicated for urgent treatment of circulatory collapse but prompt administration of adequate

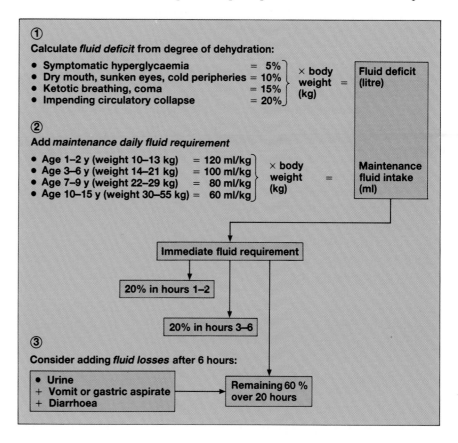

Fig. 87.6. Fluid volume replacement in ketoacidosis in children.

volumes of saline will in most cases correct hypotension and improve tissue perfusion.

INSULIN THERAPY

Insulin is best given by continuous intravenous infusion using a system separate from that delivering intravenous fluid. Soluble insulin can be diluted to 1 U/ml in isotonic saline and infused using a static syringe-driver pump through a cannula inserted into a peripheral vein or the intravenous fluid line (see pp. 822–3). A suitable starting dose is 0.1 U/kg/h and this should be altered according to the blood glucose concentration and its rate of change. Insulin delivery should be titrated to reduce the blood glucose concentration to around 10 mmol/l within 6 hours or so; faster rates of fall are unnecessary and have been implicated in the development of cerebral oedema.

COMPLICATIONS OF DIABETIC KETOACIDOSIS

The use of controlled fluid replacement, continuous low-dose insulin administration and rapid bedside blood glucose measurements have improved the management of diabetic ketoacidosis, and most children recover rapidly and are able to change to routine diabetic treatment after 24–36 hours. The commonest complications — hypoglycaemia and hypo- or hyperkalaemia — are largely avoided by frequent glycaemic and biochemical monitoring and early corrective action.

The most serious complication, and the major cause of death from ketoacidosis in childhood, is acute cerebral oedema which leads to herniation of the brain stem and cerebellar tonsils into the foramen magnum [45–47]. The pathogenesis of cerebral oedema is poorly understood but several studies suggest that rapid changes in blood osmolarity during fluid and insulin replacement may contribute. Possible mechanisms favouring transport of sodium and water into brain tissue include disruption of the blood–brain barrier by opening of the tight junctions between the endothelial cells of the cerebral capillaries [47] and activation by insulin of the Na^+/H^+ exchanger (antiport) in the neurone plasma membrane which normally pumps Na^+ ions inwards in exchange for H^+ ions [48]. Excessive vasopressin secretion [49] may cause retention of free water and cause sudden shifts in osmolarity in various compartments. These possibilities argue that dehydration,

acidosis and hyperglycaemia should be corrected in a controlled fashion over several hours.

Most children with untreated diabetic ketoacidosis have a degree of subclinical brain swelling detectable by CT scanning [50, 51]. The development of clinically significant cerebral oedema is suggested by the onset of headache or a deterioration in conscious level, which may be accompanied by papilloedema. CT scanning of the brain will confirm generalized cerebral oedema (Fig. 87.7).

At present, the treatment of established cerebral oedema is empirical. The fluid replacement regimen should be reviewed and restricted if overload seems likely. Mannitol, 1–2 g/kg infused intravenously over 20–30 minutes, or dexamethasone, 2–4 mg injected intravenously or intramuscularly every 6 hours, may sometimes reduce intracranial pressure, praticularly if given within 10 minutes of brain herniation. Despite active therapy, the mortality of clinically apparent cerebral oedema still exceeds 50%.

INVESTIGATION OF CAUSES OF KETOACIDOSIS

The management of ketoacidosis is incomplete until its cause has been identified and treated as far as possible. A major cause in children is intercurrent infection, often of the urinary or respiratory tracts, and this must be vigorously sought and treated with broad-spectrum antibiotics if suspected. Omission of insulin, either inadvertently or deliberately, seems to be a surprisingly common cause and the child's insulin regimen and ability to draw up and inject insulin must always be checked. Emotional disturbance has been cited as an important precipitant of ketoacidosis, probably because it interferes with the child's ability or desire to manage his or her own diabetes, rather than through any direct metabolic effects (see Chapters 77 and 88).

The development of ketoacidosis often indicates imperfect diabetic education; admission to hospital should be used as an opportunity to evaluate the child's understanding and to correct or reinforce it as necessary.

Hypoglycaemia

Hypoglycaemia is common in diabetic children and typically follows unusual exercise, a missed meal or an injection error. Older children are

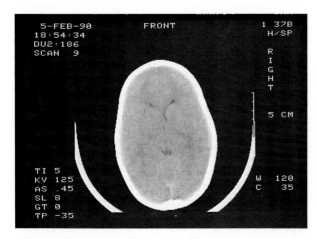 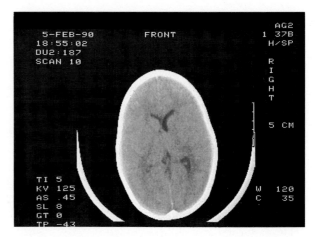

Fig. 87.7. CT scan of the brain of a child with diabetic ketoacidosis complicated by cerebral oedema, showing swelling and loss of detail of the brain substance with compression of the lateral ventricles. (Reproduced by kind permission of Dr Helen Carty, Alder Hey Hospital, Liverpool.)

usually aware of hypoglycaemia themselves or react in a way recognizable to their parents. However, some teenagers with relatively long-standing disease and autonomic neuropathy may lose their warning signs of hypoglycaemia and, in infants, symptoms may not be recognized until severe neuroglycopenia has developed. Hypoglycaemic symptoms usually appear when the blood glucose level falls below 2.5–3.0 mmol/l but the threshold varies greatly, and the features of hypoglycaemia differ considerably between children and may also be inconsistent for a given child. Common symptoms include faintness, a feeling of hunger, sweating, shivering, irritability, abdominal pain, nausea and vomiting, headache, behavioural disturbance and blurred vision. The child will usually appear pale and sweaty and may seem distant, argumentative, confused, aggressive or tearful (Fig. 87.8). Profound neuroglycopenia may result in unconsciousness and fitting.

TREATMENT OF HYPOGLYCAEMIA

Typical symptoms can be treated immediately but, if possible, the diagnosis should be confirmed by measuring the blood glucose concentration. For mild attacks, 20–40 g of oral carbohydrate (e.g. a glass of milk and two plain biscuits, a sweet fizzy drink or six glucose tablets) is usually sufficient. Carbohydrate should be immediately available at home and at school and when travelling or playing sports. Other family members, teachers and friends should know how to treat hypoglycaemia.

If these simple measures fail, glucose-containing gel (e.g. Hypostop®) or ordinary jam can be smeared inside the child's cheeks, or glucagon

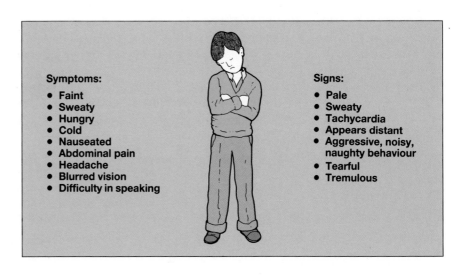

Symptoms:
- Faint
- Sweaty
- Hungry
- Cold
- Nauseated
- Abdominal pain
- Headache
- Blurred vision
- Difficulty in speaking

Signs:
- Pale
- Sweaty
- Tachycardia
- Appears distant
- Aggressive, noisy, naughty behaviour
- Tearful
- Tremulous

Fig. 87.8. Common features of hypoglycaemia in children.

(0.5 mg for children under 6 years and 1.0 mg for those over this age) given by deep subcutaneous or intramuscular injection. Parents should be instructed in the use of both and should be aware that glucagon may cause abdominal pain, sweating and malaise (sometimes resembling hypoglycaemia) 1—2 hours after injection. It should be remembered that glucagon acts by mobilizing hepatic glycogen stores and that these may rapidly become depleted with repeated glucagon administration. If the child does not begin to recover within a few minutes, medical assistance should be sought immediately.

Hypoglycaemic children who are semiconscious, comatose, fitting or slow to recover should be admitted urgently to hospital and given intravenous glucose. An initial bolus of 50—100 ml of 50% dextrose is followed if necessary by 10% dextrose infused at a rate of 100 ml/h, maintained until the child regains consciousness or the blood glucose concentration remains normal and shows no tendency to fall. Fitting due to hypoglycaemia will often settle rapidly with intravenous glucose but may be refractory to intravenous anticonvulsants. After profound hypoglycaemia, especially if due to a long-acting insulin, the intravenous cannula should be left in place and blood glucose monitoring continued for some hours in case hypoglycaemia recurs. Concentrated glucose solutions are very irritant to vein walls and, to avoid thrombosis, should only be injected into large veins.

Following correction of hypoglycaemia, most children recover quickly, although headache and abdominal pain may persist for some hours. If the child remains unconscious after the blood glucose concentration has returned to normal, the most likely cause is a post-ictal state following a hypoglycaemic fit, although other causes of coma (e.g. a head injury sustained during fitting) must be suspected if this is prolonged. Post-hypoglycaemic restlessness is often due to anxiety or discomfort, such as from a full bladder.

Hypoglycaemia may be due to an unsuitable insulin regimen or poor education, and an episode should prompt careful assessment of the child's treatment and understanding of diabetes.

LONG-TERM SEQUELAE OF HYPOGLYCAEMIA

Recovery from profound hypoglycaemia, even with fitting and prolonged unconsciousness, is usually rapid and without apparent neurological damage. Occasional patients may, however, suffer irreversible brain damage or even die during hypoglycaemia. It is not clear whether repeated mild or moderate hypoglycaemic episodes cause any cumulative, permanent intellectual or neurological damage.

Hypoglycaemia is the aspect of diabetes feared most by many patients and their families and its impact must not be underestimated. Anxiety about hypoglycaemic symptoms and the unwelcome attention which they attract may discourage some diabetic children (and adults) from trying to achieve tight glycaemic control. On the other hand, self-induced 'factitious' hypoglycaemia may be used to seek attention from the family or the diabetes care team and is a common feature of 'brittle' diabetes (see Chapter 88).

Microvascular complications

Children and teenagers who have had diabetes for several years may display a number of features, mostly asymptomatic, of incipient or established microvascular complications of the disease. These include excessive urinary albumin excretion [52—55], cardiovascular indices of autonomic neuropathy [56], sensory nerve damage [57], retinopathy [58], cheiroarthropathy [59] and reduced hyperaemic responses of the skin vasculature [60]. Microvascular complications of IDDM are broadly related to the duration of the disease (see Chapter 52) and are more likely to affect people who develop the disease in childhood rather than later in life. This is true of retinopathy and nephropathy and a recent prospective study has demonstrated that autonomic dysfunction advanced markedly during a 5-year period in postpubertal subjects with IDDM [61].

Recent epidemiological evidence suggests that the prepubertal years have little effect on the course of microvascular disease but that 'malignant microangiopathy', i.e. rapidly developing proliferative retinopathy, may appear during late adolescence in children with long-standing diabetes [62]. No specific hormonal or metabolic feature of puberty has yet been implicated.

There have been no long-term studies of the natural history of chronic diabetic complications extending throughout childhood and into adult life, and it should be emphasized to the child's parents, and to the child himself as soon as he is able to understand, that the vast majority of diabetic children (probably well over 70%) will live a long and relatively healthy life. Moreover, recent epidemiological studies suggest that the morbidity and mortality associated with diabetes are beginning to decline (see Chapter 52). This important information must be given to the patient and his parents and will help to encourage them to negotiate the difficult periods of living with diabetes.

The same optimism should apply to discussion about the effects of improved diabetic control on the development and progression of microvascular complications. Although not yet proven, the balance of evidence suggests that near-normoglycaemia may help to prevent or retard complications. Diabetic children — who will face the longest exposure to the disease — should be encouraged as soon as practicable to try to achieve the best possible control of their diabetes. At the same time, they should be reminded that the present-day target range of 4–8 mmol/l is far below the general glycaemic level of diabetic patients a decade ago and that occasional values above 8–10 mmol/l are still consistent with good control.

Organization of care for diabetic children

Paediatric diabetic clinic

As with adult diabetic care, the emphasis is shifting away from the traditional outpatient clinic [63]. A specific children's diabetic clinic should be held in a non-threatening environment, with play facilities, refreshments and videos unrelated to diabetes. All members of the diabetes care team — medical and nursing staff, specialist nurse, dietitian, paediatric social worker and the paediatric psychologist, psychiatrist or counsellor — should be available for discussion and to offer advice and support to the child and his family. This arrangement is usually welcomed by the children and attendance is generally good.

In the first year, frequent visits to the clinic will be needed to establish control and to educate the child and his family about diabetes. Clinic follow-up may usefully be backed up by home visits from medical, nursing and dietetic staff. Children with uncomplicated established diabetes probably need to be seen only 2 or 3 times per year. At each clinic visit, glycaemic control should be assessed and discussed from the child's own blood glucose records and an HbA_1 estimation taken (best measured in a finger-prick sample).

Random blood glucose measurements in the clinic are of limited use, other than to check self-monitoring technique.

Older children with diabetes of several years' standing should be reviewed annually, perhaps during a one-day admission to the ward. The blood pressure and fundi should be checked and a 24-hour urine collection taken to measure albumin excretion.

The diabetes care team should provide a constantly available advice service and a contact telephone number for emergencies; conversely, all families with a diabetic child should have access to a telephone.

Diabetic camps

These provide an informal atmosphere, much appreciated by the children, in which information and education can be provided and practical techniques taught. The first priority of a diabetic camp is to provide an enjoyable holiday, with medical help at hand if necessary. The parents will often benefit by having a rest from the constant, worrying routine of family life with diabetes. In Britain, camps were introduced by the British Diabetic Association, but are now organized locally by many diabetic clinics; encouraging the parents to participate may help them to cope more confidently with the problems posed by having a child with diabetes [64]. Specific activity and adventure holidays for diabetic children are now being developed. The British Diabetic Association can provide information about these and other camps and has suggested guidelines for the medical and nursing supervision of camps.

Diabetes teaching and education in the camps comes from informal discussion with camp staff and other children and is often reinforced by a certain degree of peer pressure. It is important not to expect too much from camps as an educational forum: there are no convincing data that attending a camp produces any improvement in coping with diabetes or in glycaemic control, and the child with 'difficult' diabetes, although usually enjoying the experience, will probably fare no better when he returns home.

Adolescence

Adolescence is a time of great physiological, emotional and behavioural changes which may dramatically influence diabetic control. Fortunately, most adolescent patients cope well with their diabetes and only a few suffer prolonged difficulties, exemplified by 'brittle' diabetes (see Chapter 88).

With many changes in life-style, the patient's motivation to look after his diabetes may be blunted. The continuing need to maintain good glycaemic control must be explained firmly but sympathetically and the risks of long-term complications must be discussed in a realistic but non-threatening fashion.

The best setting to follow patients through adolescence is probably a specific clinic to bridge the gap between the paediatrician and the adult clinic; the latter is a particularly daunting place for teenagers, which may explain their poor attendance if referred directly to a routine adult clinic [43]. Establishing such a clinic will require close cooperation between the paediatrician and the adult diabetologist and the support of other team members.

Teenagers with diabetes undoubtedly benefit from discussing their problems in coping with diabetes, school, employment and personal life with other patients of their own age. A number of schemes, such as the Diabetes Youth Project [65] have now been developed with the aim of improving facilities for young people with diabetes.

Conclusions

Diabetes in childhood presents many challenges, emotional and social as well as medical. Its treatment, whether routine or in emergencies, emphasizes the need for an integrated, carefully planned approach and close cooperation between the various members of the diabetic care team. Its correct management is vitally important as it lays the foundations to help the child and his family to cope with a lifetime of diabetes.

STEPHEN A. GREENE

References

1 Diabetes Epidemiology Research International Group. Geographic pattern of childhood insulin-dependent diabetes mellitus. *Diabetes* 1988; **37**: 1113–19.

2 Gamble DR, Taylor KW. Seasonal incidence of diabetes mellitus. *Br Med J* 1969; **3**: 631–3.

3 Patterson CC, Smith PG, Webb J, Heasman MA, Mann JI. Geographical variation of the incidence of diabetes mellitus in Scottish children during the period 1977–1983. *Diabetic Med* 1988; **5**: 160–5.

4 Waugh NR. Insulin-dependent diabetes in a Scottish region: incidence and urban/rural differences. *J Epidemiol Community Health* 1986; **40**: 240–3.

5 Stewart-Brown S, Hashim M, Butler N. Evidence for increasing prevalence of diabetes mellitus in childhood. *Br Med J* 1983; **286**: 1855–7.

6 Patterson CC, Thorogood M, Smith PG, Heasman A, Clarke JA, Mann JI. Epidemiology of Type 1 (insulin dependent) diabetes in Scotland, 1968–76: evidence of an increasing incidence. *Diabetologia* 1983; **24**: 238–43.

7 Brouhard BH. Management of the very young diabetic. *Am Dis J Child* 1985; **139**: 446–7.

8 Aynsley-Green A, Polak JM, Bloom SR *et al*. Nesidioblastosis of the pancreas: definition of the syndrome and the management of severe neonatal hyperinsulinaemic hypoglycaemia. *Arch Dis Child* 1981; **56**: 496–508.

9 Greene SA, Aynsley-Green A, Soltesz G, Baum JD. The management of diabetes mellitus following total pancreatectomy in infancy. *Arch Dis Child* 1984; **59**: 356–9.

10 Hamilton DV, Mundis SS, Lister J. Mode of presentation of juvenile diabetes. *Br Med J* 1976; **2**: 211–12.

11 Elliott RB, Crossley JR, Bergman CC, Jones AG. Partial preservation of β-cell function in children with diabetes. *Lancet* 1981; ii: 1–4.

12 Marner B, Lernmark A, Ludvigsson J *et al*. Islet cell antibodies in insulin dependent (type 1) diabetic children treated with plasmapheresis. *Diabetes Res* 1985; **5**: 231–6.

13 Shiler CR, Dupre J, Gent M *et al*. Effects of cyclosporin immunosuppression in insulin-dependent diabetes mellitus of recent onset. *Science* 1984; **223**: 1362–7.

14 Assan R, Feutren G, Debray-Sachs M *et al*. Metabolic and immunological effects of cyclosporin in recently diagnosed type 1 diabetes mellitus. *Lancet* 1985; i: 67–71.

15 International Study Group of Diabetes in Children and Adolescents (ISGD). Warning against routine use of cyclosporin for newly diagnosed diabetes. *Lancet* 1987; ii: 981.

16 Ludvigsson J, Heding LG. β-cell function in children with diabetes. *Diabetes* 1978; **26** (suppl 1): 230–4.

17 Akerblom HK, Hiekkala H. Diurnal blood and urine glucose and acetone bodies in labile juvenile diabetes on one and two injection therapy. *Diabetologia* 1970; **6**: 130–4.

18 Werther GA, Jenkins PA, Turner RC, Baum JD. Twenty-four hour metabolic profiles in diabetic children receiving insulin injections once or twice daily. *Br Med J* 1980; **281**: 414–18.

19 Dahlquist G, Blom L, Bolme P *et al*. Metabolic control in 131 juvenile-onset diabetic patients as measured by HbA$_1$c: relation to age, duration, C-peptide, insulin dose and one or two insulin injections. *Diabetic Care* 1982; **5**: 399–403.

20 Jefferson G, Marteau TM, Smith MA, Baum JD. A multiple injection regimen using an insulin injection pen and prefilled cartridged soluble human insulin in adolescents with diabetes. *Diabetic Med* 1985; **2**: 493–7.

21 McCaughey ES, Betts PR, Rowe DJ. Improved diabetic control in adolescents using the Penject syringe for multiple insulin injections. *Diabetic Med* 1986; **3**: 234–6.

22 Greene SA, Smith MA, Baum JD. Clinical application of insulin pumps in the management of insulin dependent diabetes. *Arch Dis Child* 1983; **58**: 578–81.

23 Davies AG, Price DA, Houlton CA, Burn JL, Fielding BA, Postlethwaite RJ. Continuous subcutaneous insulin infusion in diabetes mellitus. *Arch Dis Child* 1984; **59**: 1027–33.

24 Hindmarsh PC, Matthews DR, Di Silvio L, Kurtz AB, Brook CGD. Relation between height velocity and fasting insulin concentrations. *Arch Dis Child* 1988; **63**: 665–6.

25 Mortensen HB, Hartling SG, Petersen KE. A nationwide cross-sectional study of glycosylated haemoglobin in Danish children with type 1 diabetes. *Diabetic Med* 1988; **5**: 871–6.

26 Kinmonth AL, Baum JD. Dietary management of diabetes. In: Meadow R, ed. *Recent Advances in Paediatrics*. London: Churchill Livingstone, 1984.

27 Baum JD. Home monitoring of diabetic control. *Arch Dis Child* 1981; **56**: 897–9.

28 Tattersall RB. Measuring adequacy and lability of control. *Arch Dis Child* 1984; **59**: 807–9.

29 Daneman D, Wolfson DH, Becker DJ, Drash AL. Factors affecting glycosylated haemoglobin values in children with insulin-dependent diabetes. *J Paediatr* 1981; **99**: 847–53.

30 Price DA. Strict glycaemic control. *Arch Dis Child* 1984; **59**: 810–12.

31 Salardi S, Tonioli S, Tassoni P, Tellarini M, Mazzanti L, Cacciari E. Growth and growth factors in diabetes mellitus. *Arch Dis Child* 1987; **62**: 57–62.

32 Jackson RL. Growth and maturation of children with insulin dependent diabetes mellitus. *Paediatric Clin North Am* 1984; **31**: 545–67.

33 Hocking MD, Rayner PWH, Nattrass M. Residual insulin secretion in adolescent diabetes after remission. *Arch Dis Child* 1987; **62**: 1144–7.

34 Mauriac P. Gros ventre, hépatomégalie, troubles de la croissance chez des enfants diabétiques, traités depuis plusieurs années par l'insuline. *Gazette hebdomadaire de la Société Médicale de Bordeaux* 1930; **26**: 402–10.

35 Rosenbloom AL, Clarke DW. Excessive insulin treatment and the Somogyi effect. In: Pickup JC, ed. *Brittle Diabetes*. Oxford: Blackwell Scientific Publications, 1985: 103–31.

36 Stein TP, Hoyt RW, Settle RG, O'Toole M, Hiller WDB. Determination of energy expenditure during heavy exercise, normal daily activity and sleep, using the doubly-labelled-water ($^2H_2{}^{18}O$) method. *Am J Clin Nutr* 1987; **45**: 534–9.

37 Gath A, Smith MA, Baum JD. Emotional, behavioural and educational disorders in diabetic children. *Arch Dis Child* 1980; **55**: 371–5.

38 Close H, Davies AG, Price DA, Goodyear IM. Emotional difficulties in diabetes mellitus. *Arch Dis Child* 1986; **61**: 337–40.

39 Rover JF, Ehrlich RM. Effect of temperament on metabolic control in children with diabetes mellitus. *Diabetes Care* 1988; **11**: 77–82.

40 Challen AH, Davies AG, Williams RJW, Hashum MN, Baum JD. Measuring psychosocial adaptation to diabetes in adolescence. *Diabetic Med* 1988; **5**: 739–40.

41 Lindsay M. Emotional management. In: Baum JD, Kinmonth AL, eds. *Care of the Child with Diabetes*. London: Churchill Livingstone, 1985.

42 Farquhar JW. The adolescent diabetic. *Diabetic Med* 1984; **1**: 9–15.

43 Newton RW. Conference for Young Diabetics: Innovative Care 4. *Diabetic Med* 1987; **4** (suppl): 335–6.

44 Tunbridge WMG. Factors contributing to deaths of diabetics under fifty years of age. *Lancet* 1981; ii: 569–72.

45 Greene SA, Jefferson IG, Baum JD. Cerebral oedema complicating diabetic ketoacidosis. *Develop Med Child Neurol* 1990 (in press).

46 Rosenbloom AL, Riley WJ, Weber FT, Malone JI, Donelly WH. Cerebral oedema complicating diabetic ketoacidosis in childhood. *J Paediatr* 1981; **96**: 357–61.

47 Harris GD, Fiordalsi I, Finberg L. Safe management of diabetic ketoacidaemia. *J Paediatr* 1988; **113**: 65–8.

48 Van der Meulen JA, Klip A, Grinstein S. Possible mechanism for cerebral oedema in diabetic ketoacidosis. *Lancet* 1987; ii: 306–8.

49 Duck SC, Wyatt DT. Factors associated with brain herniation in the treatment of diabetic ketoacidosis. *J Paediatr* 1988; **113**: 10–14.

50 Krane EJ, Rockoff MA, Wallman JK, Wolfsdorf JI. Subclinical brain swelling in children during treatment of diabetic ketoacidosis. *N Engl J Med* 1985; **312**: 1147–51.

51 Hoffman WH, Steinhart CM, El Grammal J *et al.* Cranial CT in children and adolescents with diabetic ketoacidosis. *Am J Neuroradiol* 1988; **9**: 733–9.

52 Huttenen NP, Kaar ML, Puukar R, Akerblom HK. Exercise induced proteinuria in children and adolescents with Type 1 (insulin dependent) diabetes. *Diabetologia* 1981; **21**: 495–7.

53 Jefferson IG, Greene SA, Smith MA, Smith RF, Griffin NKG, Baum JD. Urine albumin to creatinine ratio-response to exercise in diabetes. *Arch Dis Child* 1985; **60**: 305–10.

54 Davies AG, Price DA, Postlethwaite RJ, Addison GM, Burn JL, Fielding BA. Renal function in diabetes mellitus. *Arch Dis Child* 1985; **60**: 299–304.

55 Rowe DJ, Bagga H, Betts PB. Normal variations in rate of albumin excretion and albumin to creatinine ratios in over-night and daytime urine collections in non-diabetic children. *Br Med J* 1985; **291**: 693–4.

56 Young RJ, Ewing DJ, Clarke BF. Nerve function and metabolic control in teenage diabetes. *Diabetes* 1983; **32**: 142–7.

57 Heimans JJ, Bertelsmann FW, de Beaufort CE, de Beaufort AJ, Feber Y-A, Bruining GJ. Quantitative sensory examination in diabetic children: assessment of thermal discrimination. *Diabetic Med* 1987; **4**: 251–3.

58 Burger W, Hovener G, Düsterhus R, Hartmann R, Weber B. Prevalence and development of retinopathy in children and adolescents with Type 1 (insulin dependent) diabetes mellitus. A longitudinal study. *Diabetologia* 1986; **29**: 17–22.

59 Rosenbloom AL, Malone JI, Yucha J, Van Cader TC. Limited joint mobility and diabetic retinopathy demonstrated by fluorescein angiography. *Eur J Paed* 1984; **31**: 107–17.

60 Ewald N, Tuvemo T. Reduced vascular reactivity in diabetic children and its relation to diabetic control. *Acta Paed Scand* 1985; **74**: 77–84.

61 Young RJ, Macintyre CCA, Ewing DJ, Prescott RJ, Clarke BF. Clinical neuropathy is common in young IDDM and predicted by abnormal neurophysiology 5 years earlier. Abstract 26 *British Society Paediatric Endocrinology* Meeting, September 1988.

62 Norris J, Dorman J, Orchard T *et al.* Contribution of diabetes duration before puberty to development of microvascular complications in IDDM subjects. *Diabetes Care* 1989; **12**: 686–93.

63 Working Party Report. *Organisation of Services for Children with Diabetes in the United Kingdom*. London: British Paediatric Association, 1989.

64 Marteau TM, Gillespie C, Swift PGF. Evaluation of a weekend group for parents of children with diabetes. *Diabetic Med* 1987; **4**: 488–90.

65 Newton RW, Isles T, Farquhar JW. The Firbush Project — sharing a way of life. *Diabetic Med* 1985; **2**: 217–24.

88 'Brittle' Diabetes Mellitus

Summary

• 'Brittle' diabetes can be defined as metabolic instability sufficient to cause major disruption to the lifestyle or to endanger the life of a diabetic patient.

• It occurs mostly in IDDM patients and, although rare, its management is frequently costly and results in immense physical and emotional strain on the patients, their families and the health care team.

• There are many possible causes of brittleness, including inappropriate insulin regimens (particularly over-insulinization), defective subcutaneous insulin absorption, abnormal insulin clearance, abnormalities in counter-regulatory hormones, infections and intercurrent illness, factitious disease, the effects of psychosocial stress and eating disorders. Deliberate interference with treatment is thought to be a major cause.

• In most brittle patients, no clear cause can be identified. These 'idiopathic' cases tend to present with some common features: young women predominate, with mild overweight, high subcutaneous insulin requirements, a high prevalence of family and psychosocial problems and an onset of brittleness which is temporally related to menarche.

• A treatable disorder is not usually found and management consists of ensuring that a single senior doctor is assigned to investigate and explore treatment approaches, and is available for consultation at all times. Insulin given by continuous subcutaneous infusion (CSII) or by intravenous, intramuscular or intraperitoneal infusion is not usually effective in the long-term, although totally-implanted insulin pumps have produced some improvement in a few cases.

• Psychotherapy and counselling may help to reduce hospital admissions but objective measures of glycaemic control are not usually improved.

'Brittle' diabetes can be defined as metabolic instability sufficient to cause major disruption to the lifestyle or to endanger the life of a diabetic patient. Virtually all such patients have IDDM, but many different factors may contribute to brittleness. Although brittle diabetes is rare, the condition imposes immense physical and emotional burdens on the patients, their families and the diabetes care team, and its management can be enormously expensive. It has been difficult to formulate a rational approach to brittle diabetes because there is no general agreement as to how to identify, investigate or treat these patients, and there is still debate as to the causes of brittleness and even as to whether the condition truly exists. The problems posed by brittle diabetes have aptly been described as 'frustrating, tedious and difficult' [1].

This section will attempt to review the definitions and possible causes of brittleness and will outline a scheme for the investigation and management of patients with disabling metabolic instability.

Definitions of brittle diabetes

The term was first used by Woodyatt some 15 years after the introduction of insulin [2] and has been used with great enthusiasm and inconsistency ever since. The key features of brittleness are metabolic instability and disruption of life, and both must be quantified in order to define the condition consistently.

Metabolic instability is manifested by chaotic profiles of blood concentrations of glucose and other metabolites, such as ketone bodies and non-esterified fatty acids. For convenience, metabolic control is commonly described in glycaemic terms alone (see Chapter 34). The hallmark of brittleness is variability, which may be measured simply by the number of hypoglycaemic or ketoacidotic episodes, or more rigorously by the frequency, amplitude and unpredictability of glycaemic swings. Examples of extremely unstable glycaemic profiles from a girl with brittle diabetes are illustrated in Fig. 88.1.

The measures used to quantify glycaemic behaviour are shown in Table 88.1 (see also Chapter 34) and representative 'stable' and 'brittle' values are given in Table 88.2. Average glycaemic values (measured as the mean of a series of estimations, or assessed indirectly by HbA₁ or fructosamine concentrations) are frequently high in brittle patients but provide no information about variability, which is described by parameters such as the standard deviation of a glucose series [3], M value, mean amplitude of glycaemic excursions (MAGE), fasting ascending glycaemic excursions (FAGE) and the mean of daily differences (MODD). The M value of Schlichtkrull [4] is an attempt to express the quality of glycaemic control (measured as excursions from an 'ideal' value) in a single number; its derivation is described in Chapter 34. MAGE is a measure of the amplitude of significant glycaemic excursions [5], whereas FAGE [6], indicates the magnitude of the 'dawn phenomenon' (see Chapter 51) and MODD [7] the extent of day-to-day variability. Urinary

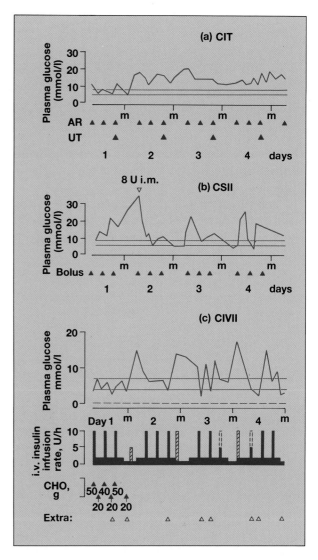

Fig. 88.1. Extremely unstable glycaemic profiles in a 14-year-old girl with brittle diabetes, treated with conventional injection treatment (CIT) with ultralente (UT) and short-acting insulin (AR) (a); CSII (b); and continuous intravenous insulin infusion (CIVII) (c). m = midnight. (Reproduced from [59] with permission of the Editor of *Diabetes Care*.)

Table 88.1. Some indices of brittleness (see text for explanation).

Average control	Glycaemic excursions	Average plus excursions	Day-to-day variability
Mean blood glucose level	SD	M value	MODD
HbA₁	Range MAGE		SD of fasting blood glucose level
Fructosamine	FAGE		
Glycosylated albumin	Frequency of hypoglycaemia Frequency of ketoacidosis		

Index	Normal	Stable diabetic	Brittle diabetic	Reference
MAGE (mmol/l)	2.5	4−5	>7.0	5
M value (4.4 mmol/l as standard)	0−1	10−30	40−300	5, 17
MODD (mmol/l)	0.5	0.5−2.0	2−9	7
SD of fasting BG	−	0.7−1.6	4.4−6.4	3

Table 88.2. Representative values for some indices of brittleness. BG = blood glucose concentration.

glucose or ketone estimations do not provide sufficiently precise information about metabolic instability.

Disruption to lifestyle can be assessed by means such as the number of emergency admissions to hospital per year, and the time absent from work or school.

Possible causes of brittle diabetes

Some possible causes of metabolic instability in insulin-treated IDDM patients are shown in Fig. 88.2. As emphasized below and in several recent large studies [8−10], the cause of brittleness remains elusive in many cases.

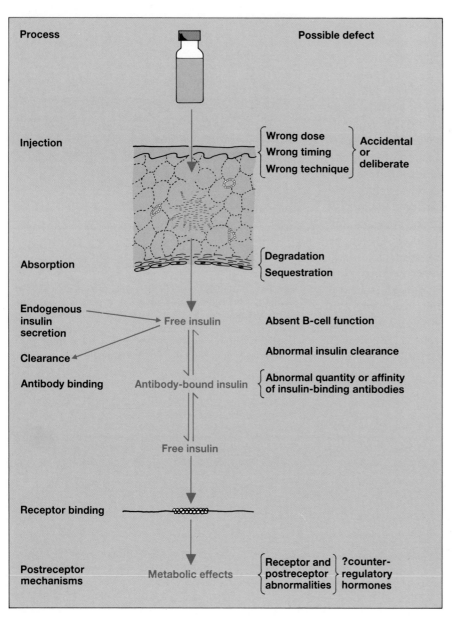

Fig. 88.2. Some possible causes of metabolic instability in insulin-treated diabetic patients.

Inappropriate insulin regimens

Iatrogenic brittleness can be due to prescribing an insulin regimen unsuited to the patient's individual needs. The proposal by Michael Somogyi and others [11–15] that wide glycaemic fluctuations might be due to excessive insulin dosages has received much attention. The 'Somogyi effect' describes hyperglycaemia following in the wake of hypoglycaemia, the latter often occurring at night and sometimes being asymptomatic. The original patients displayed cyclical glycosuria and ketonuria, and both hypo- and hyperglycaemia tended to improve when initially high insulin dosages (often >1.5 U/kg/day) were reduced [12–15]. Rebound hyperglycaemia was attributed to accentuated insulin resistance following excessive release of counter-regulatory hormones during hypoglycaemia. Although this mechanism can be demonstrated and may contribute to hyperglycaemia before breakfast and during the day following nocturnal hypoglycaemia, it is undoubtedly rarer than previously assumed. The role of the Somogyi effect and its interaction with the physiological predawn increase in insulin resistance (due mostly to growth hormone secreted during the small hours) and with the effects of increasing insulin deficiency (from the previous evening's insulin injection running out), are discussed in detail in Chapter 51.

Since Somogyi's original observations, insulin treatment and measurements of metabolic control have both been refined. The relevance of over-insulinization to patients nowadays regarded as brittle is controversial. Rosenbloom and colleagues [15, 16] argue that insulin dosages are excessive in up to 70% of diabetic children, one-third of whom may display features of the so-called 'Mauriac' syndrome of over-insulinization, such as hepatomegaly, truncal obesity, growth failure and delayed puberty (Table 88.3 and Fig. 87.3). Many of these characteristics have been described in the various groups of patients with 'idiopathic' brittle diabetes and apparent insulin resistance (see below) but, unlike patients with true over-insulinization, reducing insulin dosages in 'idiopathic' brittle patients merely exacerbates hyperglycaemia and ketosis [17, 18].

The patient may be responsible for an inappropriate insulin regimen, either accidentally through ignorance, misunderstanding or carelessness, or by deliberate interference with treatment. Factitious hyper- or hypoglycaemia due to intentional

Table 88.3. Clinical clues to the diagnosis of over-insulinization (based on Rosenbloom and Giordano [15]).

- Obvious hypoglycaemic episodes
- Polyuria, nocturia, enuresis
- Excessive appetite
- Hepatomegaly
- Headaches, relieved by food
- Weight gain
- Exercise intolerance
- Variation in glycosuria and glycaemia
- Frequent ketoacidosis
- Mood swings, irritability
- Increasing insulin dosages yet worsening control
- Ketonuria without glycosuria
- Worsening symptoms with increased insulin dosages

omission or overdosage of insulin may be commoner than suspected and may explain some cases of 'idiopathic' brittleness (see below).

Defective subcutaneous insulin absorption

Several groups have reported patients who, when treated with subcutaneous insulin injections, displayed glycaemic instability (i.e. brittleness) and/or high insulin requirements, but whose metabolic control improved markedly when conventional insulin dosages were given intravenously [19–22], intramuscularly [23], or intraperitoneally [24]. These alternative routes were presumed to bypass a 'barrier' to insulin absorption from subcutaneous tissue. The observation that subcutaneous injection of insulin mixed with the protease inhibitor, aprotinin, also improved control in some such patients [22] suggested that the 'barrier' might be due to excessive degradation of insulin at its injection site. This possibility has been supported by direct evidence in only three cases, where subcutaneous fat biopsies showed an increased ability to destroy insulin [21, 25, 26]. In other apparently similar cases, however, insulin-degrading activity of subcutaneous fat does not seem to be increased [10, 27]; the absorption-enhancing effect of aprotinin, which also occurs in non-diabetic subjects [28], may be due to its powerful stimulation of blood flow close to the injection site [29]. The postulated barrier to subcutaneous insulin absorption has also been attributed to defects in injection-site blood flow. Insulin causes prolonged hyperaemia at its subcutaneous insulin site in normal and stable diabetic subjects, but this response was significantly impaired in a group of patients with idiopathic brittle diabetes [30]. However, although subcutaneous blood flow is a major determinant of insulin absorption, subsequent studies [31, 32] found no relationship between the magnitude of injection-site hyperaemia and insulin appearance in the circulation or, indeed, any evidence that the absorption or hypoglycaemic action of insulin was impaired in brittle as compared with stable subjects. Further detailed and carefully controlled investigations, again in clinically similar subjects with unexplained metabolic instability and apparent insulin resistance, also found that the increase in plasma free insulin levels and the glycaemic fall after standardized subcutaneous insulin injection did not differ significantly from those in stable IDDM subjects [10]. These latter authors conclude that the 'syndrome of subcutaneous insulin resistance', if it exists at all, must be extremely rare even in these highly selected patients with apparent brittleness and/or insulin resistance. It seems most likely that some, perhaps all, of their patients were surreptitiously interfering with their treatment, although it could be argued that the highly artificial setting of the study might have failed to reveal a genuine defect in insulin absorption or action.

Absence of endogenous insulin secretion

Virtually all severely brittle IDDM patients have undetectable C-peptide levels after glucagon stimulation [3, 17, 18, 33]. As a group, C-peptide-negative patients show more unstable metabolic control than those with residual endogenous insulin secretion, even if this is minimal [34, 35]. However, after several years of diabetes, a large proportion of IDDM patients will have no detectable insulin secretion and yet enjoy reasonable or even good metabolic control. Absence of endogenous insulin secretion is therefore clearly not the primary cause of brittleness, although the inability to 'buffer' against periods of insulin deficiency, especially when the injection depot becomes exhausted overnight, may aggravate instability due to other causes.

Abnormal insulin clearance

Circulating free insulin concentrations are determined by the interplay between insulin entering the circulation from endogeneous secretion (if any remains) and absorption from the injected depot,

and its removal either by clearance in tissues (notably the liver and kidney) or by becoming complexed to insulin-binding antibodies (if these are present). Insulin resistance, sometimes extreme but essentially never accompanied by unpredictable metabolic instability (i.e. true brittleness), is a feature of the various syndromes characterized by congenital or acquired defects of the insulin receptor; in these subjects, impairment of receptor-mediated internalization and clearance of insulin leads to extremely high circulating insulin levels (see Chapter 29).

There is no firm evidence for insulin receptor abnormalities in brittle diabetes. However, three patients have been described with massive resistance to insulin administered by all routes, including the intravenous, implying that the cause of insulin resistance could not solely be defective subcutaneous absorption [26, 36, 37]. These patients had inappropriately low plasma insulin levels during very high rates of intravenous insulin delivery (up to 20 000 U/day) [37], which could only be explained by very rapid clearance from the circulation. The sites of clearance in these cases are not known, but as well as the liver and kidney, the vascular endothelium is a possible candidate, as it is known to be able to take up insulin [38]. One of these patients [37] also showed unpredictable and unexplained periods of apparently restored insulin sensitivity, when administration of small insulin dosages produced appropriate rises in circulating insulin levels. These episodes were signalled by sudden and profound hypoglycaemia and usually followed a period of poor control; it has been postulated that the preceding very high rates of insulin delivery may have saturated the extraction mechanism, and that hypoglycaemia might be due to re-entry into the circulation of previously sequestered, non-degraded insulin [37]. Theoretically, such a mechanism could explain insulin resistance and, if clearance were irregular, metabolic instability in other brittle patients. However, the responses of a large group of idiopathic brittle and/or insulin-resistant patients to intravenous insulin were essentially normal [10], arguing against this possibility.

Removal of free insulin by insulin-binding antibodies can cause immunological insulin resistance (see Chapter 40) and fluctuations in the avidity or capacity of antibody binding could, theoretically, cause brittleness. However, there is no evidence to support this hypothetical mechanism.

Abnormalities in counter-regulatory hormones

The counter-regulatory hormones (growth hormone, glucagon, cortisol and catecholamines) tend to aggravate hyperglycaemia and are implicated in the posthypoglycaemic insulin resistance of the Somogyi effect; nocturnal growth hormone secretion may also contribute to the fasting hyperglycaemia of the dawn phenomenon (see Chapter 51). Conversely, deficiencies of these hormones — as in patients with total pancreatectomy or hypopituitarism — may severely impair the ability to recover from hypoglycaemia, leading to profound and sometimes life-threatening hypoglycaemic attacks. Fluctuating levels of one or more counter-regulatory hormones could therefore produce brittleness, with or without insulin resistance. Growth hormone secretory peaks are exaggerated and more frequent in adolescent IDDM patients, especially those with unstable disease [39] but are apparently the result rather than the cause of poor control. IDDM patients in general may show enhanced sensitivity to the metabolic effects of various counter-regulatory hormones [40] but specific studies in brittle patients have not been performed. In one group of idiopathic brittle patients, circulating glucagon, cortisol and growth hormone levels (measured under conditions of good control achieved by the artificial endocrine pancreas) were similar to those in stable patients [41].

The role, if any, of counter-regulatory hormones is therefore uncertain. A possible effect of gonadal steroids is suggested by the very high female preponderance of 'idiopathic' brittle diabetes but this possibility has not been formally investigated.

Infections and other intercurrent events

Infections may precipitate up to 30% of all episodes of ketoacidosis in IDDM patients [42] and the metabolic response to infection could, in principle, contribute to or even provoke episodes of hyperglycaemia and ketoacidosis. However, with the exception of a few children in whom recurrent streptococcal pharyngitis was thought to explain repeated episodes of poor control [43], there is no evidence of chronic or relapsing infection in the published studies of brittle diabetic patients.

Coexisting endocrine conditions — adrenal failure or overactivity, thyroid disorders, hypopituitarism — and other diseases such as chronic pancreatitis, malabsorption, gastroparesis, drug and alcohol abuse can all disturb diabetic control, sometimes in an unpredictable way, but do not contribute significantly to the numbers of patients with long-standing, life-disrupting metabolic instability [9, 44].

Factitious disease and malingering

It has become apparent that some and possibly many patients with otherwise unexplained metabolic instability may be interfering with their treatment. Such interference may take many forms; factitious hypoglycaemia [45−47] is quite common and some other examples are illustrated in Table 88.4. This behaviour must aggravate metabolic control in many cases and in one series was held responsible for brittleness in one-half of the subjects [9]. However, some patients with indisputably 'organic' causes of brittleness may also sometimes interfere with their treatment [37], and the importance of malefaction is far from clear in many others.

Some workers have distinguished 'malingering' or 'manipulating', where patient-induced disease has a supposedly obvious motive of gain (such as avoiding school, work or responsibilities) from factitious disease, where self-destructive behaviour has no identifiable ulterior motive [8]. However, their separation may depend largely on the success of the psychiatrist in uncovering any motive and the distinction is probably not useful. It is easy to formulate plausible reasons for deliberate non-compliance, including 'cries for help', seeking attention or affection, 'testing' of parents and doctors, punishing self and others, and denial of illness [48]. However, whether these motives actually operate has not been tested and would be difficult to investigate.

Inadvertent non-compliance may arise because the patient has been badly informed, has poor understanding or is unable to execute and adjust his own treatment. Most groups have found little or no reason to think that brittle diabetes is the result of deficient education, although perhaps surprisingly, Schade et al. [8] concluded that about one-quarter of their patients with incapacitating brittle diabetes had deficits in communication skills sufficient to account for their instability. It is not clear why these patients were not improved

Example	How detected
Faked injections (under close supervision)	Injected insulin (labelled with low-activity isotope) discovered in cotton-wool swab used to clean injection site; none detectable at supposed injection site
Diluting insulin in pumps (CSII or intravenous infusion) with tap-water	Possibility suggested by recurrent septicaemia with cold-growing (tap-water) organisms; very low measured insulin levels and lack of characteristic smell of cresol insulin preservative in pump reservoir
Additional injections (under close supervision)	Insulin and syringes hidden, e.g. in lavatory cistern or under window-sill
Immobilizing pump by removal or reversal of pump batteries	Routine (unexpected) checking of pump
Disconnecting infusion cannulae; pulling out central venous catheters (tunnelled subcutaneously and stitched to the skin)	Routine checks
Simulating hypoglycaemia (in presence of inexperienced medical staff)	Normal blood glucose level on checking
Simulating hyperglycaemia	Sticky fingertips (previously dipped in fizzy glucose drink)
Fabricating home blood records	Comparison with values recorded simultaneously by a 'memory' meter

Table 88.4. Examples of interference with treatment documented in IDDM patients with unexplained brittleness. It must be emphasized that this behaviour may or may not be the underlying cause of brittleness.

by in-hospital, supervised, intensive insulin therapy if psycholinguistic difficulties were the only explanation for their poor control.

The detection of interference with treatment is often difficult, as is underlined by the ingenuity of some of the examples in Table 88.4. None of our patients has ever admitted deliberate manipulation while in hospital but a few have subsequently confirmed this, normally to fellow patients. Sadly, management of this problem is neither easy nor successful. Confronting the patient with 'being caught out' — no matter how tactfully — has a uniformly unsatisfactory outcome and usually succeeds only in alienating the patient, her family and often other members of the diabetes care team. Formal psychiatric or psychological assessment may fail to detect recognizable pathology and most patients will refuse psychotherapy or psychiatric follow-up. Orr *et al.* [45] described a group of adolescent patients with self-induced hypoglycaemia, all of whom displayed significant psychopathology including depression and suicidal behaviour; these latter features may be

relatively common in idiopathic brittle patients [44, 49].

Psychosocial influences

There is no doubt that many patients with unstable diabetes suffer much psychosocial stress, which often spills over to affect other family members [50, 51]; common problems in these patients are illustrated in Table 88.5. However, it is not clear, largely because of methodological difficulties [48], whether brittleness is the cause or effect of the psychosocial disturbance or is merely an epiphenomenon. As discussed in Chapter 77, psychosocial stress is still generally assumed to be able to cause severe metabolic instability, even though the early studies [52, 53] are difficult to interpret and have not been repeated, and recent carefully controlled acute studies (with rather unsatisfactory stressors) have failed to confirm such an effect [54].

Nonetheless, family stresses are often considerable and could indirectly lead to brittleness,

Table 88.5. Some commonly reported psychosocial associations in patients with brittle diabetes and their families.

- Single parent
- Parents or patient divorced
- Poor living conditions and/or limited financial resources
- Over-protective parents
- Inadequate or disinterested parents
- Family conflict
- Psychiatric pathology or alcoholism in family
- Illness or death in family
- Poor acceptance of diabetes by patient
- Manipulation of diabetes by patient
- Truancy or poor performance at school
- Antisocial behaviour of patient
- Depression in patient
- Decreased self-esteem of patient
- Anxiety in patient

Table 88.6. Clinical features of 'idiopathic' brittle diabetes (compiled from [8–10, 17, 18]).

- Young females (virtually exclusively)
- Onset of brittleness often closely related to puberty
- Mildly overweight
- High apparent subcutaneous insulin dosages (often >2.0 U/kg/day)
- Variable responsiveness to intramuscular, intravenous or intraperitoneal insulin administration
- Menstrual irregularities
- High incidence of psychosocial disturbances
- Deliberate interference with treatment is common

perhaps by encouraging deliberate malefaction by the patient (e.g. omitting insulin to become unwell and therefore the centre of attention), rather than through a neuroendocrine stress response.

Eating disorders

Anorexia or bulimia, especially if alternating in bouts, could clearly profoundly disturb metabolic control. Eating disorders seem to be commoner in diabetic patients than in non-diabetic subjects [55] (see Chapter 82) and their high prevalence in young women, the group most represented in patients with idiopathic brittle diabetes, suggests the need for further study of a possible association.

'Idiopathic' brittle diabetes

A large proportion of patients unresponsive to modern intensified insulin treatment regimens will have no obvious cause for their instability. Despite different demographic characteristics and rather informal diagnostic criteria, several British and North American groups have found these 'idiopathic' brittle diabetic patients to have certain common clinical features [8–10, 17, 18] (Table 88.6). Interestingly, with few exceptions, brittle diabetes has not apparently emerged as a significant clinical problem in other countries during the last decade or so.

The vast majority of these patients (indeed, 100% in some series) are young females, mostly in their teens or early twenties. Most spend several weeks or even months per year in hospital. They tend to be mildly overweight (body-mass index generally

23–25 kg/m^2), which is perhaps surprising in view of their tendency to severe hyperglycaemia and recurrent ketoacidosis. Their apparent subcutaneous insulin requirements are high, often >2.0 U/kg/day and sometimes reaching several thousand U/day, but many respond normally to very closely supervised subcutaneous, intramuscular or intravenous insulin administration, at least initially. The age at onset of brittleness was significantly correlated with that of menarche, hinting at a role for endocrine and/or emotional disturbances at this time [17] and subsequently; menstrual disorders were also common. Some patients have obvious lipohypertrophy at injection or infusion sites [17]. Most study groups suggest a very high prevalence of family and psychosocial problems, sometimes with overt psychiatric disorder, and episodes of malefaction were detected in many cases.

The cause or causes of brittleness in this group remain unknown, although deliberate malefaction seems likely in many cases [8–10, 17, 18, 49]. Despite their apparent uniformity, there is no firm evidence to suggest a well-defined pathophysiological 'syndrome'; the high prevalence of idiopathic brittle diabetes in young females may simply parallel those of other disorders with a variable element of surreptitious 'self-destructive' behaviour such as anorexia nervosa, bulimia, laxative and diuretic abuse, psychogenic vomiting and artefactual dermatitis. Few such patients have been followed up over the long term but one study suggests that most patients tend to improve metabolically, although only a minority become 'stable' [49]. Microvascular complications tend to develop after several years of brittleness. Psychosocial problems generally persist, and some patients have died unexpectedly, possibly through suicide ([49]; G.V. Gill, personal communication).

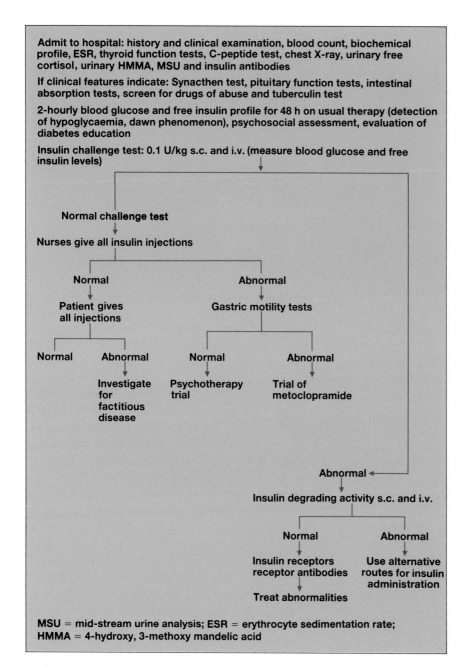

Admit to hospital: history and clinical examination, blood count, biochemical profile, ESR, thyroid function tests, C-peptide test, chest X-ray, urinary free cortisol, urinary HMMA, MSU and insulin antibodies

If clinical features indicate: Synacthen test, pituitary function tests, intestinal absorption tests, screen for drugs of abuse and tuberculin test

2-hourly blood glucose and free insulin profile for 48 h on usual therapy (detection of hypoglycaemia, dawn phenomenon), psychosocial assessment, evaluation of diabetes education

Insulin challenge test: 0.1 U/kg s.c. and i.v. (measure blood glucose and free insulin levels)

Normal challenge test

Nurses give all insulin injections

Normal

Patient gives all injections

Abnormal

Gastric motility tests

Normal

Abnormal

Investigate for factitious disease

Normal

Psychotherapy trial

Abnormal

Trial of metoclopramide

Abnormal

Insulin degrading activity s.c. and i.v.

Normal

Insulin receptors receptor antibodies

Treat abnormalities

Abnormal

Use alternative routes for insulin administration

MSU = mid-stream urine analysis; ESR = erythrocyte sedimentation rate;
HMMA = 4-hydroxy, 3-methoxy mandelic acid

Fig. 88.3. An algorithm for the investigation of brittle diabetes. (Adapted from [8–10] and [44].)

Investigation of brittle diabetes

Figure 88.3 outlines suggestions for the investigation of a patient with unstable IDDM; these guidelines have been adapted from our own experience and that of other groups [8–10, 44]. Routine tests to exclude coexistent endocrine, infective or other conditions should be followed by formal insulin challenge tests [10] under closely supervised conditions in which deliberate interference with the procedures is made as difficult as possible; a glance at Table 88.4 will confirm that this may not be a simple task. Patients should be confined to a previously checked room for 48

hours without personal possessions; insulin injections must be given by medical or nursing staff, visitors must be banned, and all food entering and leaving the room must be checked. Persuading a patient to undergo these investigations will obviously demand great tact and careful explanation if he or she is to continue to trust and have confidence in the diabetes team looking after him or her. Normal ranges for insulin challenge tests have been published by Schade and Duckworth [10]. Fig. 88.4 shows the results of a bedside locker search in a brittle diabetic.

Psychological and/or psychiatric assessment,

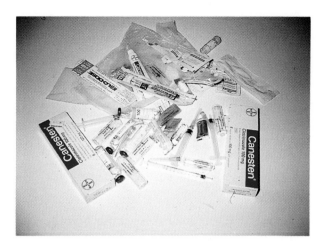

Fig. 88.4. The results of a bedside locker search of a brittle diabetic patient. (Reproduced by kind permission of Dr Geoffrey V. Gill, Arrowe Park Hospital, Wirral.)

ideally by a specialist who works closely with the diabetic team and who has experience in this area, is invaluable and should be organized early; even if no pathology is discovered, many patients will require and should be offered the opportunity of long-term follow-up to help them to cope with their disrupted lives.

Treatment approaches

In most cases, a treatable disorder will not be found. In this case, the management of brittle diabetes is 'primarily an exercise in the organization and delivery of medical care' [56]. A single senior doctor should be assigned to investigate and treat the patient and should be available by telephone at all times to advise her and her family. On-demand consultation may be able to avert hospital admissions, which are often prolonged, ultimately demoralizing for the patient and all concerned, and extremely costly in medical resources.

A number of different methods of administering insulin have been attempted; most approaches will succeed for a while in patients who are naïve to them, but metabolic control will soon deteriorate in most cases.

Continuous subcutaneous insulin infusion (CSII) (see Chapter 42)

This generally fails to improve day-to-day metabolic control or to reduce the frequency or duration of hospital admissions [23]; indeed, failure to respond to CSII has been used as a diagnostic cri-

terion for this group [17, 18]. CSII may, however, improve control in patients whose principal difficulty is with recurrent hypoglycaemia [57], and variable-rate basal CSII regimens (without prandial boosts) have been claimed to reduce but not abolish instability in a small group of highly selected patients [58].

Continuous intramuscular infusion

This uses a CSII pump delivering insulin through a cannula implanted into the deltoid, and is essentially a research procedure which has improved control in a few cases for up to several days [23]. Some patients have been treated for longer (up to 1 year) but the practical difficulties of the technique and the local hazards of infection and fibrosis preclude its routine use.

Continuous intravenous insulin infusion (CIVII)

This has been more widely used, usually employing a portable external pump infusing insulin (commonly at rates of 1–5 U/h) through a Silastic® Hickman catheter which is tunnelled subcutaneously and passed into the right atrium through the subclavian vein [22, 59]. Some patients apparently unresponsive to subcutaneous insulin administration have enjoyed short periods of satisfactory control, although far from the near-normoglycaemia which would be expected in stable IDDM patients; overall control was not improved [59]. Some patients, particularly those with difficult peripheral venous access, have been maintained with CIVII for several months. However, complications are frequent and include infection at catheter insertion sites, septicaemia and central venous thrombosis (Fig. 88.5); some of these episodes may have been due to deliberate tampering with the pump, including diluting the insulin with tap-water [59].

Implantable pumps

Implantable pumps delivering insulin into either a central vein or the peritoneal cavity [24, 60–62] have met with a certain success, perhaps because these devices are inaccessible to most tampering. The design of the Infusaid® pump and related devices is discussed in Chapter 44. Metabolic control may be improved to the point where the patient can return to school or work. Emergency admissions with ketoacidosis have been virtually

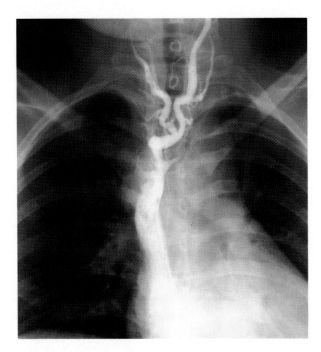

Fig. 88.5. Extensive central venous thrombosis in a brittle diabetic girl after several months' treatment with continuous intravenous insulin infusion delivered by an external pump into a subclavian vein—right atrial catheter. She subsequently admitted to having diluted the infused insulin with tap-water. (Reproduced with permission from Gill *et al.* 1985 [18].)

abolished in some cases, when the costs of the pump and materials have been rapidly offset by the savings in other hospital resources [62].

Adjunctive treatments

There are designed to enhance insulin absorption or action. As mentioned above, a few subcutaneously resistant patients have responded to aprotinin—insulin mixtures injected subcutaneously [22], but many others have not [63, 64] and life-threatening anaphylaxis has followed the use of this agent [64]. One patient with massive resistance to subcutaneously and intravenously administered insulin and increased insulin-degrading activity in subcutaneous fat showed improved insulin sensitivity when treated with oral chloroquine phosphate; this effect presumably relates to the ability of chloroquine to inhibit insulin degradation in various tissues [26].

Psychotherapy and counselling

Psychotherapy and counselling for the patient either alone or in a small group to include the patient's family or other similar patients, may be accepted by a few subjects and may help to reduce hospital admission and to improve attendance at school; objective measures of metabolic control are, however, generally unaffected [50]. A team approach involving the specialist nurse, the physician responsible for the patient, a social worker, psychologist and psychiatrist is probably the most likely to succeed.

Conclusions

A glance at the literature concerning brittle diabetes will confirm that the pendulum of medical opinion has swung several times between 'organic' and 'emotional' factors as being the likely cause of the condition. At present, attention has drifted away from possible organic causes such as defective insulin absorption, which was a popular notion a few years ago. Nonetheless, the contribution of malefaction remains uncertain as it may coexist with a 'genuine' defect [37]. Gill [44] has made the intriguing suggestion that initial tampering with treatment could lead to loss of metabolic control which, combined with iatrogenic attempts to restore normoglycaemia with ever-larger doses of insulin, could ultimately induce a self-perpetuating, uncorrectable state of insulin resistance and instability.

Brittle diabetes remains a rare and difficult enigma, but its cost to the community — well over £100 000 in the case of one patient [37] — is still considerable and the damage it inflicts on the patient and her family is incalculable. Intellectual and financial considerations suggest that brittle diabetes deserves urgent intensive research; however, given its attendant psychological problems, some would say that close investigation and attention to these patients may not be in their best interests.

JOHN C. PICKUP
GARETH WILLIAMS

References

1 Santiago JV. Another facet of brittle diabetes. *J Am Med Ass* 1986; **256**: 3263–4.
2 Woodyatt RT. Diabetes mellitus. In: Cecil R, ed. *A Textbook of Medicine*, 4th edn. Philadelphia: W.B. Saunders, 1937: 620.
3 Shima K, Tanaka R, Morishita S, Tarui S, Kumahara Y, Nishikawa M. Studies on the etiology of 'brittle diabetes'. Relationships between diabetic instability and insulino-genic reserve. *Diabetes* 1977; **26**: 717–25.

4 Schlichtkrull J, Munck O, Jersild M. The M value: an index of blood sugar control in diabetics. *Acta Med Scand* 1965; **177**: 95–102.

5 Service FJ, Molnar GD, Rosevear JW, Ackerman E, Gatewood LC, Taylor WT. Mean amplitude of glycemic excursions, a measure of diabetic instability. *Diabetes* 1970; **19**: 644–55.

6 Schmidt MI, Hadji-Georgopoulos A, Rendell M, Margolis S, Kowarski A. The dawn phenomenon, an early morning glucose rise: implications for diabetic intraday blood glucose variation. *Diabetes Care* 1981; **4**: 579–85.

7 Molnar G, Taylor WF, Ho MM. Day-to-day variation of continuously monitored glycaemia: a further measure of diabetic instability. *Diabetologia* 1972; **8**: 342–8.

8 Schade DS, Eaton RP, Drumm DA, Duckworth W. A clinical algorithm to determine the etiology of brittle diabetes. *Diabetes Care* 1985; **8**: 5–11.

9 Schade DS, Drumm DA, Duckworth WC, Eaton RP. The etiology of incapacitating, brittle diabetes. *Diabetes Care* 1985; **8**: 12–20.

10 Schade DS, Duckworth WC. In search of the subcutaneous insulin resistance syndrome. *N Engl J Med* 1986; **315**: 147–53.

11 Somogyi M. Exacerbation of diabetes by excess insulin action. *Am J Med* 1959; **26**: 169–91.

12 Perkoff GT, Tyler FH. Paradoxical hyperglycemia in diabetic patients treated with insulin. *Metabolism* 1954; **3**: 110–17.

13 Bloom ME, Mintz DH, Field JB. Insulin-induced posthypo-glycemic hyperglycemia as a cause of 'brittle' diabetes. *Am J Med* 1969; **47**: 891–903.

14 Bruck E, MacGillivray MH. Posthypoglycemic hyper-glycemia in diabetic children. *J Pediatr* 1974; **84**: 672–80.

15 Rosenbloom AL, Giordano BP. Chronic overtreatment with insulin in children and adolescents. *Am J Dis Child* 1977; **131**: 881–5.

16 Rosenbloom AL, Clarke DW. Excessive insulin treatment and the Somogyi effect. In: Pickup JC, ed. *Brittle Diabetes*. Oxford: Blackwell Scientific Publications, 1985: 103–31.

17 Pickup JC, Williams G, Johns P, Keen H. Clinical features of brittle diabetic patients unresponsive to optimised sub-cutaneous insulin therapy (continuous subcutaneous insulin infusion). *Diabetes Care* 1983; **6**: 279–84.

18 Gill GV, Husband DJ, Walford S, Marshall SM, Home PD, Alberti KGMM. Clinical features of brittle diabetes. In: Pickup JC, ed. *Brittle Diabetes*. Oxford: Blackwell Scientific Publications, 1985: 29–40.

19 Schneider AJ, Bennett RH. Impaired absorption of insulin as a cause of insulin resistance (abstract). *Diabetes* 1975; **24**: 443.

20 Henry DA, Lowe JM, Citrin D, Manderson WG. Defective absorption of injected insulin (letter). *Lancet* 1978; ii: 741.

21 Paulsen EP, Courtney JW, Duckworth WC. Insulin resistance caused by massive degradation of subcutaneous insulin. *Diabetes* 1979; **28**: 640–5.

22 Freidenberg GR, White NH, Cataland S, O'Dorisio TM, Sotos JF, Santiago JV. Diabetes responsive to intravenous but not subcutaneous insulin: effectiveness of aprotinin. *N Engl J Med* 1981; **305**: 363–8.

23 Pickup JC, Home PD, Bilous RW, Keen H, Alberti KGMM. Management of severely brittle diabetes by continuous subcutaneous and intramuscular insulin infusions: evidence for a defect in subcutaneous insulin absorption. *Br Med J* 1981; **282**: 347–50.

24 Campbell IW, Kritz H, Najemnik G, Hagmueller G, Irsigler K. Treatment of type 1 diabetic with subcutaneous insulin resistance by a totally implantable insulin infusion device ('Infusaid'). *Diabetes Res* 1984; **1**: 83–8.

25 Maberly GF, Wait GA, Kilpatrick JA, Loten EG, Gain KR, Stewart RDH, Eastman CJ. Evidence for insulin degradation by muscle and fat tissue in an insulin resistant patient. *Diabetologia* 1982; **23**: 333–6.

26 Blazar BR, Whitely CB, Kitabchi AE *et al*. In vivo chloroquine-induced inhibition of insulin degradation in a diabetic patient with severe insulin resistance. *Diabetes* 1984; **33**: 1133–7.

27 Williams G, Pickup JC. Subcutaneous insulin degra-dation. In: Pickup JC, ed. *Brittle Diabetes*. Oxford: Blackwell Scientific Publications, 1985: 154–66.

28 Berger M, Cüppers HJ, Halban PA, Offord RE. The effect of aprotinin on the absorption of subcutaneously injected regular insulin in normal subjects. *Diabetes* 1980; **29**: 81–3.

29 Williams G, Pickup JC, Bowcock S, Cooke E, Keen H. Subcutaneous aprotinin causes local hyperaemia: a poss-ible mechanism by which aprotinin improves control in some diabetic patients. *Diabetologia* 1983; **24**: 91–4.

30 Williams G, Pickup J, Clark A, Bowcock S, Cooke E, Keen H. Changes in blood flow close to subcutaneous insulin injection sites in stable and brittle diabetics. *Diabetes* 1983; **32**: 466–73.

31 Williams G, Pickup JC, Collins ACG, Keen H. Subcutaneous insulin absorption and glycaemic responses in brittle dia-betes (abstract). *Diabetic Med* 1986; **3**: 6A.

32 Williams G. Blood flow at insulin injection sites. In: Pickup JC, ed. *Brittle Diabetes*. Oxford: Blackwell Scientific Publi-cations, 1985: 132–53.

33 Gill GV, Home PD, Massi-Benedetti M *et al*. Clinical and metabolic characteristics of patients with 'brittle' diabetes (abstract). *Diabetologia* 1981; **21**: 507.

34 Fukuda M, Tanaka A, Tahara Y, Yamamoto Y, Kumahara Y, Shima K. Relationship between residual B-cell function and A-cell response to hyperglycemia (abstract). *Diabetes* 1987; **36** (suppl 1): 97A.

35 Yue DK, Baxter RC, Turtle JR. C-peptide secretion and insulin antibodies as determinants of stability in diabetes mellitus. *Metabolism* 1978; **27**: 35–44.

36 McElduff A, Eastman CJ, Haynes SP, Bowen KM. Apparent insulin resistance due to abnormal enzymatic insulin degradation: a new mechanism for insulin resistance. *Aust NZ J Med* 1980; **10**: 56–61.

37 Williams G, Pickup JC, Keen H. Massive insulin resistance apparently due to rapid clearance of circulating insulin. *Am J Med* 1987; **82**: 1247–52.

38 Jialal I, King GL, Buchwald S *et al*. Processing of insulin by bovine endothelial cells in culture. Internalisation with-out degradation. *Diabetes* 1984; **33**: 794–800.

39 Molnar GD, Taylor WF, Langworthy A, Fatourechi V. Diurnal growth hormone and glucose abnormalities in un-stable diabetics: studies of ambulatory-fed subjects during continuous blood glucose analysis. *J Clin Endocrinol* 1972; **34**: 837–46.

40 Shamoon H, Hendler R, Sherwin RS. Altered responsiveness to cortisol, epinephrine, and glucagon in insulin-infused juvenile onset diabetics. *Diabetes* 1980; **29**: 284–91.

41 Home PD, Gill GV, Husband DJ, Massi-Benedetti M, Marshall SM, Alberti KGMM. Hormonal and metabolic abnormalities. In: Pickup JC, ed. *Brittle Diabetes*. Oxford: Blackwell Scientific Publications, 1985: 167–80.

42 Nattrass M, Hale PJ. Clinical aspects of diabetic ketoacido-sis. *Rec Adv Diabetes* 1984; **1**: 231–8.

43 White NH, Santiago JV. Clinical features and natural history of brittle diabetes in children. In: Pickup JC, ed. *Brittle Diabetes*. Oxford: Blackwell Scientific Publications, 1985: 19–28.

44 Gill GV, Walford S, Alberti KGMM. Brittle diabetes — present concepts. *Diabetologia* 1985; **28**: 579–89.

45 Orr DP, Eccles T, Lawlor R, Golden M. Surreptitious insulin administration in adolescents with insulin-dependent diabetes mellitus. *J Am Med Ass* 1986; **256**: 3227–30.

46 Schade DS, Drumm DA, Eaton RP, Sterling WA. Factitious brittle diabetes mellitus. *Am J Med* 1985; **78**: 777–84.

47 O'Brien IAD, Lewin IG, Frier BM, Rodman H, Genuth S, Corrall RJM. Factitious diabetic instability. *Diabetic Med* 1985; **2**: 392–4.

48 Williams G, Pickup JC, Keen H. Psychological factors and metabolic control: time for reappraisal? *Diabetic Med* 1988; **5**: 211–15.

49 Williams G, Pickup JC. The natural history of brittle diabetes. *Diabetes Res* 1988; **7**: 13–18.

50 Orr DP, Golden MP, Myers G, Marrero DG. Characteristics of adolescents with poorly controlled diabetes referred to a tertiary care center. *Diabetes Care* 1983; **6**: 170–5.

51 White K, Kolman ML, Wexler P, Polin G, Winter RJ. Unstable diabetes and unstable families: a psychosocial evaluation of diabetic children with recurrent ketoacidosis. *Pediatrics* 1984; **73**: 749–55.

52 Hinkle LE, Wolf S. Importance of life stress in course and management of diabetes mellitus. *J Am Med Ass* 1952; **148**: 513–20.

53 Baker L, Barkai A, Kaye R, Haque N. Beta adrenergic blockade and juvenile diabetes: acute studies and long-term therapeutic trial. *J Pediatr* 1969; **75**: 19–29.

54 Kemmer FW, Bisping R, Steingruber HJ, Baar H, Hardtmann F, Schlaghecke R, Berger M. Psychological stress and metabolic control in patients with type 1 diabetes mellitus. *N Engl J Med* 1986; **314**: 1078–84.

55 Rodin GM, Daneman D, Johnson LE, Kenshole A, Garfinkle P. Anorexia nervosa and bulimia in female adolescents with insulin dependent diabetes mellitus: a systematic study. *J Psychiatr Res* 1985; **19**: 381–4.

56 Gale EAM. Basic principles in the management of unstable diabetic control. In: Pickup JC, ed. *Brittle Diabetes*. Oxford: Blackwell Scientific Publications, 1985: 183–99.

57 Ng Tang Fui S, Pickup JC, Bending JJ, Collins ACG, Keen H, Dalton N. Hypoglycemia and counterregulation in insulin dependent diabetic patients: a comparison of continuous subcutaneous insulin infusion and conventional injection therapy. *Diabetes Care* 1986; **9**: 221–7.

58 Nathan DM. Successful treatment of extremely brittle, insulin-dependent diabetes with a novel subcutaneous insulin pump regimen. *Diabetes Care* 1982; **5**: 105–10.

59 Williams G, Pickup JC, Keen H. Continuous intravenous insulin infusion in the management of brittle diabetes: etiologic and therapeutic implications. *Diabetes Care* 1985; **8**: 21–7.

60 Husband DJ, Marshall SM, Walford S, Hanning I, Wright PD, Alberti KGMM. Continuous intraperitoneal insulin infusion in the management of severely brittle diabetes — a metabolic and clinical comparison with intravenous infusion. *Diabetic Med* 1984; **1**: 99–104.

61 Gill GV, Husband DJ, Wright PD *et al*. The management of severe brittle diabetes with 'Infusaid' implantable pumps. *Diabetes Res* 1986; **3**: 135–7.

62 Buchwald H, Chute EP, Goldenburg FJ *et al*. Implantable infusion pump management of insulin diabetes mellitus. *Ann Surg* 1985; **202**: 278–82.

63 White NH, Santiago JV. Enhancing subcutaneous insulin absorption. In: Pickup JC, ed. *Brittle Diabetes*. Oxford: Blackwell Scientific Publications, 1985; 241–53.

64 Pickup JC, Bilous RW, Keen H. Aprotinin and insulin resistance. *Lancet* 1980; ii: 93–4.

89   Diabetes Mellitus and Old Age

Summary

• In old age, diabetes and glucose intolerance are more frequent and are increasing in frequency.

• Fasting blood glucose concentrations increase by 0.05 mmol/l per decade and levels 1−2 h after an oral glucose load by 0.4−0.7 mmol/l.

• Postreceptor insulin resistance (which reduces glucose uptake into muscle) and impaired insulin secretion are the main causes of glucose intolerance in old age.

• Diabetic symptoms are often non-specific and vague; presentation is often because of cardiovascular disease and other associated conditions, or through biochemical screening.

• Diabetic old people frequently have significant cardiovascular and other complications.

• Cardiovascular disease in old age may present with atypical symptoms, such as painless myocardial infarction or lower limb ischaemia without claudication.

• Ketoacidosis is rare but its mortality is high; non-ketotic hyperosmolar coma almost always occurs in old age and also carries a high mortality.

• Weight reduction has a very low success rate in elderly people.

• Shorter-acting 'second generation' sulphonylurea drugs are preferred in old people, whose impaired glucose homeostasis and renal function increase the risks of hypoglycaemia.

• Metformin is best avoided in elderly people because of their increased tendency to lactic acidosis.

• The benefits and disadvantages of insulin treatment must be carefully considered in older NIDDM patients, in whom insulin can often be safely withdrawn.

• Drug interactions, non-compliance and inappropriate prescription are particular hazards of drug treatment in elderly people.

There is no clear definition of 'elderly' but 'old age' is often taken to begin at 65 years, when men generally retire and pensions become payable. However, most people aged 65−75 years do not feel or seem 'old', or make use of health and social services facilities for the elderly. Beyond the age of 75 years, people become increasingly frail and susceptible to multiple chronic diseases, leading to disability and increasing dependence on others. Of particular relevance are the 'oldest old' (those aged 85 years and over), who are not only most liable to the problems of old age but are also the most rapidly increasing age group in Western countries [1].

One of the most important features of old age is variability, both within and between individuals, which apparently increases with advancing age. Chronological age is therefore a poor criterion for deciding medical care in the elderly. The characteristics of old age are general trends; medical care plans must be made for each individual and not based on arbitrary rules.

Frequency and social impact of diabetes in old age

There are two main problems in interpreting studies on diabetes and impaired glucose tolerance (IGT) in old age. First, most data were gathered before the introduction of the WHO classification of diabetes (see Chapter 6) and secondly, many studies have assumed that the criteria for the diagnosis of diabetes do not vary with age.

NIDDM, the commoner type of diabetes in old age, is often asymptomatic and is diagnosed on the basis of arbitrary glycaemic criteria. Determination of the true frequency of diabetes therefore requires special surveys and clear definitions, which should take account of the 'glucose intolerance of ageing' described below.

Despite these caveats, it is clear that both diabetes and glucose intolerance become more frequent with advancing age. Although 2.4% of adult Americans have known diabetes, the prevalence rises to 8.0% for those aged 65 years and over and to 17% for those aged 65−74 [2]. The Framingham study, which used rather inexact diagnostic criteria, found a prevalence of diabetes of 10% in those aged 70 years and over, with an annual incidence of 0.8% in the same age group [3]. Even higher prevalence rates of diabetes in old people have been reported from Finland, where (according to the WHO criteria) 30% of men aged 65−84 years had diabetes and a further 30% had IGT [4]. In this study, the prevalence was higher in those aged 75−79 years than in those aged 80−84. In England, 36% of people aged 85 and over had abnormal glucose tolerance [5]. The prevalence of diabetes in old people appears to be increasing with time, perhaps because obesity is becoming more frequent or because people with diabetes are surviving for longer.

Patients with known diabetes spend 2−3 times more time in hospital than the general population of the same age, the excess being almost entirely due to insulin-treated patients [6] (see Chapter 5). Older diabetic patients are particularly heavy users of hospital beds. In the age group 60−74 years, the average number of admissions per diabetic patient per year was 0.47 for males and 0.50 for females, but was 1.12 for insulin-treated patients. The average number of bed days occupied per diabetic patient per year was 6.8 for men and 8.2 for women [7].

Complications of diabetes are common in old people. Severe uncontrolled diabetes is more common in those aged over 50 years and in one study carried a mortality of 43% compared with 3.4% in younger patients [8]. The increased mortality in older patients is due largely to associated conditions, of which cardiovascular disease is by far the most important [6]. Hypertension, retinopathy, cataracts, neuropathy and lipid abnormalities are also frequent in older diabetic patients [3, 9].

In people aged 85 years and over, pre-existing diabetes is associated with reduced survival, although newly diagnosed diabetes seems to have no effect on mortality [10]. The annual mortality in insulin-treated diabetic patients diagnosed after age 65 years was 11%, compared with 6% in those treated with diet and/or oral agents [11].

Although IDDM can occur at any age, diabetes in old age is most often non-insulin-dependent. The peak prevalence of IDDM is 11−13 years, whereas that of NIDDM is 65−69 years for men and 70−74 years for women. Only 4.8% of subjects diagnosed diabetic after age 55 years have IDDM [12, 13] and true insulin dependence is very rare in patients older than 65 years at diagnosis [11]. IDDM patients commonly have an HLA-DR3 phenotype, a history of ketonuria, significant titres of thyroid and parietal cell antibodies and a past history of endocrine disease [13].

The effect of age on carbohydrate metabolism

In 1921, a significant year in the history of diabetes, Spence reported that five men over the age of 60 had hyperglycaemia and decreased glucose tolerance compared with younger men and suggested that 'the carbohydrate storage mechanism tends to become impaired as age advances' [14]. Since then, the finding of glucose intolerance in elderly people has been repeatedly confirmed. Both fasting and postchallenge glucose levels increase slightly but significantly with advancing age, fasting glucose concentration by about 0.05 mmol/l per decade and levels 1 and 2 h after a glucose challenge by 0.38−0.72 mmol/l per decade [15] (Fig. 89.1). These glycaemic increases do

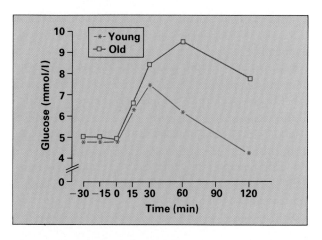

Fig. 89.1. Blood glucose levels following 50-g oral glucose load in young and old subjects (data from McConnell *et al.* 1982 [23]).

not bring older people within the definition of diabetes, although some may enter the category of IGT (see Chapter 6). Glycosylated haemoglobin levels also rise with age [16].

The mechanism of the glucose intolerance of ageing has been intensively studied and is apparently multifactorial (Fig. 89.2). The principal abnormality is insulin resistance, which is directly related to the severity of carbohydrate intolerance [17–22] and which evidently occurs at a postreceptor level, as the number and affinity of insulin receptors in muscle and other peripheral tissues are unchanged by age [19–21, 23]. The defect may lie in the glucose transporters on the cell surface (see Chapter 12), whose numbers decline with age although individual units continue to function normally [24, 25]. The main effect of insulin resistance is to reduce insulin-mediated glucose uptake into muscle [19, 26].

A separate abnormality is impaired insulin secretion, with a delay in the initial insulin rise following glucose stimulation [22, 26]. Paradoxically, postglucose blood insulin levels are normal or even elevated [23, 27], probably because of reduced clearance of insulin from the circulation

[27, 28]. The impairment of insulin secretion means that the compensatory hyperinsulinaemia necessary to overcome the insulin resistance cannot be achieved. The defective insulin secretory response to glucose probably accounts for the failure of glucose loading to suppress hepatic glucose output, another factor contributing to glucose intolerance in old age [20, 26].

There is no evidence that age-related glucose intolerance is due to excessive activity of the counter-regulatory hormones [29–31], although hepatic sensitivity to glucagon may be enhanced [31]. In old age, glucose absorption from the gut is slightly delayed [22, 26], opposing the general tendency to worsening postprandial glucose tolerance. The abnormal carbohydrate metabolism of ageing could be secondary to several possible age-related factors, although none satisfactorily explains the phenomenon. Obesity is associated with insulin resistance and glucose intolerance and, although body weight may not change in older people, a higher proportion of the body mass consists of fat. However, a possible effect of increased adiposity has been excluded by several studies of age-related glucose intolerance [21, 27,

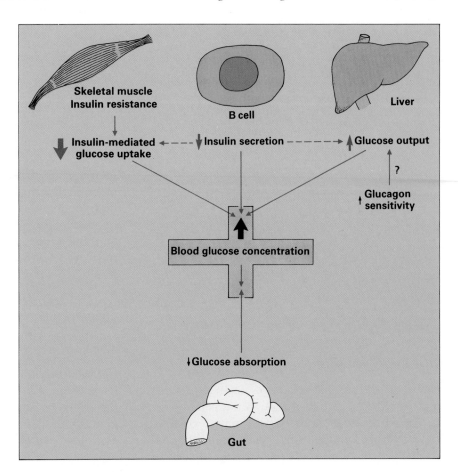

Fig. 89.2. Age-related changes in carbohydrate metabolism and the pathogenesis of glucose intolerance in elderly people.

32]. Other possible factors which may contribute to hyperglycaemia in individual cases but do not seem to be of general importance, include physical inactivity, inadequate carbohydrate intake (which can cause glucose intolerance [33]), renal impairment, and hypokalaemia (especially as a side-effect of treatment with diuretics, the most commonly prescribed drugs in the elderly).

The glucose intolerance of ageing has three practical consequences. First, as discussed below, it may cause diagnostic difficulty, although fasting blood glucose concentration is little changed and the use of fasting hyperglycaemia as the diagnostic criterion should avoid confusion. Secondly, the glucose intolerance of ageing makes the older person more susceptible to diabetogenic influences, particularly drugs such as thiazides, β-adrenoceptor antagonists and phenothiazines (see Chapter 79). Thirdly, hyperglycaemia may be of sufficient degree to increase the risk of heart disease and stroke [34], even when blood glucose levels are below those generally associated with specific diabetic complications [35].

Relationship of diabetes to ageing

The increasing prevalence of diabetes with advancing age and the demonstration of age-related hyperglycaemia have led to the suggestion that ageing and diabetes may be related. A number of other features are common to both conditions and may be relevant to certain chronic diabetic complications. Physico-chemical changes in collagen associated with ageing occur prematurely in diabetes [36, 37] and glycosylation of collagen and other tissue proteins is increased in both ageing and diabetes [38, 39]. Furthermore, skin fibroblasts grown from diabetic tissue have impaired plating efficiency and limited replicative lifespans, defects similar to those of ageing [40–4].

These and other findings have led to a hypothesis that diabetes may promote survival under conditions of nutritional deprivation but may accelerate ageing under conditions of plenty [45].

Diabetes in old age

Diabetes may present in old age, when it is almost always NIDDM [12] even though the patient may be insulin-treated; rarely, IDDM may develop in old age [13]. Although life expectancy is reduced in diabetes, patients with pre-existing NIDDM or IDDM often survive into old age, frequently with complications of the disease.

Diagnosis of diabetes in old age

The 1980 WHO criteria (see Chapter 6) are not age-related but are conservative enough to exclude age-related glucose intolerance; age-related diagnostic criteria are therefore no longer necessary. The WHO criteria distinguish diabetes from normality, with the intermediate category of IGT. Although IGT may be associated with an increased risk of cardiovascular disease, it is not a precursor to diabetes nor does it predispose to chronic diabetic complications. In old people, therefore, it seems reasonable to restrict attention to the diagnosis of diabetes. As postchallenge glucose levels in particular rise with increasing age, glucose tolerance testing is not indicated in clinical diagnosis. Diabetes in old age should be diagnosed when the fasting blood glucose level exceeds 7.0 mmol/l.

Clinical features of diabetes in old age

Elderly people do not usually present with the classical clinical features of the disease shown by younger patients, but often attend the doctor for some other condition, sometimes diabetes-related, such as cardiovascular disease or a urinary tract infection. The widespread use of biochemical screening in patients attending hospital may have increased the detection of diabetes in older people.

In older people, symptoms are often non-specific. Lassitude, lack of energy, a change in mental state, falls, impaired mobility and urinary incontinence may all be related to diabetes. A high index of clinical suspicion is therefore necessary for all doctors managing the elderly, and the blood glucose concentration should be measured following any change of health status in older people.

Complications of diabetes in older people

ACUTE METABOLIC COMPLICATIONS

Ketoacidosis is rare in the older diabetic person. Its features and management do not differ from those in younger people but its mortality is greatest in old age [8], particularly because of associated cardiovascular disease [46]. Hyperosmolar coma almost always occurs in old people.

Both these complications are discussed in detail in Chapter 49.

CHRONIC DIABETIC COMPLICATIONS

The chronic complications of diabetes — cardiovascular disease, neuropathy, retinopathy and nephropathy — are the same in old age as in the young. These long-term complications may never develop when diabetes presents in old age but are commonly established in patients with pre-existing diabetes when they enter old age. Cardiovascular disease is very common in old people without diabetes and is extensive in many older diabetic patients, irrespective of the duration of the diabetes.

Cardiovascular disease may present in old age without typical symptoms [47]. Myocardial infarction may be painless, and manifested instead by cardiac failure, falls or lassitude. Lower-limb ischaemia may occur without claudication, and present first as gangrene. Diabetes may worsen the prognosis of both myocardial infarction [48] and stroke [49]. Whether this is due to more extensive atherosclerosis, the harmful effects of hyperglycaemia on the ischaemic heart and brain, or an abnormal stress response is unknown.

Management of the older diabetic patient

As with any older patient, the whole person must be treated in the context of his overall health, lifestyle, environment and wishes. Multiple pathology is common in old age; diabetes may be only one of a number of health problems with which the older person has to contend, and mild diabetes may not demand a high priority in the total health care of the patient.

Treating the elderly patient with any drug poses a number of particular problems [50]. These include:
1 Inappropriate drug treatment. Drugs are sometimes used for problems which are mainly environmental or social rather than medical, or are used to treat minor complaints (e.g. ankle oedema); the effects of the treatment may be worse than the symptoms.
2 Multiple drug prescribing. This may be due to multiple pathology, but drugs are sometimes prescribed by several doctors who are not individually aware of the patient's other medications.
3 Poor drug compliance. This may be due to deficits in memory, sight or hearing, because the drug has unacceptable side-effects or because of confusion between multiple drugs.
4 Drug interactions. These are particularly common with multiple prescribing.
5 Unwanted effects of drugs. Pharmacokinetics and pharmacodynamics are altered in old age, the most important change being decreased clearance of drugs normally eliminated through the kidneys. Drug toxicity is therefore commoner in elderly people.

Before any drug is prescribed to an elderly patient, the doctor must satisfy himself that the drug is essential, must review all the drugs prescribed for the patient, and must take measures to ensure that the patient takes the prescribed medication (if necessary, by asking a relative or other suitable person to undertake responsibility for this).

Why treat diabetes in old age?

The reasons for treating diabetes at any age are to relieve its symptoms and to prevent its acute and chronic complications. Symptoms are most likely to occur when fasting glucose levels exceed 11 mmol/l, when the risks of hyperosmolar coma and ketoacidosis are also increased. There are good reasons, therefore, to treat elderly people with fasting blood glucose concentrations above 11 mmol/l.

The issue of preventing complications is more contentious because of the time required for their development and because some, particularly cardiovascular disease, are commonly present in older people anyway. There is also little evidence so far that treatment of diabetes prevents complications. The management of the older person whose fasting blood glucose is between 8 and 11 mmol/l is therefore open to debate. In such people, other health problems may take priority, although many are overweight and attempts to reduce weight are appropriate in the interests of their general health.

Diet

In NIDDM, dietary modification aims to reduce calorie intake and weight and in the overweight elderly diabetic patient, a low-calorie diet with restricted saturated fat and cholesterol is appropriate [51]. However, weight reduction is difficult at any age and has a very low success rate in old people. Even if initial enthusiasm produces some weight loss and hence a fall in blood glucose levels, weight will frequently be regained.

Oral hypoglycaemic agents

Oral agents are used in elderly people when dietary treatment has not reduced glycaemia adequately. Because dietary treatment is often ineffective or inappropriate in old people, prolonged trials of diet alone are not indicated and oral agents should be used more readily. The shorter-acting sulphonylureas such as tolbutamide or gliclazide are preferable in older patients, whose impaired homeostatic ability renders them particularly susceptible to severe and prolonged hypoglycaemia. The longer-acting drugs such as chlorpropamide and glibenclamide (which has an unexpectedly prolonged circulating half-life in some individuals) should generally be avoided. Nevertheless, it would be meddlesome to change the medication of an old person who has long been well controlled by one of the longer-acting sulphonylureas, simply because of these theoretical considerations. Renal impairment prolongs the activity of drugs cleared through the kidneys, and patients with significant renal failure should be treated either with a sulphonylurea which is metabolized mainly in the liver (e.g. gliclazide, gliquidone), or with insulin.

The biguanide, metformin, carries a small risk of lactic acidosis, particularly in the presence of renal or circulatory failure. These risks are greater in old people, in whom metformin should be avoided.

Insulin

This is the most effective means of lowering blood glucose. Its only major side-effect is hypoglycaemia, which is particularly undesirable in old people with their vulnerable cerebral function. The practical difficulties of administering insulin may limit its use in old people. Self-injection may be rendered impossible by arthritis, impaired vision or dementia. Insulin treatment also demands dietary regulation and regular monitoring of blood glucose levels. Nevertheless, if insulin is required to reduce glucose to the desired levels, the age of the patient alone should not be a contraindication. If self-injection is impracticable, arrangements should be made to have the insulin given by a relative or community nurse. When insulin administration is difficult, it is reasonable to use once-daily insulin regimens and to accept suboptimal blood glucose control.

Withdrawing insulin therapy

As mentioned above, true insulin dependency is very rare in old age [11]. It has been estimated that at least 15% of diabetic patients may be unnecessarily treated with insulin [52]. Acute illness or hyperosmolar coma may have been temporarily treated with insulin, which has not subsequently been discontinued. The potential benefits of withdrawal of insulin therapy include greater freedom for the patient, a more flexible diet, reduced risk of hypoglycaemia, sometimes weight loss in overweight patients, improved diabetic control, and an increased feeling of well-being [52]. The advantages of not being restricted to insulin in old age are obvious and withdrawal of insulin should be actively considered in older patients, particularly if overweight. Fasting C-peptide levels may indicate whether insulin treatment is unnecessary (see Chapter 36). Insulin can be withdrawn gradually on an out-patient basis, or more rapidly if the patient is closely supervised as an in-patient.

Monitoring treatment

As in other age groups, diabetic treatment is best monitored by assessing the patient's general health, with special reference to diabetic complications, and by measuring blood glucose concentrations. Self-monitoring may be difficult for the disabled old person who lives alone. Because the renal threshold for glucose reabsorption increases with age, glycosuria may be an unreliable indicator of control. The best compromise is often to check blood glucose levels in general practice or hospital out-patient clinics, no more often than is strictly necessary.

Community and social support

As with any older person, the aim must be to achieve the greatest possible degree of independence. The whole patient and his environment must therefore be carefully considered and any management intervention, whether treatment or attendance at a clinic, must only be used if it clearly benefits the patient. Multiple pathology often means multiple doctors and attendance at multiple clinics. This must be avoided, and one doctor should take overall charge of the patient's management. Ideally this should be the general practitioner, with hospital attendance reserved only for well-defined reasons.

Diabetes and its complications, together with other chronic diseases and the impaired mobility, vision, mental capacity and self-care abilities of old age, may cause loss of independence. It is important, however, to aim to continue care in the community for as long as possible, not for economic or political reasons, but because this is what old people themselves desire. Support in the community must therefore be well-organized and co-ordinated. The type of support will depend on need, and may range from help with household duties and personal care to arranging admission to residential or nursing homes [53].

ROBERT W. STOUT

References

1 Stout RW, Crawford V. Active-life expectancy and terminal dependency: trends in long-term geriatric care over 33 years. *Lancet* 1988; i: 281–3.

2 Bennett PH. Diabetes in the elderly: diagnosis and epidemiology. *Geriatrics* 1984; **39**: 37–41.

3 Wilson PWF, Anderson KM, Kannell WB. Epidemiology of diabetes mellitus in the elderly. The Framingham Study. *Am J Med* 1986; **80** (suppl 5A): 3–9.

4 Tuomilehto J, Nissinen A, Kivela S-L, Pekkanen J, Kaarsalo E, Wolf E, Aro A, Punsar S, Karvonen MJ. Prevalence of diabetes mellitus in elderly men aged 65 to 84 years in eastern and western Finland. *Diabetologia* 1986; **29**: 611–5.

5 Smith MJ, Hall MRP. Carbohydrate tolerance in the very aged. *Diabetologia* 1973; **9**: 387–90.

6 Damsgaard EM, Froland A, Green A. Use of hospital services by elderly diabetics: the Frederica Study of diabetic and fasting hyperglycaemic patients aged 60–74 years. *Diabetic Med* 1987; **4**: 317–22.

7 Harrower ADB. Prevalence of elderly patients in a hospital diabetic population. *Br J Clin Pract* 1980; **34**: 131–3.

8 Gale EAM, Dornan TL, Tattersall RB. Severely uncontrolled diabetes in the over-fifties. *Diabetologia* 1981; **21**: 25–8.

9 Nathan DM, Singer DE, Godine JE, Perlmuter LC. Non-insulin-dependent diabetes in older patients. Complications and risk factors. *Am J Med* 1986; **81**: 837–42.

10 Kaltiala KS, Haavisto MV, Heikinheimo RJ, Mattila KJ, Rajala SA. Blood glucose and diabetes mellitus predicting mortality in persons aged 85 years or above. *Age Ageing* 1987; **16**: 165–70.

11 Kilvert A, Fitzgerald MG, Wright AD, Nattrass M. Newly diagnosed, insulin-dependent diabetes mellitus in elderly patients. *Diabetic Med* 1984; **1**:115–18.

12 Laakso M, Pyörälä K. Age of onset and type of diabetes. *Diabetes Care* 1985; **8**: 114–17.

13 Kilvert A, Fitzgerald MG, Wright AD, Nattrass M. Clinical characteristics and aetiological classification of insulin-dependent diabetes in the elderly. *Q J Med* 1986; **60**: 865–72.

14 Spence JC. Some observations on sugar tolerance, with special reference to variations found at different ages. *Q J Med* 1921; **14**: 314–26.

15 Davidson MB. The effect of aging on carbohydrate metabolism: a review of the English literature and a practical approach to the diagnosis of diabetes in the elderly. *Metabolism* 1979; **28**: 688–705.

16 Arnetz BB, Kallner A, Theorell T. The influence of aging on hemoglobin A1c (HbA1c). *J Gerontol* 1982; **37**: 648–50.

17 DeFronzo RA. Glucose intolerance and aging. Evidence for tissue insensitivity to insulin. *Diabetes* 1979; **28**: 1095–101.

18 Robert J-J, Cummins JC, Wolfe RR, Durkot M, Matthews DE, Zhao XH, Bier DM, Young VR. Quantitative aspects of glucose production and metabolism in healthy elderly subjects. *Diabetes* 1982; **31**: 203–11.

19 Jackson RA, Blix PM, Matthews JA, Hamling JB, Din BM, Brown DC, Belin J, Rubenstein AH, Nabarro JDN. Influence of ageing on glucose homeostatis. *J Clin Endocrinol Metab* 1982; **55**: 840–8.

20 Fink RI, Kolterman OG, Griffin J, Olefsky JM. Mechanisms of insulin resistance in aging. *J Clin Invest* 1983; **71**: 1523–35.

21 Rowe JW, Minaker KL, Pallotta JA, Flier JS. Characterization of the insulin resistance of aging. *J Clin Invest* 1983; **71**: 1581–7.

22 Chen M, Bergman RN, Pacini G, Porte D Jr. Pathogenesis of age-related glucose intolerance in man: insulin resistance and decreased B cell function. *J Clin Endocrinol Metab* 1985; **60**: 13–20.

23 McConnell JG, Buchanan KD, Ardill J, Stout RW. Glucose tolerance in the elderly: the role of insulin and its receptor. *Eur J Clin Invest* 1982; **12**: 55–61.

24 Fink RJ, Kolterman OG, Kao M, Olefsky JM. The role of the glucose transport system in the postreceptor defect in insulin action associated with human aging. *J Clin Endocrinol Metab* 1984; **58**: 721–4.

25 Fink RI, Wallace P, Olefsky JM. Effects of aging on glucose-mediated glucose disposal and glucose transport. *J Clin Invest* 1986; **77**: 2034–41.

26 Jackson RA, Hawa MI, Roshania RD, Sim BM, DiSilvio L, Jaspan JB. Influence of aging on hepatic and peripheral glucose metabolism in humans. *Diabetes* 1988; **37**: 119–29.

27 Minaker KL, Rowe JW, Tonnino R, Pallotta JA. Influence of age on clearance of insulin in man. *Diabetes* 1982; **31**: 851–5.

28 Reaven GM, Greenfield MS, Mondon CE, Rosenthal M, Wright D, Reaven EP. Does insulin removal rate from plasma decline with age? *Diabetes* 1982; **31**: 670–3.

29 Elahi D, Muller DC, Tzankoff SP, Andres R, Tobin JD. Effect of age and obesity on fasting levels of glucose, insulin, glucagon, and growth hormone in man. *J Gerontol* 1982; **37**: 385–91.

30 McConnell JG, Alan MJ, O'Hare MMT, Buchanan KD, Stout RW. The effect of age and sex on the response of enteropancreatic polypeptides to oral glucose. *Age Ageing* 1983; **12**: 54–62.

31 Simonson DC, DeFronzo RA. Glucagon physiology and aging: evidence for enhanced hepatic sensitivity. *Diabetologia* 1983; **25**: 1–7.

32 Rosenthal M, Doberne L, Greenfield M, Widstrom A, Reaven GM. Effect of age on glucose tolerance, insulin secretion, and *in vivo* insulin action. *J Am Geriatr Soc* 1982; **30**: 562–7.

33 Brunzell JD, Lerner RL, Hazzard WR, Porte D Jr, Bierman EL. Improved glucose tolerance with high carbohydrate feeding in mild diabetes. *N Engl J Med* 1971; **284**: 521–4.

34 Fuller JH, Shipley MJ, Rose G, Jarrett RJ, Keen H. Mortality from coronary heart disease and stroke in relation to degree of glycaemia: the Whitehall study. *Br Med J* 1983; **287**: 867–70.

35 Pettitt DJ, Knowler WC, Lisse JR, Bennett PH. Development of retinopathy and proteinuria in relation to plasma-glucose concentrations in Pima Indians. *Lancet* 1980; ii: 1050–2.

36 Hamlin CR, Kohn RR, Luschin JH. Apparent accelerated aging of human collagen in diabetes mellitus. *Diabetes* 1975; **24**: 902–4.

37 Monnier VM, Kohn RR, Cerami A. Accelerated age-related browning of human collagen in diabetes mellitus. *Proc Natl Acad Sci USA* 1984; **81**: 583–7.

38 Schnider SL, Kohn RR. Glucosylation of human collagen in aging and diabetes mellitus. *J Clin Invest* 1980; **66**: 1179–81.

39 Cerami A, Vlassara H, Brownlee M. Glucose and aging. *Sci Am* May 1987: 82–8.

40 Goldstein S, Littlefield JW, Soeldner JS. Diabetes mellitus and aging: diminished plating efficiency of cultured human fibroblasts. *Proc Natl Acad Sci USA* 1969; **64**: 155–60.

41 Goldstein S, Moerman EJ, Soeldner JS, Gleason RE, Barnett DM. Chronologic and physiologic age affect replicative life-span of fibroblasts from diabetic, prediabetic and normal donors. *Science* 1978; **199**: 781–2.

42 Goldstein S, Moerman EJ, Soeldner JS, Gleason RE, Barnett DM. Diabetes mellitus and genetic prediabetes. Decreased replicative capacity of cultured skin fibroblasts. *J Clin Invest* 1979; **63**: 358–70.

43 Vracko R, Benditt EP. Restricted replicative life-span of diabetic fibroblasts *in vitro*: its relation to microangiopathy.

44 Rowe DW, Starman BJ, Fujimoto WY, Williams RH. Abnormalities in proliferation and protein synthesis in skin fibroblast cultures from patients with diabetes mellitus. *Diabetes* 1977; **26**: 284–90.

45 Goldstein S. Analytical review: the pathogenesis of diabetes mellitus and its relationship to biological ageing. *Humangenetik* (Berlin) 1971; **12**: 83–100.

46 Barnett DM, Wilcox DS, Marble A. Diabetic coma in persons over 60. *Geriatrics* 1962: 327–36.

47 Pathy MS. Clinical presentation of myocardial infarction in the elderly. *Br Heart J* 1967; **29**: 190–9.

48 Oswald GA, Smith CCT, Betteridge DJ, Yudkin JS. Determinants and importance of stress hyperglycaemia in non-diabetic patients with myocardial infarction. *Br Med J* 1986; **293**: 917–22.

49 Power MJ, Fullerton KJ, Stout RW. Blood glucose and prognosis of acute stroke. *Age Ageing* 1988; **17**: 164–70.

50 Caird FI, ed. *Drugs for the Elderly*. Geneva: World Health Organisation, 1985.

51 Wilson EA, Hadden DR, Merrett JD, Montgomery DAD, Weaver JA. Dietary management of maturity-onset diabetes. *Br Med J* 1980; **280**: 1367–9.

52 Cohen M, Crosbie C, Cusworth L, Zimmet P. Insulin — not always a life sentence: withdrawal of insulin therapy in non-insulin dependent diabetes. *Diabetes Res* 1984; **1**: 31–4.

53 Hodkinson E, McCafferty FG, Scott JN, Stout RW. Disability and dependency in elderly people in residential and hospital care. *Age Ageing* 1988; **17**: 147–54.

Fed Proc 1975; **34**: 68–70.

90   Diabetes Mellitus in the Third World

Summary

• Some 50 million diabetic patients live in the Third World, where the health problem of diabetes is seriously underestimated and ineffectively addressed.
• Diabetic microvascular complications are quite common but significant macrovascular disease relatively rare; end-stage complications are rare, probably because of the short survival of diabetic patients in the Third World.
• 50% of diabetic patients in developing countries die from potentially treatable causes, mainly hyperglycaemic comas or infections.
• An effective diabetes care programme depends on accurately assessing the size of the problem; promoting diabetes health education and recruiting and training staff; securing supplies of insulin and essential drugs; and developing appropriate technology for the prevention, early diagnosis and treatment of the disease.

Diabetes mellitus was recognized in India and Egypt centuries before Christ but even now, relatively little is known about diabetes in Third-World countries, where the fight against communicable diseases has attracted most attention. Although many gaps remain, recent descriptive studies have started to build up a global picture of the particular aetiopathogenesis, social and prognostic features of diabetes in developing countries.

Diabetes may be one of the most underestimated public health problems in the Third World, which accommodates some two-thirds of the human race, including an estimated 50 million diabetic patients. It is indeed true that 'the poor also have

diabetes' [1]. Although not formally costed (see Chapter 5), the social and financial burden of diabetes in developing countries must be enormous.

The epidemiology of diabetes is discussed in detail in Chapter 7. The purpose of this chapter is to outline some of the particular problems posed by diabetes in the Third World and the medical and social impact of the disease.

Chronic diabetic complications in the Third World

Very few population-based studies on the prevalence of long-term diabetic complications have been conducted in the Third World although clinic and hospital series have provided some useful (albeit limited) information. Studies such as the large multinational investigation based in three centres (Havana, Hong Kong and New Delhi) under the auspices of the WHO [2] should provide much valuable data about the prevalence of micro- and macrovascular disease in diabetes in developing countries.

Ocular complications

In Western countries, diabetes is the commonest cause of blindness in the working population. In tropical countries, however, blindness due to diabetes is overshadowed by that resulting from trachoma, vitamin A deficiency and other conditions. The pattern of retinopathy probably resembles that of Caucasian populations except that proliferative changes are unusual, possibly because of the rarity of early-onset diabetes and the limited survival of the patients [3]. The reported prevalence rates of retinopathy in Africa vary greatly from 0.6% to 48% [3], whereas the WHO Multinational Study's preliminary data suggest that (with few exceptions) the rates in Cuba, Hong Kong and India are similar to those in Europe and North America. Not surprisingly, the frequency and severity of retinopathy increases with increasing duration of diabetes.

In the developing countries, the main threat to vision posed by diabetes is cataract, which appears to be very common [3].

Nephropathy

The WHO study [2] and others have suggested that the prevalence of diabetic nephropathy (defined as proteinuria, with or without hypertension) in the Third World is probably similar to that in Western countries, and that its frequency and severity are greater with increasing duration of the disease. Reported frequencies of proteinuria in African diabetic clinic populations vary from 1% to 30% [3]. End-stage renal failure is rarely described, probably because of early death.

Neuropathy

All types of diabetic neuropathy are encountered in the Third World and may even be the first manifestation of the disease [4]. The relatively fragmentary data from Africa, South America and Asia suggest frequencies as high as 50% [3, 5].

Hypertension and macrovascular disease

As in Caucasian populations, hypertension is associated with diabetes in Third World patients, particularly those with NIDDM, in whom the frequency of hypertension ranges from 19 to 50% [6]. An increasing prevalence with age (especially in females) and with duration of diabetes has recently been confirmed by the WHO Multinational Study [2]. In New Delhi, 21% of male and 33% of female diabetic patients were hypertensive; the corresponding figures for Hong Kong were 28% of males and 31% of females and for Havana, 31% of males and 40% of females. The clear-cut female preponderance is similar to that in many Caucasian populations. The close correlation in Natal Indians and Africans between hypertension and glucose intolerance has led Seedat [7] to suggest that all hypertensive Africans should be screened for diabetes.

Atherosclerosis is relatively rare in African and Oriental diabetic patients — as is the case in these populations in general. In Hong Kong, fewer than 1% of Chinese diabetic patients showed major electrocardiographic (ECG) abnormalities [2]. Using the same WHO protocol, macrovascular disease was also found to be relatively rare in middle-aged Ethiopian diabetic patients in Addis Ababa; 14% had ECG evidence of coronary heart disease and only 5% had significant clinical disease (angina, myocardial infarction, stroke or limb ischaemia) [8]. However, the protection against atheroma enjoyed by these populations seems to disappear when they move to urbanized or Westernized environments. Although not yet formally confirmed, preliminary data suggest that urbanized East Indians (both diabetic and non-diabetic) are highly susceptible to coronary heart disease. More information is awaited on the prevalence of this major problem and associated risk factors (such as hyperlipidaemia) in this expanding population.

Mortality from diabetes in the Third World

The mortality due to diabetes in the Third World has undoubtedly been underestimated, largely because of incomplete data collection and under-reporting of the disease on death certificates. Nonetheless, diabetes has been suspected to carry a high mortality in Africa, South America, Asia and the Middle East. The highest diabetes-related mortality rates reported to the WHO between 1976 and 1983 were from Mauritius, Mexico, Venezuela, Singapore and Malta [9]. In all countries, mortality associated with diabetes rose with increasing age.

Life expectancy, already poor in developing countries, may be considerably shortened by diabetes: Ethiopian diabetic patients, for example, survive on average for only 11 years after diagnosis and only 5% live for more than 25 years [10].

Tragically, the causes of death are all too often potentially treatable. In principle, the discovery of insulin over 65 years ago should have dramatically improved the quality of life and prognosis of diabetic patients the world over. However, Third World patients are still threatened by the lethal problems of the preinsulin era: acute metabolic complications (ketoacidotic and hyperosmolar coma) and infections (especially due to pyogenic organisms and tuberculosis) are cited as immediate causes of death in over 50% of diabetic people in the developing countries [3, 10]. Tuberculosis in particular seems to be considerably commoner in diabetic patients than in the general population, with prevalence rates varying from 0.9% to 8% being reported from different diabetic clinics [3]. Renal or vascular complications account for relatively few deaths in Third World diabetic patients.

Diabetes may well be implicated in the very high perinatal mortality rates in developing countries, although the outcome of diabetic pregnancy in the Third World has not yet been systematically studied.

Specific problems in managing diabetes in the Third World

Despite increasing awareness of the growing problem of non-communicable diseases such as diabetes and hypertension, the developing countries still face major problems in managing diabetes. Provision of general health care is difficult in the Third World countries which, irrespective of their individual racial, religious and cultural identities, all share the same burdens of widespread poverty, malnutrition, illiteracy, poor sanitation and unsafe drinking water, often complicated by political instability and natural catastrophes. Health care is generally inadequate and often inaccessible to the vast majority of people. The overstretched and understaffed public health services are further restricted by the lack of equipment and laboratory support. Scarce health resources are often diverted to treat infectious diseases and malnutrition and, against the background of these large-scale problems, diabetes often assumes a low priority. This neglect is compounded by ignorance about the extent of the disease and its repercussions; possible ways of tackling the problem under these conditions have not been rigorously studied. Fortunately, some governments are now incorporating diabetes control programmes into their existing primary health care plans [3, 11].

Epidemiological assessments of diabetes

The first step, not yet undertaken by many countries, is to define the size of the problem posed by diabetes and its complications. Large-scale epidemiological surveys are expensive, and Third World countries may find an integrated examination of other conditions (e.g. hypertension, cardiovascular disease) as well as diabetes to be more cost-effective. Such an approach is currently being evaluated in Tanzania.

In developing countries, diabetes is diagnosed from obvious clinical features: in practical terms, the precise criteria of the WHO (Chapter 6) are less relevant than in Western countries where formal glucose tolerance testing can be easily performed as a screening procedure or in case of clinical suspicion. Diabetes often remains undiagnosed in the Third World, where severe hyperglycaemia is apparently tolerated with few symptoms or complaints.

Organization of diabetic care in the Third World

There is no doubt that creating specific diabetes centres within the existing health-care framework will increase early detection of the disease and improve the quality of care delivered to diabetic patients in the Third World. However, even the few existing diabetes centres have to contend with the lack of resources and of trained physicians which is common to all poor countries. Another major problem, widespread throughout Africa, Asia and South America, is that of diabetic patients defaulting from follow-up and treatment [3, 12]. The reasons for this apparently include the high costs of prolonged treatment (insulin and oral hypoglycaemic agents are all expensive in these countries), the patients' reliance on traditional treatment methods, and their reluctance to accept the fact that diabetes cannot be cured permanently. As a result, patients often move from one source of medical help to another, and many die prematurely from acute metabolic complications or untreated infection.

Various solutions to these problems can be proposed. First, the price of drugs and insulin in a developing country could be revised and fixed at a realistic level, perhaps according to the country's gross national product. Because of many factors — ranging from the prices demanded by the drug manufacturers to black-market dealing within the country — this suggestion may not be feasible, but the support of Western diabetes associations could be very valuable in implementing such a policy. Drugs could also be salvaged from the vast quantities wasted in industrialized countries, where large stocks of outdated insulin are destroyed every year. Such insulin may have variably reduced biological activity but is otherwise safe and could be life-saving in the many parts of the world where insulin is not obtainable at all. Even when available, insulin may be difficult to store safely in the tropics: those unable to afford a refrigerator can be instructed to keep insulin vials in the dark in pots half-full of cool water which is renewed periodically. Finally, the crucial importance of education in the management of diabetes cannot be overemphasized, even though social and cultural customs may impede the success of the programme.

The prerequisites for the establishment of a diabetes care programme in a developing country can be summarized as follows:

1 Accurate assessment of the size of the problem posed by diabetes and its complications in a defined geographical area.

2 Promotion of diabetes health education: this is essential and should aim both to inform the community and to increase recruitment and training of doctors and nurses.

3 Maintenance of supplies of insulin and other essential drugs.

4 Development of appropriate technology for the prevention, early diagnosis and treatment of diabetes and its complications.

Such plans will be greatly assisted by international co-operation and it is to be hoped that many will follow the example of the WHO, whose collaborative diabetes centres have begun to make the expertise of the industrialized countries available to the Third World.

JEAN-MARIE EKOÉ

References

1 Krall LP. The wide world of diabetes. In: Krall LP, ed. *World Book of Diabetes in Practice*, vol 2. Amsterdam: Elsevier, 1986: 209−12.

2 The World Health Organization Multinational Study of vascular disease in diabetics. Prevalence of small and large vessel disease in diabetic patients from 14 centres. *Diabetologia* 1985; **28** (suppl): 615−40.

3 McLarty D. Diabetes in Africa. In: Krall LP, ed. *World Book of Diabetes in Practice*, vol 2. Amsterdam: Elsevier, 1986: 218−28.

4 Osuntokun BO. *The Neurology of Diabetes Mellitus in Nigerians*. MD Thesis, University of London, 1971.

5 Keen H, Ekoé JM. The geography of diabetes mellitus. *Br Med Bull* 1984; **40**: 359−65.

6 Ekoé JM. Diabetic complications in Africa. *Int Diab Fed Bull* 1987; **32**: 138−41.

7 Seedat YK, Seedat MA. An inter-racial study of the prevalence of hypertension in an urban South African population. *Trans R Soc Trop Med Hyg* 1982; **76**: 62−71.

8 Lester FT, Keen H. Macrovascular disease in middle-aged diabetic patients in Addis Ababa, Ethiopia. *Diabetologia* 1988; **31**: 361−7.

9 *World Health Statistics Annals, 1978−83*. Geneva, Switzerland: World Health Organization, 1984.

10 Lester FT. Diabetes mellitus in Ethiopians. *Ethiop Med J* 1984; **22**: 61−6.

11 Morrison EYSt-A. Problems of diabetes in the Caribbean. In: Krall LP, ed. *World Book of Diabetes in Practice*, vol 2. Amsterdam: Elsevier, 1986: 244−7.

12 Zhi-Sheng C. Some aspects of diabetes in the People's Republic of China, Part 1. A perspective from Beijing. In: Mann JI, Pyörälä K, Teuscher A, eds. *Diabetes in Epidemiological Perspective*. Edinburgh: Churchill Livingstone, 1984: 78−86.

91   Diabetes Mellitus in Ethnic Communities in the UK

Summary

• The prevalence of diabetes (mainly NIDDM) in British Asians is high — about 20% of those aged 60 y or more are known to have diabetes.

• Presentation is at an earlier age than in Europeans.

• Although comparably prone to complications, the large number of Asian patients and their long exposure to diabetes may result in high future morbidity and mortality in this population.

• The cause of the high prevalence is unknown, but genetic factors are probably important.

• Similar problems may exist within the UK Afro-Caribbean community, but few data are available at present.

Over two million British citizens in the 1981 census belonged to ethnic minority groups, with approximately 1.2 million 'Asians' originating from the Indian subcontinent and East Africa, and 600 000 'Afro-Caribbeans', principally from the West Indies. Patients from these two groups form a substantial proportion of many diabetic clinics in the UK. The high prevalence of diabetes now documented within the Asian population has stimulated considerable interest over recent years, although diabetes within the Afro-Caribbean community has so far attracted less attention.

Diabetes in British Asians

Prevalence

It is well established that diabetes prevalence in Indian Asian migrant groups in South Africa, Fiji,

Trinidad and Singapore is unduly high. The British Asian community is larger than any of these groups, and recent studies have shown that they also have a high prevalence. The Southall Diabetes Survey examined by house-to-house enquiry a mixed Asian (predominantly Punjabi Sikh) and European population of over 65 000 in West London. The age-adjusted prevalence of known diabetes was approximately 4 times higher in Asians than in Europeans (Fig. 91.1), with a five- to sevenfold excess in subjects aged 40–64 years [1]. 18% of Asians aged 60–69 years were known to be diabetic, with presumably many more undiagnosed subjects. Broadly similar results have been reported from Leicester, Coventry and East London, in predominantly Gujerati, Punjabi and Bangladeshi communities respectively. Thus

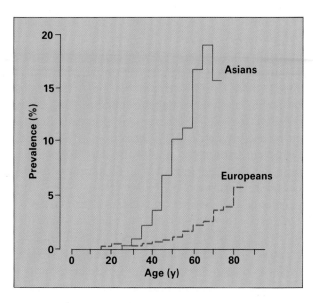

Fig. 91.1. Prevalence of known diabetes in Asians and Europeans in Southall, West London. (Adapted from Mather and Keen 1985 [1] with permission from the publishers.)

909

the prevalence seems high in the major subgroups of British Asians.

There are approximately 25 000 known Asian diabetic patients in Britain, living mainly in London, the Midlands and north-west England [2]. The age-structure of the Asian population is relatively young, with proportionately more young adults and fewer elderly. Thus, a marked increase in the total number of diabetic patients can be anticipated over the next few years, as the population ages and a disproportionate number of adults enter middle-age. It is important to anticipate this when planning health care in districts with a substantial Asian community.

The vast majority of Asian diabetic subjects are non-insulin-dependent, although approximately 20% require insulin for adequate glycaemic control. They generally present at an earlier age than in Europeans, with a striking excess of patients diagnosed in their thirties, reaching a peak at 40–54 years [1]. By contrast, classical insulin-dependent diabetes is uncommon and may indeed be less common than in Europeans, although this has not been strictly proven.

Chronic diabetic complications

Large cross-sectional studies have shown that Asian diabetic patients are as prone to complications as are Europeans [3]. Ischaemic heart disease seems equally common in the two groups, and diabetes may be an important factor contributing to the high prevalence of this complication within the Asian population as a whole. Nephropathy, assessed by either the degree of microalbuminuria [4] or the presence of Albustix-positive proteinuria [5], seems more common in Asian than European patients, and increasing numbers of Asian diabetic patients are being referred for renal replacement therapy. Retinopathy is probably equally common in Asian and European patients (although the data are conflicting) as are lens opacities and neuropathy. By contrast, peripheral vascular disease and foot problems may be less common in Asian patients.

Overall, therefore, with the possible exception of nephropathy, complication rates are not increased in Asian diabetic patients. However, because of the strikingly higher diabetes prevalence within Asians and its earlier onset and potentially longer exposure, the future morbidity and mortality from diabetic complications may be considerable in Asian populations.

Factors contributing to the high prevalence

The aetiology of non-insulin-dependent diabetes (NIDDM) is multifactorial and is considered elsewhere (see Section 7). The various genetic and environmental influences may assume differing degrees of importance in different ethnic groups and locations. Until recently, it had been generally assumed that the diabetes prevalence in Asian migrant groups was higher than in India, emphasizing the role of environmental factors. However, a recent study found a remarkably similar prevalence of known diabetes in Delhi to that in Southall Asians [6]. Thus, genetic factors probably contribute markedly to the high prevalence of NIDDM within Asians. Attempts to identify a genetic marker have so far been unsuccessful. There is preliminary evidence that Asian subjects (both diabetic and non-diabetic) have increased insulin resistance as compared with their European counterparts and it is speculated that this might explain the Asian predisposition to both diabetes and ischaemic heart disease. The influence of environmental factors such as obesity, diet and exercise has not been adequately studied in British Asians but the available evidence suggests that obesity does not play an all-important role. The search for avoidable or remediable risk factors is particularly urgent within this community, because of their high susceptibility. However, no environmental factors have yet been identified with sufficient certainty to justify a community-based prevention programme.

Practical aspects of management

DIABETES EDUCATION

Communication and comprehension problems due to language difficulties may occur, especially in middle-aged or elderly women. Although a younger, bilingual relative is often brought to the clinic, the need for a proficient interpreter is obvious. To help with these problems, a wide range of educational aids have been produced in several Asian languages. Written material is occasionally useful but is ultimately of limited value because of literacy problems. However, audio and video cassette tapes are now available, and are extremely popular with patients. Details can be obtained from the British Diabetic Association.

DIET

The traditional Asian diet is rich in saturated fat and refined carbohydrate and remains so in many diagnosed diabetic patients [7]. Many are overweight and attempts at weight reduction are often unsuccessful. Compliance with dietary advice may be poor for a variety of reasons. It may be impractical to modify the diet of the entire extended family. Some patients also equate obesity with health and prosperity. Nevertheless, simple practical measures to reduce saturated fat and refined carbohydrate intake may be effective. These include the use of measured quantities of oil and ghee in cooking, and a reduced consumption of fried snacks, Asian sweetmeats (e.g. jalebi) and 'gur' (unprocessed rock sugar) [8]. This advice should be given by an Asian dietitian, who will have the detailed knowledge required to adapt it to individual patients, as well as the necessary linguistic skills. Details of appropriate diet sheets and other teaching aids can be obtained from the British Diabetic Association.

INSULIN TREATMENT

Only moderate glycaemic control is achieved in many patients and some remain poorly controlled despite dietary advice and treatment with sulphonylureas. Approximately 20% require insulin, and most cope remarkably well even when communication seems difficult. In the elderly, insulin injections may be given by younger relatives and the tradition of the extended family usually ensures reliable insulin therapy without the need for a district nurse.

Diabetes in British Afro-Caribbeans

Much less is known about diabetes within this population. So far, there are virtually no prevalence data although some pointers suggest a higher prevalence than in Europeans. Roughly 9000 of these patients attend hospital clinics in the UK [2]. As with the Asians, they are mainly non-insulin-dependent and present at a relatively early age compared with Europeans; true insulin-dependent diabetes seems relatively uncommon [9]. They are prone to both obesity and hypertension, and may be predisposed to develop hyperosmolar coma. Lens opacities seem more common, and retinopathy equally common compared with Europeans [10]. More effort is required to define and provide for the special educational and dietary needs of this group of patients.

HUGH M. MATHER

References

1 Mather HM, Keen H. The Southall Diabetes Survey: prevalence of known diabetes in Asians and Europeans. *Br Med J* 1985; **291**: 1081−4.
2 Goodwin AM, Keen H, Mather HM. Ethnic minorities in British Diabetic Clinics: a questionnaire survey. *Diabetic Med* 1987; **4**: 266−9.
3 Nicholl CG, Levy JC, Mohan V, Rao PV, Mather HM. Asian diabetes in Britain: a clinical profile. *Diabetic Med* 1986; **3**: 257−60.
4 Allawi J, Rao PV, Gilbert R, Scott G, Jarrett RJ, Keen H, Viberti GC, Mather HM. Microalbuminuria in non-insulin dependent diabetes: its prevalence in Indian compared with Europid patients. *Br Med J* 1988; **296**: 462−4.
5 Samanta A, Burden AC, Feehally J, Walls J. Diabetic renal disease: differences between Asian and white patients. *Br Med J* 1986; **293**: 366−7.
6 Verma NPS, Mehta SP, Madhu S, Mather HM, Keen H. Prevalence of known diabetes in an urban Indian environment: the Darya Ganj diabetes survey. *Br Med J* 1986; **293**: 423−4.
7 Peterson DB, Dattani JT, Baylis JM, Jepson EM. Dietary practices of Asian diabetics. *Br Med J* 1986; **292**: 170−1.
8 Baylis J, Dattani J. Dietary advice for Asian diabetics. *Practical Diabetes* 1986; **3**: 194−5.
9 Nikolaides K, Barnett AH, Spiliopoulos AJ, Watkins PJ. West Indian diabetic population of a large inner city diabetic clinic. *Br Med J* 1981; **283**: 1374−5.
10 Cruickshank JK, Alleyne SA. Black West Indian and matched white diabetics in Britain compared with diabetics in Jamaica: body mass, blood pressure and vascular disease. *Diabetes Care* 1987; **10**: 170−9.

SECTION 16
LIVING WITH DIABETES

92   Employment, Life Insurance, Smoking and Alcohol

Summary

• Insulin-treated diabetic patients are barred from only a few occupations where hypoglycaemia poses particular hazards to themselves or others (e.g. public transport, Armed Forces).
• Non-insulin-treated patients without complications should enjoy the same job prospects as non-diabetic people.
• Special life insurance policies are available for diabetic people.
• The risks of developing coronary heart and other macrovascular disease are markedly increased by diabetes and by smoking, and almost certainly further increased by smoking and diabetes together. Diabetic patients must be strongly discouraged from smoking.
• Alcohol readily provokes hypoglycaemia in diabetic patients. Daily alcohol intake should not exceed three equivalents (e.g. three small glasses of wine) for diabetic men or two equivalents for diabetic women.

Employment

From the employers' point of view, the main problem of diabetes is the risk of impaired performance and possibility of injury to the diabetic patient or others through hypoglycaemia. Accordingly, diabetic patients treated by diet alone or by diet and oral hypoglycaemic agents, and who are free from complications, should experience few problems with finding employment. On the other hand, insulin-treated diabetic patients may find that employment presents a major hurdle. Fortunately, this hurdle can be overcome in all but a few cases and, with determination and the help and support of the diabetic care team, insulin-treated patients in good general health can be successfully placed in most occupations [1, 2].

Insulin-dependent diabetes is, however, a bar to certain occupations. By international treaty, insulin-treated patients are not allowed to hold a commercial pilot's licence or, following an agreement between British Rail and the transport unions, to drive a passenger train in the United Kingdom. They are also effectively excluded from joining the Armed or Police Forces, although established members who come to need insulin treatment may be allowed to continue to serve, usually in a relatively undemanding post. Certain other employers, such as the Merchant Navy and the offshore oil industry, apply similarly rigid rules. It is difficult, although not illegal, for insulin-treated patients to obtain or keep licences for Heavy Goods Vehicles or Public Service Vehicles (see Chapter 93).

Employers are frequently anxious about absenteeism and poor performance at work. Several studies have shown that this particular concern is unfounded: as a group, diabetic patients lose slightly more time than average off work through sickness but compensate for this by their generally good performance records. Nowadays, there is little evidence of discrimination against people with diabetes, although individual employers still raise objections, which are sometimes absurd [3].

It is important for the diabetes care team to ensure that employers judge diabetic people by their individual qualities rather than their disease, and to deal with misconceptions where necessary. In the UK, consultation with the British Diabetic Association (who provide a useful and inexpensive leaflet entitled *Looking for Work*) and with

915

similar organizations in other countries (see Chapter 102) may be of considerable help.

Life insurance

Insurance companies calculate life insurance policy premiums on the basis of current life expectancy statistics. The shortened life expectancy of diabetic patients reflects the standard of diabetic care over the last few decades and may therefore not be predictive of the future [4]. Life insurance premiums are usually unaffected if agreed before diabetes is diagnosed. However, patients with established diabetes applying for a new life insurance policy are likely to have to pay 10–40% more than non-diabetic applicants, even when free from complications, and may have their application refused if complications are present [5]. It is essential to compare quotations from several insurance companies and the diabetic associations can once again be very helpful: the British Diabetic Association, for example, has special arrangements with a firm of insurance brokers. Low-cost endowment policies, such as for a mortgage, do not usually carry an increased premium for diabetes.

Smoking and diabetes

Atherosclerosis of the coronary, cerebral and peripheral arteries is an important cause of morbidity and a major cause of premature death in diabetes (see Chapter 68). Smoking is well recognized as an independent risk factor for atheroma formation in men and women. Diabetic patients who smoke are at a considerably increased risk of atherosclerotic complications, particularly ischaemic heart disease. A recent large-scale study (based on 120 000 nurses in North America) found that coronary heart disease was 8 times more frequent in diabetic patients overall (both smokers and non-smokers) than in non-diabetic subjects, with an even higher risk of fatal and non-fatal myocardial infarction in diabetic patients who smoked more than 15 cigarettes per day [6]. Additional evidence that smoking further increases the risks of cardiovascular disease in diabetes has been provided by other studies from California [7] and Sweden [8], although the Bedford study in the UK found no relationship between smoking and increased cardiovascular mortality in diabetic patients [9].

The possible relationship of smoking to diabetic complications other than large-vessel atheroma is less clear, although some reports have suggested that smoking may worsen and possibly accelerate the development of retinopathy, nephropathy and the soft-tissue complications of the diabetic hand [10–12]. The deleterious effects of smoking in diabetes have recently been extensively reviewed [13, 14].

There is convincing evidence that non-diabetic subjects who abstain from smoking for several years can progressively reduce their risk of developing coronary heart disease towards that of life-long non-smokers. Although the effects of stopping smoking have not yet been systematically studied in a diabetic population, preliminary evidence suggests that stopping smoking is also beneficial for diabetic patients [8], and the weight of available evidence demands that every effort must be made to discourage diabetic patients from smoking. Diabetic patients should be routinely asked about their smoking habits and advised accordingly, although the results of recent intensive educational programmes targetted at heavy smokers are far from encouraging [15, 16]. Various leaflets and posters are available to reinforce anti-smoking programmes in the clinic.

Alcohol and diabetes

Ethanol is a potent inhibitor of gluconeogenesis and can cause hypoglycaemia in fasting normal subjects, despite their very low circulating insulin concentrations. Where the normal negative feedback mechanisms which suppress endogenous insulin secretion during hypoglycaemia fail to operate, as in diabetic patients treated with insulin or sulphonylureas, alcohol may precipitate severe hypoglycaemia. This is the most important way in which alcohol affects diabetic management. Alcohol intake should therefore be moderate, and always accompanied by food. Low-carbohydrate lagers (especially pilsener) and beers have been marketed by their manufacturers as being particularly suitable for diabetic patients, but because of their relatively high alcohol contents (increasing the risk of hypoglycaemia) and cost, these cannot be recommended. As well as provoking hypoglycaemia, the effects of alcohol may mask hypoglycaemic symptoms. Conversely, many sober but hypoglycaemic diabetic patients have been mistakenly assumed to be drunk, sometimes with disastrous consequences. It is, therefore, essential to check the blood glucose concentration immediately whenever a diabetic patient is thought to be intoxicated by alcohol. High-carbohydrate alcoholic drinks and mixers should also be avoided by non-insulin-dependent patients because of the increased risk of reactive hypoglycaemia. The calorie content of drinks (which is derived from both sugars and alcohol itself) may be considerable and must be taken into account by patients following a weight-reducing diet.

Alcohol ingestion may elevate blood triglyceride levels and abstinence should be recommended for patients with persistent hypertriglyceridaemia. The same advice applies to hypertensive patients. Alcohol also increases plasma lactate concentrations and may have been a contributory factor in the development of lactic acidosis during phenformin treatment. It may, therefore, be prudent to avoid prescribing metformin to patients who are unable to restrict their alcohol intake to only the occasional drink. Alcohol ingestion can cause embarrassing and sometimes uncomfortable facial flushing in a proportion of patients treated with chlorpropamide.

Excessive alcohol consumption has long been associated with large-fibre peripheral nerve damage and may also exacerbate neuropathic symptoms in diabetic patients [17]. Abstention from alcohol should therefore be considered for patients with distressing neuropathic symptoms. In the general diabetic population, however, alcohol consumption seems to have no independent effect on peripheral nerve function as judged by vibration perception threshold measurements in a large clinic population [18].

Table 92.1 shows an abbreviated list of the recommendations of the British Diabetic Association regarding alcohol intake in diabetic patients [19]. The guidelines suggested by the American Diabetes Association [20] are similar, except for

their more cautious advice to limit alcohol intake to two 'equivalents' once or twice per week (one 'equivalent' represents a single measure of spirits, a small glass of wine, or a half-pint of beer).

ANDREW MACLEOD

Table 92.1. The British Diabetic Association's recommendations regarding alcohol consumption by diabetic patients. (Modified from Connor and Marks 1985 [19]. One equivalent = a single measure of spirits, a small glass of wine, or a half-pint of beer.)

- Maximum daily intake = three equivalents for men, or two equivalents for women
- Never take alcohol without food, or before driving
- Include calorie contents of drinks in weight-reducing diets; avoid sweet wines, liqueurs and 'mixers'
- Patients taking sulphonylureas should limit their alcohol intake, and those with neuropathic symptoms or hypertriglyceridaemia should abstain completely

References

1 Lister J. The employment of diabetics (editorial). *Br Med J* 1983; **287**: 1087–8.
2 Sönksen PH. The employment of diabetics. *Br Med J* 1984; **288**: 239.
3 Ardron M, MacFarlane I, Robinson C. Educational achievements, employment and social class of insulin-dependent diabetics: a survey of a young adult clinic in Liverpool. *Diabetic Med* 1987; **4**: 546–8.
4 Fuller JH. Causes of death in diabetes mellitus. *Horm Metab Res* (suppl) 1985; **15**: 3–9.
5 Frier BM, Sullivan FM, Stewart EJ. Diabetes and insurance: a survey of patient experience. *Diabetic Med* 1984; **1**: 127–30.
6 Willett WC, Green A, Stampfer MJ *et al.* Relative and absolute excess risks of coronary heart disease among women who smoke cigarettes. *New Engl J Med* 1987; **317**: 1303–9.
7 Suarez L, Barrett-Connor E. Interaction between cigarette smoking and diabetes mellitus in the prediction of death attributed to cardiovascular disease. *Am J Epidemiol* 1984; **120**: 760–5.
8 Rosengren A, Welin L, Tsipogianni A *et al.* Impact of cardiovascular risk factors on coronary heart disease and mortality among middle aged diabetic men. *Br Med J* 1989; **299**: 1127–31.
9 Jarrett RJ, McCartney P, Keen H. The Bedford Survey: ten year mortality rates in newly diagnosed diabetics, borderline diabetics and normoglycaemic controls; and risk indices for coronary heart disease in borderline diabetics. *Diabetologia* 1982; **22**: 79–80.
10 Mühlhauser I, Sawicki P, Berger M. Cigarette-smoking as a risk factor for macroproteinuria and proliferative retinopathy in Type 1 (insulin-dependent) diabetes. *Diabetologia* 1986; **29**: 500–3.
11 Telmer S, Christiansen JS, Andersen AR, Nerup J, Deckert T. Smoking habits and prevalence of clinical diabetic microangiopathy in insulin-dependent diabetics. *Acta Med Scand* 1984; **215**: 63–8.
12 Eadington DW, Patrick AW, Collier A, Frier BM. Limited joint mobility, Dupuytren's contracture and retinopathy in type 1 diabetes: association with cigarette smoking. *Diabetic Med* 1989; **6**: 152–7.
13 Mühlhauser I. Smoking and diabetes. *Diabetic Med* 1990; **7**: 10–15.
14 Rana BS, Botha JL. Should diabetics be advised not to smoke? A review of the epidemiological evidence. *Practical Diabetes* 1990; **7**: 61–6.
15 Ardron M, MacFarlane IA, Robinson C, van Heyningen C, Calverley PMA. Anti-smoking advice for young diabetic smokers: is it a waste of breath? *Diabetic Med* 1988; **5**: 667–70.
16 Jones RB, Hedley AJ. Prevalence of smoking in a diabetic population: the need for action. *Diabetic Med* 1987; **4**: 233–6.

17 McCulloch DK, Campbell IW, Prescott RJ, Clarke BF. Effect of alcohol intake on symptomatic peripheral neuropathy in diabetic men. *Diabetes Care* 1980; **3**: 245−7.

18 Williams CD, Till S, Macleod AF, Lowy C. Biothesiometry in diabetic patients. *Diabetic Med* 1988; **5** (suppl) 1: 78.

19 Connor H, Marks V. Alcohol and diabetes. *Diabetic Med* 1985; **2**: 413−6.

20 American Diabetes Association. Nutritional recommendations and principles for individuals with diabetes mellitus. *Diabetes Care* 1986; **10**: 126−32.

93   Driving and Diabetes Mellitus

Summary

- Diabetes (especially IDDM) presents several potential hazards to the driver, although there is little evidence that diabetic drivers suffer more traffic accidents than other drivers.
- In the UK, all drivers are legally required to notify diabetes to the Driver and Vehicle Licensing Centre and to their own insurance company.
- Diabetic drivers in the UK can hold Public Service or Heavy Goods Vehicle licences, but in practice those treated with insulin are barred from driving vehicles which carry passengers.
- Hypoglycaemia must be avoided while driving by careful planning and blood glucose testing; a supply of glucose must be kept in the car.
- The minimum legal requirement for a driver's vision (reading a standard number plate at 23 m; roughly 6/10) does not take account of many visual problems caused by diabetes, which require separate assessment.
- All diabetic patients must be asked if they drive; those who do must be given appropriate advice.

Table 93.1. Advice to diabetic drivers.

- Inform the licensing authority (UK: DVLC) and motor insurer (these are legal requirements)
- Always keep a supply of glucose in the car
- Avoid long journeys without rest periods and meals, and check blood glucose levels frequently
- If hypoglycaemic, stop driving and leave the driver's seat
- Do not drive if eyesight deteriorates suddenly (e.g. after vitreous haemorrhage), or if corrected visual acuity is less than 6/12 in both eyes

Driving a car is an everyday activity which demands skill, co-ordination and a high level of concentration; almost half of the population of the UK possess a driving licence. Diabetes presents several potential problems for the driver. These include the development of hypoglycaemia and the effects of long-term complications such as cataract or retinopathy causing visual impairment, or peripheral neuropathy, vascular disease and amputation which can interfere mechanically with driving. In most countries, the diabetic driver is therefore subject to specific statutory regulations for the issue and renewal of a driving licence and has to undergo a regular assessment of medical fitness to drive. Information and advice about diabetes and driving should be a fundamental part of patient education (Table 93.1).

Diabetes and the driving licence

In the UK, diabetes is designated as either a 'prospective' or a 'relevant' disability for driving (Road Traffic Act, 1972, Part III, amended by Schedule 3, 1974). Applicants for a driving licence must inform the Driver and Vehicle Licensing Centre (DVLC) that they have diabetes when applying afresh, or if diabetes develops while already holding a licence. This is a legal requirement, irrespective of the type of diabetes or the treatment required, because the severity of the disorder may increase with time and serious complications are not confined to patients treated with insulin. A restricted driving licence is granted for a maximum period of 3 years and is reissued (at no cost to the diabetic driver) provided that the medical report is satisfactory. When medical reports are required, these are usually obtained from the patient's general practitioner, but some cases require a more detailed report from a hospital specialist.

The onus to declare diabetes is entirely on the patient, and failure to inform the DVLC, whether through lack of knowledge or deliberate concealment, is breaking the law and could incur a fine. Moreover, motor insurance cover can be invalidated regardless of whether diabetes has been declared independently to the motor insurer. Many drivers do not appreciate that claims following road traffic accidents often involve motor insurance companies other than their own or that repudiation of insurance liability may have major financial repercussions, especially when serious personal injury is involved. Doctors who look after diabetic patients are not legally obliged to inform them of the statutory regulations on driving, but it is important to advise patients to comply for their own protection. The revelation that motor insurance protection may be jeopardized by failing to notify diabetes often concentrates the minds of those reluctant to declare this material fact to the DVLC.

Scottish surveys of insulin-treated and non-insulin-dependent diabetic drivers revealed that many fail to notify both the DVLC and motor insurers [1–3], although increased awareness of the regulations and improved education have subsequently increased the rate of notification [4]. The problem does not lie entirely with the diabetic driver: many general practitioners have poor knowledge of the statutory requirements and of the type of practical advice required for diabetic drivers [5].

Vocational driving licences

Public Service Vehicle (PSV) licences are issued to diabetic drivers but in practice, the transport companies (airlines, rail, coach and bus companies) do not allow insulin-treated diabetic patients to drive vehicles which carry passengers. Patients taking oral hypoglycaemic therapy (particularly biguanides) may be allowed to operate certain types of public transport vehicles, but medication which could induce hypoglycaemia is usually considered a major contraindication. Medical fitness to drive with a PSV licence is assessed more rigorously by the transport companies than an application to the DVLC for an ordinary driving licence, as are applications to local authorities for taxi licences. At present, in-

sulin-treated diabetic drivers are permitted to drive minibuses using an ordinary licence, but the regulations governing this type of vehicle are currently under review and possession of a PSV licence may become necessary.

The Heavy Goods Vehicle (HGV) licence and the insulin-treated diabetic driver present a thorny problem. The European Economic Community (EEC) Driving Licence Directive (80/1263/EEC), which became effective in 1983, specified that HGV licences should not be granted to diabetic drivers requiring insulin, and this policy was implemented by the Department of Transport. It was challenged successfully in a legal action on behalf of an individual diabetic driver and the precedent was established that a HGV driving licence cannot be withheld from a diabetic applicant without consideration of individual circumstances [6]. Individual insulin-treated diabetic drivers are currently granted an HGV licence on a discretionary basis, but this situation may change.

Problems of the diabetic driver

Advice for diabetic drivers is summarized in Table 93.1.

Hypoglycaemia

Hypoglycaemia is probably the single greatest hazard for the diabetic motorist and, in patients treated with insulin, is relatively common while driving. One-third of a group of 250 insulin-treated diabetic drivers in Edinburgh had experienced hypoglycaemia while driving in a 6-month period. Road traffic accidents may be caused by hypoglycaemia [1, 4, 7–9], and subclinical hypoglycaemia, causing cognitive dysfunction and impaired judgement, can occur without provoking acute autonomic symptoms of hypoglycaemia [10], and may produce automatism. Some patients have described irrational and compulsive behaviour with inability to stop driving despite being aware of concurrent hypoglycaemia. Patients with hypoglycaemic unawareness are probably at greatest risk of being involved in road traffic accidents [4], although there is virtually no evidence available to establish that the overall accident rate of diabetic drivers is greater than that of the non-diabetic driving population [4, 6, 7–9]. The estimated accident rate may have been reduced through a process of self-selection by diabetic drivers who have advancing complications or recurrent hypoglycaemia, who had ceased driving of their own volition [4, 8].

All insulin-treated drivers should keep glucose or other carbohydrate to hand in their vehicles; disturbingly, many do not [11]. Each car journey, no matter how short, must be planned in advance and attention paid to unexpected events such as delays in traffic jams or having to change a wheel, which increase the risk of hypoglycaemia. Measurement of capillary blood glucose before and during long journeys, together with frequent rests and meals, is advisable. If symptomatic hypoglycaemia occurs during driving, the diabetic driver should stop the car, switch off the engine and leave the driver's seat, as a charge can be made of driving while under the influence of a drug (insulin) even if the car is stationary. Press reports appear with monotonous regularity of semiconscious, hypoglycaemic diabetic drivers being taken into police custody under the mistaken impression that they are drunk or suffering from some other acute illness. Diabetic drivers should therefore carry a card or bracelet stating that they suffer from the disease. Some newly diagnosed IDDM patients may have to stop driving temporarily until their glycaemic control is stable, but no established guidelines exist and advice should be tailored to individual circumstances [12].

Vision

Monocular vision alone is accepted for driving in the UK where the minimum legal requirement is the ability to read a number plate with letters 3.5 in (8.9 cm) high from 75 feet (22.9 m), wearing spectacles if necessary. This corresponds approximately to 6/10 on the Snellen chart. The number plate test is difficult to perform under clinical conditions and does not assess night vision, the ability to see moving objects, or the visual fields which may be severely reduced by

extensive photocoagulation for diabetic retinopathy. In some cases, the DVLC now requests assessment of visual fields by perimetry as part of the medical report. Cataract formation may accentuate glare from headlights and affected patients should not drive at night. Many patients stop driving voluntarily when they notice deteriorating vision [4, 8] and previous surveys have identified few active diabetic drivers who would fail the eyesight tests [1, 2, 4, 8]. More practical tests of vision are required for the routine assessment of the diabetic driver.

BRIAN M. FRIER

References

1 Frier BM, Matthews DM, Steel JM, Duncan LJP. Driving and insulin-dependent diabetes. *Lancet* 1980; i: 1232−4.
2 Steel JM, Frier BM, Young RJ, Duncan LJP. Driving and insulin-independent diabetes. *Lancet* 1981; ii: 354−6.
3 Frier BM, Sullivan FM, Stewart EJC. Diabetes and insurance: a survey of patient experience. *Diabetic Med* 1984; **1**: 127−30.
4 Eadington DW, Frier BM. Type 1 diabetes and driving experience: an eight year cohort study. *Diabetic Med* 1989; **6**: 137−41.
5 Fisher BM, Storer AM, Frier BM. Diabetes, driving and the general practitioner. *Br Med J* 1985; **291**: 181−2.
6 Cockram CS, Dutton T, Sönksen PH. Driving and diabetes: a summary of the current medical and legal position based upon a recent Heavy Goods Vehicle (HGV) case. *Diabetic Med* 1986; **3**: 137−40.
7 Songer TJ, Laporte RE, Dorman JS, Orchard TJ, Cruickshank KJ, Becker DJ, Drash AL. Motor vehicle accidents and IDDM. *Diabetes Care* 1988; **11**: 701−7.
8 Stevens AB, Roberts M, McKane R, Atkinson AB, Bell PM, Hayes JR. Motor vehicle driving among diabetics taking insulin and non-diabetics. *Br Med J* 1989; **299**: 591−5.
9 Ratner RE, Whitehouse FW. Motor vehicles, hypoglycemia and diabetic drivers. *Diabetes Care* 1989; **12**: 217−22.
10 Pramming S, Thorsteinsson B, Theilgaard A, Pinner EM, Binder C. Cognitive function during hypoglycaemia in type 1 diabetes mellitus. *Br Med J* 1986; **292**: 647−50.
11 Clarke B, Ward JD, Enoch BA. Hypoglycaemia in insulin-dependent diabetic drivers. *Br Med J* 1980; **281**: 586.
12 Alexander W. Initiation of insulin treatment and driving. *Diabetes Update*. London: British Diabetic Association. March 1988; **12**: 3.

94 Travel and Diabetes Mellitus

Summary

- Diabetes is not a bar to travel, even over long distances, but careful planning, adequate supplies of medication and sensible self-monitoring are essential.
- Patients must be fully instructed in what to do during diarrhoea, vomiting or other intercurrent illness.
- Insulin can be kept safely at warm room temperature for at least 1 month.
- Extended 'days' during long westward air journeys often require an additional dose of short-acting insulin followed by a meal.

Where to find information

Diabetic people can and do travel throughout the world. The journal of the British Diabetic Association, *Balance*, frequently records amazing feats of adventure undertaken successfully by diabetic patients. Useful advice can be found in several patients' guides [1, 2]. The British Diabetic Association's Diabetes Care Department provides general information. It produces excellent printed travel guide booklets giving information about food and drink, types of insulin and oral hypoglycaemic agents available, health agreements and useful phrases for the most commonly visited European countries. Supplementary travel sheets are also available for various other destinations (e.g. India), on which information is available, mainly from the National Diabetic Associations. The Department also has up-to-date information from the insulin manufacturers about the availability of types and strengths of insulins throughout the world. Those planning to travel should be encouraged to contact the head of this Department. The specific topic of 'outward bound' adventure holidays is discussed in a recent book [3].

There are a few simple rules which should be followed and several topics which can usefully be discussed with diabetic people planning a holiday.

Food

Holidays do not always go exactly as planned. Trains, buses and aeroplanes can be late; cars can be caught in traffic jams; or the expected buffet car or café can be closed. These unforeseen eventualities should not, however, present a serious problem to the well-prepared. Diabetic patients should always carry dextrose tablets or other rapidly absorbed carbohydrate, whether on holiday or not, and additional carbohydrate such as a packet of biscuits is also advisable (ginger biscuits are particularly suitable as they do not crumble). For long journeys, further supplies of carbohydrate should be packed in a reasonably accessible place.

When travelling abroad, the patient should check on the basic form of carbohydrates eaten in the country to be visited, and with foods such as rice or pasta, they might usefully learn to judge the quantities of these containing 10 g of carbohydrate. While on holiday, it should be possible to select from the local menus and to supplement carbohydrate if necessary with bread, biscuits or fruit.

Drinks

In most places, coffee, tea and table water are available. In Britain and America, there is rarely difficulty in obtaining low-calorie drinks but in

922

parts of Europe this can be a problem; it is often forgotten that fresh or cartoned orange juice contains 10 g of carbohydrate per 100 ml. Those who dislike drinking plain or soda water can use lemon juice with a sweetener or flavoured, effervescent vitamin C tablets, or can take with them a supply of low-calorie cola or other flavoured concentrates. Alcohol is discussed in Chapter 92.

Insulin and syringes

Diabetic patients should be advised to take an ample supply of insulin and syringes and to divide them between two different bags (one can be carried by a relative or friend) in case of loss. If insulin is lost, it is almost always possible to obtain replacement supplies, but not necessarily of the usual strength and type. The British Diabetic Association list of the preparations available in different countries is generally a very good guide, but it is difficult to keep this information completely up to date and there can be quite marked variations in the type of insulin available within a country. Whereas America, Australia and the UK use exclusively 100-U preparations, parts of Europe and some countries further afield still use 40-U insulin. If 40-U insulin is used, it is easiest to measure it with a 40-U syringe, now unfamiliar to many patients in the UK. It is clearly desirable to avoid any danger of running into such problems. A general practitioner in the UK can prescribe a three months' supply of insulin, enough to cover most holidays.

Patients occasionally ask for a letter for the customs officer to prove that they are diabetic and not drug addicts. A diabetic identity card, necklace or bracelet is also adequate for this purpose.

Storage of insulin while on holiday may give rise to concern. When travelling by air, insulin should not be put in luggage which is to go into the hold, not only because this may be lost but also because sub-zero temperatures in the hold can denature the insulin. For the same reason, insulin should never be put in the freezer compartment of a refrigerator or in a cold bag where it could freeze.

People tend to worry, generally unnecessarily, about keeping insulin cool. Insulin can be damaged by high temperatures and insulin manufacturers (who are naturally anxious to avoid problems due to loss of activity) emphasize the importance of keeping insulin in a refrigerator.

The biological stability of insulin at different temperatures varies with the insulin formulation, deterioration occurring more rapidly in bright light than in the dark. Generally, however, all insulin preparations can be kept at 25°C for several months with a loss of only 2% of biological potency, and for at least 10 months at that temperature before potency is reduced by 5%. Insulin can even be maintained at 40°C for several weeks and lose only 5% of its potency [4–6].

When travelling in moderate climates, insulin can safely be stored out of a refrigerator as long as it is not exposed to direct sunlight (e.g. on the back ledge of a car), close to a fire or directly above a radiator. In hot climates, patients are usually advised to store insulin in a cool bag or hotel refrigerator. Because of the risks of loss or theft, an additional supply should be stored in the coolest part of the room, covered with a wet flannel if it is very warm. Insulin can be kept safely at up to 25°C for at least 1 month and, even in hot Third World countries without electricity, insulin usually retains adequate activity for 6 months [7].

When damaged by heat, soluble insulin usually becomes cloudy whereas insulin suspensions may show changes such as a granular appearance, and occasionally a brownish colour. Insulin displaying any of these appearances should obviously not be used.

Insurance

When travelling in countries of the European Community (EC), medical attention is completely or substantially free to EC members but patients from the UK should be advised to obtain certificate E111 from their local Social Security office to simplify any claim. Some other countries offer free or reduced-cost medical treatment for EC members. These include Australia, Austria, the Channel Islands, Hong Kong, Iceland, New Zealand, Norway, Poland, Rumania, Sweden, the USSR and Yugoslavia. Leaflet SA30 *Medical Costs Abroad* gives details about the care available in these countries and can be obtained from travel agents, Social Security Offices or the Department of Health. The British Diabetic Association also provides information given by the diabetic associations in several countries.

Patients should be advised to obtain full health insurance with comprehensive cover as, in some countries, particularly North America, health care can be extremely expensive. It is advisable to shop around several insurance companies or agents as premiums can vary widely.

Immunization

Some diabetic patients believe that it may be dangerous in some way for them to receive immunization. It is of course just as important, if not more so, that they receive the recommended protection. Very occasionally, a severe reaction to the typhoid vaccine may cause a temporary increase in insulin requirements, but the others rarely cause any problems. Malaria prophylaxis should be taken if recommended. The Department of Health leaflet SA23 (in the UK) gives detailed and up-to-date recommendations for different countries.

Illness while travelling

Any patient prone to travel sickness should be advised to take anti-sickness tablets prophylactically to avoid the problems associated with vomiting in diabetes.

In countries where the water is not safe, bottled water only should be drunk, and water for brushing teeth or washing food should be sterilized by boiling or by adding sterilizing tablets. Ice cubes should be avoided as they may be made from contaminated water.

Should vomiting or diarrhoea develop, the patient must understand the importance of continuing to take insulin injections, with carbohydrate in the form of drinks and adequate fluid replacement, while carefully monitoring blood glucose levels and testing for urinary ketones.

Monitoring diabetic control

It is quite understandable that many diabetic patients on holiday also wish to have a holiday from blood and urine tests. However, as holiday activity and lifestyle may be very different from usual, monitoring is particularly important. Some people take more exercise on holiday and may try new sporting activities while others do less than usual, so it is important to understand the effect of activity on blood glucose. Diabetic people should always take some glucagon on holiday in addition to dextrosol, glucose drinks and perhaps glucose gel (e.g. Hypostop®). Glucagon can be given simply and safely by a friend or relative, thus avoiding the problem of finding medical assistance and sometimes risking prolonged hospital admission for severe hypoglycaemia.

Extremes of temperature

In the heat, insulin absorption occurs more rapidly. Sunburn can be dangerous and those with neuropathy should be specifically warned to avoid this. If a diabetic person is hyperglycaemic, dehydration can occur rapidly in a hot climate and large amounts of fluid may be needed.

In a very cold climate, the rate of insulin absorption is slower but on warming up later it may suddenly be absorbed. The energy output associated with shivering reduces the blood glucose level. The main danger for a diabetic person in a cold climate is that if hypoglycaemia does occur, it inhibits thermoregulatory shivering and hypothermia can occur [8, 9]. Diabetic patients should be warned about this possibility and about the danger of frostbite. Patients with neuropathy should be specifically instructed about the prevention of frostbite if visiting a cold climate. Diabetic people should also appreciate the need to keep their blood glucose strips warm and dry, as cold may produce falsely low readings by inhibiting the enzymes in the strips.

Air travel

The airline should be informed that a client is diabetic at the time of booking. Some will provide special meals and enquire if they can do anything to help. All airlines tend to produce meals at fairly frequent intervals but these can be rather small, and even official 'diabetic' meals can contain as little as 15 g of carbohydrate [10]. Patients should carry their own supplies of carbohydrate to make up the deficit, if necessary.

The number of people travelling abroad has increased enormously over recent years and it is no longer only the very wealthy who cross the Atlantic or the Equator. Journeys across time zones can mean that adjustments in insulin regimens are necessary. Individual cases should be discussed in detail but, in general, changes of less than 4 h do not require major alterations in the injection schedule. If the day is extended, extra carbohydrate should be taken. A common example would be a flight to New York, which adds 5 or 6 h to the 'day'. Planes usually leave at about noon. A diabetic patient taking short- and intermediate-acting insulin twice daily should take his or her morning insulin, breakfast, lunch and snacks as normal. On arrival at about 1400 h local time (1900 h British time), a small extra dose of short-acting insulin followed by a meal will cover the extra hours, and the usual evening dose of insulin followed by a meal (at 1800–1900 h American time) will bring the patient into phase with the new time zone. If it is planned to go to sleep and miss the late-night snack, the evening dose of intermediate-acting insulin should be reduced. On the return journey (West to East), 5 or 6 h are lost. Flights are usually in the evening; by omitting the evening dose of intermediate-acting insulin, it is possible to arrive at 0200 h American time and switch back into phase with British time (0700 h) by taking the morning dose of insulin and breakfast. If the patient plans to go to sleep and miss lunch, both insulins should be cut back considerably.

The exact instructions will obviously vary with the journey to be taken, the timing of the journey and the insulin regimen which the patient is taking. A logical schedule can be devised from the times of the journey and the time-zone changes, by dividing the day into 6-h periods and adding, omitting or reducing insulin dosages as indicated. In making these adjustments, it is wise to aim on the side of slightly high blood glucose levels to avoid the risk of hypoglycaemia.

Those taking oral agents should have no particular problem. It is not necessary to take extra tablets to cover an extended day but one dose of tablets can be omitted on a particularly short day in the case of a long West to East journey.

Holiday and travel are opportunities for the unexpected to arise and it is impossible to anticipate every problem that the patient may encounter. It is therefore essential that every diabetic patient is educated in the basic principles of his own management so that he can react sensibly to any eventuality.

JUDITH M. STEEL

References

1 Day JL. Insulin dependent diabetes. In: *The British Diabetic Association Diabetes Handbook*. Wellingborough, New York: Thorsons Publishing Group, 1986: 125–32.

2 Steel JM, Dunn M. *Coping with Life on Insulin*. Edinburgh: W&R Chambers, 1987.

3 Hillson R. *Diabetes. A Beyond Basics Guide*. London: Optima, 1986.

4 Pingel M, Volund A. Stability of insulin preparations. *Diabetes* 1972; **21**: 805–13.

5 Brange J. *Galenics of Insulin*. Berlin: Springer-Verlag, 1987: 52–6.

6 Blakeman K. The characteristics and storage requirements of modern insulins. *Pharmaceut J* 1983; 711–13.

7 Steel JM, Mngola EW. Diabetes in Kenya. *Tropical Doctor* 1974; **4**: 184–7.

8 Gale E, Bennett T, Green JH et al. Hypoglycaemia, hypothermia and shivering in man. *Clin Sci* 1981; **61**: 463–9.

9 Hillson R. Hypoglycaemia and hypothermia. *Diabetes Care* 1983; **6**: 211.

10 Johnston RV, Neilly IJ, Lang JM, Frier BM. The high flying diabetic: dietary inadequacy of airline meals (abstract). *Diabetic Med* 1986; **3**: 580A.

95 Adjustment to Life with Diabetes Mellitus

Summary

• Each patient's ability to live with and adjust to diabetes depends on his or her beliefs and attitudes concerning the disease and health in general. Time must be taken to explore these in detail and to correct any misconceptions.

• Misconceptions about diabetes and its complications often encourage fatalism. By contrast, many others acknowledge the potential gravity of the disease but do not perceive themselves as vulnerable to its effects.

• Self-care is clearly essential in diabetes but is contrary to the expectations of many newly diagnosed patients.

• Hypoglycaemia is an important cause of patients losing confidence in their ability to control their own diabetes.

• The effect of relatives and other influential people must not be overlooked.

• Physicians must fully discuss with the patient all monitoring test results − including 'discrepant' HbA$_1$ or fructosamine values and any necessary changes in treatment. Failure to do this will encourage non-compliance.

It is difficult to explain why some people with diabetes are able to accept and comply with the major adjustments in lifestyle demanded by the physician, whereas others are not. This chapter aims to examine some of the factors which determine whether a diabetic patient will adhere to or reject the recommended treatment regimen.

The expectations of the newly diagnosed patient should first be considered. Most people believe that the responsibility for their treatment lies with the medical team. In the case of diabetes, this belief is counterproductive as it is essential for the patient to undertake his own management. The fact that many fail to do this is self-evident in everyday practice: even those with long-standing diabetes often expect their physician to adjust their insulin dosage and regard the suggestion that they should do this themselves as a revolutionary concept. Even patients who claim to adjust their own treatment seem reluctant to do this, as is apparent from the constancy of the insulin dosages which they report at clinic visits. Similar beliefs may explain the frequent failure of home blood glucose monitoring to improve glycaemic control: patients may rely on the technique itself and neglect the need to react to the results [1, 2].

An individual's attitudes about what might affect his future health have been formalized as the 'locus of control'; an 'internal' locus denotes someone who feels that he himself is able to influence the outcome of his illness, whereas an 'external' locus implies that the future is determined by forces over which he has no control, such as chance, or the medical team. The locus of control may partly determine patients' responses to suggested treatment, as exemplified by recent studies on IDDM patients undertaking continuous subcutaneous insulin infusion (CSII) treatment [3]. Subjects with an external locus of control may regard the insulin pump as a 'black box' which will control their diabetes for them, and they may persist with this belief even if their glycaemic control is manifestly poor. Such views may explain some patients' enthusiasm for 'new technology' devices such as glucose monitors and insulin pumps. These beliefs, and particularly a nearly total reliance on the diabetic care team, may be very difficult to alter but the first step is for the doctor or nurse concerned to try to recognize them.

Another important factor in determining whether the subject will follow the doctor's recommendation is his knowledge of diabetes, whether correct or incorrect [4]. This must be ascertained early to allow any misconceptions to be corrected. Mythology may be rampant: for example, anxieties about amputation may be reinforced all too often by seeing wheelchair-bound amputees waiting in the clinic for their transport home. Patients under the impression that all diabetic people become blind may see little purpose in self-monitoring or adjusting their insulin regimens. Many young diabetic men fear impotence: as this is most commonly due to psychogenic factors, even in the diabetic population, this expectation may be self-fulfilling. These attitudes emphasize the crucial importance of honest and complete discussion of the disease and its complications, soon after diagnosis and whenever necessary thereafter, to prevent fatalism from holding sway.

Other reasons why subjects fail to follow recommendations include lack of appreciation of the need to change their behaviour, reluctance to undertake adequate self-monitoring and fear of hypoglycaemia. Motivation may be poor in those who do not perceive themselves as threatened by diabetes or its complications. Bradley's studies of the health beliefs held by IDDM patients [5] have revealed wide discrepancies between their rating of the severity of various disease outcomes (including heart disease and cancer as well as the short- and long-term diabetic complications) and the extent to which they considered themselves vulnerable to them. Denial is particularly frequent among teenagers. The physician's demand for monitoring of control is a frequent bone of contention and an important barrier to effective self-management. Blood glucose testing does hurt and is inconvenient. The request for intensified testing will only be accepted by patients who perceive this as necessary and not by those who already consider themselves well controlled even if this is hopelessly optimistic [6]. This misconception may be due to the physician's reluctance to tell the patients how far short of ideal they really fall and may be corrected by routinely informing them of their HbA$_1$ or fructosamine results. Patients reluctant to test may fabricate records to increase the number of tests apparently done or to improve on the results obtained; studies with 'memory meters' suggest that these practices are surprisingly common [7, 8].

'Learned hopelessness' may be another reason for failing to self-monitor, especially if the results vary in a haphazard way. Many patients may have fallen prey to this, perhaps after learning that their adjustments and those recommended by their physicians have little effect. Even patients who monitor themselves often fail to make any adjustments in insulin, meals or lifestyle. The availability of an instant response to results may be a great motivator. Highly intensified regimens with immediate adjustment to allow individuals to eat quite freely are an example [9]. The role of important other people must not be overlooked and must be identified. The persuasive effect, positive or negative, of a close friend or relative may be more potent than hours of professional counselling.

The powerful effect of hypoglycaemia and ignorance about its outcome cannot be overemphasized. Many patients are afraid of dying during hypoglycaemia. Lack of warning symptoms can be particularly devastating and can shatter the individuals' confidence in their capacity to manage their own diabetes.

Ultimately, patients' decisions may be determined by their perception of the balance between the benefits of and the barriers to treatment. Barriers other than hypoglycaemia and frequent testing include the need for regular meals, the attitudes and behaviour of others, and prohibition of particular activities. Some apparently feel that the price of commitment is too high: they agree to attend a yearly examination but not daily blood tests. On balance, however, most patients perceive more benefits than barriers; many patients are gratified by achieving normal results and feeling in control of their diabetes.

The impact of diabetes is modified by the free range of an individual's personality and people's responses will therefore be varied. This has been emphasized by Dunn's work [10], which used a general attitude questionnaire designed to examine several attributes identified as stress, feelings of coping, guilt, alienation or co-operation, rejection or acceptance, and tolerance. Individuals' responses to a diabetes education programme could be related to their initial attitudes. Patients showing strongly co-operative attitudes but low coping skills had reasonably good metabolic control initially which improved after the programme, whereas control in those with generally 'imbalanced' attitudes was poor before and even worse after the programme. A further group with uniformally poor adjustment, except for high tolerance scores, had the worst control initially but improved the most after the programme.

These problems can only be solved by paying much more attention to the patient's attitudes and beliefs, not only at diagnosis but throughout his diabetic life. Beliefs can be changed for the good, but only if opportunities are provided for them to be expressed and explored. The traditional diabetic clinic is often an inappropriate environment for these discussions. The informal atmosphere of the diabetes day centre or group discussions (either formal or on a self-help basis) may be valuable in facilitating this process [11, 12].

JOHN L. DAY

References

1 Worth R, Home PD, Johnson DG et al. Intensive attention improves glycaemic control in insulin-dependent diabetes without further advantage from home blood glucose monitoring: results of a controlled trial. Br Med J 1982; 285: 1233–9.
2 Mazze RS, Pasmantier R, Murphy JA, Shamoon H. Self-monitoring of capillary blood glucose: changing the performance of individuals with diabetes. Diabetes Care 1985; 8: 207–13.
3 Bradley C et al. The use of diabetes-specific perceived control and health belief measures to predict treatment choice and efficacy in a feasibility study of continuous subcutaneous insulin infusion pumps. Psychol Health 1987; 1: 133–46.
4 Lockington TJ, Meadows KA, Wise PH. Complaint behaviour: relationships to attitudes and control in diabetic patients. Diabetic Med 1987; 4: 56–61.
5 Bradley C, Brewin CR, Gamsu DS, Moses JL. Development of scales to measure perceived control of diabetes mellitus and diabetes-related health beliefs. Diabetic Med 1984; 1: 213–18.
6 Burfield R, Walker R, Day JL. Good diabetes control. The role of patients, perceptions and beliefs (abstract). Diabetologia 1986; 29: 523A.
7 Smith MA, Greene SA, Kuykendall VG, Baum JD. Memory blood glucose reflectance meter and computer: a preliminary report of its use in recording and analysing blood glucose data measured at home by diabetic children. Diabetic Med 1985; 2: 265–8.
8 Mazze RS, Shamoon H, Pasmentier R et al. Reliability of blood glucose monitoring by patients with diabetes mellitus. Am J Med 1984; 77: 211–17.
9 Howorka K. Funktionelle, nahenormoglykämische Insulinsubstitution. Berlin: Springer-Verlag, 1987.
10 Dunn SM. Reaction to educational techniques: coping strategies for diabetics and learning. Diabetic Med 1986; 3: 419–26.
11 Day JL, Johnson G, Rayman G, Walker R. The feasibility of a potentially 'ideal' system of integrated diabetes care and education based on a day centre. Diabetic Med 1988; 5: 70–5.
12 Tattersall RB, McCulloch DK, Aveline M. Group therapy in the treatment of diabetes. Diabetes Care 1985; 8: 180–8.

96   A Patient's View of Diabetes

I got diabetes in 1973, when I was 21. Being told about it was almost a relief because I had been feeling so worn down for so long. A lot of new diabetics feel like that and cope with the news well if they are told about the problems and dangers of the condition gently, so they can take it in at their own pace. Everyone has his or her own pace of adjustment. I like being told everything, including the worst bits, straight away, but most people seem to prefer taking the news in little by little. It is the doctor who has to decide when to tell the patient the next thing he or she needs to know, and in my experience, hospital doctors are insensitive about the time and the way to do this. For instance, when you first realize you are diabetic the most horrifying news is that you will have to inject yourself every day for the rest of your life, but this news is usually delivered point-blank, confirming the general impression that the doctor is in a hurry to move on to more serious cases. General practitioners seem to be better at understanding how much a small thing of no medical importance, like frequent injecting, can upset the person who has to do it.

When you leave hospital, you meet people full of horror stories about diabetes. It is reassuring if you understand, however simply, what diabetes is and what causes its side-effects; this takes the mystique out of the horror stories and makes you feel it must be possible to work out a good balance. It also cheers up your family to know about the condition and realize that they can help by doing something as simple as making a sugary drink.

The more people who know about your diabetes and what it involves, the easier your life becomes. This is especially true of work, where a lot of problems are caused by employers panicking when they see a diabetic employee having a 'hypo' which — to their eyes at least — is often spectacular and always alarming. Work would be much less fraught if you could feel, as you soon feel at home and with friends, that your employers are not frightened of the condition because they know how to alleviate its effects.

Without any doubt, the worst thing about diabetes, for the diabetic and for outsiders, is hypoglycaemia. As time goes by, bad 'hypos' feel worse and worse, developing new dimensions of mental nightmare to go with all the physical humiliations. Not surprisingly, outsiders are appalled by them and they increase the diabetic's sense of living in a different world, not of illness but of continual unease, waiting for trouble. However, you quickly get used to living under a pall of weariness with hypos and with knowing that they hang over every moment of your life. When someone is nice to you after a hypo, and believes your description of how ghastly they are, it is wonderfully comforting. Doctors are usually rather brusque and clinical about hypos, and if you meet one who is understanding about them, you get a close doctor–patient relationship straightaway. Patients need to be warned about hypos, however lightly, from the start.

Dietitians never have any inhibitions about giving patients warnings. They are the most forthcoming of hospital diabetic care teams, so much so that you often end up feeling more like a victim than a patient. It is hard giving an exact account of what you eat and it is made all the harder when the account has to be given to a thin, efficient, uniformed dietitian writing everything down and looking disapproving. They usually explain the carbohydrate side of the diabetic diet well, but grimly. I think diet is one of the few areas of diabetic care where written lists and booklets are as useful as spoken instruction. They give you time to work out for yourself what you have to eat and how best you can fit it in with your lifestyle.

On the subject of weight, women are always sensitive, and dietitians and doctors tend to upset them by being a bit brutal. I know they are right (medically speaking) but one of the most upsetting things about diabetes is having to eat when you don't want to; being scolded about the weight this produces only adds to the misery. Food stops being a pleasure when you are diabetic; it is a compulsory, routine bore, with all spontaneity lost.

Hospital diabetic doctors are usually tired after a long clinic when they see you, and make little effort to look interested in your version of events. The most common complaint among diabetic patients is that doctors don't listen to them; they work from standard questions which make no allowance for the miseries and worries that have been building up inside the patient for weeks. It helps if you know the doctor. That makes him easier to talk to, but it is difficult to develop that sort of relationship in the depressing atmosphere of a hospital clinic.

Clinics are better than they used to be. They now have posters and children's toys, but they could be greatly cheered up by a few simple touches. Last year's magazines are particularly dispiriting; maybe there could be boxes left in public waiting-rooms and shops for people to fill with magazines they have finished reading, which hospitals could collect each week. The hospital clinic I go to has no food or drink. Surely diabetic clinics more than any others need a coffee, fruit juice and biscuits machine? Boredom is the main enemy, in clinics and in hospitals generally, and life could be improved out of sight by having more shops or trolleys selling books, magazines, newspapers, cards, writing materials and simple things to do.

The best way to get to know a diabetic doctor is at a non-hospital clinic, in a local surgery or health centre. These are smaller, more friendly and less intimidating because they are free of the equipment, uniform and timetable atmosphere that makes hospitals so daunting.

TERESA MCLEAN

SECTION 17
THE ORGANIZATION OF DIABETES CARE

97 Diabetes Education

Summary

• Education is essential to ensure effective patient self-management and improved diabetes control, and to help to prevent long-term complications.

• Education involves a major behavioural change. Long-term reinforcement is essential if motivation is to be maintained.

• Educational programmes must use well-trained teachers; diabetes nurse specialists are particularly valuable.

• Teaching methods and timetables must match the needs of the individual patient.

• Programmes should be based on objectives which are agreed by the whole team and adapted for and decided with each individual patient. Basic objectives lists have been produced by the British Diabetic Association and other bodies.

• Learning about diabetes and its management is difficult for patients in traditional diabetic clinics. Purpose designed units combining clinical and educational facilities are more appropriate.

• Individual patients' progress and the performance of the programme itself must be evaluated regularly.

Education is undoubtedly essential to achieve the high standards of self-management on which good diabetic control depends. This was acknowledged in the 1920s with the development of the Joslin Clinic in the USA and in the doctrine of R.D. Lawrence in the UK [1, 2]. The pivotal role of education and the vital need for its further development has been emphasized by numerous studies in the last 15 years [3−9]. These have demonstrated that educational measures such as formal instruction programmes, 24-h telephone advice services and the introduction of nurse practitioners significantly improved various endpoints including glycaemic control, hospital admission rates for diabetic patients and the frequency of amputations.

The cost benefits of education are now well recognized in children, adolescents and adults. Nonetheless, general standards of glycaemic control remain disappointingly low and admission rates for ketoacidosis, hypoglycaemia and foot ulceration — all theoretically preventable — are consistently too high [10]. Much of the blame for this may be due to failure of provision of effective instruction to both enable and persuade individuals to take the necessary steps to achieve higher standards. The existence of the 'behaviour gap', i.e. the difference between what people know and do, emphasizes that such programmes cannot be confined to provision of information alone, but must encompass the much more complicated task of persuading individuals to adopt and maintain all those steps required to put theory into practice [11, 14]. Beliefs of the individual which may alter with time are important determinants of behaviour and consequently glycaemic control [15−17].

The principles of educational programmes

Various educational curricula have been used, largely determined by the local health system. The units in Düsseldorf [18] and Geneva, and many in the USA, use 1−2 week programmes, after which care of the patients reverts to their private physician. British and Australian practice

933

favours out-patient curricula spread over weeks, months or years as part of routine clinical follow-up [19, 20]. Domiciliary education is also employed, especially for children [21].

The curriculum's format is determined by practical factors and other considerations, including the well-demonstrated waning effect of intensive programmes with time [22, 23]; the level of training of members of the clinical care team; and the need to match programmes to the wide range of individual patients' abilities and beliefs. The crucial importance of educating team members has been elegantly demonstrated by Mazucca and colleagues [24], who found that separate programmes directed at patients and their physicians had additive benefits. The need for individual flexibility is highlighted by the work of Dunn, which suggests that each patient's attitude determines their response to and benefit from educational programmes [20]. It is therefore becoming clear that education must involve the 'educators' as well as the patients, and that the process is inextricably involved in clinical management [10, 19].

Structuring an educational programme

The need for objectives

Diabetic education is complicated and unlikely to succeed without a formal list of clear-cut objectives. This is particularly true in longer-term, out-patient-based systems, in which items demanding immediate attention are likely to appear unpredictably. Without these, omission is virtually guaranteed, which may explain, for example, the scanty basic knowledge of long-standing diabetic subjects [25] and the widespread failure to report diabetes to driving licence authorities [26].

The objective list should not simply itemize subjects for discussion, but should also identify the outcome expected of the individual [27]. This immediately helps the teacher to select the learning methods which match the patient's needs and will indicate appropriate means of evaluation. In formulating these lists, it immediately becomes apparent that different behaviours (knowledge, skills and attitudes) require different learning methods (e.g. practical demonstrations, written material, counselling, small group sessions). Moreover, the time-scale for different objectives will vary considerably: some 'first aid' measures must

be learned in the first few days after diagnosis, whereas others can be acquired over much longer periods. Such differentiation permits more rational planning of staff time.

All educational team members must determine and agree their objectives. Attitudes to various objectives (e.g. foot care [28]) diverge considerably both between and within different professional groups, some items being rated as very important by some and of little significance by others. Such conflict is easily perceived by the patients, who become confused and may even reject the team's advice.

Lists of objectives are best drawn up in consultation with the patient, so that each outcome can be discussed and its relevance to the individual determined. Objectives must be adapted to the individual and must consider the age of the subject, presence or absence of complications, social factors, previous knowledge or mythology about diabetes, treatment and special circumstances such as pregnancy. To improve their chances of being realized, they should be fully agreed between teacher and learner, perhaps almost on a 'contractual' basis. Basic objective lists have been produced by the British Diabetic Association and the Diabetes Education Study Group of the European Association for the Study of Diabetes [29, 30].

Choice of learning method

Learning methods may be influenced by the availability of staff, the health care setting and the local population characteristics but must also be appropriate to the individuals concerned. Out-patient-based systems generally rely on 'one-to-one' tuition with a doctor, nurse or dietitian.

Some structure is necessary to avoid omissions, especially as clinical problems may demand priority. The need for lists of objectives has already been stressed. The initial interview should seek to identify the patient's existing knowledge and beliefs about diabetes and his expectations, and to correct these if mistaken. The necessity for self-assessment and self-management should be stressed early. Open-ended questions should be substituted for didactic statements to ensure that the patient's needs are identified and met [31]. Timing is also vitally important. For example, new cases of non-insulin-dependent diabetes will require several sessions concerning diagnosis, future management, self-testing, dietary recommendations and so on; if possible, these should be separated, to avoid overloading the patient with information and also to make best use of staff time (Table 97.1). Furthermore, the immediate emotional response to the diagnosis may prevent the patient from learning all but a few very simple messages and skills.

Use of group teaching

Group learning can provide important advantages for those of all ages with diabetes [32]. Lecturing to groups may apparently save teachers' time but assumes that all the learners have similar baseline knowledge. The greatest value of groups is that they provide an interactive system which enables each individual to explore and learn from his or her peers' experiences and to discuss beliefs which might not be expressed in a 'one-to-one' encounter with a teacher. Accordingly, the teacher must positively withdraw from the dominant position of 'lecturer', and instead help to ensure that all group members participate fully in the discussion.

As the agenda for each session may be unpredictable and set by the individuals themselves, those topics which are inadequately covered should be earmarked by the group leader for future discussion. It takes time to acquire first-hand experience of diabetes, and sessions are best scheduled a few weeks after diagnosis. Group learning generally contributes more to the longer-term rather than the 'first-aid' objectives.

As well as these 'task-orientated' sessions, self-help groups may serve additional psychotherapeutic purposes in enabling subjects to share concerns and express beliefs; they may increase long-term motivation and improve morale [33], but are difficult to maintain.

Diabetic children and adolescents can also derive great pleasure and learning from group teaching, particularly in the context of summer camps such as that at Firbush in Scotland [34]. An instructive example of the value of group discussion in younger patients is provided by the video *Sugar Mountain Blues* [35].

Groups may be particularly useful for reinforcing and recapitulating knowledge in the years following diagnosis. Patients' spouses should also be encouraged to attend.

Audiovisual materials

Many leaflets, handbooks, audio- and videotapes designed to help patients to learn about diabetes are now available, but must be carefully selected.

Table 97.1. Suggested programme for insulin-dependent and non-insulin-dependent patients after initial medical interview.

Week 1 Day 1	*Insulin-dependent diabetes* Demonstration of:	*Non-insulin-dependent diabetes* Diagnostic interview	40 minutes
	• First injection (diabetes nurse specialist)	Interview with diabetes nurse specialist	30 minutes
	• Blood glucose measurement • 'First aid' diet and advice (dietitian)	Interview with dietitian	30 minutes
Day 2	Telephone contact (diabetes nurse specialist)		
Day 3	Further review (diabetes nurse specialist) Dietary advice (dietitian)		
Day 5	Telephone contact (diabetes nurse specialist)		
Week 2 Day 8	Control check (diabetes nurse specialist)		
Day 11	Home visit (diabetes nurse specialist)		
Week 3 Day 15	Control check (doctor, diabetes nurse specialist, dietitian) Telephone contact if necessary	*Weeks 4–6* Three group sessions *Week 7* Follow-up session	90 minutes (each) 20 minutes
Weeks 12–21	Group meeting		

The diabetes nurse specialist or a medical team member should ideally be available by telephone at all times.

Many are over-complex, frankly misleading or unsuitable for their target audience. Literature containing contradictory statements or unacceptable recommendations (such as several leaflets on foot care) should be avoided [28]. Indexed handbooks which can easily be searched for answers to specific questions are useful home reference sources. Examples include the handbooks for IDDM and NIDDM patients and the many single-topic leaflets published by the British Diabetic Association [36–39]. Diet sheets translated for use by immigrant groups are also essential.

Most current videotapes are too long, containing several topics lasting 15–20 min. They are often targetted at professional as well as patient audiences and so fail to be effective teaching instruments. Short videotapes can certainly enliven educational programmes [40], but are probably best used to prime group discussions. Computer-based interactive learning programmes (discussed fully in Chapter 101) are probably best viewed as part of an integrated teaching curriculum.

Curriculum planning

Timetables must be carefully planned, both to provide the patient with relevant information at the appropriate time and to optimize the use of medical and supporting staff.

Individuals are best fitted into a preplanned weekly programme, with back-up services available on demand. Education can safely be delayed for a couple of days in most IDDM patients and a scheduled programme for NIDDM subjects can begin 1–3 weeks after diagnosis. Examples for non-residential programmes are given in Table 97.1.

Education in diabetes must be lifelong; regular follow-up sessions, perhaps every 1–2 years, will help to maintain the original standards and to introduce new objectives as appropriate. Opportunities should be provided to update, evaluate and reinforce the need for continued care. A possible forum is a half-day workshop of perhaps 30 patients working in groups of half-a-dozen to revise their practical skills and discuss their own ways of adjusting to the disease.

The setting for delivering education is important. Many education units have been established separately from the clinic [10], but it seems illogical to divorce education from care. Specialized day centres allow education sessions to run in parallel with routine follow-up clinics, so making

maximum use of diabetes nurse specialists and other staff [19].

It may be easier to learn about living with diabetes in an informal, non-clinical setting; the clinic proper should possibly be reserved for dealing with specific medical complications.

Evaluation of learning

Monitoring success and failure is an essential component of all educational programmes but at present, the evaluation of diabetes care is generally inadequate. Many units do not undertake any evaluation and simply assume the outcomes to be favourable. Chosen indicators of performance may be inappropriate as, for example, the use of HbA_1 as the only end-point in assessing the effect of changing aspects of diabetes care; specific strategies, perhaps aiming to reduce hypoglycaemic episodes or increase flexibility in the choice and timing of food, may not necessarily alter overall glycaemic control [41].

Effective evaluation helps to ensure that educational activity is not wasted and that important objectives are not overlooked. Both individual and group education programmes should be evaluated, as they serve quite different purposes [42]. Individual assessments aim to identify the patient's skills and deficiencies and to determine whether his performance improves. On the other hand, group evaluation reflects the outcome of the programme as a whole.

Individual assessment

A patient's performance can be assessed simply by periodically checking the outcome of his checklist of objectives. Multiple-choice questionnaires may identify major gaps in knowledge but must be adequately validated and well designed [25, 43, 44].

Evaluation lists can be compiled for individual patients by selecting and updating appropriate objectives from a source list, perhaps using a computerized database.

As mentioned above, there is often a considerable behaviour gap between theory and practice. Attitudes and self-management behaviour, although most important, are difficult to assess. Questionnaires have also been used to evaluate patients' attitudes to their diabetes and its treatment, but probably have a relatively limited role [45]. However, good open-ended interviews with subsequent completion of a checklist may provide reasonably accurate assessment of most important outcomes. More information may be obtained by observation of patients in groups.

Evaluation of the educational programme

The overall effectiveness of the programme itself should be monitored from time to time to determine whether modification is needed. This may be done by compiling the results of individual patients' assessments (most simply in a representative sample rather than the whole clinic population), using validated multiple-choice questionnaires relating to knowledge of diabetes, attitudes and health beliefs and 'satisfaction scales' [15, 25, 44−47]. It is helpful to analyse and store the results by computer for long-term assessment of the programme. Many other outcomes may be examined, e.g. admission rate for ketoacidosis or measures of glycaemic control, but it must be remembered that these may be only partly determined by education. The literature is replete with conclusions that education has failed because HbA_1 is unchanged, yet many educational objectives have little to do with glycaemic control *per se* and other, more appropriate end-points should also be considered.

Reinforcing and maintaining learning

Despite considerable effort and carefully designed education programmes, early achievements undoubtedly wane with time, usually within 12−18 months. Strenuous efforts must therefore be made to ensure that the initial gains are not lost.

After starting treatment, follow-up in most units is in routine out-patient clinics, whose environment, atmosphere and organization may be poorly suited to maintaining the necessary high level of motivation. Common problems include difficulty in access, long waiting times, short consultations, poor continuity of care and crowded, depersonalized waiting areas. Many nursing and junior medical staff have received no formal training in diabetes education. Purpose-designed units combining clinical and educational functions and using diabetes nurse specialists to provide much of the routine follow-up and advice may address some of these problems.

Self-help groups may be particularly useful in helping to sustain motivation, especially in certain groups such as parents, children, teenagers and weight-reducers. However, these groups tend to be self-selected and may omit those most in need of education and reinforcement.

The importance of the annual review should be stressed to the patient, and the reasons for its performance and the preventative gains of good control should be discussed. Detection of complications should prompt new objectives: for example, the finding of early neuropathy should lead to discussion about foot care.

As discussed above, the educational as well as the clinical follow-up should be structured. Each patient's educational check-list should be regularly examined and updated and 1−2 yearly 'refresher' courses may be useful. The patient's long-term compliance, which is crucial to the outcome of treatment, is a complex process discussed in Chapter 95.

Providing time

Readers faced with large and overcrowded clinics might be forgiven for regarding the aspirations outlined above as unrealistic. However, careful organization can save enough time and resources for these objectives to be achieved. The clear definition of objectives and the confidence that they will be dealt with by specific team members will avoid considerable duplication of work. Spacing the weekly programme may allow appointments to be allocated to different team members, so avoiding overcrowding or gaps in clinic attendance.

Conclusions

No diabetic care programme will be successful without considerable time, energy and skill being devoted to developing and providing education. Like diabetes itself, the educational programme is a lifelong commitment. As with any other 'therapy', this must be effectively organized and delivered. All team members should receive at least some basic educational training, and curricula should be well planned but remain flexible to individual needs. Clearly defined objectives agreed by the team members and with the patients themselves are imperative. Learning methods should be appropriate for the objectives of the individuals concerned. Regular, valid evaluation is essential. The setting for learning about diabetes should be as favourable as possible; the best place is not the traditional diabetic clinic.

JOHN L. DAY

References

1 Joslin EP, Gray H, Root HF. Insulin in hospital and home. *J Metab Res* 1922; **2**: 651–99.

2 Lawrence RD. *The Diabetic Life*. London: J & A Churchill, 1925.

3 Miller LV, Goldstein J, Nicolaisen G. Evaluation of patient's knowledge of diabetes self care. *Diabetes Care* 1978; **1**: 275–80.

4 Runyan JW. The Memphis chronic disease program. *J Am Med Ass* 1975; **231**: 264–7.

5 Nersesian W, Zaremba M. Impact of diabetes outpatient education program — Maine. *Morbid Mortal Weekly Rep* 1982; **31** (No. 23): 307–414.

6 Geller J, Butler K. Study of educational deficits as the cause of hospital admissions for diabetes mellitus in a community hospital. *Diabetes Care* 1981; **4**: 487–9.

7 Scott RS, Brown LJ, Clifford P. Use of health services by diabetic persons. II. Hospital admissions. *Diabetes Care* 1985; **8**: 43–7.

8 Assal J-Ph, Gfeller R, Ekoé J-M. Patient education in diabetes. In: *Recent Trends in Diabetic Research*. Stockholm: Almqvist & Wiksell International, 1982: 276–89.

9 Mülhauser I, Jörgens V, Graninger W et al. Bicentric evaluation of a teaching and treatment programme for Type 1 (insulin dependent) diabetic patients: improvement of metabolic control and other measures of diabetes care for up to 22 months. *Diabetologia* 1983; **25**: 470–6.

10 Day JL, Spathis M. District diabetes centres in the United Kingdom. *Diabetic Med* 1988; **5**: 372–80.

11 Terént A, Hagfall O, Cederholm V. The effect of education and self-monitoring of blood glucose on glycosylated haemoglobin in Type 1 diabetes. *Acta Med Scand* 1985; **217**: 47–53.

12 Graber AL, Christman BG, Alogna MT, Davidson JK. Evaluation of diabetes patient education programmes. *Diabetes* 1977; **26**: 61–4.

13 Beggan MP, Cregan D, Drury MI. Assessment of the outcome of an educational programme of diabetes self care. *Diabetologia* 1982; **23**: 246–51.

14 Germer S, Campbell IW, Smith AWM, Sutherland JD, Jones IG. Do diabetics remember all they have been taught? A survey of knowledge of insulin-dependent diabetics. *Diabetic Med* 1986; **3**: 343–5.

15 Bradley C et al. The use of diabetes-specific perceived control and health belief measures to predict treatment choice and efficacy in a feasibility study of continuous subcutaneous insulin infusion pumps. *Psychol Health* 1987; **1**: 133–46.

16 Burfield R, Walker R, Day JL. Good diabetic control — The role of patients' perceptions and beliefs. *Diabetologia* 1986; **29**: 523A.

17 Sjöberg S, Carlson A, Rosenqvist U, Östman J. Health attitudes, self-monitoring of blood glucose, metabolic control and residual insulin secretion in Type 1 diabetic patients. *Diabetic Med* 1988; **5**: 449–53.

18 Mühlhauser I, Bruckner I, Berger M et al. Evaluation of an intensified insulin treatment and teaching programme as routine management of Type 1 (insulin-dependent) dia-

betes. *Diabetologia* 1987; **30**: 681–90.

19 Day JL, Johnson G, Rayman G, Walker R. The feasibility of a potentially 'ideal' system of integrated diabetes care and education based on a day centre. *Diabetic Med* 1988; **5**: 70–5.

20 Dunn SM. Reaction to educational techniques: coping strategies for diabetics and learning. *Diabetic Med* 1986; **3**: 419–26.

21 Walker J. The clinical management of the diabetic adolescent. *Postgrad Med J* 1970; **46**: 625–9.

22 Lawrence PA, Cheely J. Deterioration of diabetic patients' knowledge and management skills as determined during outpatient visits. *Diabetes Care* 1980; **3**: 214–18.

23 Korhonen T et al. A controlled trial on the effects of patient education in the treatment of insulin-dependent diabetes. *Diabetes Care* 1983; **6**: 256–60.

24 Mazucca SA, Moorman NH, Wheeler ML, Norton JA, Vinicor F, Cohen SJ, Clark CM. The diabetes education study: a controlled trial of the effects of diabetes patient education. *Diabetes Care* 1986; **9**: 1–10.

25 Farrant S, Dowlatshahi D, Ellwood-Russell M, Wise PH. Computer based learning and assessment for diabetic patients. *Diabetic Med* 1984; **1**: 309–15.

26 Frier BM, Steel JM, Matthews DM, Duncan LJP. Driving and insulin dependent diabetes. *Lancet* 1980; **ii**: 1232–4.

27 Mager RF. *Preparing Instructional Objectives*. California: Fearon, 1967.

28 Day JL. Patient education — how may recurrence be prevented? In: Connor H, Boulton A, Ward J, eds. *The Foot in Diabetes*. London: John Wiley and Sons, 1986: 135–43.

29 *Minimal Educational Requirements for the Care of Diabetes in the UK*. London: British Diabetic Association, 1987.

30 Check-list for diabetes patient education. In: *The Teaching Letter*. Paris: Diabetes Education Study Group, 1988: 89–94.

31 Fox CJ, Gillespie CR, Kilvert A. Can the medical consultation be made more effective in diabetes care? *Diabetologia* 1986; **29**: 538A.

32 Tattersall RB, McCulloch DK, Aveline M. Group therapy in the treatment of diabetes. *Diabetes Care* 1985; **8**: 180–8.

33 Groen JJ, Pelser HE. Newer concepts of teaching, learning and education and their application to the patient–doctor cooperation in the treatment of diabetes mellitus. *Pediatr Adolesc Endocrinol* 1982; **10**: 168–77.

34 Newton RW, Isles T, Farquhar JW. The Firbush Project — sharing a way of life. *Diabetic Med* 1985; **2**: 217–24.

35 *Sugar Mountain Blues*. Videotape, Boehringer Corporation, London.

36 *The Diabetes Handbook — Insulin Dependent Diabetes*. Wellingborough: Thorsons, 1986.

37 *The Diabetes Handbook — Non-Insulin Dependent Diabetes*. Wellingborough: Thorsons, 1986.

38 *Countdown*. London: British Diabetic Association, 1988.

39 *Catalogue of British Diabetic Association publications*. London: British Diabetic Association, 1988.

40 Ward JD et al. Video cassette programmes in diabetes education. *The Diabetes Educator* 1984; **10** Spec No: 48–50.

41 Sjöberg S, Carlson A, Rosenqvist U, Ostman J. Health attitudes, self-monitoring of blood glucose, metabolic control and residual insulin secretion in type 1 diabetic patients. *Diabetic Med* 1988; **5**: 449–53.

42 Evaluating diabetes education. In: *The Teaching Letters*. Paris: Diabetes Education Study Group, 1988: 67–71.

43 Dunn SM, Bryson JM, Hoskins PL, Alford JB, Handlesman DJ, Turtle JR. The development of diabetes knowledge (DKN) scales: forms DKNA, DKNB and DKNC. *Diabetes Care* 1984; **7**: 36–41.

44 Lockington TJ, Meadows KA, Wise PH. Compliant behaviour: relationships to attitudes and control in diabetic patients. *Diabetic Med* 1987; **4**: 56–61.

45 Dunn SM, Smartt HH, Beeney LJ, Turtle JR. The measurement of emotional adjustment in diabetic patients: validity and reliability of the ATT39. *Diabetes Care* 1986; **9**: 480–9.

46 Hess GE, Davis WK. The validation of a diabetic patient knowledge test. *Diabetes Care* 1983; **6**: 591–5.

47 Bradley C, Brewin CR, Gamsu DS, Moses JL. Development of scales to measure perceived control of diabetes mellitus and diabetes-related health beliefs. *Diabetic Med* 1984; **1**: 213–18.

98 Organization of Diabetes Care in the Hospital

Summary

• Deficiencies in staffing and facilities for diabetes care in the UK have led to recommendations for the provision of physicians with specialist training, diabetes nurse specialists, dietitians and chiropodists, and for annual retinal screening and ready access to treatment for diabetic eye disease.

• A team leader is required whose agreed responsibility is to organize diabetes care within a hospital and its district.

• Purpose-designed diabetes day centres provide a focus and a suitable environment for the team approach to diabetes care.

• Traditional clinics serve mainly to identify medical problems, screen for complications and assess metabolic control.

• It is valuable to establish clinics for specific groups, e.g. children and adolescents, antenatal care and preconception counselling, foot problems, retinal screening and renal impairment.

• In-patient care is improved by routine referral of diabetic emergencies for a specialist opinion, written protocols, and combined care of diabetes (e.g. during surgery, pregnancy or for foot problems).

• Frequent team meetings maintain communication, education and motivation.

What is included in 'diabetes care'?

'*Care*' implies an interested concern for an individual's total well-being which extends beyond the usual definition of *treatment*. It begins by meeting the immediate emotional and practical needs following diagnosis and continues as a life-long commitment to inform, support and motivate the patient so that he can effect the life changes required for long-term health (Table 98.1).

The size of the task

In the UK, care must be provided for at least 1 million diabetic patients in more than 200 geographical health districts. Each district's diabetic population ranges from about 1500 to 5000.

Who is responsible for organizing diabetes care?

Successful services on this scale will not happen by accident. An efficient organization requires an organizer. The many aspects of providing diabetes care require skills in communication, vision, leadership and energy which will have to be maintained over many years.

This role of development manager/team leader

Table 98.1. The nature of diabetes care.

1 *Caring for the patient*
• Immediate measures:
Diagnosis; initial clinical and laboratory assessment
Assessment of family, socio-economic factors, personality and knowledge
Reassurance, education, building relationships with the diabetes care team
Metabolic stabilization
• Continuing measures:
Monitoring of 'control'
Further education
Screening for complications
Treatment of complications
Emergency management
2 *Caring for the carers*
Formal education
Mutual team support

940

should naturally fall to the consultant physician with a special interest in diabetes, at least one of whom is required for each NHS district. In most places, this requirement has been fulfilled, but more often through poorly defined hopes on the part of Health Authorities rather than a clearly stated intent. In larger districts with more than one diabetologist, an agreement is required as to who shall be responsible for the overall organization of diabetes care for the district.

Who provides diabetes care?

No single person can provide all that is involved in diabetes care. Indeed, the very size of the team required may overwhelm the newly diagnosed patient with advice, sympathy and instruction coming from many directions at once. To be effective, the team must speak with one voice, both on matters of overall clinical policy and on minute practical detail.

Despite the size of the complete team, the number of members involved in looking after an individual patient at any one time may be small. For practical convenience, we may consider an inner core team, and an outer team of others whose specific contributions to the care of an individual may be needed relatively infrequently.

Figure 98.1 demonstrates the complicated interrelationships of the members of an ideal diabetes care team. As with the pieces of a jigsaw, the individual members must link neatly with each other. Every piece has its own place and importance: a missing piece will produce an incomplete picture and a piece failing to join comfortably with its neighbours will upset the whole.

Although the task of co-ordinating this diverse and scattered group may appear formidable, there is scope for a number of linked services between departments and a sharing of the tasks between hospital and primary care teams. With tact and determination, there is every possibility of creating an effective organization for the benefit of those with diabetes.

Minimal staffing requirements

The report by the Royal College of Physicians of London and the British Diabetic Association in 1984 [1] demonstrated the woeful inadequacy of diabetes care facilities in terms of manpower, materials and space, in many parts of the UK (Table 98.2).

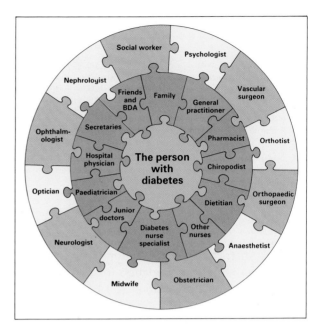

Fig. 98.1. The diabetes care team and how it fits together.

Table 98.2. Gross staffing deficiencies — hospital diabetes services in the UK in 1984 [1].

Out of 234 health districts in the UK:
- 30 districts had no physician with a special interest in diabetes; in 13 the need was recognized by other consultants, in 17 the need was unrecognized
- 68 districts had a single consultant with a special interest in diabetes or endocrinology, but recognized a need for a further consultant

Out of 428 respondents to an enquiry covering 234 districts:
- 53% had no diabetes nurse specialist or community liaison nurse
- 20% had no dietitian available in the out-patient clinic
- 60% had no chiropodist available in the out-patient clinic, and 11% had no chiropodist available at all
- 83% had no secretarial help available for diabetic work

Gross staffing deficiencies prompted the joint recommendations shown in Table 98.3 to be made.

By January 1988, however, only limited progress had been achieved. The number of districts without a diabetologist had only fallen to 26 (W.M.G. Tunbridge, personal communication). The number of districts without a nurse specializing in adult diabetes had fallen to 23%, with a further 4% of districts having a diabetes nurse specialist caring only for children. However, only 31% of districts had two or more diabetes nurse specialists [2].

Table 98.3. Staffing recommendations for district diabetes services, 1984 [1].

- One physician with specialist training in diabetes is required per 100 000 of the population. This physician should have at least five sessions per week for diabetes
- Two diabetes nurse specialists (full-time) are required per 100 000 population
- A dietitian should be present at every diabetic clinic
- A chiropodist should be present at every diabetic clinic
- Adequate facilities should be available for annual retinal screening and there should be easy access to retinal treatment expertise

As most districts have populations well in excess of 100 000, the recommendation for two specialist nurses per 100 000 population is a long way from fulfilment.

Facilities and equipment

Facilities in hospital clinics

In addition to staffing deficiencies, the 1984 report also highlighted the grossly inadequate provision of other facilities in many clinics in the UK. The most serious was the fact that 30 districts did not even have a specialist clinic. Table 98.4 indicates the major problems revealed. The level of provision was extremely patchy. Large populations sometimes seemed better served but this advantage was usually offset by the excessive size of the population covered. Large clinics often need to rely more heavily on junior medical staff, which in itself should be regarded as undesirable. Overall, an urgent need to increase resources for diabetes care was identified.

Table 98.4. Deficiencies in diabetes facilities in the UK in 1984, reported by 428 respondents from 234 districts.

No combined clinics with obstetricians	80%
No combined clinics with ophthalmologists	92%
No dietitian available in clinic	20%
No chiropodist available	11%
No specialist nurse available	53%
Blood glucose results unavailable at clinic	19%
HbA$_1$ unavailable at any time	22%
Inadequate examination facilities	10%
No dark-room for retinal examination	48%
No access to any type of photocoagulation	11%
No access to argon laser	26%
No facilities for educational displays	51%
No educational sessions	84%

The inherent disadvantages of the traditional diabetic clinic

Even with generous staffing levels and unlimited resources, many will admit that the traditional diabetic clinic cannot cope with all the needs of those with diabetes (see Chapter 97). The problems are familiar to all: long waiting times, short consultation time, frequent changes in staff and a small chance of seeing the same doctor. The bustling clinical environment is not conducive to receptive learning. When the deficiencies in staffing, material facilities and space still prevailing in most clinics are added to this, the impossibility of providing a complete service is only too obvious. Radical changes are required, and it is not surprising that the establishment of district diabetes centres is so appealing [3–5].

However, the idea of the diabetes centre did not originate solely in the failures of the traditional clinic; other factors have contributed. In the last 10 years, the growing conviction that better metabolic control results in fewer complications has awakened the resolve to educate patients more professionally (Chapter 97). Blood glucose self-monitoring, glycosylated haemoglobin estimations, and improved insulin formulations and delivery systems have all enabled control to be measured more accurately and sometimes improved. The need to equip diabetic people with this new technology first stimulated the emergence of the diabetes nurse specialist (Chapter 100). Working alongside the physician, the diabetes nurse specialist has drawn in dietitian and chiropodist colleagues to form the inner core team. The diabetes centre is all-important as it provides the ideal base from which the team may operate.

Diabetes centres

The concept of a purpose-designed area to meet the educational needs of diabetic patients and their families is not new. Elliot Joslin described such a facility in his textbook, *Treatment of Diabetes Mellitus* [6]:

'We must have islands of safety, available all the year round and at a low cost. Each hospital in the country treating diabetics should have a classroom — Hospital Teaching Clinics to which ambulant patients may go. They do not need elaborate nursing care. Diet kitchens may be utilised without hospitalisation. It has far exceeded our expectation — never have we had patients learn so much in so short a time.'

In 1977, a diabetes day centre was established in Dublin [7] and by 1986 at least six further day centres were operational in the British Isles [3, 5]. Since then, their numbers have increased dramatically: a survey in 1988 revealed that there were 39 fully operational district diabetes centres in the UK, with a further 20 scheduled to open by the end of 1989 [8].

PURPOSE OF DIABETES CENTRES

Diabetes centres will vary in size and the number of functions that they can serve. Some may be little more than an education room, others will provide all the space and facilities required to bring under one roof most of the hospital diabetes care activities. Centres obviously provide a better environment for staff and patients, improved facilities for teaching and treating and easier communication and organization of the district service. However, their most significant advantage is that they promote a team approach.

The functions of a comprehensive diabetes centre therefore mirror those of the district diabetes service itself, and will either take place in the centre or be organized and co-ordinated from it.

SETTING UP A CENTRE

Acquiring a district diabetes centre is a long and arduous task for which enthusiasm is the primary requirement. The process may be summarized in Fig. 98.2.

PLANNING, RUNNING AND STAFFING

Operational arrangements must be clearly understood at an early stage of planning a diabetes centre. These will depend upon geography, population size and many other local factors and above all, upon the ideas and abilities of the existing members of the diabetes care team. A fundamental and early decision must be whether to maintain the diabetic clinic in the out-patient department, with the diabetes centre as an additional facility, or whether to incorporate all diabetes follow-up into the work load of the centre. Either option can be successful, but the design of the centre is dependent on the system chosen. Fig. 98.3 shows

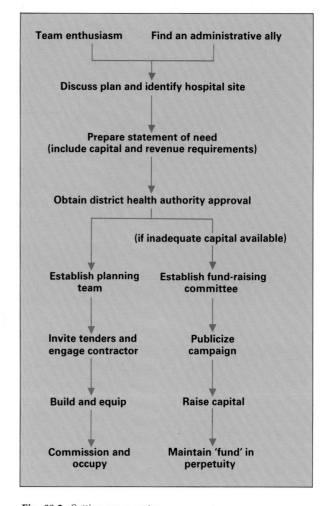

Fig. 98.2. Setting up a centre.

the floor plan at Stoke Mandeville Hospital.

The staffing of the centre need not exceed the basic staffing requirements for the district diabetes service (with the possible exception of a receptionist). This is important, as most of the perceived costs of a diabetes centre consist of staff salaries. The argument should be that the staff are necessary to run a district diabetes service, whether or not there is a centre; the costs of the centre should be confined to heating, lighting, cleaning and the maintenance of furnishing and building.

The exact weekly programme for a diabetes centre will differ from place to place. The nursing staff, dietitian and chiropodist will need time to carry out their educational work, whether on a one-to-one basis with patients or by group teaching. Medical staff will need time for certain specialized clinics such as for children, adolescents, and pregnant women. Specific events may be incorporated into the calendar, such as

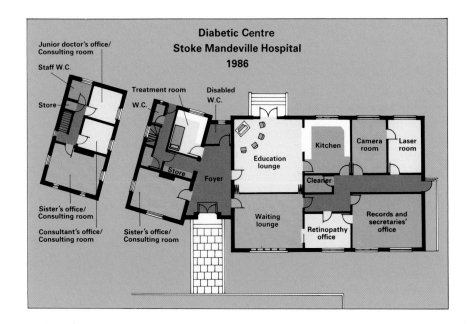

Diabetic Centre
Stoke Mandeville Hospital
1986

Junior doctor's office/ Consulting room

Staff W.C.

Store

Treatment room

W.C.

Disabled W.C.

Store

Foyer

Education lounge

Kitchen

Camera room

Laser room

Cleaner

Sister's office/ Consulting room

Consultant's office/ Consulting room

Sister's office/ Consulting room

Waiting lounge

Retinopathy office

Records and secretaries' office

Fig. 98.3. Floor plan of the diabetes centre, Stoke Mandeville Hospital: an example of a new purpose-built centre.

'cook-ins' or education days for groups of certain ages or specific needs. In addition to these programmed activities, staff should make available 'open-door' and 'phone-in' advice services which are very reassuring to diabetic patients and their families.

Medical staff need to be readily available, but the specialist nursing staff soon develop considerable (and appropriate) skills in decision-making. Where the existing out-patient diabetic clinic is maintained following the establishment of a diabetes centre, its prime purpose will be to identify medical problems, to screen for complications, and to assess metabolic control and health attitudes. Any complications identified should be managed in a specialist clinic (e.g. foot, ophthalmic or renal), although many other diabetic problems may be best solved in the diabetes centre.

All the facilities of a district diabetes centre should also be readily available to patients supervised by the primary health care team, and to diabetes organizations which meet out of hours, such as the local diabetic association branch, parents' and young people's groups.

Organizing the diabetes care systems

Hospital care, general practitioner care and shared care

Quite apart from the well-stated arguments for involving general practitioners in the care of many of their diabetic patients [9] (see Chapter 99), any hospital clinic would soon become overwhelmed and self-defeated if it failed to collaborate with the local primary care teams. Many clinical parameters must be checked annually, and wherever this is done, it must be both well organized and well documented. The annual review visit, whether carried out by the hospital team or by the primary care team, must be built into the long-term plan for each patient.

Special categories and clinic stratification

There are advantages in subdividing the clinic into a number of groups either by age or by special requirement, such as the following categories.

CHILDREN AND ADOLESCENTS

Most children below the age of 14 years come under the care of a paediatrician. The management of adolescents, however, offers an ideal opportunity for combined care which allows the paediatrician to maintain interest and involvement to adulthood, and the expertise of the adult physician to be utilized from an early stage. The gradual change-over, perhaps spread over 8 or more years, avoids the trauma of an abrupt change of supervision at puberty. The diabetes centre, with its more relaxed and less threatening atmosphere, is an ideal venue for both paediatric and adolescent diabetic activities (see Chapter 87).

ANTENATAL CLINICS AND
PRECONCEPTION COUNSELLING

Integrated multidisciplinary management is essential during diabetic pregnancy. The importance of strict metabolic control to the successful outcome of pregnancy has also identified the need for preconception counselling (see Chapter 83). Both these functions would be well served in the environment of the diabetes centre.

DIABETIC FOOT CLINICS AND
CHIROPODY SERVICES

Diabetic patients with potentially serious foot problems may be referred by the diabetes physician to vascular or orthopaedic surgeons, but combined clinics offer many advantages (Chapter 70). Any district will have a sufficient case load of diabetic patients with 'feet at risk' to more than justify this approach. The expertise of physician, surgeon, chiropodist, shoe-fitter (orthotist) and diabetes nurse specialist should all be simultaneously available in such a clinic. As well as collaborating with specialist diabetic foot clinics, the district chiropody service must integrate well with the diabetes service, in both hospital and the community, and chiropodists must play a continuous role in education, and in assessing and treating foot problems.

RETINAL SCREENING AND TREATMENT OF
RETINOPATHY

The provision of adequate retinal screening of all the district's diabetic patients is vital and must be the responsibility of the hospital diabetes physician. Whatever the detailed arrangements, the entire diabetic population must be examined annually, either directly through dilated pupils or by non-mydriatic retinal photography (see Chapter 59).

This must be carried out by competent senior personnel who can ensure continuity of service. Any abnormality found then requires expert assessment, with rapid access to treatment where necessary. Although this latter function will normally involve an ophthalmologist or specifically trained and experienced clinical assistants, initial retinal screening must be carried out or be supervised by the diabetes team, who will need adequate medical time and full nursing and secretarial support. All personnel require adequate

Table 98.5. Requirements for primary retinal screening.

Total district diabetic population	1500
Primary screening visits per annum	1500
Doctor's time per week	2 sessions
Nurse's time per week	2 sessions
Secretarial time per week	10 h

training; this task is too important to be allowed to slip into unskilled hands [10]. A modestly sized district with a diabetic population of 1500 will eventually require the provisions set out in Table 98.5.

An alternative strategy is to utilize the services of ophthalmic opticians [11, 12]. This bases the service outside the hospital and therefore requires considerable communication skills to ensure that no patients slip through the net.

Retinal treatment. It is at the stage of assessment that co-operation with the ophthalmologist must be particularly close to ensure rapid management of treatable retinopathy. Alternatively, ophthalmically trained clinical assistants can be attached to the diabetes care team to carry out primary retinal screening and also to assess and treat retinopathy. The ophthalmologist is then required to deal only with the more resistant retinopathies or the surgical management of advanced diabetic eye disease. This approach has also been shown to be effective [10].

RENAL IMPAIRMENT

Special grouping of patients with renal impairment concentrates expertise in hypertension, diet and renal failure and may also be beneficial by facilitating referral to the services dealing with end-stage renal failure, which are usually organized at regional level. The report of a joint working party of the British Diabetic Association, Renal Association and Royal College of Physicians [13] emphasized the need to increase the availability of resources for diabetic patients in renal failure, in both diabetic and renal units. In view of the relative costliness and complexity of managing diabetic renal failure, the report also encouraged joint management between renal and diabetes physicians (see Chapter 67).

APPOINTMENT TIMING, WAITING TIME,
RECALL, NON-ATTENDANCE

Aspects of clinic organization require periodic scrutiny. Analysis of appointment times, transport arrangements, waiting times and patient through-put, may lead to relatively simple remedies for some of the worst features of life in the clinic. Procedural 'necessities' and traditional 'essentials' need to be challenged periodically. For example, might it not be better to spend time enquiring about cigarette consumption rather than measuring a random blood glucose level? Non-attenders are not just an administrative nuisance; they constitute the most worrying group of all. Follow-up and recall must obviously be attempted, but more searching enquiry into the causes of non-attendance is required, since this group eventually return, often with chronic complications.

Evening clinics for working people

Wherever such facilities are provided for those with daytime commitments, there is no shortage of patients willing to attend. The problem is to provide and fund the staff for such a service from a work force that is largely made up of part-time employees.

Secretarial support

All these logistic considerations highlight the vital need for full secretarial support. Secretarial hours, office space and facilities are hardly ever adequate within the Health Service. In a purpose-built diabetes centre, the secretarial space should be second only to the educational lounge space.

Record-keeping and computers

The complex organization of the district service lends itself to computerization. This is more fully discussed in Chapter 101. Computer-held district diabetes registers, with limited and largely static data for each individual, could undoubtedly assist in planning future developments. However, the more extensive use of computers is more questionable. Even without computers, efficiency can reach a high level, especially when (as in purpose-built diabetes centres) secretaries are personally involved in appointment making and assist at clinics and when records are held in their office. Automatic letter generation and the handling of large-scale data for research are usually cited as the trade-off for the considerable effort in entering data. Written hospital records have in the past been poorly designed and poorly kept, but need not be so. The author has for 6 years used a purpose-designed, total diabetes record book for each patient [14], kept within the hospital record folder, which has proved highly efficient, easy to use by all members of the diabetes care team and adaptable to new practices. This format strongly encourages the multidisciplinary approach and competes very favourably with computerized registers in terms of efficiency, individual data retrieval and ease of use.

Shared care, with a co-operative scheme between hospital and primary care teams, will work best where communication is efficient. This may be computer-assisted and/or operate through a co-operation card or booklet [15, 16].

Hospital services for diabetic in-patients

The hospital-based diabetes team has an important role in ensuring good care for all diabetic patients admitted to hospital. The UK study on diabetic deaths under the age of 50 years revealed an alarming frequency of mismanagement of keto-acidosis in hospital. Delays in diagnosis and treatment, inadequate or excessive replacement measures and poor supervision all contributed to fatal outcomes [17]. Such cases should always be notified to the most experienced diabetes opinion available and not left to the luck of those whose skills lie in other fields. Written protocols for diabetic emergencies should be formulated by the diabetes team.

For similar reasons, surgical teams should notify and take advice from the diabetes team for diabetic patients undergoing surgery. Co-operation with the obstetric department must be provided at the most experienced level, and will be a natural continuation of the co-operative out-patient antenatal care scheme. Diabetic foot problems involve considerable use of hospital beds and again demand a combined medical and surgical approach, ideally involving close liaison with a single vascular and/or orthopaedic surgeon, which will streamline the service. The diabetes team has an important educational task in maintaining standards of care in all disciplines and departments of the hospital: the diabetes nurse specialist with her colleagues on the wards and the school of nursing, the dietitian with ward and kitchen staff, and the doctors with their colleagues. Quality control of blood glucose monitoring, chart discipline, catering services and prescribing practices also require continuous vigilance.

Links between the accident and emergency department and the diabetes team must also be fostered. Although the common emergency of hypoglycaemia will usually be managed entirely by the casualty officers, some occasions will require the attendance of a medical member of the diabetes team. In all cases, the diabetes team should at least be informed of the occurrence of hypoglycaemia, to enable appropriate early follow-up arrangements to be made.

Telephone advice service

The hospital-based diabetes nurse specialist invariably provides a telephone advisory service, which is extremely valuable, especially in offering timely advice to prevent ketoacidosis. It may be difficult to provide such a facility for 24 hours every day, although the service could be linked to a medical ward out of hours.

Communications, morale and staff education

The organization of diabetes care must always consider the team members themselves and should foster team accord. There should be frequent 'protected' meetings of the inner core team and less frequent, but none the less regular, meetings of all involved in diabetes care throughout the district. Communication between different disciplines and between hospital and community-based team members must also be efficient, and should promote free debate but result in common policies. The multidisciplinary approach, however, must never imply lack of leadership, and ultimate responsibility must be assumed by the leader when necessary.

In conclusion, every piece of the diabetes care jigsaw must be looked after; there is nothing more frustrating than a jigsaw with a piece missing.

ANTHONY H. KNIGHT

References

1 Royal College of Physicians of London and British Diabetic Association. *The Provision of Medical Care for Adult Diabetic Patients in the United Kingdom (1984)*. London: Royal College of Physicians of London, 1985.
2 Redmond S. Analysis of Diabetes Specialist Nurse questionnaire — British Diabetic Association (1988). *Unpublished statistics.*
3 Ling P, Lovesay JM, Mayon-White VA, Thomson J, Knight AH. The diabetic clinic dinosaur is dying: will diabetic day units evolve? *Diabetic Med* 1985; **2**: 163–5.
4 Brown KGE. Integrated district care based in a diabetes centre. *Diabetic Med* 1987; **4**: 330–2.
5 Day JL, Spathis M. District diabetes centres in the United Kingdom. *Diabetic Med* 1988; **5**: 372–80.
6 Joslin ED, Root HF, White P, Marble A. *Treatment of Diabetes Mellitus*, 10th edn. Philadelphia: Lea and Febiger, 1959: 16.
7 Drury MI, Cregan D. Ten years experience in a diabetic day centre. *Diabetic Med* 1988; **5**: 288–9.
8 Knight AH, Redmond S. District diabetes centres in the United Kingdom and Eire. *Diabetic Med* 1989; **6**: 639–42.
9 Thorne PA, Russell RG. Diabetic clinics today and tomorrow: mini-clinics in general practice. *Br Med J* 1973; **2**: 534–6.
10 Mayon-White VA, Jenkins LM, Knight AH. A district screening and treatment service for diabetic retinopathy. *Diabetic Med* 1986; **3**: 253–6.
11 Burns-Cox CJ, Dean Hart JC. Screening of diabetics for retinopathy by ophthalmic opticians. *Br Med J* 1985; **290**: 1052–4.
12 Hill RD. Primary health care screening programme for diabetic eye disease (abstract). *Diabetologia* 1981; **20**: 670.
13 British Diabetic Association, Renal Association and Royal College of Physicians. Care of diabetics with renal failure. *Diabetic Med* 1988; **5**: 79–84.
14 Brown LA, Brown RS, Chiverton NA, Green JE, Hull RP, Knight AH, List M, Mayon-White VA, McGough NI, Stratford J, Thackray J, Turner EV. The Stoke Mandeville diabetes record system — effective management and teamwork without a computer. *Practical Diabetes* 1988; **5**: 253–5.
15 Hill RD. The community care service for diabetics in the Poole area. *Br Med J* 1976; **2**: 1137–9.
16 Paterson KR, McDowell J. A passport to improved diabetes care. *Diabetic Med* 1988; **5**: 285–7.
17 Tunbridge WMG. Factors contributing to deaths of diabetics under fifty years of age. *Lancet* 1981; **ii**: 569–72.

99 General Practice and the Community

Summary

• 'Shared care' schemes, combining the skills of the general practitioner and the hospital physician, are an effective use of resources.
• Most diabetic patients can be managed largely by general practitioners, although specific groups (children, adolescents, pregnant women and those with specific complications or poor control) will require hospital review.
• Diabetic care in general practice, as elsewhere, is best delivered by an integrated team, coordinated by the doctor but with the practice nurse as the patient's main contact.
• All patients should have a full annual review, including assessments of the cardiovascular system and feet and a fundal examination performed by an experienced person.
• Good record keeping is essential; a 'co-operation card' or booklet provides effective communication between the practice and the hospital.
• Patient education is essential to good diabetes management; initial 'survival' information must be followed up by a continuing educational programme.

Diabetes is a common, chronic condition which (including undiagnosed cases) probably affects an estimated 6% of adults in the USA and about 1–2% of the British population [1]. The prevalence of diabetes is higher in the elderly (one person in six over the age of 65 years) and the long-term complications of the condition become more common as the average age of the population rises [2]. In Britain, the average general practice list will include about 30 diabetic patients and, because diabetes impinges on many aspects of

medicine, a significant part of the general practitioner's workload can involve diabetes. General practitioners have a crucial part to play in the successful management of the condition: it is important, for instance, to know whether the woman seeking contraceptive advice, the toddler with an upper respiratory tract infection, or the older patient in heart failure has diabetes.

Hospital diabetic clinics clearly cannot and should not have to deal with all diabetes. General practitioners must accept the clinical challenge of the disease; indeed, many would argue that they should supervise most aspects of the diabetic patient's life, only referring to the local specialist those patients who have complications or particular problems with control.

Successful general practice management depends on a joint team approach involving the patient, his relatives, a specialist nurse, dietitian, chiropodist and the doctor, who should co-ordinate activities. There is now evidence that the diabetic patient's attitude and behaviour are crucial to good metabolic control [3, 4], and education about diabetes and its treatment is a vital part of the health-care plan. Each team member must decide the various components of the education programme for which he is responsible, and the information given must be uniform and consistent.

Organizational aspects of diabetic care in general practice

The team members

Diabetic care in general practice — as everywhere — must aim to maintain the patient in as nearly a normoglycaemic state as possible in the

hope of minimizing the risks of long-term complications, and to identify and treat these should
they arise. Many different diabetic management
plans have evolved, ranging from total hospital
clinic care to total general practice care. Only a
few patients will need the former but many, including those who are insulin-dependent (and especially children, adolescents and pregnant
women) will need to be reviewed at intervals by
hospital-based diabetes specialists. One of the
most exciting current developments in diabetic
management is the concept of 'shared care', which
combines the expertise of the diabetes specialist
with the general practitioner's detailed knowledge
of the patient's general and social well-being. The
organization of the shared care scheme is outlined
in Fig. 99.1.

The first requirement is that patients must be
able to identify a focal person in the practice
diabetic team. This should be the practice nurse,
who is best able to provide consistent continuity
of care. She can have overall responsibility for
patient education, and maintain registers and a
recall system. Secondly, other diabetes services
such as dietary advice (ideally, provided by a
community-based dietitian) and chiropody should
also be available at community level. There should
be clear guidelines as to the role of the hospital
clinic and the two teams should meet regularly to
discuss professional education and ways of optimizing care. Specific issues raised by transferring
care from the hospital to the community include
hospital discharge policies, the ability of the community dietetic and chiropody services to cope
with the increased workload, and the vitally im-

portant question of who carries out retinal screening. General practitioners are responsible for the
day-to-day management of their patients and thus
have to be familiar with the acute metabolic complications of hyper- and hypoglycaemia and
understand the action to be taken during illness.

The requirements for a successful general practice clinic

Diabetic care has to be both practical and well-
managed. Looking after people with diabetes requires 'protected time' (such as a specific session
devoted only to diabetes), because time must be
set aside for the team to meet and discuss individual management plans and because patient
education is time-consuming and impossible to
separate from clinical management.

Many different systems are evolving, shaped
largely by local circumstances. Over 10 years ago,
Thorn and Russell [5] in Wolverhampton pointed
out that the function of the hospital clinic should
be to stabilize difficult patients, and suggested
plans for 'mini-clinics' in general practice. Hill [6]
has developed a shared-care scheme in Poole
(Dorset) in which the general practitioner is responsible for everyday diabetic care, leaving
the hospital to screen for complications. A co-
operation booklet serves as a link between the
hospital clinic and the general practitioner. In
King's Lynn, we have maintained a 'protected-
time' clinic for almost 10 years, independent of
the local hospital clinic, which currently serves
about 400 patients [7]. However, all these systems
depend heavily upon the practitioner's enthusiastic interest in the condition and upon there
being enough patients to provide the necessary
experience in dealing with the wide range of
problems encountered. One criticism of this system is that those practitioners who do not participate may lose their own skills in dealing with
diabetic problems. The requirements for a successful clinic are summarized in Fig. 99.2.

Clinical care

The cornerstone of organized diabetic care must
be a register of all known diabetic patients in the
practice. In the absence of a disease index, compiling such a register is a formidable task, but diabetic patients can be identified from memory, by
scanning requests for repeat prescriptions, and
by screening: blood or urine glucose should be

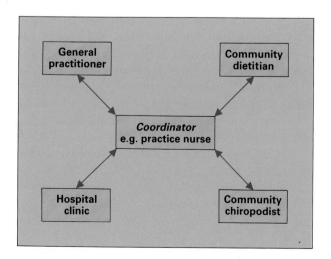

Fig. 99.1. The shared care team in general practice.

- An interested and enthusiastic general practitioner

- An easily accessible practice nurse

- A regular clinic session (protected time)

- A specialized record card

- Secretarial facilities which identify defaulters

- Close cooperation with the local hospital diabetic clinic and biochemistry laboratory

Fig. 99.2. Requirements for general practice care of diabetic patients.

- Lying and standing blood pressure

- Visual acuity with refraction through a pin-hole

- Examination of fundi (dilate pupils after checking acuity)

- Foot examination

- Examination of peripheral pulses

- Screening of peripheral sensory nervous system (reflexes, light touch, pin prick); full examination if symptoms are present

- Urinalysis (a) ketones,
  (b) protein

- Blood (a) urea, creatinine, electrolytes,
  (b) fasting lipids

Fig. 99.3. A suggested annual review for general practice.

routinely checked in all newly registered patients and in those with obesity, septic lesions of any sort or leg ulceration, or a family history of diabetes.

Within general-practice-based clinics, the doctor must take the overall responsibility for routine clinical care, although it is important that the doctor and practice nurse work together. Consultations are frequent soon after diagnosis, but thereafter are determined by the patient's confidence in self-management, his degree of control and various other medical and social factors. At each visit, routine evaluation should include the patient's weight, assessment of home glycaemic control (ideally using self-recorded results), and measurements of blood glucose and HbA$_1$ concentrations, if appropriate. The feet should be examined in patients with a current or previous history of foot problems.

All patients should undergo an annual review, to enable any complications to be identified at an early stage. A suitable plan is shown in Fig. 99.3. Much of this examination can be performed by the practice nurse, except for fundoscopy. General practitioners involved in diabetic care must be confident in their ability to examine the eyes; if not, alternative arrangements must be made for all patients to have expert retinal examinations once a year. Fundoscopy must be carried out through a dilated pupil unless the patient is very long-sighted. With practice and experience, background and proliferative retinopathy can be identified, but it must be remembered that diminished visual acuity without

extensive retinopathy may signify macular oedema, which is often difficult to detect by direct fundoscopy and can progress rapidly and cause blindness. Patients whose visual acuity is worse than 6/9 or deteriorates by more than 1 line on the Snellen chart (e.g. from 6/5 to 6/9) must be referred immediately to an ophthalmologist.

Record keeping

A diabetic record card is mandatory if vital current data are not to be lost. Record cards are best designed after experience has been gained in running a clinic, and the information they carry will depend entirely on local circumstances. Some centres use a co-operation booklet, carried by the patient, which serves mainly as communication between the general practitioner and his hospital colleagues and can also contain essential educational material.

Administrative staff should document clinic and annual review attendance and also maintain registers of the type of diabetes seen. This information can also be used for audit purposes.

Education within general practice

Diabetes education in general practice must be

well planned and effectively delivered, ideally by a practice nurse with a special knowledge of diabetes (or the local diabetic health visitor), who is crucial to its success. Another essential requirement in education is time. Newly diagnosed diabetic patients are stressed and often exhibit anger, denial and possibly grief, which all increase the time taken to become receptive to education. Shortly after diagnosis, one-to-one teaching — and listening — is essential to inform and reassure the patient and correct any misconceptions. Group teaching for people sharing similar experiences and difficulties can be a useful adjunct to the individual approach (see Chapter 97). Education is a continuing process, as individual needs alter and early information, concepts and opinions change or are forgotten.

'Survival' education is the first stage in the continuing learning process. The patient has to be told the diagnosis, taking into account any knowledge which he already possesses. During this consultation, a treatment plan is devised, emphasizing the need for the patient's participation. The basic fundamentals of care, including metabolic complications such as hypoglycaemia and what to do during intercurrent illness must be taught early in the programme.

Thereafter, continuing education is as vital to the patient as it is to all other members of the health care team; it is alarming how complacent patients can become over the years, having been lulled into a false sense of security by their feeling of well-being. There is therefore a continuing need to reinforce information and to keep up to date with new technology and forms of treatment.

Conclusions

Close involvement with diabetic patients has many rewards. Within general practice, there is enormous potential to improve the care of patients without having to rely heavily on the hospital services. A successful practice-based service depends on improved education and close co-operation between all members of the health-care team. Transferring diabetic care to the community in this way allows the hospital clinics to concentrate on those patients who truly need their attention, particularly those with specific problems of control or complications.

PETER R.W. TASKER

References

1 World Health Organization. Technical Reports Series, 1980; Editorial 646.
2 Sönksen PH, Judd SL, Lowy C et al. Home monitoring of blood glucose. Method for improving diabetic control. Lancet 1978; ii: 729−32.
3 Nessesian W, Zaremba M. Impact of diabetes out-patient education programme — Maine. Morbid Mortal Weekly Rep 1982; 31 (No 23): 307−414.
4 Mülhauser I, Jörgens V, Groninger W et al. Bicentric evaluation of a teaching and treatment programme for Type I (insulin dependent) diabetic patients. Improvement of metabolic control and other measures of diabetes care for up to 22 months. Diabetologia 1983; 25: 470−6.
5 Thorn PA, Russell RG. Diabetic clinics today and tomorrow. Mini clinics in general practice. Br Med J 1973; 2: 534−6.
6 Hill RD. Community care service for diabetes in the Poole area. Br Med J 1976; 1: 1137−9.
7 Tasker PRW. Is diabetes a disease for general practice? Practical Diabetes 1984; 1: 21−4.

100 The Role of the Diabetes Specialist Nurse

Summary

• Diabetes specialist nurses have essential roles to play in educating, advising and counselling people with diabetes, in teaching their colleagues about the disease, and in co-ordinating the delivery of diabetes care by the hospital and/or the community.
• The Royal College of Physicians has recommended that, in the UK, there should be at least one diabetes specialist nurse per 100 000 population.
• In the UK, training as a diabetes specialist nurse begins with 6 months basic training in diabetes followed by a short course under the auspices of the English National Board. Various advanced courses for specialist nurses are now available.
• Home visits by the specialist nurse to supervise the initiation or stabilization of insulin treatment, or to tackle specific topics such as self-monitoring, can often avoid the need for hospital admission or out-patient attendance. Specialist nurses can therefore save considerable hospital resources and are very cost-effective.

It is now generally accepted that diabetic people must understand their diabetes and how to manage it in order to achieve sufficiently good control to avoid the acute metabolic problems of the disease and, it is hoped, its chronic complications. It is also now acknowledged that the diabetes specialist nurse has a valuable role to play in providing education, advice and support to diabetic patients [1]. The primary objective of the diabetes specialist nurse is to educate people with diabetes so that they can regain as much independence as possible and to live life to the full within the constraints of their disease. This task often requires patience, tact and tenacity as well as sound theoretical and practical knowledge of diabetes. In addition to being an educator, the nurse will have to develop skills as an advisor in emergencies, a counsellor and — as she is often the 'interface' between the patient and other members of the diabetic care team — a general coordinator of diabetes management [2, 3].

This chapter will outline the training of diabetes specialist nurses and their various functions within and beyond the diabetes care team.

Training of diabetes specialist nurses

Until recently, diabetes specialist nurses had little or no formal training, relying on learning from daily experience, reading and — when finances allowed — attendance at a limited number of conferences and courses [4]. Formal, nationally recognized training schemes are now established throughout North America and are becoming popular in Europe. In the UK, basic training in diabetes is provided by a minimum period of 6 months working in a designated area of diabetes care, often under the direct instruction of a specialist nurse, followed by a short diabetes course under the auspices of the English National Board [5]. Nurses with special experience or interests, such as in community nursing or paediatrics, may wish to concentrate on these areas. Further courses in counselling and teaching skills may be available at the hospital or at a local university or college of further education, and several advanced courses for diabetes specialist nurses are now available. The latter are particularly valuable for nurses who have worked in the field for some time, to reinforce and update their knowledge and practice.

Details of courses in the UK may be obtained from the local Department of Nurse Education

Professional Development Section or the Nursing Adviser at the British Diabetic Association [6]. Funding to attend these courses may be difficult to obtain in the UK, but individual nurses should be able to participate in those which will most benefit their knowledge and professional development; the short-term costs will generally soon be outweighed by the organizational and financial advantages to the diabetes care programme.

Nurses and the organization of care

The local diabetes care system will be moulded by its geography, resources and personnel and may range from the traditional diabetes clinic organized by a hospital physician to a 'shared care' scheme operated jointly by general practitioners and the physician [7] or a purpose-built diabetes centre combining facilities for follow-up, education and research [8] (see Chapters 98 and 99). Accordingly, specialist nurses may be based predominantly in the hospital or the community and must remain flexible enough in approach to be able to provide a service in both environments. Their role should be clearly defined in the contractual job description but may need regular review to reflect changing needs. Together with medical and other members of the diabetic team, nurses should play an important part in designing and organizing the scheme to deliver diabetes care.

The diabetes specialist nurse has an important function in ensuring close liaison between the various agencies providing care for diabetic people. Her unique position between the hospital and the community means that she can help to maintain clear and free communication. At a practical level, she can be involved in establishing and maintaining shared-care schemes and with training practice nurses in educational or practical procedures.

Another important aspect of the specialist nurse's work is visiting patients at home, initially to help with education or self-monitoring or with starting or stabilizing insulin treatment. Relatively few patients require admission to hospital to begin insulin treatment, provided that an effective system for home visiting and follow-up exists; such a system will rapidly become cost-effective by sparing expensive hospital resources. The person with newly diagnosed IDDM will initially require daily visits but these can soon be spaced out at intervals of several days, with telephone contact maintained in between. After the initial visit,

patients with NIDDM often need only weekly visits until they are able to manage. After 3 months or so, most diabetic patients should be relatively independent and able to cope with everyday events. Home visits can be carried out in conjunction with the district nurse.

Home visiting is essential in the care of young children with diabetes; parents gain much support and confidence from being able to discuss freely all aspects of their child's condition. The patient's home is an easier and less intimidating environment than the diabetic clinic in which to discuss problems such as school, adolescence and eventual transfer to the adult diabetic clinic with the child and other family members.

The independence with which specialist nurses operate outside hospitals has important implications for their clinical responsibility, particularly with regard to insulin treatment. Although insulin is not legally a prescription-only drug, it is best that the decision to begin or stop insulin treatment should be made by a physician although, if specified in her job description, an appropriately trained diabetes specialist nurse can alter insulin regimens [9].

The functions of the diabetes specialist nurse

Co-ordinating care

The specialist nurse is well placed to be able to co-ordinate the services provided by the entire diabetes care team and is often crucial in ensuring continuity of care. Effective coordination can only be achieved by free and clear communication between the specialist nurse and her colleagues [6]. She should be easily accessible through an efficient open-referral system which avoids delays in home visiting and in turn should keep her colleagues informed through various means such as formal lectures, seminars, computer-assisted learning programmes or written material. She should also draw up an educational 'package' for newly diagnosed and other patients which other team members can use in her absence.

Diabetes education

The specialist nurse can become largely responsible for teaching the theory and practice of diabetes management to diabetic patients, the health care professionals and the community at large. Her first obligation is, of course, to her patients and their families, who must learn how to look after themselves and their diabetes. People with diabetes must understand enough about their condition to be able to eat a sensible diet, take any medication correctly and avoid its side-effects as far as possible, and cope with any unexpected events ranging from mild hypoglycaemia to severe intercurrent illness with loss of appetite and vomiting. They must also know how to monitor their diabetic control, using blood or urine testing for glucose or ketones in a way appropriate to their diabetes and life-style and how to interpret and act upon the results.

The specialist nurse can also advise about many aspects of life which may be affected by diabetes, ranging from the value of exercise to the need for regular inspection and care of the feet in patients at risk, the hazards of smoking in diabetic people and problems encountered during pregnancy. Education needs to be well planned, and the content and format of the information presented to an individual patient must be carefully chosen to suit his own particular requirements

(see Chapter 97). Check-lists of essential items — which should also be tailored to individual needs — may be useful to avoid repetition and omission but it must be remembered that completion of a check-list does not necessarily imply completion of teaching or of learning. Basic check-lists for patients with IDDM or NIDDM are shown in Tables 100.1–100.4. The specialist nurse is well placed to be able to choose the best education style for each patient: initially, 'one-to-one' sessions with the patient on his own are generally the most effective but certain topics — for example, discussion about fears of complications or practical day-to-day difficulties in coping with diabetes — lend themselves to group discussions. Guidelines for setting up and maintaining groups are discussed further in Chapter 97.

It must be appreciated that the acquisition, updating and application of knowledge is a lifelong process and that the patient — and indeed, the educator — will never cease to learn. The practical consequence of this is that each patient's educational needs and the success or failure of efforts

Table 100.1. 'First aid' knowledge check-list for patients with IDDM.

1 Simple explanation of IDDM and need for insulin

2 The patient's own insulin regimen:
- Type(s) of insulin; mixing technique if necessary
- Number of injections; timing relative to meals
- Syringe: site, and special aids (pen device, 'click-count', etc.)
- Injection technique, sites and rotation
- Insulin storage and where to obtain supplies

3 Diabetic control:
- Define and explain normal, too high and too low values
- Self-monitoring using blood or urine glucose testing
- When to test
- Recording of results
- What to do if values are too high or too low
- Use of Ketostix if needed

4 The patient's own diet:
- Choice of unrefined carbohydrate, high-fibre and low-fat foods
- Recognition of amounts of carbohydrate
- Regular spacing of meals
- Ideal body weight

5 Hypoglycaemia:
- Recognizing symptoms
- Corrective action; need to carry sugar and identification
- How to avoid hypoglycaemia

6 Keeping in contact:
- Written or taped instructions
- Contact telephone number and next planned contact

Table 100.2. More advanced knowledge check-list for patients with IDDM.

1 Insulin regimen:
  • Action profile and time-course of patient's insulin(s)
  • Reasons why blood glucose levels rise or fall
  • How and when to alter the dose

2 Intercurrent events:
  • Exercise, parties
  • Minor illness; major illness with fever, anorexia, vomiting
  • How to recognize ketoacidosis
  • Warning signs to call for help

3 Chronic complications of diabetes:
  • Long-term complications
  • Positive action to try to avoid these
  • Specific complications and their treatment, e.g. foot care
  • Need for annual review and what to expect

4 Miscellaneous:
  • Driving
  • Insurance
  • Employment
  • Smoking and alcohol
  • Holidays and travel
  • Genetic counselling, contraception, pregnancy
  • Membership of British Diabetic Association or other national associations and patient groups
  • New advances in diabetes care or research

Table 100.3. 'First aid' check-list for patients with NIDDM.

1 Simple explanation of NIDDM

2 The patient's own diet:
  • Choice of unrefined carbohydrate, high-fibre and low-fat foods
  • Recognition of amounts of carbohydrate
  • Regular spacing of meals
  • Ideal body weight and targets for weight loss

3 The patient's own drug treatment
  • Mode of action
  • Possible side-effects
  • Dosage and schedule

4 Diabetic control ⎤
5 Hypoglycaemia ⎬ as for IDDM (Table 100.4).
6 Keeping contact ⎦

Table 100.4. More advanced knowledge check-list for patients with NIDDM.

1 Treatment regimen:
  • Reasons why blood glucose levels fall or rise
  • How to recognize need for a change in dosage

2 Intercurrent events ⎤
3 Chronic complications of diabetes ⎬ as for IDDM (Table 100.2)
4 Miscellaneous ⎦

ingly responsible for teaching other health care professionals about the disease.

Learner nurses will benefit greatly from having a source of specialist knowledge about diabetes readily available as they learn to nurse patients in a variety of settings such as acute metabolic emergencies, during and after surgery, in old age or childhood, or during pregnancy. Certain departments of nurse education do not allow specialist nurses to teach formally if they do not hold a teaching certificate: in this case, the tutors should be able to consult the specialist nurse for up-to-date information.

Trained nurses should be fully familiar with how to give an insulin injection and able to measure blood glucose concentration accurately using test

to teach him must be reviewed as regularly as his medical condition and attempts made to correct any deficiencies whenever recognized.

It is obvious that the educational role of the specialist nurse extends far beyond the simple demonstration of basic skills such as injection and blood glucose monitoring techniques. Diabetes specialist nurses are also becoming increas-

strips; several recent studies have shown that many nurses (and junior hospital doctors) are unfamiliar with even simple blood glucose measurements. The specialist nurse can arrange demonstrations of these essential skills and can also check periodically that the techniques are being performed correctly in the daily ward routine. Trained nurses should also be given enough information so that they can discuss diabetes and its basic self-management with their patients, and can also learn how to use practical aids such as scale magnifiers, preset syringes and pen injectors. Community nurses, school nurses and health visitors will often appreciate the opportunity to discuss individual patients.

Many other health care professionals, both within and beyond the diabetes care team, will find the advice and support of the specialist nurse useful in dealing with diabetic problems in hospital or in the community. She can also help to educate the community at large about diabetes through agencies such as the local diabetic association, voluntary first-aid organizations and schools.

Advice

The specialist nurse is often the fixed point of the diabetes team whom patients find easiest to contact for advice about problems they encounter. She should be prepared to be available to patients and their families at short notice and ideally, perhaps on a shared rota with other team members, outside working hours. Patients with free access to advice tend to become independent more rapidly and many avoid the need for hospital admission with acute metabolic problems; however, a constantly available advice service must be closely monitored to ensure that it is not abused.

Newly diagnosed patients may need repeated advice before they are able to assimilate the information and act upon it, as may those people with established diabetes who encounter a new problem such as a chronic complication. Initially, advice should be given freely but, thereafter, independence should be encouraged by testing the patient's understanding and correcting or reinforcing his knowledge as appropriate. Positive reinforcement, by acknowledging and praising periods of good control or correct action taken during an intercurrent problem will encourage the patient's motivation much more than criticizing errors or episodes of poor control. The latter

are inevitable in most cases; the ways in which the patient reacted and which may have contributed to loss of control must be fully but sympathetically explored and guidelines should be provided about managing similar problems should they arise again. Recurrent or chronic episodes of poor control may indicate an underlying medical problem, inappropriate treatment, misunderstanding or ignorance on the part of the patient, or poor emotional adaptation to having diabetes, which can lead to denial, anger, depression and other psychological problems (see Chapter 77). The specialist nurse may be crucial in helping to determine the cause of poor control and in offering corrective advice or counselling. The nurse specialist will often enjoy the confidence of her patients and may be consulted about problems which are felt to be too sensitive or trivial to be discussed with doctors. These problems may include practical difficulties with injections or glucose monitoring, lapses in diet or compliance with treatment, or fears about the future; the nurse's knowledge of these difficulties may be extremely valuable in planning how to tackle them.

Counselling

Counselling may be defined as 'a process through which one person helps by purposeful conversation in an understanding atmosphere'. It seeks to establish a helping relationship in which the person counselled can express his thoughts and feelings in such a way as to clarify his own situation, come to terms with some new experience, see his difficulty more objectively and face his problem with less anxiety and tension. Its basic purpose is to assist the individual to make his own decision from the choices available to him [10].

As discussed in Chapter 77, the emotional adaptation following the diagnosis of diabetes is in some ways similar to that in bereavement, with grieving for the loss of health and lifestyle. This is often complicated by anxiety or depression about the disease, its treatment and its long-term complications and outcome. Fortunately, most patients pass through this phase successfully and are able to accept their disorder, but others are unable to restore these feelings. Maladaptation may result in anger or fear, sometimes preventing the patient from taking on personal responsibility for managing his own diabetes, or denial, which may be seen as an attempt to protect himself from the burden of the disorder [10]. These emotional difficulties make it difficult for the patient to recognize and learn what is relevant to his own management, and careful counselling may be needed before he is able to come to terms with the problem and accept advice and information.

In counselling, the emphasis should be on how the person feels about his own problem [11], which allows him to accept his condition and learn to live comfortably with it. This approach requires a break from the traditional 'nurse–patient' relationship which tends to concentrate on the disease rather than the person and so reduces his sense of independence. It is essential that the person with diabetes is actively involved in setting the goals of his own management.

Many specialist nurses find that some formal knowledge of counselling techniques can greatly help their delivery of diabetes care. Counselling courses are now available through many hospitals and universities.

Conclusions

Diabetes specialist nurses have much to offer in teaching patients and those involved in managing diabetes and in ensuring that the delivery of diabetes care is as efficient and well coordinated as possible. Their integral role in the diabetes management team has been recognized by the Royal College of Physicians, which in 1985 [1] recommended that there should be at least one diabetes specialist nurse per 100 000 population; there are, however, still many areas within the UK where this quota is not fulfilled. It must be emphasized that employing a specialist nurse makes sound economic sense, as the costs of training and employing her will soon be offset by reductions in the numbers of hospital admissions and out-patient attendances. This point will, how-

ever, only be proved by keeping accurate records of the diabetes work load and by calculating the savings that result.

The place of the diabetes specialist nurse has become clearer, but her time must be used efficiently [12] and teaching other colleagues to teach will remain an important means of sharing her burden of responsibility. By bridging the gap between primary and secondary care, the diabetes specialist nurse can help to obtain the best possible health for people with the disorder.

PATRICIA M. JOHNS

References

1 Royal College of Physicians of London and British Diabetic Association. *The Provision of Medical Care for Adult Diabetic Patients in the United Kingdom, 1984.* London: Royal College of Physicians of London, 1985.
2 Anderson R. The personal meaning of having diabetes. Implications for patient behaviour and education. *Diabetic Med* 1986; **3**: 13–15.
3 Kyne D. The role of the diabetic nurse specialist. *Treat Diabetes* 1986; **3**: 13–15.
4 Mallow C. The training of the nurses in the care of diabetes. *Practical Diabetes* 1985; **3**: 230.
5 Craddock S, West D, Downham D, Shaw K. The E.N.B. short course in diabetic nursing. *Practical Diabetes* 1985; **2**: 29–31.
6 Clarke P. The role of the diabetes nurse specialist. *Practical Diabetes* 1985; **3**: 229.
7 Thorn PA, Russell RG. Diabetic clinics today and tomorrow. Mini clinics in general practice. *Br Med J* 1973; **2**: 534–6.
8 Roberts S. Developments at North diabetes resource centre. *Diabetic Med* 1989; **6**: 363–5.
9 The extending role of the clinical nurse — legal implications and training requirements. *Department of Health and Social Security Circular* HG77/11. DHSS, 1977.
10 Nichols KA. *Psychological Care in Physical Illness.* Beckenham: Croom Holm, 1984: 142–6.
11 Royal College of Nursing Working Party. *Counselling in Nursing.* London: Royal College of Nursing, 1978: 14.
12 Waine C. Shared care in diabetes — a view from general practice. *Treat Diabetes* 8–12.

101 Computers in Diabetes Management

Summary

• Computer-based registers can easily store and process the clinical and administrative data from a busy diabetic clinic. Such systems are increasingly cheap, cost-effective and easy to use and can be interfaced to transfer information between other computers within or outside the hospital.

• Blood glucose meters incorporating a 'memory' microchip can record blood glucose data at the time of measurement, for subsequent analysis.

• Algorithms stored in microcomputers or pocket calculators can be used to adjust insulin treatment schedules.

• Computerized systems can be used successfully to teach patients and others about diabetes management, and to evaluate their knowledge of diabetes.

Thanks to cheaper capital costs and the general spread of computing skills, computers now play an important part in many areas of diabetes care and research. Their high operating speed, limitless storage power and decreasing size will undoubtedly increase their future uses in administrative, clinical and research settings. Four major current applications will be dealt with in this chapter.

Computer-based diabetes registers and management systems

Patient registers, the earliest application of computers in diabetes management [1], were a response to the increasing problems of collecting, storing and manipulating clinical data. The need to provide statistical information concerning clinical diabetic activity [2] may soon dictate that all diabetic clinics will have to operate registers of patient numbers and visits, even if only to justify staffing requirements. Currently available systems can hold enough information to satisfy the Körner minimum data set shown in Table 101.1 [3], can accumulate both clinical and laboratory information [4] for cross-sectional or longitudinal analyses, and can cover such divergent applications as audit of clinic performance and epidemiological studies of the clinic population. An application of great practical importance is the automatic generation of recall letters for clinic defaulters who might otherwise be lost to follow-up. This simple manoeuvre may substantially reduce the morbidity from those complications which frequently suffer severely from lapses in care, such as retinopathy and foot problems.

The quality of the resulting data will, of course, be no better than the clinical acumen, ability and care of the user. Much effort has been expended in minimizing the risk of logging incorrect information. Data can be entered directly through a keyboard at the consulting desk, using an interactive program which provides the necessary prompts on a visual display unit (VDU). Theoretical arguments that this system is impersonal as it reduces eye-to-eye contact between doctor and patient have been largely refuted [5]. An alternative method is to enter data in batches at the end of the clinic, using preprinted forms filled out for each patient at the time of the visit. This obviously demands more clerical time: it has been estimated that a half-time clerical officer would be needed to operate a batch-entry system, for an average clinic population of 2000–4000 patients. However, these costs can be largely offset against the savings

Table 101.1. The Körner minimum dataset: the ideal diabetes database should at least include out-patient variables.

In-patient		Out-patient
On admission	—	District patient number
	Sex	Sex
	Post code	Post code
	Date of birth	Date of birth
	Marital status	Marital status
	GP code	GP code
	Category of patient	Category of patient
	Date of admission	Date of all appointments made
	Method of admission	If appointment took place and reasons, if not
	Source of admission	Source of initial attendance
	Need to admit date	Consultant's clinic code
	Management intention	Code location of clinic
		Date discharged from clinic
At start of each episode	Consultant/GP code (specialty)	Name of clinic
		Number of clinics which took place in each period
Ward stay	Ward code	Number of clinics cancelled in each period
Discharge	Date of discharge	Number of patients seen:
	Method of discharge	(a) Referrals
	Destination of discharge	(b) Consultant initiated
		Number of private patients
		Number of patients who failed to attend
End of consultant episode	Codes of diagnoses	
	Codes of operations	

in secretarial time previously devoted to typing clinic and recall letters.

All systems will benefit from being interfaced with an existing computerized administration system, which reduces the need for re-entering basic personal details. Similarly, interfacing with a computer-based pathology reporting system should avoid errors in transcribing results. The ideal system would comprise a multi-user network with terminals in the diabetic clinic, day-care centre, dietetic department, pharmacy and appointments desk. Many existing systems already allow physicians to make appointments for their patients directly on-line to the computer (Table 101.2).

Efficiency can be further improved by using computer-generated letters, not only to recall patients to clinics but also to keep the general practitioner or other doctors up to date. Early systems produced a rather rigid and impersonal format, but experienced programmers can now generate letters which read well and also provide for free text which can be entered either by hand or via the computer. Computers are increasingly

used in general practice and can be linked to the diabetic clinic through the telephone network, so that information about the patient can be rapidly and accurately transmitted to the general practitioner. Ideally, access should be reciprocal: general practitioners should also be able to retrieve information from the hospital-based register and to enter their own data concerning the patient. Diagnostic listings and recall letters could also be transmitted in this way. These possibilities are technically feasible but so far have been neglected. As diabetic care is being progressively devolved into the community, computer-based communication between general practitioners and hospitals should be given a high priority.

The issue of confidentiality is particularly important in all databases containing information about people's health. Registration under the United Kingdom Data Protection Act (in force since November 1987) is obligatory, and only a minimum of free text should be stored.

Nearly 20 years have now elapsed since the first computerized registers were installed, and precise information about their relative costs and

Table 101.2. A selection of currently available diabetes management systems.

System name	Facilities	Compatability	Source
DLB Diabetes System	Stand alone or multi-user network, statistics, appointments, recall letters	IBM	DLB Systems, Unit 151, Cambridge Science Park, Milton Road, Cambridge CB4 4GG, UK
CDS System	Appointments, graphics, letter generation for recall and communication, remote (telephone) modem capability	IBM	Clinical Computing Ltd, 10 Barley Road Passage, London W4 4PH, UK
CPDS	Appointment and follow-up	IBM	C.P. Pharmaceuticals, Ash Road (North), Wrexham Industrial Estate, Wrexham, Clwyd, Wales LL13 9UF, UK
Diabeta	Comprehensive: interactive or batch data entry	IBM	Diabetic Unit, St Thomas' Hospital, London SE1 7EH, UK
Ames Data Register	Comprehensive facility for data storage and letter generation	IBM	Ames Division, Miles Laboratories Ltd, PO Box 37, Stoke Poges, Slough SL2 4LY, UK
Micro-DM	Data storage and patient recall and letter generation	BBC	Micro-DM, Novo Laboratories, Ringway House, Bell Road, Daneshill East, Basingstoke, Hants RG24 0QN, UK

benefits must be gathered to encourage their wider use. Health authorities have been reluctant to fund such systems and will require very convincing financial justification before they support the routine installation of diabetic registers. Further work will hopefully prove the value of computer-based registers in reducing total costs and improving patient care [6].

Applications of computers to blood glucose monitoring

Inexpensive microchip memories have recently been incorporated into a variety of blood glucose meters, allowing storage of up to 80 blood glucose readings which can be subsequently recalled in sequence. Studies in patients unaware of the presence of the memory chip have revealed that the blood glucose values written down by the patients tend to be more 'normal' than the true, electronically recorded results. This finding suggests that, convenience apart, such memory meters are essential for any research which depends on self-monitored blood glucose measurements, and indeed questions the validity of previous studies which employed only the patients' own records.

It is, of course, still possible to fabricate blood glucose data using a memory meter, by inserting previously exposed test strips with the desired reading.

Several systems [7, 8] now allow memory meters to be coupled directly to clinic-based computers for retrospective analysis of glycaemic control when the patient attends the clinic. Blood glucose values can, for example, be categorized by time of day or day of week and displayed numerically as mean values, or graphically by scattergram or histogram; 'event markers' indicating meals and insulin injections can also be incorporated. Printed copies of this information can provide a valuable objective record of control, which in simplified form can be useful for educating the patient. These systems have not yet been critically assessed, but such complete and accurate documentation is likely to benefit both patient and physician. Blood glucose data can now be transmitted directly from the patient's meter to the hospital computer via telephone lines and a modem interface, and the patient can then be telephoned back with advice or suggestions. This approach has obvious advantages where attendance at a central diabetic clinic is difficult for geographical or other reasons. It is likely that memory meters will in due course also incorporate insulin dosage guides, as described in the following section.

Computer-assisted adjustment of insulin dosages

The ability to adjust insulin regimens differs greatly between patients, and clearly depends on the intelligence, interest and educational background of the patient. Written guidelines have been devised to adjust insulin dosage and diet in response to glycaemic changes. Algorithms can similarly be constructed for use in microcomputers which store series of glucose values [9], or incorporated into the memory of pocket calculators [10] for use with either insulin injection or infusion regimens [11] (see Chapter 43). Insulin dosage or infusion rate can be altered in response to variables such as exercise profile, diet and a sequence of entered blood glucose values. Studies have revealed that the use of such systems can lead to better blood glucose control and fewer hypoglycaemic episodes, although it is notable that improved control depends upon continuing use of the 'guidance system'; patients do not apparently learn to better their performance from the advice itself which they are given [12]. The final acceptability of these systems will depend on the magnitude of long-term improvement in control as well as the patients' perception of the benefits of removing some of the uncertainties in adjusting food and insulin schedules. It seems that only highly motivated patients willing to monitor blood glucose 3–4 times daily will benefit. However, the high cost of blood glucose monitoring (approximately 10 times that of urine glucose testing) can only be justified if the test results lead to logical decisions and appropriate corrective action. The type of system already available commercially would appear to satisfy this objective.

The quality of life of diabetic patients under algorithmic control may need careful evaluation, as has already been done for patients treated with continuous subcutaneous insulin infusion (CSII). Studies have shown that many patients derive satisfaction and self-confidence from making decisions about their own management and may therefore feel uneasy at having to depend on computed insulin dosages.

Greater experience with algorithm design has enabled the mathematical modelling of glucose–insulin responses to be further refined. This will be invaluable when improvements in glucose

sensors lead to the development of totally implantable, autonomous insulin delivery devices.

Computer-based diabetes education

The escalating costs of diabetic health care, together with the increasing desire for patient independence, have demanded a new look at the ways in which education is provided for diabetic patients and for the diabetes care team.

It is clear that a one-to-one relationship between educator and patient best provides the all-important emotional support and personal guidance at the time of diagnosis. Thereafter, however, the newly diagnosed patient needs to be equipped with a considerable bank of information which is both factual and procedural. The patients' widely differing educational levels require a flexible approach to education. Computer-based learning is one method whose use is likely to increase as computer equipment costs fall and as more innovative programs become available. Computers are currently applied to diabetes education in two main ways.

Computer-based instruction

Animated graphics can portray many simple or even complex biological functions, including the mode of action of insulin, the concept of the renal threshold, the procedures of urine and blood testing, and the glycaemic effects of food and exercise. Some systems (Table 101.3) use a visual presentation followed by a multiple-choice questionnaire which assesses whether the patient (or other operator) has understood the concept. Success at a given stage leads on to presentation of the next concept, whereas failure results in a re-run of the previous instructional sequence (Fig. 101.1). Such programmed learning can be made enjoyable by the use of high-quality colour graphics and can systematically cover the important principles of diabetes management. The patient can proceed at his or her own pace, without the fear of embarrassment or inhibition which can sometimes arise during group teaching sessions. It has been shown that both knowledge and diabetic control improve as a result of using these systems, over and above those achieved by conventional personal instruction [13]. The popular 'game' image of computers appeals particularly to children, and teaching programs have been compiled in the form of video

Table 101.3. A selection of computer-based diabetes education systems.

System name	Facilities	Compatability	Availability
Diabetes Key Facts	Information provision and assessment in ten separate areas of knowledge	IBM	Miles Laboratories, PO Box 37, Stoke Poges, Slough, S22 4LY, UK
Diabetalog	Knowledge analysis (MCQ) with on-screen and printer feedback and scoring	BBC Spectrum	John Wiley and Sons, Baffins Lane, Chichester Sussex, PO19 1UD, UK
Diabetes: a program for healthy living	Information provision, programmed instruction and basic diabetes knowledge, problem simulation	BBC Spectrum	Dunitz Software 154 Camden High Street London, NW1
Diabase	Children's diabetes computer game: self-challenging	BBC	Diabase Ltd 42 Hightrees House, Nightingale Lane, London, SW12 8QA, UK

games which provide competitive objectives for young diabetic patients (Table 101.3).

Problem simulation represents another method of harnessing the processing power of the com-puter. A problem (e.g. increasing thirst and polyuria) is presented to the patient in textual form and a choice of strategies is provided on the screen [14]. Correct decisions lead stepwise to

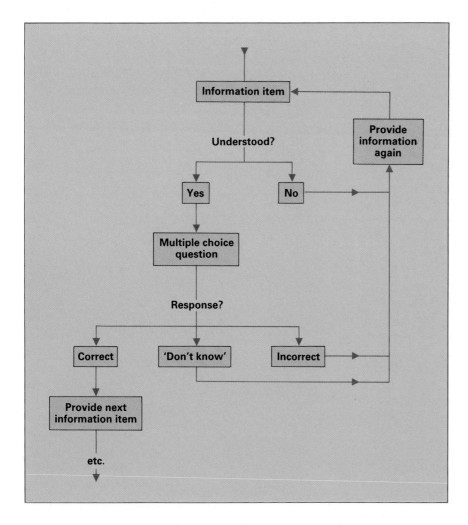

Fig. 101.1 Basic concept of standard teaching/assessment loop in computer-based instruction program.

'recovery', whereas wrong decisions may lead ultimately to 'hospitalization', with a number of opportunities for 'saving' the situation. In this way, real-life situations can be modelled very accurately. This computer-based learning strategy has been applied to teach medical students and clearly lends itself to instructing paramedical staff. Its evaluation in educating diabetic patients is awaited.

Computer-based knowledge assessment

Knowledge assessment is now considered adjunctive or even fundamental to evaluating diabetes education. The simple end-point of poor diabetic control provides, of itself, little guidance as to which area the patient finds difficult. For several years following diagnosis, diabetic patients require methodical re-evaluation of knowledge; unless identified and corrected, faulty concepts can persist for many years and adversely affect not only metabolic control but also other important areas such as foot health.

Early systems for knowledge assessment were cumbersome and expensive, especially as they required an intermediate operator [15]. The development of simplified, telephone-style keypads and an overall increase in keyboard literacy has led to 'user-friendly' systems which do not need either intermediate operators or supervision, and are therefore much more cost-effective.

Most systems use an interactive, multiple-choice format which presents question stems and answer options on the screen [16]. Simple responses are typed in, appear on the screen, and are categorized by the computer as correct, incorrect or missed. Such questionnaires help the patient to learn and are readily analysed by the health educator. The computer can print out all feedback responses and prepare a series of statements which highlight for the patient his areas of ignorance and provide some understanding of why his responses were incorrect. Various 'domains' of knowledge (e.g. foot care, insulin dosage adjustment, complications) can be identified and scored separately by computer to provide the health educator with an immediate profile of the patient's knowledge. Use of such systems has been shown to be associated with improvements in both diabetic knowledge and quality of control [13].

Similar analyses can be performed retrospectively on printed questionnaires which are edgemarked by the patient and scored by an optical mark-reader interfaced with a computer. The computer identifies areas of weakness and prints out corrective statements appropriate to the patient. This uses computers more efficiently than the interactive on-line system described above [16].

Although apparently effective, these systems require more widespread evaluation. At present, they represent the only way of profiling knowledge 'domains' within an entire clinic, in such a way as to identify educational targets and provide greater emphasis where it is needed. At an individual level, each patient's areas of ignorance can be highlighted and then tackled in specific teaching sessions to make the best use of limited educational resources. Computerized systems may ultimately prove essential in the difficult area of continuing care and evaluation of the diabetic patient.

PETER H. WISE

References

1 Levy RP, Cammarn MR, Smith MJ. Computer handling of clinic records. *J Am Med Ass* 1964; **190**: 1033–7.
2 Jones R, Hedley A, Gale E. Identification of diabetic patients treated with insulin or oral hypoglycaemics within a defined population. *Commun Med* 1986; **8**: 104–10.
3 Körner E. First report of the NHS/DHSS Health Services Information, London: Department of Health, 1982.
4 Watkins GB, Sutcliffe T, Pyke DA, Watkins PJ. Computerisation of diabetic clinic records. *Br Med J* 1980; **281**: 1402–3.
5 Higgins E, Oakley NW. A cheap microcomputer network for diabetic clinic management. *Practical Diabetes* 1988; **4**: 293–7.
6 Jones RB, Nutt RA, Hedley AJ. Incorporating the quality of data in a computerised patient master index: implications for costs and patient care. *Effect Health Care* 1984; **2**: 97–102.
7 Mazze RS, Lucido D, Langer O, Hartmann K, Rodbard D. Ambulatory glucose profile: representation of verified self-monitored blood-glucose data. *Diabetes Care* 1987; **10**: 111–17.
8 Zimmet P, Gerstman M, Raper LR, Cohen M, Crosbie C, Kuykendall V, Michaels D, Hartmann K. Computerised assessment of self-monitored blood-glucose results using a Glucometer reflectance photometer with memory and microcomputer. *Diab Res Clin Pract* 1985; **1**: 55–63.
9 Pernich NL, Rodbard D. Personal computer to assist with self-monitoring of blood glucose and self-adjustment of insulin dosage. *Diabetes Care* 1986; **9**: 61–9.
10 Schiffrin A, Mihic M, Leibel BS, Albisser AM. Computer-assisted insulin dosage adjustment. *Diabetes Care* 1985; **8**: 545–22.
11 Peterson CM, Jovanovic L, Chanoch H. Randomised trial of computer-assisted insulin delivery in patients with type-I diabetes beginning pump therapy. *Am J Med* 1986; **81**: 69–72.
12 Albisser AM, Beyer J. Meeting report: first international symposium on computer systems for insulin adjustment in

diabetes mellitus. *Diabetes Care* 1986; **9**: 208−9.

13 Wise PH, Dowlatshahi DC, Farrant S, Fromson BS, Meadows KA. Effect of computer-based learning on diabetes knowledge and control. *Diabetes Care* 1986; **9**: 504−8.

14 Wise PH, Farrant S. *Diabetes: A Program for Healthy Living.* (Spectrum Computer Cassette) Dunitz Software, 1982.

15 Miller LV, Goldstein J, Nicolaisen G. Evaluation of patients' knowledge of diabetes self-care. *Diabetes Care* 1978; **1**: 275−80.

16 Meadows KA, Fromson B, Gillespie C, Brewer A, Carter C, Lockington T, Clark G, Wise PH. Development, validation and application of computer-linked knowledge questionnaires in diabetes education. *Diabetic Med* 1988; **5**: 61−7.

102 Helping People with Diabetes to Help Themselves: A History of the Diabetic Associations

Summary

• The first diabetic organization was the Portuguese Association for the Protection of Poor Diabetics, formed in 1926.

• The British Diabetic Association (BDA), formed in 1934, was the first patient-oriented association for people suffering from a particular disease.

• The first international symposium on diabetes was in Brussels in 1949 and the International Diabetes Federation (IDF) was founded in 1950.

• The foremost diabetes association in Europe is the European Association for the Study of Diabetes (EASD), founded in 1964.

• Several associations have been formed primarily to represent the interests of special groups of diabetic patients, e.g. the Juvenile Diabetes Foundation International.

Early development

The introduction of insulin treatment in 1923 not only extended life for people with diabetes, but also created new challenges concerning the quality of that life. Amongst the first to witness the miracle of insulin therapy was a Portuguese doctor, Ernesto Roma, who was visiting Boston. On his return to his native Lisbon in 1926, Dr Roma determined to make the new drug available to those who could not afford it and formed the world's first diabetic organization, the Portuguese Association for the Protection of Poor Diabetics, which provided insulin free of charge. Even at this early stage, Dr Roma recognized the vital importance of education, not only for patients, but also for their relatives and for the members of the medical and paramedical teams; the courses which he started for all these groups continue to this day.

The initiative for the Diabetic Association in the UK came from an appeal for funds to expand the Diabetic Clinic at King's College Hospital in London, by Dr R.D. Lawrence (Fig. 102.1), himself a diabetic whose life had been saved by the introduction of insulin. Lawrence was disappointed at the response of one of his eminent patients, the writer, H.G. Wells (Fig. 102.2). When tackled on the paucity of his donation, Wells pleaded poverty but offered to write to *The Times* seeking public contributions. The overwhelming response to his letter — not only from London, but all parts of the UK — suggested that there might be enough motivation within the diabetic community to form an organization to protect their own interests. Wells therefore wrote again to *The Times* to suggest the formation of a Diabetic Association, or more accurately, an Association of Diabetics, with the aim of helping each other through their experiences.

Thus, in 1934, was created the first patient-oriented association of people suffering from a particular disorder: a combination of patients and their medical advisers, with the valued support of almoners and dietitians. Its intention was not to become a 'pressure group', but it believed that, through contact with those in authority and in government, the needs of the diabetic community would not be overlooked. Its basic aims were:

1 To provide an organization for the benefit of and service to the diabetic community and those interested in the disease.

2 To act as an authoritative and advisory body to safeguard the social and economic interests of patients with diabetes.

3 To publish educational material and to promote

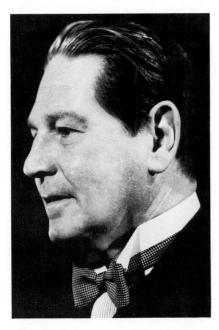

Fig. 102.1. Dr R.D. Lawrence (1892−1968) who was himself diabetic and played a leading part in the formation of the British Diabetic Association in 1934.

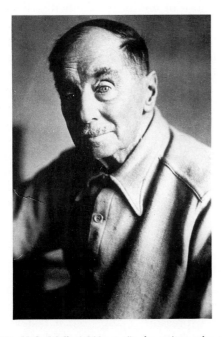

Fig. 102.2. H.G. Wells (1866−1946), the writer, who was a diabetic patient of R.D. Lawrence and who wrote to *The Times* suggesting the formation of an 'association of diabetics'.

lectures and discussions for the information and benefit of diabetic people and their relatives, of their medical advisers and involved paramedical personnel, and of the general public.

4 To promote the study of the causes and treat-

ment of diabetes mellitus and the diffusion of information concerning the same amongst all those concerned with the care of diabetic people at home or in hospital.

The success of the Diabetic Association in the UK (which became the British Diabetic Association (BDA) in 1954) was noted by colleagues in other countries. In 1938, the French formed a similar association, consisting of doctors and patients working together for the benefit of the diabetic community. Despite the war — or perhaps because of it — similar associations were formed in Belgium, Sweden and the Netherlands (1942, 1943 and 1945 respectively). After the war, new societies blossomed throughout Europe and further afield, including Canada, Australia and Uruguay. Meanwhile in the USA, an association of physicians and scientists interested in diabetes had been formed in 1940, with lay interests represented by State Associations. The resulting American Diabetes Association (ADA) changed in the late 1960s (probably for tax advantages) to a voluntary health organization which was obliged to admit diabetic lay people to the national organization.

Although some diabetic associations may have been formed by individuals motivated by the possibility of personal financial gain, the paramount concern of the vast majority has been the patients' best interests.

Diabetic associations and the patient

The central theme of most associations has been education, which in recent years has been developed as though it were new. In fact, its place in treatment was fully recognized by such physicians as Joslin, Roma, Lawrence, J.P. Hoët of Belgium, George Graham in London, and many others. It is somewhat ironic that the BDA has recently formed an Education Section, although this trend evidently reflects the renewed recognition of the importance of the subject and the new technology and methodology which are available.

Other practical ways of helping the patient have been developed. Within a year of its foundation, the BDA had made available beds for convalescence, where diabetic patients could receive correct diet and treatment. A holiday home and annual summer camps were established for children with diabetes. The BDA also tackled the widespread prejudice against diabetic people in employment and managed to arrange life insurance for diabetic patients, which previously had been virtually impossible.

An important development has been the publication of news-sheets or magazines designed to help the patient manage and cope with diabetic life at home. That published by the BDA first appeared in 1935 and is now called *Balance*; similar magazines are produced by innumerable diabetic associations, often under the rather bland title of *Diabetes* but sometimes with stirring names which reflect the intentions of these groups, such as *Victory* and *Conquest*. They aim to give the diabetic reader new information about research, and more important, encouragement to lead a full and active life through stories of those who have achieved much despite diabetes. They also provide useful and often tasty recipes to provide variety in the diet. More weighty volumes covering every aspect of diabetes appear with increasing frequency, and sometimes add to confusion and disinterest. Nonetheless, there are some well written and useful publications on many aspects of diabetes, ranging from patients' guides to foot care and self-monitoring to vegetarian and ethnic dietary advice.

Other vital activities of the diabetic associations include local patient groups, fund-raising to improve clinical services or for research, and drawing attention to problems such as the lack of UK government funding for plastic syringes, needles and blood glucose testing sticks (issues which are now happily resolved).

Diabetic associations and the medical and scientific community

Initially, the support of research was not a primary aim of the diabetic associations, although most now have a strong commitment in this area: for example, the BDA, which first granted £50 for 6 months' assistance in 1936, now spends over £1 million annually on research.

In 1949, an international symposium on diabetes was held in Brussels and united some 75 patients and doctors from 11 countries to discuss their mutual problems in managing diabetes. Lay people were excluded from the scientific sessions but ideas and ideals were freely exchanged and led to a meeting in Amsterdam the following year at which the International Diabetes Federation (IDF) was founded. The main activity of the IDF has been to sponsor triennial congresses, which bring together doctors and patients, relatives and allied health personnel. These have gradually increased in popularity; as the number of national associations and therefore the complexities of ethnic variation and language barriers have expanded, the IDF has had to create seven Regional Councils, each of which is represented on the IDF Executive Board. The addresses of the Councils, and of the Associations within each region, can be obtained from the headquarters of the IDF at 40 Washington Street, Brussels, Belgium.

One early intention of the IDF, however, has not been fulfilled. It was originally assumed that the union of the Associations would encompass both patients and doctors working together. For various reasons, this has not always been practical, and many separate groups representing different interests have been formed. The Juvenile Diabetes Foundation came into being primarily because of a belief that the ADA was not doing enough for children with diabetes. Similarly, the American Association of Diabetes Educators was created in part because of a feeling amongst paramedical personnel that their interests and concerns were neglected by the ADA. In the UK, the interests of doctors and scientists were recognized by the formation of the Medical and Scientific Section of the BDA, whose twice-yearly meetings, serviced and organized by the permanent BDA secretariat, concentrate on advances in scientific and clinical research. A similar Professional Services Section was later formed to represent the interests of all those involved in the care of patients at home or in hospital.

Many associations now publish scientific journals devoted to diabetes research. The longest established is *Diabetes*, published by the ADA. The foundation of its European counterpart, *Diabetologia*, first demanded the establishment of an authoritative and responsible organization to co-ordinate its activities at an international level and ensure scientific quality. The result, in 1964, was the European Association for the Study of Diabetes (EASD), which was based initially in Geneva under the able and effective leadership of the late Professor Albert E. Renold, its first Honorary Secretary. The EASD has rapidly become the foremost diabetes association in Europe and its annual meetings, held in different European cities, attract participants from all over the world. *Diabetologia* was launched in 1967 and has been published monthly since 1978, its Editor-in-Chief being appointed by the General Assembly of EASD.

Conclusions

The growth of diabetic associations is in itself a recognition of diabetes as a major public health problem. The activities of such associations cover the whole range of diabetes from childhood to old age, and their work has been invaluable in improving the quality of life for people with the disease and for funding research into its causes and treatment. There is, however, a need for these societies to continue to combat the remaining ignorance about diabetes and the prejudice against people who suffer from the disease.

JAMES G.L. JACKSON

SECTION 18
FUTURE DIRECTIONS FOR DIABETES RESEARCH AND MANAGEMENT

103 Prevention of Insulin-Dependent Diabetes Mellitus

Summary

• Immunosuppression with azathioprine or cyclosporin (with or without high-dose glucocorticoids) started soon after presentation of IDDM can induce clinical remission lasting many months, often without the need for insulin, in a proportion of patients.

• B-cell function (measured as fasting or glucagon-stimulated C-peptide levels) also shows sustained improvement.

• Not all IDDM patients respond to immunosuppression, and those who achieve remission generally relapse during or after stopping immunotherapy.

• Subjects at increased risk of developing IDDM can be recognized by HLA-typing, the presence of autoimmune markers and abnormal insulin responses to intravenous glucose, but those who will become diabetic cannot yet be confidently identified; the use of immunosuppression or other treatment in the primary prevention of IDDM is therefore not yet feasible.

In theory, IDDM could be prevented either by aborting the B-cell damage which leads ultimately to the disease, or by preventing environmental factors from triggering the disease process in susceptible individuals. This chapter emphasizes the first of these possibilities and particularly the possible role of immunosuppressive drugs in modifying the presumed autoimmune destruction of the B cells which precedes the appearance of the clinical disease. These drugs have so far only been used in 'secondary intervention' trials, i.e. in patients with established but recent-onset IDDM, and their use in this indication will be discussed as a basis for the possible place of im-

munotherapy in 'primary intervention', i.e. in preventing the disease from developing in high-risk individuals, and in ameliorating its long-term complications.

Environmental agents undoubtedly contribute to the pathogenesis of IDDM as is evidenced by the low concordance rates of the disease in identical twins, the wide geographical and temporal variations in its incidence and the observation that migrants assume the risk of IDDM characteristic of their new location. Immunogenetically and environmentally orientated strategies should therefore also be considered in the prevention of IDDM, but will not be discussed further here, as specific environmental triggers for human IDDM have not yet been convincingly identified.

Effects of immunosuppressive treatments in IDDM

Transient and partial recovery of B-cell function (the 'honeymoon period' — Chapter 3) occurs in many IDDM patients during the first few months of conventional insulin treatment [1], and is manifested by increased circulating C-peptide concentrations, symptomatic remission and a decline in insulin requirements [1]. The rationale for immunotherapy in established IDDM is that such remissions might be enhanced and prolonged by suppressing the putative autoimmune B-cell damage (see Chapter 15). It has indeed been shown that immunosuppressive drugs can induce partial remission of recent-onset IDDM, an effect associated with improved B-cell function. The encouraging results from initial uncontrolled studies using a variety of agents [2] — and particularly the striking improvement and preservation of B-cell function in patients receiving cyclosporin [3] — indicated the need for formal clinical trials.

Controlled trials with azathioprine

In the first such study, azathioprine was administered to 13 of 24 alternately-presenting patients (mean age 25 years), within 12 weeks of the onset of symptoms [4]. When the drug was discontinued after 1 year, seven of the 13 were in clinical remission without requiring insulin, whereas only one such remission occurred in the placebo-treated group. This study prompted a randomized, placebo-controlled, double-blind trial in which the same dose of azathioprine was employed in 49 patients of mean age 11 years, starting within 20 days of diagnosis [5]. Although there was a modest and transient increase in fasting plasma C-peptide concentrations in the azathioprine-treated group, there were no significant effects on insulin dosage or on the plasma C-peptide responses to a standard meal. The apparently low efficacy of azathioprine in this second study may have been due to inadequate immunosuppression in these younger patients.

In a further controlled study, azathioprine dosage was adjusted to depress leucocyte and lymphocyte counts to within defined safety limits and high dosages of methylprednisolone were given intravenously on alternate days for 4 days from entry, followed by oral prednisone in reducing dosage during the following 10 weeks [6]. This combination therapy significantly increased mean plasma C-peptide levels and reduced mean insulin dosages in the immunosuppressed group.

Overall, these results suggest that effective immunosuppression with azathioprine improves B-cell function in recent-onset IDDM, and that administration of high-dose glucocorticoids soon after diagnosis may confer additional benefit.

Controlled trials with cyclosporin

The first reported controlled trial of cyclosporin in IDDM, conducted in France [7], involved 122 patients whose mean duration of symptoms was 10 weeks and whose mean age was 16 years. Cyclosporin was administered in predetermined dosages based on organ transplantation protocols. 'Non-insulin-receiving' (NIR) remission was defined as preprandial blood glucose levels maintained at <7.8 mmol/l with HbA$_1$ concentration < 7.5%, without insulin treatment, and 'partial

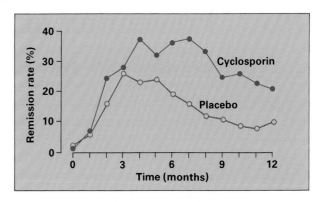

Fig. 103.1. Rates of non-insulin-receiving (NIR) remission in IDDM patients receiving either cyclosporin, or placebo for 12 months. Data from the Canadian−European Randomized Control Time Group. (Reproduced from [8].)

remission' as similar levels of metabolic control achieved with <0.25 U/kg/day of insulin. The rate of NIR remission at 9 months was significantly higher in the cyclosporin-treated group (24%) than in the placebo-treated group (6%); B-cell function was not studied in this trial.

In the Canadian−European Randomized Control Trial of cyclosporin, 187 patients (mean age 22 years) were entered within 14 weeks of onset of symptoms [8]. The initial cyclosporin dose (10 mg/kg/day) was similar to that employed in the French study but was subsequently adjusted to maintain target blood drug levels. NIR remission with preprandial blood glucose concentrations <7.8 mmol/l before meals was significantly commoner in the cyclosporin-treated group, occurring in 38% of cyclosporin-treated patients and 19% of placebo-treated subjects at 6 months and in 24% and 9% of these respective groups at 12 months. B-cell function (measured as the plasma C-peptide response to glucagon) was significantly greater in the cyclosporin-treated patients than in those receiving placebo by 3 months. Improved B-cell function was preserved for 1 year in the cyclosporin-treated group, whereas in the placebo-treated group, glucagon-stimulated C-peptide responses had fallen to entry levels by 6 months and continued to decline thereafter.

The doses of cyclosporin employed in these studies caused a mean reduction in glomerular filtration rate of approximately 20%, reversible on stopping the drug. Follow-up of cyclosporin-treated patients in remission has shown that interrupting immunotherapy after 1 year or more is likely to be followed within weeks by the renewed need for insulin therapy [9]. It is also clear that clinical relapse may occur during cyclosporin treatment, even though the improvement in B-cell function is maintained. For example, of the NIR remissions obtained at approximately 4 months in the Canadian–European trial, 37% were lost by 12 months from entry, although mean glucagon-stimulated C-peptide levels did not change significantly [8]. The possible reason for this is discussed in the next section.

Discussion of immunomodulatory treatment in overt IDDM

These studies provide convincing evidence that immunomodulatory treatment started soon after diagnosis can improve B-cell function and modify the course of IDDM. The results virtually prove the autoimmune hypothesis for the immediate process of B-cell damage. The endocrine and metabolic status of patients in NIR remission resembles that of the prodromal or prediabetic phase of IDDM in siblings of patients with IDDM [10]. Insulin responses to glucose are grossly obtunded but near-normoglycaemia is maintained under physiological conditions, presumably because the B cells remain responsive to stimuli other than glucose [11]. The relapse of clinical remissions in immunosuppressed patients is disappointing but may be explained by preliminary evidence which suggests that improvements in insulin sensitivity as well as in B-cell function are necessary for NIR remission, and that deterioration in either can lead to relapse [12]. As insulin therapy alone may improve both insulin sensitivity [13] and B-cell function [14], secondary interventions combining intensive insulin therapy with immunosuppression might further improve and preserve these functions and so extend remission.

Adverse effects of immunosuppression

The clinical and biochemical adverse effects of immunosuppression with azathioprine or cyclosporin in these studies were generally no greater than in the treatment of other conditions. However, the reversible functional nephrotoxicity of cyclosporin mentioned above was accompanied in some cases by histological damage in renal biopsies [8]. Subsequent open studies using lower initial doses of cyclosporin (5 mg/kg/day) and maintenance regimens which did not affect creatinine clearance induced clinical remissions at rates similar to those observed in the higher-dose studies, with no deleterious histological effects after 1 year [15].

Predictability of response to immunosuppression

In the Canadian–European study, clinical remissions were largely confined to patients with less than 6 weeks of symptoms, including no more than 2 weeks of insulin therapy. Indeed, a relatively short duration of symptoms was the sole predictor of clinical response among several possibly relevant characteristics at entry, including HLA-type, presence or absence of islet-cell antibodies, plasma C-peptide levels and the age or sex of the patients [8].

Preventative treatment of IDDM

Future approaches to the primary prevention of IDDM might include the elimination of specific environmental risk factors from selected or general populations and the use of immunomodulatory treatments in susceptible individuals before evidence of the active disease process appears. Because of remaining uncertainties in these areas, neither approach is currently feasible. Conventional immunotherapy has only a limited ability to induce sustained, non-insulin-requiring remissions, but the encouraging effects on B-cell function suggest that immunomodulatory treatment might be beneficial if employed in the prodromal phase, when the autoimmune disorder is detectable. Although subtle abnormalities in insulin secretion and/or insulin sensitivity are present even at this early stage, effective immunosuppression might prevent progression to clinically significant metabolic disorder. Treatment in the prodromal phase would depend critically on the development of adequate techniques to detect and monitor the disease process. The concept of preventative treatment might be further broadened to include interventions at later stages, with ultimate aims of eliminating insulin dependence or the long-term complications associated with current therapy. These considerations are discussed further below.

Predictability of clinical IDDM

Interest in the disease process in prodromal IDDM has focused attention on the siblings and first-degree relatives of IDDM patients, whose risk of developing the disease is greatly increased. Even within this group, it remains impossible to predict confidently those individuals who will become diabetic. HLA-typing is not currently predictive but might be used in this setting to exclude persons at very low risk. It has been suggested that autoimmune markers, such as circulating islet-cell antibodies or insulin antibodies, may identify particularly high-risk patients and that serial intravenous glucose tolerance tests can detect a characteristic impairment of B-cell function which heralds overt diabetes. A model for predicting the interval to the onset of overt IDDM has been derived from such studies [16]. Further refinement of this approach, and its extension to population screening in the typical sporadic case, will be essential for the development of preventative treatment. However, it is not yet clear whether the disease process advances consistently or is subject to temporary or long-term interruption. The latter possibility is suggested by findings

in discordant identical twins of diabetic siblings [17, 18], some of whom do not progress to overt diabetes even though they show both metabolic dysfunction and autoimmune abnormalities. This encourages belief that the condition is arrestable at this stage, and also emphasizes the importance of including appropriate 'controls' in future trials. The hope that immunotherapy might serve to maintain B-cell function in patients with active autoimmune disease is supported by the findings that administration of monoclonal antibodies directed against a T-cell helper population can induce long-term remissions of IDDM in the NOD mouse (see Chapter 17), despite continuing insulitis [19]. The possible relevance of this to human IDDM is indicated by the findings of analogous T-cells with HLA-restricted cytotoxicity in the peripheral blood of patients with recent-onset IDDM [20].

Nevertheless, at present, monitoring of the prodromal phase has not yet developed to the

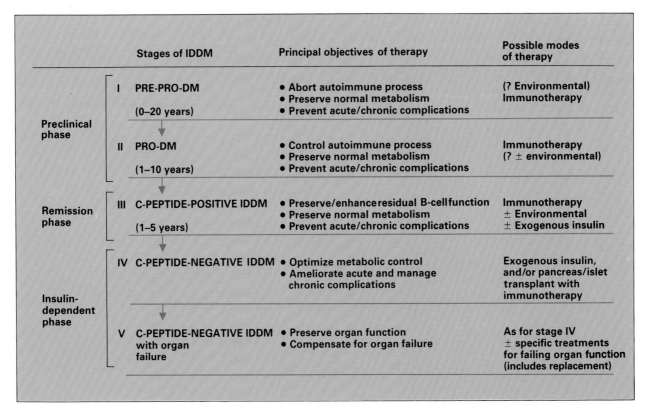

Fig. 103.2. The figure identifies five stages of the disease process in IDDM and suggests appropriate objectives of therapy at each stage. The term 'immunotherapy' covers any kind of intervention that would modify the immune process in a beneficial way. The abbreviation 'PRO-DM' indicates prodromal diabetes, i.e. that stage of the disease preceding the overt metabolic disorder in which autoimmune abnormalities are detectable. 'PRE-PRO-DM' represents the interval from conception to the stage of detection of the abnormalities defining prodromal diabetes.

point where experimental interventions can be timed with the confidence necessary in clinical trials.

Overview and conclusions

Continuing studies of immunomodulatory treatments in prodromal or overt IDDM are clearly experimental, and will remain so until clinical benefits and improved long-term prognosis of the disease can be unequivocally demonstrated. Safer and more effective modes of immunosuppression are likely to be developed for controlling allograft rejection, and new protocols will thus become available for trials in autoimmune disease. Because of the present difficulties in staging the prodromal phase, the use of experimental therapies in overt IDDM of very recent onset should be further explored.

Some possible treatment modalities and their objectives at different stages of the disease are illustrated in Fig. 103.2. Effective preventative interventions may be developed as a result of improved ascertainment and better understanding of the relative contributions of environmental and immune factors in the prodromal phase, especially in the very early shifting target of 'preprodiabetes'. However, intervention later in the course of the disease, with or without replacement of insulin or insulin-secreting tissue, may be able to reduce the excess morbidity and mortality currently associated with IDDM. Therefore, recent advances in understanding the disease process itself demand that the search continues for more effective immunomodulatory treatments and that these are tested for possible clinical benefit. The ultimate goal must be to define plausibly safe and effective treatments that could be tested for clinical benefit in long-term controlled trials.

JOHN DUPRÉ

J.L. MAHON

C.R. STILLER

References

1 Wallensteen M, Dahlquist G, Persson B, Landin-Olsson M, Lernmark A, Sundkvist G, Thalme B. Factors influencing the magnitude, duration, and rate of fall of B-cell function in Type I (insulin-dependent) diabetic children followed for two years from their clinical diagnosis. *Diabetologia* 1988; **31**: 664–9.

2 Stiller CR, Dupré J. Immune intervention in diabetes: state of the art and future directions in autoimmunity and the pathogenesis of diabetes. In: McEvoy RC, ed. *Endocrinology*

and Metabolism: Basic Science in the Clinical Arena. Berlin: Springer Verlag (in press).

3 Stiller CR, Dupré J, Gent M, Jenner MR, Keown PA, Laupacis A, Martell R, Rodger NW, von Graffenried B, Wolfe BMJ. Effects of cyclosporine immunosuppression in insulin-dependent diabetes mellitus of recent onset. *Science* 1984; **223**: 1362–7.

4 Harrison LC, Colman PG, Dean B, Baxter R, Martin FIR. Increase in remission rate in newly diagnosed type I diabetic subjects treated with azathioprine. *Diabetes* 1985; **34**: 1306–8.

5 Cook JJ, Hudson I, Harrison LC, Dean B, Colman PG, Werther GA, Warne GL, Court JM. A double-blind controlled trial of azathioprine in children with newly diagnosed type I diabetes. *Diabetes* 1989; **38**: 779–83.

6 Silverstein J, MacLaren N, Riley W, Spillar R, Radjenovic D, Johnson S. Immunosuppression with azathioprine and prednisone in recent onset IDDM. *N Engl J Med* 1988; **319**: 599–604.

7 Feutren G, Papoz L, Assan R, Vialettes B, Karsenty G, Vexiau P, Du Rostu H, Rodier M, Sirmai J, Lallemand A, Bach JF. Cyclosporin increases the rate and length of remissions in insulin-dependent diabetes of recent onset. *Lancet* 1986; ii: 119–23.

8 Canadian–European Diabetes Study Group. Cyclosporin-induced remission of IDDM after early intervention: association of 1 year of cyclosporin treatment with enhanced insulin secretion. *Diabetes* 1988; **37**: 1574–82.

9 Dupré J, Stiller CR, Gent M, Donner A, von Graffenreid B, Heinrichs D, Jenner MR, Keown PA, Laupacis A, Mahon J, Martell R, Rodger NW, Wolfe BM. Effects of immunosuppression with cyclosporine in insulin dependent diabetes mellitus of recent onset. The Canadian Open Study at 44 months. *Transplant Proc* 1988; **20** (suppl 3): 184–92.

10 Srikanta S, Ganda OP, Rabizadeh A, Soeldner JS, Eisenbarth GS. Pre-type I diabetes: linear loss of beta cell response to intravenous glucose. *Diabetes* 1984; **33**: 717–20.

11 Dupré J, Stiller CR, Jenner M, Mahon J, Keown P, Rodger NW, Wolfe BM. Responses to nutrients in non-insulin requiring (NIR) remission of type I diabetes during administration of cyclosporin (abstract). *Diabetes* 1987; **36** (suppl 1): 74A.

12 Hramiak I, Finegood D, Dupré J. Insulin sensitivity in cyclosporine treated type I diabetes in remission (abstract). *Diabetes* 1988; **37** (suppl 1): 16A.

13 Shirish C, Shah MD, John I, Malone MD, Simpson NE. A randomized trial of intensive insulin therapy in newly diagnosed insulin-dependent diabetes mellitus. *N Engl J Med* 1989; **320** (9): 550–8.

14 Yki-Järvinen H, Koivisto VA. Natural course of insulin resistance in type I diabetes. *N Engl J Med* 1986; **315**: 224–30.

15 Bougnères PF, Carel JC, Castano L, Boitard C, Gardin JP, Landais P, Hors J, Mihatsch MJ, Paillard M, Chaussain JL, Bach JF. Factors determining very early remission of type I diabetes in children treated with cyclosporin A. *N Engl J Med* 1988; **318**: 663–71.

16 Bleich D, Jackson RA, Soeldner JS, Eisenbarth GS. Analysis of metabolic progression to type 1 diabetes in ICA⁺ relatives of patients with type 1 diabetes. *Diabetes Care* 1990; **13**: 111–18.

17 Millward BA, Alviggi L, Hoskins PJ et al. Immune changes associated with insulin dependent diabetes may remit without causing the disease: a study in identical twins. *Br Med J* 1986; **292**: 793–6.

18 Heaton DA, Millward BA, Gray P, Tun Y, Hales CN, Pyke

DA, Leslie RDG. Evidence of B cell dysfunction which does not lead on to diabetes: a study of identical twins of insulin dependent diabetics. *Br Med J* 1987; **294**: 145–6.

19 Shizuru JA, Taylor-Edwards C, Banks BA, Gregory AK, Fathman CG. Immunotherapy of the nonobese diabetic mouse: treatment with an antibody to T-helper lymphocytes. *Science* 1988; **240**: 659–62.

20 De Berardinis P, James RFL, Wise PH, Londei M, Lake SP, Feldman M. Do CD4-positive cytotoxic T cells damage islet beta cells in type I diabetes? *Lancet* 1988; ii: 823–4.

104   New Drugs in the Management of Diabetes Mellitus

Summary

• Soluble dietary fibres such as guar impair intestinal glucose absorption and reduce post-prandial glycaemic rises. Chronic treatment may slightly reduce fasting glycaemia, possibly by increasing insulin sensitivity, and slightly lowers cholesterol levels. Dietary fibre supplements have variable efficacy, significant gastrointestinal side-effects and poor palatability.

• Starch digestion may be blocked by inhibitors of either α-amylase (e.g. tendamistate) or α-glucosidase (e.g. acarbose). These compounds reduce postprandial blood glucose, insulin and triglyceride levels. Troublesome gastrointestinal side-effects are due to carbohydrate malabsorption.

• Novel hypoglycaemic drugs include agents which stimulate insulin secretion, improve insulin sensitivity, inhibit counterregulatory hormone secretion, or inhibit gluconeogenesis or lipolysis.

• Anti-obesity agents, potentially useful in NIDDM, include the serotonergic drug D-fenfluramine, and β₃-adrenoceptor agonists which stimulate energy expenditure.

• Immunosuppressive drugs may be able to limit autoimmune B-cell damage and perhaps prevent IDDM and the rejection of pancreatic transplants. Newer drugs are less toxic to pancreatic B cells than cyclosporin.

• Somatostatin analogues suitable for subcutaneous or intranasal administration can improve metabolic control in insulin-treated diabetic patients but not in NIDDM patients who are not receiving insulin. Somatostatin analogues may improve both postural hypotension and diarrhoea in diabetic autonomic neuropathy.

• Aldose reductase inhibitors can prevent or reverse many biochemical defects and some functional and structural features of chronic diabetic complications in experimental diabetes. No consistent benefits have yet been demonstrated in human diabetic complications, possibly because treatment is started too late.

• Newer lipid-lowering agents suitable for use in diabetic patients include gemfibrozil and other fibrates, inhibitors of hydroxymethylglutaryl coenzyme A reductase ('statins') and the nicotinic acid derivative, acipimox.

• Essential fatty acids (EFAs) have many key metabolic and cellular functions. N-3 (ω-3) EFAs lower triglyceride levels and blood pressure but may raise LDL-cholesterol and blood glucose levels in NIDDM. N-6 (ω-6) EFAs lower blood lipid and glucose levels and are reported to have beneficial effects on diabetic cataracts, retinopathy and neuropathy.

This chapter will deal with a number of therapeutic approaches to diabetes and its complications which have been developed or have found new applications relatively recently. At the time of writing, most were still being actively investigated, a few had been abandoned and some had undergone clinical trials; none had found an accepted place in the treatment of diabetes.

These drugs may be subdivided broadly into those intended to improve metabolic control in diabetes (dietary fibre, starch digestion inhibitors, novel hypoglycaemic agents, insulin analogues and anti-obesity drugs) and those which may prevent or slow the progression of diabetic complications (aldose reductase inhibitors and other agents). Some drugs, such as essential fatty acids and somatostatin analogues, have been suggested to benefit both these aspects of diabetic management.

Dietary fibre

Dietary fibre comprises various polysaccharides derived from plants. Although generally held to be 'indigestible', some types of fibre may undergo fermentation by bacteria in the colon and the products may be partially absorbed (see Chapter 20). Dietary fibre is classified as either soluble or insoluble. The soluble fibres, such as guar, pectin, ispaghule, konjac and carrageenan, form gels with water and exert variable metabolic effects. Insoluble fibre, such as bran, increases stool bulk but has little metabolic activity.

Metabolic effects of soluble fibre

The principal soluble fibre is guar, a flour extracted from the Indian cluster bean (*Cyamopsis tetragonoloba*) which is very rich in galactomannan polysaccharide. Guar given with food reduces postprandial glycaemic rises, apparently by delaying or reducing glucose absorption from the jejunum. The physical properties of the guar−food mixture in the gut lumen may impede diffusion of glucose across the unstirred layer next to the mucosa [1−4]. Guar lowers postprandial blood glucose levels more effectively than other fibres, possibly because of its high viscosity [1]. Postprandial insulin levels in non-diabetic or NIDDM subjects are also reduced [5]; with chronic treatment, fasting blood glucose levels may fall slightly, possibly through improved insulin sensitivity and increased glucose uptake and utilization by the peripheral tissues [1, 6, 7].

Guar has a modest cholesterol-lowering action, predominantly affecting the LDL−cholesterol fraction; the fibre may bind bile salts in the gut and so prevent their enterohepatic circulation, and may directly inhibit hepatic cholesterol synthesis. HDL-cholesterol and triglyceride levels are essentially unaffected [7−10].

Clinical effects in diabetes

Many 'field' studies of fibre supplements have been less successful than those performed under close supervision. This is probably because of differences in patient selection and the dosages and physical properties of the various preparations used, and in the tenacity with which patients adhere to their treatment.

Beneficial glycaemic effects, with a reduction of up to 50% in postprandial glycaemic area and/or a modest fall (1−2 mmol/l) in fasting blood glucose concentrations, have been reported in some studies of NIDDM patients [6, 7, 11] but not in others [10, 12]. Insulin-treated patients (both NIDDM and IDDM) have been reported to show slightly improved glycaemic control, sometimes allowing a minor reduction in insulin dosage [9].

Most studies agree that total and LDL-cholesterol levels fall by 5−15% during long-term guar treatment, with little or no change in HDL-cholesterol so that the LDL:HDL-cholesterol ratio predictive of coronary heart disease decreases [6−10]. A recent long-term study demonstrated a sustained 7% reduction in LDL-cholesterol, which from epidemiological data may correspond to a 15% reduction in the risks of developing coronary heart disease [10]. Xanthan gum has similar glucose- and cholesterol-lowering properties to guar [13].

An important negative finding is the apparent failure of long-term guar treatment to reduce body weight, despite initial reports that the perception of hunger might be reduced.

Adverse effects

Soluble fibres have major gastrointestinal side-effects — notably abdominal bloating, excessive flatus production and sometimes diarrhoea — and are notoriously unpalatable. These problems account for the very high drop-out rate (up to 20%) from clinical trials and the undoubtedly poor compliance with long-term treatment, which probably explains the apparent failure of some trials.

The absorption of some drugs such as penicillin, digoxin and paracetamol may be modified or impaired but sulphonylureas are not affected and clinically significant malabsorption of nutrients, vitamins or trace elements does not occur with guar treatment [14, 15]. Guar preparations must not be taken dry as, with the addition of water, the gum forms an expanding mass which may obstruct or even perforate the oesophagus [16].

Indications and dosage

Dietary fibre supplements should theoretically be most useful for poorly controlled NIDDM patients but have not found favour because of their variable clinical efficacy and problems with compliance. They are not indicated for the treatment of obesity *per se*.

The recommended dosage of guar is 10–15 g/day, divided into mealtime dosages. The starting dose should be low (e.g. 2.5 g once daily) and increased slowly to avoid gastrointestinal side-effects. Guar granules sprinkled on to food seem to be relatively well tolerated [6], as are ingenious examples of gastronomic subterfuge such as guar-enriched crispbread, snack bars, pasta and bread rolls and xanthan gum muffins [13]; however, guar-containing snack bars have an excessively high carbohydrate content [17].

Inhibitors of starch digestion

Starch consists of glucose molecules combined into two basic patterns. α-Amylose comprises a single, helical chain of glucose subunits connected end to end through $\alpha(1-4)$ glucosidic linkages, whereas amylopectin has a dendritic structure with side-branches arising from $\alpha(1-6)$ linkages (Fig. 104.1).

The different glucosidic linkages are hydrolysed by two distinct enzymes which are both required for the complete digestion of starch and oligosaccharides. α-Amylase, secreted in saliva and pancreatic juice, hydrolyses the $\alpha(1-4)$ linkages and α-glucosidase, found in the brush border of the small intestinal villi, cleaves the $\alpha(1-6)$ linkages (Fig. 104.1).

Inhibitors of either enzyme prevent polysaccharides from being hydrolysed to the monosaccharides which are absorbed from the small intestine, and therefore reduce the glycaemic rise after meals. Several competitive, completely reversible inhibitors have now been isolated and characterized. These 'starch digestion blockers', mostly derived from bacteria or moulds, are substituted mono- or oligosaccharides. Most experience has been gained with α-glucosidase inhibitors, although preliminary studies with α-amylase inhibitors such as tendamistate [18] and trestatin [19] have demonstrated broadly similar properties.

α-glucosidase inhibitors

The two principal compounds currently undergoing clinical evaluation are acarbose (Bay g 5421), a pseudotetrasaccharide of microbial origin, and

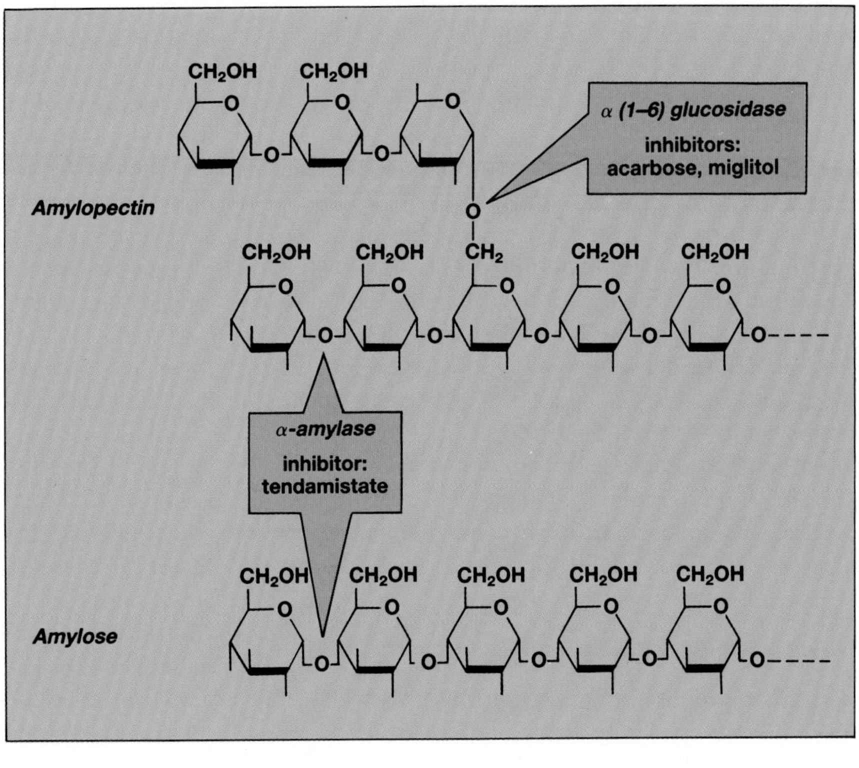

Fig. 104.1. Hydrolysis of starch. $\alpha(1-6)$ glucosidic linkages are cleaved by $\alpha(1-6)$ glucosidase and $\alpha(1-4)$ linkages by α-amylase.

miglitol (Bay 1099m), a glucose analogue (N-hydroxyethyl-1-desoxynojirimycin) derived from *Streptomyces* moulds [20–22].

As predicted from their action, both compounds reduce postprandial hyperglycaemia in normal subjects [21–23] and patients with IDDM [24–26] or NIDDM [26–29], but fasting blood glucose levels are not reduced. The postprandial hypoglycaemic action is relatively modest but is apparently maintained during chronic treatment [28]; one short-term study, however, failed to demonstrate any significant lowering of blood glucose levels [30]. Consistent with this mild effect during only a few hours each day, HbA_1 levels fall only slightly if at all during long-term treatment.

In parallel with the reduced blood glucose levels, postprandial insulin and C-peptide responses are flattened [23–29]. One report has claimed that miglitol improved insulin sensitivity in normal subjects [23] but this has not been confirmed by a recent study in poorly controlled NIDDM patients [29]. Long-term treatment with α-glucosidase inhibitors also reduces serum triglyceride levels to a moderate degree, probably because of the reduced insulin response [27–29].

The main adverse effects of the starch digestion inhibitors are due to iatrogenic carbohydrate malabsorption. Undigested oligo- and disaccharides pass to the colon where they are fermented by bacteria, producing flatulence and diarrhoea. These symptoms are common and often prominent and are probably an obstacle to compliance; however, they may settle spontaneously in patients who persevere with treatment, possibly because of adaptation by the gut flora. Acarbose was previously linked with renal tumours in rats but the association now appears spurious [31].

At the time of writing (1990), neither acarbose nor miglitol were available for clinical use in the UK although acarbose had been licensed for clinical use in Europe. The most obvious indication for the use of these compounds would be as adjunctive treatment in NIDDM patients, especially those poorly controlled by diet and maximal dosages of oral hypoglycaemic agents. However, their limited efficacy, unfavourable side-effects profile and possible compliance problems suggest that they may be useful in only a minority of such cases.

Novel hypoglycaemic agents

Many compounds operating through a variety of mechanisms are being evaluated for their hypoglycaemic properties [32].

Several *insulin secretagogues* apparently act similarly to the sulphonylureas by closing potassium channels in the B-cell membrane, so causing depolarization and an influx of extracellular calcium which triggers insulin release. Such agents include HB699, which structurally resembles the non-sulphonylurea portion of the glibenclamide molecule [33], and adamantane derivatives [34]. Midaglizole, an inhibitor of the α2-adrenoceptors which tonically restrain insulin secretion, causes dose-dependent hypoglycaemia lasting several hours in normal subjects [35], and in NIDDM patients lowers fasting and postprandial blood glucose levels by up to 3mmol/l [36].

Improved insulin sensitivity is an effect of several drugs including the investigational drug, ciglitazone [37], phenobarbitone and other inducers of hepatic microsomal enzymes [38], and the anti-obesity drugs, fenfluramine and BRL 26830A, which are discussed below. Insulin action is also improved by drugs which suppress the secretion of the counterregulatory hormones. Glucagon secretion is specifically inhibited by M&B 39890A [39] and that of glucagon and growth hormone by somatostatin (see below). Pirenzepine, a muscarinic cholinergic receptor antagonist, can reduce nocturnal growth hormone secretory spikes and, like somatostatin, is reported to reduce pre-breakfast hyperglycaemia in IDDM patients [40, 41].

Hepatic glucose output, the main source of fasting hyperglycaemia in NIDDM, may be reduced by *inhibitors of gluconeogenesis* such as benfluorex [42]. The interactions between glucose and free fatty acid metabolism have attracted increasing interest. According to the 'glucose fatty-acid cycle' proposed by Randle [43], high free fatty acid levels may impair insulin-stimulated uptake of glucose into tissues; they may also promote gluconeogenesis in the liver by directly stimulating pyruvate carboxylase [44]. Consistent with these hypotheses are the observations that *antilipolytic agents* such as nicotinic acid and its derivative, acipimox, and the adenosine receptor agonist, phenylisopropyladenosine, have glucose-lowering actions in experimental and human diabetes [45, 46]. Reduced free fatty acid levels as a result of increased insulin secretion and diminished lipolysis have also been suggested to contribute to the hypoglycaemic action of glibenclamide [47].

A number of *traditional plant medicines* have documented hypoglycaemic properties (Table 104.1), although many of the 400 or so

Table 104.1. Hypoglycaemic agents from traditional diabetic remedies. (Adapted from Bailey & Day [48].)

Plant and source	Origin	Active principles	Mechanisms	Active in
Karela fruit (*Momordica charantia*)	Asia	• ? Charantin (glycoside)	• Insulin secretagogue • Inhibits gluconeogenesis • Decreases glucose absorption	• Diabetic rabbits • Human NIDDM
Cluster bean seeds (guar) (*Cyamopsis tetragonoloba*)	Asia	• Galactomannan (polysaccharide)	• Decreases glucose absorption • ? Increases insulin sensitivity	• Human NIDDM • Human IDDM
Ginseng root (*Panax ginseng*)	Asia	• Oryzarans (polysaccharides)	• Unknown	• Diabetic mice
Tecoma stans leaf	Africa, South America	• Tecomine (alkaloid) • Saccharan C (polysaccharide)	• Insulin secretagogues	• Diabetic rabbits

plant extracts ascribed antidiabetic actions are ineffective and/or toxic. Some active principles have been isolated and characterized and are being investigated for possible use in diabetes [48, 49]. The use of any agent — natural or synthetic — should obviously not be sanctioned until controlled trials of its efficacy and safety have been performed.

Anti-obesity agents

Obesity is a major factor contributing to NIDDM and the inability of overweight patients to lose weight is a common cause of treatment failure. The management of obesity is difficult in diabetic and non-diabetic people alike [50]. Of the established drugs, the serotonergic drug D,L-fenfluramine is widely used and often enhances weight loss during an energy-restricted diet, although patients who fail to respond to diet alone will only rarely approach their ideal body weight. D-fenfluramine, currently undergoing clinical trials, may have fewer side-effects than the racemic D,L-fenfluramine [51]. As mentioned above, fenfluramine improves insulin sensitivity and may have an additional beneficial effect in NIDDM patients [52].

A new approach to the treatment of obesity is with thermogenic agents which act on atypical 'β3' adrenoceptors to increase energy expenditure [53]. In adult man, thermogenesis is probably activated in skeletal muscle and other tissues rather than the brown adipose tissue which is of primary

importance in rodents [54]. Of the β3-agonists being evaluated, BRL 26830A has augmented weight loss during a restricted diet in non-diabetic obese subjects [55]. These agents may enhance both insulin secretion (a β-adrenoceptor mediated effect) and insulin action in animal models of NIDDM [56]; studies in human NIDDM are awaited. Side-effects such as tremulousness, presumably due to stimulation of β2-adrenoceptors, are generally mild [55].

Immunosuppressive drugs

These agents are being evaluated both as a means of limiting autoimmune B-cell damage, with the ultimate aim of preventing IDDM (Chapter 103), and for preventing rejection of pancreatic transplants (Chapter 106). Cyclosporin, which is undergoing extensive trials for both these potential applications, adversely affects B-cell function, causing both an acute reduction in insulin secretion [57] and chronic or even permanent functional and structural damage with long-term administration [58, 59]. Alternative drugs, such as lobenzarit, which can prevent experimental autoimmune insulitis in mice [60], may be less toxic to the B cell.

Insulin preparations with improved action profiles

The available 'short-acting' insulin preparations have an excessively long duration of action, whereas the 'long-acting' formulations do not last long enough to provide steady background insulin levels. The absorption of short-acting insulin can be significantly accelerated by addition of local hyperaemic agents such as prostaglandin E_1 [61] but this approach has been rendered obsolete by the development of synthetic monomeric insulin analogues which are absorbed more rapidly and probably with less variability than conventional preparations [62]. Other analogues may be suitable for use as a basal supplement; one such is soluble at its formulation pH of 3.0 but crystallizes at pH 7.4 after injection into the tissues and is absorbed considerably more slowly and with less intra-individual variation than ultralente insulin [63]. These analogues are described further in Chapters 37, 38 and 39.

Somatostatin analogues

The many properties of somatostatin include potent antidiabetic actions — suppression of growth hormone and glucagon secretion and impairment of glucose absorption from the gut — which are opposed by its inhibition of insulin release (Table 104.2) [64, 65].

Native somatostatin, a 14-residue peptide, is unsuitable for therapeutic use because of its short circulating half-life, which means that it must be given by continuous intravenous infusion, and its lack of selectivity which causes a wide range of potential side-effects (Table 33.2). Several truncated analogues based on the active tetrapeptide sequence of somatostatin have been synthesized and have extended action profiles and somewhat greater selectivity (Fig. 104.2) [66].

The octapeptide analogue, octreotide, has a half-life of 45–70 minutes and can be given by subcutaneous injection and even orally [67–69]. Another hexapeptide analogue is effective by the intranasal route [70]. Somatostatin analogues have been investigated both as a possible means of improving metabolic control and as a potential

Table 104.2. Metabolic actions of somatostatin.

Diabetogenic action
- Inhibition of insulin secretion

Antidiabetogenic actions
- Inhibition of glucagon secretion
- Inhibition of growth hormone secretion
- Inhibition of monosaccharide absorption from gut

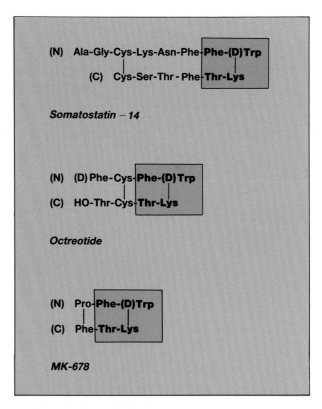

Fig. 104.2. Native somatostatin and two analogues. The active tetrapeptide sequence is shown in the shaded area. Octreotide (Sandostatin®, or SMS 201–995 — Sandoz Ltd) and MK-678 (Merck, Sharp and Dohme Ltd) are shown.

treatment for retinopathy and autonomic neuropathy in diabetic patients.

Metabolic effects of somatostatin in diabetes

The ability of somatostatin to inhibit glucagon and growth hormone secretion carries particular promise in diabetes, as circulating levels of both hormones are increased (especially in IDDM) and have adverse metabolic effects [64, 65]. This is discussed further in Chapters 33 and 51.

In IDDM patients receiving insulin, inhibition by somatostatin of any remaining endogenous insulin secretion is unimportant. Somatostatin analogues injected subcutaneously before meals rapidly suppress growth hormone and glucagon secretion and postprandial glucose absorption is retarded. Overall, postprandial glycaemic rises are flattened and match more closely the time course of insulin injected preprandially (Fig. 104.3) [71–75]. Intranasal administration of a hexa-peptide analogue at bedtime has been reported to abolish nocturnal GH surges and the 'dawn phenomenon' [70], and somatostatin may also

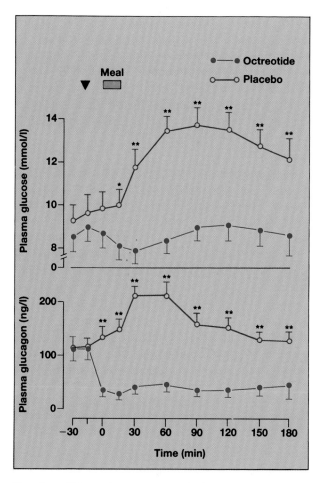

Fig. 104.3. Effects of octreotide or placebo injected 15 min before eating (▼) in 10 insulin-treated IDDM patients. Plasma glucagon levels are rapidly suppressed by octreotide (lower panel) and the postprandial glycaemic rise is significantly flattened. Error bars represent SEM; *:$P<0.05$; **:$P<0.01$. (Reproduced from [73], with permission of the Editor of *Diabetes Care*.)

prevent pre-breakfast hyperglycaemia if insulin runs out overnight [76]. Some indices of glycaemic variability may be improved. Daily insulin requirements can be reduced by up to 30%. This may reduce the risk of hypoglycaemia, although recovery from hypoglycaemia might be delayed by blockade of the growth hormone and glucagon counterregulatory responses [64]. Lower insulin dosages may also reduce peripheral hyperinsulinaemia, an inevitable consequence of non-portal insulin administration which may be a risk factor for hypertension and vascular disease [77]. Other metabolic benefits, due mainly to glucagon suppression, include decreased plasma levels of free fatty acids, glycerol, triglycerides and ketone bodies [64, 73].

Somatostatin analogues similarly improve

glycaemic control in insulin-treated NIDDM patients [78] but native somatostatin worsens hyperglycaemia in non-insulin-treated NIDDM patients [79, 80]. This suggests that their metabolic control depends critically on remaining endogenous insulin secretion and that only highly selective, insulin-sparing analogues are likely to be beneficial. Existing analogues are not sufficiently selective. Octreotide, for example, inhibits insulin secretion at low dosage in man, and when injected before meals, it delays but does not reduce the postprandial glycaemic peak (Fig. 104.4) [81, 82].

Somatostatin and diabetic complications

The most obvious possible application for somatostatin analogues is in proliferative retinopathy, in which excessive growth hormone and IGF-1 levels have been implicated and where abolition of growth hormone secretion by pituitary ablation can prevent and even reverse neovascularization [64, 83]. Octreotide at high dosages suppresses growth hormone secretion in normal and acromegalic subjects but seems on preliminary evidence to be ineffective in patients with proliferative retinopathy [84]; this may reflect specific

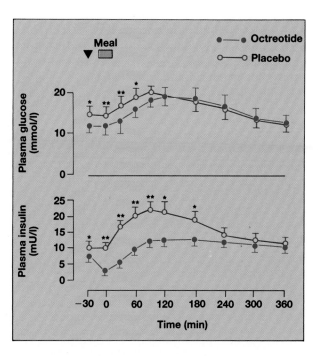

Fig. 104.4. Effects of octreotide or placebo injected 30 min before eating (▼) in 7 NIDDM patients. Octreotide flattens the postprandial insulin response and the glycaemic rise is delayed, but not reduced in area. Format as for Fig. 104.3. (Reproduced from [82], with permission of the Editor of *Hormone and Metabolic Research*.)

abnormalities in the regulation of growth hormone secretion in this group of patients [64].

Octreotide is reported to improve both postural hypotension and diarrhoea in diabetic autonomic neuropathy [85]. These actions are unexplained but the non-specific antisecretory effects of somatostatin on the gut may contribute.

Side-effects and indications

Gastrointestinal symptoms are very common and include colicky abdominal pain, flatulence, diarrhoea and occasionally steatorrhoea. These side-effects are attributable to the generally inhibitory effects of somatostatin on gut motility and nutrient absorption [64, 75]. Currently available analogues have to be given every few hours for optimal metabolic effects.

Overall, somatostatin analogues may ultimately be useful as adjunctive therapy in insulin-treated patients, but the available analogues are still too non-selective and short-acting to be used clinically.

Aldose reductase inhibitors and the polyol pathway

Aldose reductase is the first and rate-limiting enzyme of the polyol pathway, which converts glucose and other monosaccharides to their corresponding polyols (sugar alcohols), for example glucose to sorbitol and galactose to galactitol (dulcitol). The enzyme is widely distributed throughout the body and is found in those tissues

susceptible to chronic diabetic complications. In the eye, aldose reductase has been localized to the capillary pericytes, Müller cells and pigment epithelium of the retina, and to the cellular layers of the cornea and lens. It also occurs in the Schwann cells of peripheral nerves, in the glomeruli (epithelial and mesangial cells) and renal tubules, and in aortic endothelium [86, 87].

The actions of aldose reductase and the metabolic consequences of increased glucose flux through the polyol pathway are discussed in detail in Chapter 54. Aldose reductase has a low affinity for glucose which, at physiological concentrations, is preferentially phosphorylated by hexokinase to glucose-6-phosphate and channelled into either the glycolytic or pentose phosphate pathways. Under high glucose concentrations, however, glucose is diverted into the polyol pathway and converted to sorbitol in those tissues which contain aldose reductase (Fig. 104.5). Sorbitol is poorly diffusible and only slowly metabolized to fructose and so accumulates within these tissues. Several other metabolic disturbances are associated with these changes, although their precise relationships with each other and with the development of diabetic complications remain uncertain [88]. These abnormalities are described in Chapter 54 and are summarized in Table 104.3.

Aldose reductase inhibitors

Aldose reductase activity can be blocked by a number of compounds such as the non-competi-

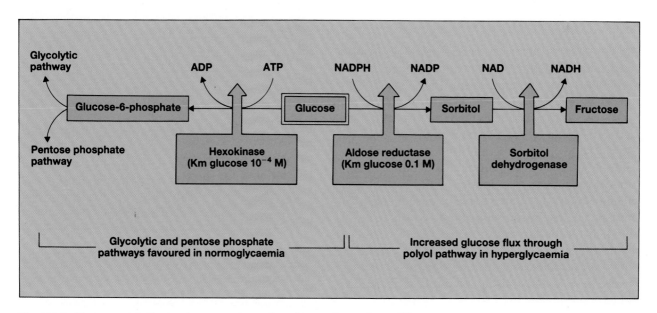

Fig. 104.5. Glucose metabolism under normoglycaemic and hyperglycaemic conditions.

Table 104.3. Metabolic and functional abnormalities in diabetic tissues.

Abnormality	Possible causes	Possible effects	References
• Increased sorbitol	• Increased glucose flux through polyol pathway	• Attracts water by osmosis	88,98,99
• Increased water	• Sorbitol accumulation	• Swelling of lens and peripheral nerves	87,88,98,99
• Increased sodium	• Altered membrane permeability • Reduced $Na^+-K^+-ATPase$	• ?Aggravates lens swelling • Slows nerve conduction	87
• Reduced myo-inositol	• Reduced myoinositol uptake (? competition with glucose, or impaired $Na^+-K^+-ATPase$-mediated transport)	• Impairs membrane phospho-inositide turnover and protein kinase C activity • Early structural defects in nerves	88,100
• Reduced membrane Na^+-K^+ ATPase activity	• Reduced phosphoinositide turnover, causing reduced protein kinase C activity	• Slows nerve conduction	88,100
• Fall in reduced glutathione (GSH)	• Altered redox state due to increased flux through polyol pathway	• Permits oxidative damage	88,100
• Reduced conduction velocity	• Reduced $Na^+-K^+-ATPase$ activity	• Impaired nerve function	88,100
• Impaired axonal transport	• Unknown	• Impaired nutrition of nerves and reduced neurotransmitter turnover	101

tive inhibitors, sorbinil (a spirohydantoin) and ponalrestat (a carboxylic acid) (Fig. 104.6) [87]. These and similar compounds inhibit the enzyme in various tissues *in vitro* and *in vivo* and, in experimental animals, have reversed or prevented many biochemical and certain early structural abnormalities associated with diabetes (Table 104.4). Even in experimental diabetes, however, aldose reduction inhibition does not necessarily imply a

beneficial effect on microvascular complications. For example, functional and structural features of nephropathy still develop in diabetic rats despite a significant fall in sorbitol concentrations in the kidney [89]. Other effects of aldose reductase inhibitors which may be relevant to microvascular complications are a reduction in the abnormally increased vascular permeability [90] and improved filterability of red blood cells, attributed to reversal of a membrane sodium pump defect, which might reduce microcirculatory sludging [91].

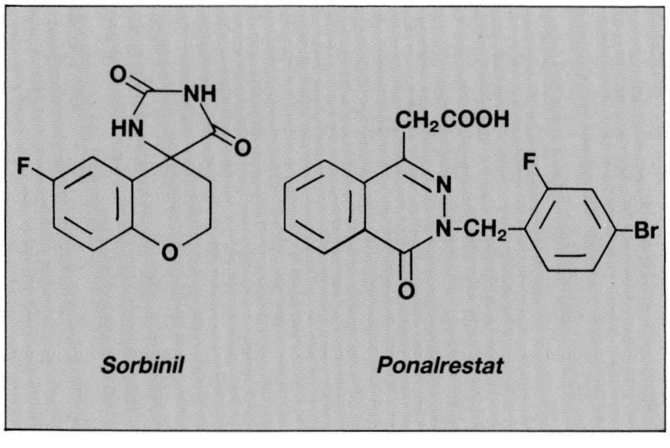

Aldose reductase inhibitors and diabetic complications in man

Clinical trials of aldose reductase inhibitors in human diabetes have not yet demonstrated consistently convincing benefits in any of the chronic complications. Most studies have been performed in diabetic neuropathy; the findings of some trials are summarized in Table 104.5. Initial claims of dramatic symptomatic improvement in patients with painful diabetic neuropathy were based on short-term, open, uncontrolled trials which are inappropriate for conditions such as diabetic neuropathy, which displays both a highly variable

Fig. 104.6. Structures of sorbinil and ponalrestat, two aldose reductase inhibitors. (Sorbinil: CP 45,634 — Pfizer Ltd; Ponalrestat: 'Statil' — ICI plc).

Nerve
- Increased sorbitol content [88,98]
- Reduced myoinositol [88, 100]
- Reduced $Na^+-K^+-ATPase$ activity [88]
- Reduced conduction velocity [88,102]
- Reduced axonal transport (fast anterograde) [101]
- Early structural lesions [103]

Kidney
- Increased sorbitol [89,104]
- Reduced myoinositol [89, 104]
- Reduced glomerular Na^+-K^+ ATPase [105]
- Increased proteinuria [106] (NB: lack of effect also observed [89])

Eye
- Increased sorbitol in lens [107]
- Reduced myoinositol in lens [107]
- Cataract formation [107]
- Retinal capillary basement membrane thickening [108]
- Deterioration of electroretinogram [109]

Table 104.4. Biochemical abnormalities in experimental diabetes which are partly or totally corrected by aldose reductase inhibitors.

Effects on pain and symptoms:
- Some improvement:
  Jaspan 1983 [110] (uncontrolled study)
  Young 1983 [111]
- No improvement:
  Lewin 1984 [112]
  Fagius 1984 [113]

Effects on objective measurements of nerve function:
- Some improvement:
  Jaspan 1983 [110] (uncontrolled study)
  Judzevitsch 1983 [93] (asymptomatic patients)
  Fagius 1984 [113]
- No improvement:
  Martyn 1987 [94] (asymptomatic patients)
  Jennings 1990 [95]

Effects on nerve regeneration:
- Some improvement:
  Sima 1988 [92]

Table 104.5. Results of clinical trials of aldose reductase inhibitors in human diabetic neuropathy.

course and frequent placebo responses. Subsequent and more rigorous trials have shown occasional improvements in symptom score or certain objective measurements of nerve function, and one study has suggested that nerve regeneration may be stimulated by long-term aldose reductase inhibition [92]. However, none of the agents tested so far has been consistently effective.

The discrepancies between these trials are probably due in part to differences in study design and patient selection. Aldose reductase inhibitors may inhibit the enzyme in animal tissues or human red cells but their activity in the tissues susceptible to diabetic complications in man is largely unknown. Moreover, they may be introduced too late in the natural history of the condition, at a stage where restoration of biochemical normality may be unable to reverse established structural and functional damage. The possible

benefits of aldose reductase inhibitors on electrophysiological indices in early, asymptomatic neuropathy are disputed [93, 94]. Most animal studies suggest that these agents can prevent diabetic complications rather than reverse them. It may therefore be necessary to begin treatment soon after the diagnosis of diabetes, an option which is not acceptable at present.

The results of large-scale, controlled trials of aldose reductase inhibitors in human diabetic retinopathy and nephropathy are awaited. Preliminary studies have suggested possible beneficial effects on microalbuminuria and abnormally exaggerated platelet reactivity [95], corneal injury [96] and, perhaps unexpectedly, on limitation of joint mobility [97].

Aldose reductase inhibitors are still being actively developed and tested. Early compounds caused frequent toxicity [87]; sorbinil has caused hypersensitivity reactions including skin rashes in about 10% of patients treated, whereas ponal-restat seems relatively free from important side-effects. Until their efficacy is proven, these drugs should be used only in rigorously designed trials.

Miscellaneous drugs in diabetic complications

Various other agents may have effects on certain diabetic complications. Aminoguanidine is thought to reduce cross-linking and irreversible 'browning' of glycosylated proteins in experimental diabetes and may represent a means of modifying the basic biochemical mechanisms of chronic tissue damage [114].

In patients with background retinopathy, 3 years of treatment with platelet aggregation inhibitors — either aspirin alone or aspirin with dipyridamole — significantly (but only slightly) reduced the appearance rate of microaneurysms as compared with placebo [115]. The non-steroidal anti-inflammatory agent, sulindac, may help to preserve the integrity of the retinal—blood barrier in background retinopathy, perhaps by interfering with prostaglandin metabolism or by inhibiting aldose reductase, which is a further property of sulindac [116]. The calcium channel inhibitor, verapamil, may prevent cataract formation in rats [117]; the mechanism is unknown.

Nerve function in diabetic neuropathy may be improved by prostaglandin E_1 analogues, possibly through vasodilation and inhibition of platelet aggregation which could improve the microcirculation in nerves [118]. Gangliosides, which may become incorporated into axon membranes and activate $Na^+-K^+-ATPase$, may promote nerve regeneration in experimental diabetes [119] and are reported to improve neuropathic symptoms and some electrophysiological abnormalities in patients with painful neuropathy [120]. In some cases, chronic neuropathic pain and dysthaesiae may respond to nortriptyline plus fluphenazine [121], intravenous lignocaine [122] or oral administration of the lignocaine derivative, mexiletine [123]. Novel treatments for foot ulcers include the patient's own serum, possibly containing growth factors which may help healing, and dimethyl-sulphoxide, a highly polar agent which readily penetrates tissues and may improve oxygen delivery [124]. Gastrointestinal symptoms due to autonomic neuropathy are often refractory to treatment, but vomiting may be improved by metoclopramide [125] or cisapride [126], and diar-

rhoea by clonidine [127], phenytoin [128] or somatostatin analogues [85].

The benefits of antihypertensive agents in slowing the progression of diabetic nephropathy are now undoubted. ACE inhibitors are claimed to have a specific action in lowering urinary albumin excretion, both at the subclinical stage of microalbuminuria and in patients with heavy proteinuria. This topic is discussed in detail in Chapter 67.

Lipid-lowering drugs

Hyperlipidaemia in diabetes is discussed in Chapter 68. The treatment of lipid abnormalities in diabetic patients differs in some respects from that in non-diabetic subjects and has been facilitated by newer lipid-lowering drugs. The long-established drugs, cholestyramine and nicotinic acid, may be unsuitable in some cases. Cholestyramine causes gastrointestinal side-effects which may be exacerbated by autonomic neuropathy and may also aggravate hypertriglyceridaemia [113, 114]. Nicotinic acid may transiently lower blood glucose levels by inhibiting lipolysis but 'rebound' hyperglycaemia tends to occur after this action wears off and can cause an overall worsening of glycaemic control [131]. As mentioned below, fish oils rich in N-3 (ω-3) essential fatty acids are unsuitable for diabetic patients, particularly those with NIDDM.

Alternative agents suitable for use in diabetic patients include certain fibrates, the 'statins' and the nicotinic acid derivative, acipimox. Newer fibrates such as gemfibrozil, bezafibrate and feno-fibrate lower plasma triglycerides and sometimes raise HDL-cholesterol levels; side-effects are uncommon and include gastrointestinal symptoms, gallstones (rarer than with the prototype fibrate, clofibrate) and a very rare myositic syndrome [131, 132]. 'Statins' inhibit hydroxymethylglutaryl coenzyme A reductase, the rate-limiting enzyme of cholesterol synthesis in the liver and intestine. These drugs include lovastatin, simvastatin and pravastatin, all of which effectively lower LDL-cholesterol levels and may also reduce triglycerides and raise HDL-cholesterol to moderate degrees [133, 134]. Side-effects are rare; rhabdomyolysis has been reported in a few cases [135]. Acipimox inhibits lipolysis in adipose tissue [45, 136] but, unlike nicotinic acid, does not appear to cause rebound hyperglycaemia and so tends to improve glycaemic control in NIDDM patients [137].

The combination of gemfibrozil with lovastatin seems effective treatment for the common clinical problem of NIDDM patients with hypertriglyceridaemia (often accompanied by reduced HDL-cholesterol levels) which persists after overweight and hyperglycaemia have been improved as far as possible [138].

Essential fatty acids, fish and vegetable oils

The essential fatty acids (EFAs) are polyunsaturated fatty acids which cannot be synthesized in the body and must therefore be obtained from food. EFAs are classified into two groups, N-6 (or ω-6) and N-3 (ω-3), depending on whether the first double bond in the molecule occurs at the third or sixth carbon atom (Fig. 104.7). N-6 EFAs, notably gamma-linolenic acid, are derived from vegetable sources such as corn and evening prim-rose oils and the N-3 EFAs (eicosapentaenoic and docosahexaenoic acids) from cold-water fatty fish; the two synthetic pathways are independent.

EFAs serve many metabolic functions. They are important constituents of cell membranes and may determine properties such as permeability, the activity of membrane-associated enzymes and re-ceptors and the deformability of red blood cells. They are also precursors for the prostaglandins and leukotrienes which influence many functions, including vascular reactivity and permeability, platelet aggregability and nerve conduction [139]. The rationale for EFA treatment in diabetes derives from observations suggesting that the diabetic metabolic *milieu* interferes with their metabolism [139].

N-3 essential fatty acids

Fish oils rich in N-3 fatty acids have been used to treat hypertriglyceridaemia in non-diabetic and diabetic people [140]. Triglyceride levels are lowered by direct suppression of hepatic tri-glyceride secretion, although high dosages of fish oils (5−30 g/day) are often needed. At these dos-ages, blood pressure may fall slightly due to de-creased vascular sensitivity to vasoconstrictors, and platelet aggregability is reduced [140]. Other potentially beneficial effects include a reduction in transcapillary albumin escape rate in diabetic patients [141] and improved cardiac performance in diabetic rats [142].

However, N-3 EFAs have several adverse effects.

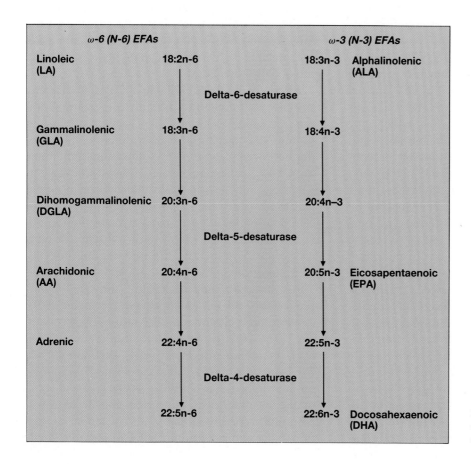

Fig. 104.7. Biosynthetic pathways of the N-3 (ω-3) and N-6 (ω-6) essential fatty acids.

Total cholesterol levels in most studies fall slightly or are unchanged but this may conceal a rise in LDL-cholesterol and/or a fall in HDL-cholesterol, changes which are associated with increased risk of atherogenesis [140]. Furthermore, glycaemic control deteriorates in many NIDDM patients, especially if treated with diet alone, with a rise in fasting and postprandial glycaemia and in HbA1 levels [143, 144]. This is apparently due to increased hepatic glucose production which overcomes a slight improvement in insulin sensitivity [145]. The high energy content of effective dosages of N-3 EFA preparations (up to 300 kcal/day) is also undesirable in obese NIDDM patients. Despite their promising effects on hypertriglyceridaemia and hypertension, these compounds are therefore probably best avoided in NIDDM.

N-6 essential fatty acids

N-6 EFAs have several beneficial metabolic actions, including lowering of blood total cholesterol, triglyceride, glucose and HbA_1 levels. Platelet aggregability may be reduced, perhaps improving microcirculatory blood flow [139].

Several striking effects on diabetic complications have been attributed to N-6 EFAs. In diabetic rats, cataract formation has been completely prevented despite persistently raised sorbitol levels in the lens [146, 147] and nerve conduction velocity is maintained, again without altering polyol concentrations in the nerve [148]. In human diabetes, retinopathy has been reported to improve or to progress more slowly in patients treated with N-6 EFA-rich vegetable oils [149–151]. A preliminary study has suggested an improvement in various electrophysiological indices in patients with diabetic neuropathy [152, 153].

Gamma-linolenic acid preparations are generally innocuous but occasionally cause headaches, nausea and loose stools, especially at high dosages; they may also exacerbate the epileptogenic potential of phenothiazine and other drugs. Further studies of N-6 EFAs in diabetic complications are in progress.

GARETH WILLIAMS

JOHN C. PICKUP

References

1 Jenkins DJA, Wolever TMS, Leeds AR et al. Dietary fibres, fibre analogues and glucose tolerance: importance of viscosity. Br Med J 1978; 1: 1992–4.

2 McIvor ME, Cummings CC, Leo TA, Mendeloft AI. Flat-tening postprandial blood glucose responses with guar gum: acute effects. Diabetes Care 1985; 8: 274–8.

3 Blackburn NA, Redfern JS, Jarjis H. The mechanism of action of guar gum in improving glucose tolerance in man. Clin Sci 1984; 66: 329–36.

4 Eisenhans B, Zenker D, Caspary WR, Blume R. Guaran effect on rat intestinal absorption. A perfusion study. Gastroenterology 1984; 86: 645–53.

5 Jenkins DJA, Leeds AR, Gassul MA. Decrease in postprandial insulin and glucose concentrations by guar and pectin. Ann Int Med 1977; 86: 20–3.

6 Füessl HS, Williams G, Adrian TE, Bloom SR. Guar sprinkled on food: effect on glycaemic control, plasma lipids and gut hormones in non-insulin dependent diabetic patients. Diabetic Med 1987; 4: 463–8.

7 Aro A, Uusitupa M, Voutilainen E, Hersio K, Korhonen T, Siitonen O. Improved diabetic control and hypocholesterolaemic effect induced by long-term dietary supplementation with guar gum in Type 2 (insulin-independent) diabetes. Diabetologia 1981; 21: 29–33.

8 Smith U, Holm G. Effect of a modified guar gum preparation on glucose and lipid levels in diabetics and healthy volunteers. Atherosclerosis 1982; 45: 1–10.

9 Ebeling P, Yki-Järvinen H, Aro H, Helve E, Sinisalo M, Koivisto VA. Glucose and lipid metabolism and insulin sensitivity in type 1 diabetes: the effect of guar gum. Am J Clin Nutr 1987; 48: 98–103.

10 Uusitupa M, Siitonen O, Savolainen K, Silvasti M, Penttila I, Parviainen M. Metabolic and nutritional effects of long-term use of guar gum in the treatment of non-insulin-dependent diabetes of poor metabolic control. Am J Clin Nutr 1989; 49: 341–51.

11 Ray TK, Mansell KM, Knight LC, Malmud LS, Owen OE, Boden G. Long-term effects of dietary fiber on glucose tolerance and gastric emptying in non-insulin-dependent diabetic patients. Am J Clin Nutr 1983; 37: 376–81.

12 Holman RR, Steemson J, Darling P, Turner RC. No glycemic benefit from guar administration in NIDDM. Diabetes Care 1987; 10: 68–71.

13 Osilesi O, Trout DL, Glover EE et al. Use of xanthan gum in dietary management of diabetes mellitus. Am J Clin Nutr 1985; 42: 597–603.

14 Huupponen R, Seppala P, Iisalo E. Effect of guar gum, a fibre preparation, on digoxin and penicillin absorption in man. Eur J Clin Pharmacol 1984; 26: 279–81.

15 Huupponen R, Karhuvaara S, Seppala P. Effect of guar gum on glipizide absorption in man. Eur J Pharmacol 1985; 28: 717–19.

16 Peterson DB, Mann JI. Guar: pharmacological fibre or food fibre? Diabetic Med 1985; 2: 345–7.

17 Van Duyn MAS, Leo TA, McIvor ME, Behall KM, Michnowski JE, Mendeloft AI. Nutritional risk of high-carbohydrate, guar gum dietary supplementation in non-insulin-dependent diabetes mellitus. Diabetes Care 1986; 9: 497–503.

18 Meyer BH, Muller FO, Clur BK. Effects of tendamistate (α-amylase inactivator) on starch metabolism. Br J Clin Pharmacol 1983; 16: 145–8.

19 Eichler HG, Korn A, Gasic S. The effect of a new specific α-amylase inhibitor on post-prandial glucose and insulin excursions in normal subjects and Type 2 (non-insulin dependent) diabetic patients. Diabetologia 1984; 26: 278–81.

20 Puls W, Keup V, Krause HP, Thomas G, Hoffmeister F. Glucosidase inhibition. A new approach to the treatment of diabetes, obesity and hyperlipoproteinaemia. Naturwissenschaften 1977; 64: 536–7.

21 Jenkins DJA, Taylor RH, Goff DV. Scope and specificity of acarbose in slowing carbohydrate absorption in man. *Diabetes* 1981; **30**: 951–4.

22 Joubert PH, Venter CP, Joubert HF, Hillebrand I. The effect of a 1-deoxynojirimycin derivative on post-prandial blood glucose and insulin levels in healthy black and white volunteers. *Eur J Clin Pharmacol* 1985; **28**: 705–8.

23 Joubert PH, Foukaridis GN, Bopape ML. Miglitol may have a blood glucose lowering effect unrelated to inhibition of alpha glucosidase. *Eur J Clin Pharmacol* 1987; **31**: 723–4.

24 Walton RJ, Sheriff IT, Noy GA, Alberti KGMM. Improved metabolic profiles in insulin-treated diabetic patients given an alpha-glucosidase inhibitor. *Br Med J* 1979; **1**: 220–1.

25 Dimitriadis GD, Tessari P, Go VLW, Gerich JE. α-glucosidase inhibition improves post-prandial hyperglycemia and decreases insulin requirements in insulin-dependent diabetes mellitus. *Metabolism* 1985; **34**: 261–5.

26 Sachse G, Willms B. Effect of the alpha-glucosidase-inhibitor Bay g 5421 on blood glucose control of sulphonylurea-treated diabetics and insulin-treated diabetics. *Diabetologia* 1979; **17**: 287–90.

27 Lardinois CK, Greenfield MS, Schwartz HC, Vreman HJ, Reaven GM. Acarbose treatment of non-insulin-dependent diabetes mellitus. *Arch Int Med* 1984; **144**: 345–7.

28 Uttenthal LO, Ukponmwan OO, Wood SM *et al.* Long-term effects of intestinal alpha-glucosidase inhibition on post-prandial glucose, pancreatic and gut hormone responses and fasting serum lipids in diabetics on sulphonylureas. *Diabetic Med* 1986; **3**: 155–60.

29 Schnack C, Prager RJF, Winkler J, Klauser RM, Schneider BG, Schernthaner G. Effects of 8-wk α-glucosidase inhibition on metabolic control, C-peptide secretion, hepatic glucose output, and peripheral insulin sensitivity in poorly controlled type II diabetic patients. *Diabetes Care* 1989; **12**: 537–43.

30 Vierhapper H, Bratusch-Marrain A, Waldhäusl W. Alpha-glucoside hydrolase inhibition in diabetes. *Lancet* 1978; ii: 1386.

31 Schluter G. In: Creutzfeldt W, ed. *Acarbose for the Treatment of Diabetes Mellitus*. Berlin: Springer-Verlag, 1988; 5–14.

32 Bailey CJ, Flatt PR, Marks V. Drugs inducing hypoglycemia. *Pharmac Ther* 1989; **42**: 361–84.

33 Garrino MG, Schmeer W, Henquin M, Meissner HP, Henquin JC. Mechanism of the stimulation of insulin release in vitro by HB699, a benzoic acid derivative similar to the non-sulphonylurea moiety of glibenclamide. *Diabetologia* 1985; **28**: 697–703.

34 Garrino MG, Henquin JC. Adamantane derivatives: a new class of insulin secretagogues. *Br J Pharmacol* 1987; **90**: 583–91.

35 Kawazu S, Suzuki M, Negishi K, Watanabe T, Ishii J. Studies of midaglizole (DG-5128), a new type of oral hypoglycemic drug in healthy subjects. *Diabetes* 1987; **36**: 216–20.

36 Kawazu S, Suzuki M, Negishi K *et al.* Initial phase II clinical studies on midaglizole (DG-5128), a new hypoglycemic agent. *Diabetes* 1987; **36**: 221–6.

37 Diani AR, Peterson T, Sawada GA, Wyse BM, Gilchrist BJ, Hearron AE, Chang AY. Ciglitazone, a new hypoglycemic agent. 4. Effect on pancreatic islets of C57BL/6J-*ob*/*ob* and C57BL/KsJ-*db*/*db* mice. *Diabetologia* 1984; **27**: 225–34.

38 Lahtela JT, Arranto AJ, Sotaniemi ED. Enzyme inducers improve insulin sensitivity in non-insulin-dependent diabetic subjects. *Diabetes* 1985; **34**: 911–16.

39 Tadayyon M, Green I, Cook D, Pratt J. Effect of a hypoglycaemic agent M&B 39890A on glucagon secretion in isolated rat islets of Langerhans. *Diabetologia* 1982; **30**: 41–5.

40 Atiea JA, Creagh F, Page M, Owens DR, Scanlon MF, Peters JR. Early morning hyperglycemia in IDDM. Acute effects of cholinergic blockade. *Diabetes Care* 1989; **12**: 443–8.

41 Page MD, Kopperschaar HPF, Dieguez C, Gibbs JT, Hall R, Peters JR, Scanlon MF. Cholinergic muscarinic receptor blockade with pirenzepine abolishes slow-wave sleep-related growth hormone release in young patients with insulin-dependent diabetes mellitus. *Clin Endocrinol* 1987; **26**: 355–9.

42 Brindley DN, Akester H, Derrick GP *et al.* Effects of chronic administration of benfluorex to rats on the metabolism of corticosterone, glucose, triacylglycerols, glycerol and fatty acids. *Biochem Pharmac* 1988; **37**: 695–705.

43 Randle PLJ, Hales CN, Garland PB, Newsholme EA. The glucose fatty-acid cycle. Its role in insulin sensitivity and the metabolic disturbances of diabetes mellitus. *Lancet* 1963; i: 785–9.

44 Ruderman NB, Toeus CJ, Shafrir E. Role of free fatty acids in glucose homeostasis. *Arch Int Med* 1969; **123**: 299–313.

45 Gey KF, Carlson LA, eds. *Metabolic Effects of Nicotinic Acid and its Derivatives*. Bern: Huber, 1970.

46 Reaven GM, Chang H, Ho H, Jeng C-Y, Hoffman BB. Lowering of plasma glucose in diabetic rats by antilipolytic agents. *Am J Physiol* 1988; **254**: E23–E30.

47 Jeng C-Y, Hollenbeck CB, Wu M-S, Chen Y-DI, Reaven GM. How does glibenclamide lower plasma glucose concentration in patients with type 2 diabetes? *Diabetic Med* 1989; **6**: 303–8.

48 Bailey CJ, Day C. Traditional plant medicines as treatments for diabetes. *Diabetes Care* 1989; **12**: 553–64.

49 Swanston-Flatt SK, Day C, Flatt PR, Gould BJ, Bailey CJ. Glycaemic effects of traditional European plant treatments for diabetes. Studies in normal and streptozotocin diabetic mice. *Diabetes Res* 1989; **10**: 69–73.

50 Carpenter MA, Bodansky HJ. Drug treatment of obesity in type 2 diabetes mellitus. *Diabetic Med* 1990; **7**: 99–104.

51 Guy-Grand B, Apfelbaum M, Crepaldi G, Gries A, Lefèbvre P, Turner P. International trial of long-term dexfenfluramine in obesity. *Lancet* 1989; ii: 1142–5.

52 Pestell RG, Crock RA, Ward GM, Alford FP, Best JD. Fenfluramine increases insulin action in patients with NIDDM. *Diabetes Care* 1989; **12**: 252–8.

53 Arch JRS, Ainsworth AT, Cawthorne MA *et al.* Atypical β-adrenoceptor on brown adipocytes as target for anti-obesity drugs. *Nature* 1984; **309**: 163–5.

54 Cunningham S, Leslie P, Hopwood D *et al.* The characterization and energetic potential of brown adipose tissue in man. *Clin Sci* 1985; **69**: 343–8.

55 Connacher AA, Jung RJ, Mitchell PEG. Weight loss in obese subjects on a restricted diet given BRL 26830A, a new atypical B adrenoceptor agonist. *Br Med J* 1988; **296**: 1217–20.

56 Cawthorne MA. Does brown adipose tissue have a role to play in glucose homeostasis? *Proc Nutr Soc* 1989; **48**: 207–14.

57 Gillison SL, Bartlett ST, Curry DL. Synthesis-secretion coupling of insulin. Effect of cyclosporin. *Diabetes* 1989; **38**: 465–70.

58 Alejandro R, Feldman EC, Bloom AD. Effects of cyclosporin on insulin and C-peptide secretion in healthy beagles.

Diabetes 1989; **38**: 698−703.

59 Helmchen U, Schmidt WE, Siegel EG, Creutzfeldt W. Morphological and functional changes of pancreatic B cells in cyclosporin A-treated rats. *Diabetologia* 1984; **27**: 416−18.

60 Iwakiri R, Nagafuchi S. Inhibition of streptozocin-induced insulitis and diabetes with lobenzarit in CD-1 mice. *Diabetes* 1989; **38**: 558−61.

61 Williams G, Pickup JC, Collins AGC, Keen H. Prostaglandin E_1 accelerates subcutaneous insulin absorption in insulin-dependent diabetic patients. *Diabetic Med* 1984; **1**: 109−12.

62 Vora JP, Owens DR, Dolben J *et al.* Recombinant DNA derived monomeric insulin analogue: comparison with soluble human insulin in normal subjects. *Br Med J* 1988; **297**: 1236−9.

63 Jørgensen S, Vaag A, Langkær L, Hougaard P, Markussen J. NovoSol Basal: pharmacokinetics of a novel soluble long acting insulin analogue. *Br Med J* 1989; **299**: 415−19.

64 Davies RR, Turner SJ, Alberti KGMM, Johnston DG. Somatostatin analogues in diabetes mellitus. *Diabetic Med* 1989; **6**: 103−11.

65 Williams G, Bloom SR. Regulatory peptides, the hypothalamus and diabetes. *Diabetic Med* 1989; **6**: 472−85.

66 Moreau JP, DeFeudis FV. Minireview. Pharmacological studies of somatostatin and somatostatin-analogues: therapeutic advances and perspectives. *Life Sci* 1987; **40**: 419−37.

67 Bauer W, Briner U, Doepfner W, Haller R, Huguenin R, Marbach P, Petcher TJ, Pless J. A very potent and selective octapeptide analogue of somatostatin with prolonged action. *Life Sci* 1982; **31**: 1133−40.

68 Füessl HJ, Domin J, Bloom SR. Oral absorption of somatostatin analogue SMS 201−995: theoretical and practical implications. *Clin Sci* 1987; **72**: 255−7.

69 Williams G, Ball JA, Burrin JM, Joplin GF, Bloom SR. Effective and lasting growth-hormone suppression in active acromegaly with oral administration of somatostatin analogue SMS 201−995. *Lancet* 1986; ii: 774−8.

70 Campbell PJ, Bolli GB, Gerich JE. Prevention of the dawn phenomenon (early morning hyperglycemia) in insulin-dependent diabetes mellitus by bedtime intranasal administration of a long-acting somatostatin analog. *Metabolism* 1988; **37**: 34−7.

71 Dimitriadis G, Tessari P, Gerich J. Effects of a long-acting somatostatin analog on postprandial hyperglycemia in insulin-dependent diabetes mellitus. *Metabolism* 1983; **32**: 987−92.

72 Dimitriadis G, Gerich J. Effect of twice daily subcutaneous administration of a long-acting somatostatin analog on 24 hour plasma glucose profile in patients with insulin-dependent diabetes. *Horm Met Res* 1985; **17**: 510−11.

73 Spinas GA, Bock A, Keller U. Reduced post-prandial hyperglycemia after subcutaneous injection of a somatostatin analog (SMS 201−995) in insulin-dependent diabetes mellitus. *Diabetes Care* 1985; **8**: 429−35.

74 Serrano-Rios M, Navascues I, Saban J, Ordonez A, Sevilla F, Del Pozo E. Somatostatin analog SMS 201−995 and insulin needs in insulin-dependent diabetic patients studied by means of an artificial pancreas. *J Clin Endoc Metab* 1986; **63**: 1071−4.

75 Osei K, O'Dorisio TM, Malarkey WB, Craig EL, Cataland S. Metabolic effects of long-acting somatostatin analog (Sandostatin) in type 1 diabetic patients on conventional therapy. *Diabetes* 1989; **38**: 704−9.

76 Scheen AJ, Krzentowski G, Castillo M, Lefèbvre PJ, Luykcx AS. A 6-hour nocturnal interruption of a continuous subcutaneous insulin infusion: 2. Marked attenuation of the metabolic deterioration by somatostatin. *Diabetologia* 1983; **24**: 319−25.

77 Stout RW. Insulin and atheroma — an update. *Lancet* 1987; i: 1077−9.

78 Candrina R, Coppini A, Graffeo M, Zuccato F, Giustina G. SMS 201−995 improves glucose tolerance in insulin-treated type II diabetic patients. *Diabetes Care* 1987; **10**: 534−5.

79 Christensen S, Hansen A, Lundbaek K. Somatostatin in maturity-onset diabetes. *Diabetes* 1978; **27**: 1013−16.

80 Tamborlane WJ, Sherwin RS, Hendler M, Felig P. Metabolic effects of somatostatin in maturity-onset diabetes. *N Engl J Med* 1977; **297**: 181−5.

81 Davies RR, Miller M, Turner SJ, Watson M, McGill A, Ørskov H, Alberti KGMM, Johnson DG. Effects of somatostatin analogue SMS 201−995 in non-insulin-dependent diabetes. *Clin Endocrinol* 1986; **25**: 739−47.

82 Williams G, Füessl HS, Burrin JM, Chilvers E, Bloom SR. Postprandial glycaemic effects of a long-acting somatostatin analogue (SMS 201−995) in non-insulin dependent diabetes mellitus. *Horm Metab Res* 1988; **2**: 168−70.

83 Sharp PS, Fallon TJ, Brazier OJ, Sandler L, Joplin GF, Kohner EM. Long-term follow-up of patients who underwent Yttrium-90 pituitary implantation for treatment of proliferative retinopathy. *Diabetologia* 1987; **33**: 199−207.

84 Sharp PS, Hyer SL, Brooks RA, Burrin JM, Kohner EM. Somatostatin analogue and diabetic retinopathy (abstract). *J Endocrinol* 1987; **112** (suppl): 124a.

85 Dudl RJ, Anderson DS, Forsythe AB, Ziegler MG, O'Dorisio TM. Treatment of diabetic diarrhea and orthostatic hypotension with somatostatin analog SMS 201−995. *Am J Med* 1987; **83**: 584−8.

86 Wirth HP, Wermuth B. Immunohistochemical localization of aldehyde and aldose reductase in human tissues. In: Flynn TG, Weiner H, eds. *Enzymology of Carbonyl Metabolism* 2: Aldehyde Dehydrogenase, Aldo-Keto Reductase and Alcohol Dehydrogenase. New York: Alan Ross, 1985; 231−9.

87 Harrison HE, Stribling D, Armstrong FM, Perkins CM. Aldose reductase in the etiology of diabetic complications: I. Introduction. *J Diabetic Complic* 1989; **3**: 6−11.

88 Greene DA, Lattimer SA, Sima AAF. Sorbitol, phosphoinositides, and sodium-potassium-ATPase in the pathogenesis of diabetic complications. *N Engl J Med* 1987; **316**: 599−606.

89 Daniels BS, Hostetter TH. Aldose reductase inhibition and glomerular abnormalities in diabetic rats. *Diabetes* 1989; **38**: 981−6.

90 Williamson JR, Chang K, Rowold E *et al.* Sorbinil prevents diabetes-induced increases in vascular permeability but does not alter collagen cross-linking. *Diabetes* 1985; **34**: 703−5.

91 Kowluru R, Bitensky MW, Kowluru A, Dembo M, Keaton PA, Buican T. Reversible sodium pump defect and swelling in the diabetic rat erythrocyte: effects on filterability and implications for microangiopathy. *Proc Natl Acad Sci USA* 1989; **86**: 3327−31.

92 Sima AAF, Bril V, Nathaniel V *et al.* Regeneration and repair of myelinated fibers in sural-nerve biopsy specimens from patients with diabetic neuropathy treated with sorbinil. *N Engl J Med* 1988; **319**: 548−55.

93 Judzewitsch RG, Jaspan JB, Plonosky KS *et al.* Aldose reductase inhibition improves nerve conduction velocity in diabetic patients. *N Engl J Med* 1983; **308**: 119−25.

94 Martyn CN, Reid W, Young RJ, Ewing DJ, Clarke BF. Six-month treatment with sorbinil in asymptomatic diabetic neuropathy. Failure to improve abnormal nerve function. *Diabetes* 1987; **36**: 987–90.

95 Jennings PE, Nightingale S, Le Guen C et al. Prolonged aldose reductase inhibition in chronic peripheral diabetic neuropathy: effects on microangiopathy. *Diabetic Med* 1990; **7**: 63–8.

96 Ohashi Y, Matsuda M, Hosotani H et al. Aldose reductase inhibitor (CT-112) eyedrops for diabetic corneal epitheliopathy. *Am J Ophthalmol* 1988; **105**: 233–8.

97 Eaton RP, Sibbit WL, Harsh A. The effect of an aldose reductase inhibiting agent on limited joint mobility in diabetic patients. *J Am Med Assoc* 1985; **10**: 1437–40.

98 Gabbay KH, Merola LO, Field RA. Sorbitol pathway: presence in nerve and cord with substrate accumulation in diabetes. *Science* 1966; **151**: 209–10.

99 Van Heyningen R. Formation of polyols by the lens of the rat with sugar cataracts. *Nature* 1959; **184**: 194–5.

100 Carroll PB, Thornton BM, Greene DA. Glutathione redox state is not the link between polyol pathway activity and myoinositol-related Na-K-ATPase defect in experimental diabetic neuropathy. *Diabetes* 1986; **35**: 1282–5.

101 Tomlinson DR, Townsend J, Fretten P. Prevention of defective axonal transport in streptozocin-diabetic rats by treatment with 'Statil' (ICI 128436), an aldose reductase inhibitor. *Diabetes* 1985; **34**: 970–2.

102 Kikkawa R, Hatanaka I, Yasuda H, Kobayashi N, Shigeta Y. Prevention of peripheral nerve dysfunction by an aldose reductase inhibitor in streptozotocin-diabetic rats. *Metabolism* 1984; **33**: 212–15.

103 Schmidt RE, Plurad SB, Sherman WR, Williamson JR, Tilton RG. Effects of aldose reductase inhibitor sorbinil on neuroaxonal dystrophy and levels of myo-inositol and sorbitol in sympathetic autonomic ganglia of streptozocin-induced diabetic rats. *Diabetes* 1989; **38**: 569–79.

104 Beyer-Mears A, Ku L, Cohen MP. Glomerular polyol accumulation in diabetes and its prevention by oral sorbinil. *Diabetes* 1984; **33**: 604–7.

105 Cohen MP, Dasmahapatra A, Shapiro E. Reduced glomerular sodium/potassium adenosine triphosphatase activity in acute streptozocin diabetes and its prevention by oral sorbinil. *Diabetes* 1985; **34**: 1071–4.

106 Beyer-Mears A, Cruz E, Edelist T, Varagianuis E. Diminished proteinuria in diabetes mellitus by sorbinil, an aldose reductase inhibitor. *Pharmacology* 1986; **32**: 52–60.

107 Beyer-Mears A, Cruz E. Reversal of diabetic cataract by sorbinil, an aldose reductase inhibitor. *Diabetes* 1985; **35**: 15–21.

108 Chakrabarti S, Sima AAF. Effect of aldose reductase inhibition and insulin treatment on retinal capillary basement membrane thickening in BB rats. *Diabetes* 1989; **38**: 1181–6.

109 MacGregor LE, Matschinsky FM. Treatment with aldose reductase inhibitor or with myo-inositol arrests deterioration of the electroretinogram of diabetic rats. *J Clin Invest* 1985; **76**: 887–9.

110 Jaspan J, Maselli R, Herold K, Bartkus C. Treatment of severely painful diabetic neuropathy with an aldose reductase inhibitor. Relief of pain and improved somatic and autonomic nerve function. *Lancet* 1983; **ii**: 758–62.

111 Young RJ, Ewing DJ, Clarke BF. A controlled trial of sorbinil, an aldose reductase inhibitor in chronic painful diabetic neuropathy. *Diabetes* 1983; **32**: 938–42.

112 Lewin IG, O'Brien IAD, Morgan MH, Corrall RJM. Clinical and neurophysiological studies with the aldose reductase

inhibitor, sorbinil, in symptomatic diabetic neuropathy. *Diabetologia* 1984; **26**: 445–8.

113 Fagius J, Brattberg A, Jameson S, Berne C. Limited benefit of treatment of diabetic polyneuropathy with an aldose reductase inhibitor: a 24-week controlled trial. *Diabetologia* 1985; **28**: 323–29.

114 Brownlee M, Vlassara H, Kouney A, Ulrich P, Cerami A. Aminoguanidine prevents diabetes-induced arterial wall protein cross-linking. *Science* 1986; **232**: 1629–32.

115 DAMAD Study Group. Effect of aspirin alone and aspirin plus dipyridamole in early diabetic retinopathy. A multicenter randomized controlled clinical trial. *Diabetes* 1989; **38**: 491–8.

116 Cunha-Vaz JG, Mota CC, Leite EC, Abreu JR, Ruas MA. Effect of sulindac on the permeability of the blood-retinal barrier in early diabetic retinopathy. *Acta Ophthalmol* 1985; **103**: 1307–11.

117 Pierce GN, Afzal N, Kooeger EA et al. Cataract formation is prevented by administration of verapamil to diabetic rats. *Endocrinology* 1989; **125**: 730–5.

118 Yasuda H, Sonobe M, Yamashita M et al. Effect of prostaglandin E1 analogue TFC 612 on diabetic neuropathy in streptozotocin-induced diabetic rats. Comparison with aldose reductase inhibitor ONO 2235. *Diabetes* 1989; **38**: 832–8.

119 Triban C, Guidolin D, Fabris M et al. Ganglioside treatment and improved axonal regeneration capacity in experimental diabetic neuropathy. *Diabetes* 1989; **38**: 1012–22.

120 Crepaldi G, Fedele D, Tiengo A et al. Ganglioside treatment in diabetic peripheral neuropathy: a multicenter trial. *Acta Diabetol Lat* 1983; **20**: 265–78.

121 Gomez-Perez FJ, Rull JA, Dies H, Rodriguez-Rivera JG, Gonzalez-Barranco J, Lozano-Castaneda O. Nortriptyline and fluphenazine in the symptomatic treatment of diabetic neuropathy. A double-blind cross-over study. *Pain* 1985; **23**: 395–400.

122 Kastrup J, Angelo HR, Peterson P, Dejgard A, Hilsted J. Treatment of chronic painful diabetic neuropathy with intravenous lidocaine infusion. *Br Med J* 1986; **292**: 173.

123 Dejgard A, Peterson P, Kastrup J. Mexiletine for treatment of chronic painful diabetic neuropathy. *Lancet* 1988; **i**: 9–11.

124 Fishner M, Lang R, Kedar I, Ravid M. Treatment of diabetic perforating ulcers (mal perforant) with local dimethylsulfoxide. *J Am Geriatr Soc* 1985; **33**: 41–3.

125 Loo FO, Palmer DW, Soergel KH, Kalbfleisch JH, Wood CM. Gastric emptying in patients with diabetes mellitus. *Gastroenterology* 1984; **86**: 484–94.

126 Horowitz M, Maddox A, Harding PE et al. Effect of cisapride on gastric and esophageal emptying in insulin-dependent diabetes mellitus. *Gastroenterology* 1987; **92**: 1899–907.

127 Fedorak RN, Field M, Chang EB. Treatment of diabetic diarrhea with clonidine. *Ann Int Med* 1985; **102**: 197–9.

128 Thomas M, Verges B. Treatment of diabetic diarrhoea with phenytoin. *Presse Méd* 1986; **15**: 11–14.

129 Lipid Research Clinics Program. The relationship of reduction in incidence of coronary heart disease to cholesterol lowering. *J Am Med Ass* 1984; **251**: 365–74.

130 Lees AM, McClusky MA, Lees RS. Results of colestipol therapy in Type II hyperlipoproteinaemia. *Atherosclerosis* 1976; **24**: 129–40.

131 O'Connor P, Feely J, Shepherd J. New drugs. Lipid lowering drugs. *Br Med J* 1990; **300**: 667–72.

132 Vega GL, Grundy SM. Gemfibrozil therapy in primary hypertriglyceridemia associated with coronary heart

disease. Effects on metabolism of low-density lipoproteins. *J Am Med Ass* 1985; **253**: 2398–403.

133 The Lovastatin Study Group. II: Therapeutic response to lovastatin (mevinolin) in nonfamilial hypercholesterolemia: a multicenter study. *J Am Med Ass* 1986; **256**: 2829–34.

134 Garg A, Grundy SM. Lovastatin for lowering cholesterol levels in non-insulin dependent diabetes mellitus. *N Engl J Med* 1988; **318**: 81–6.

135 East C, Alivizatos PA, Grundy SM, Jones PH, Farmer JA. Rhabdomyolysis in patients receiving lovastatin after cardiac transplantation. *N Engl J Med* 1988; **318**: 47–8.

136 Stirling C, McAleer M, Reckless JPD *et al*. Effects of acipimox, a nicotinic acid derivative, on lipolysis in human adipose tissue and on cholesterol synthesis in human jejunal mucosa. *Clin Sci* 1985; **68**: 83–8.

137 Bain SC, Jones AF, Barnett AH. Acipimox and hypertriglyceridaemia. *Br J Hosp Med* 1990; **43**: 182.

138 Garg A, Grundy SM. Gemfibrozil alone and in combination with lovastatin for treatment of hypertriglyceridemia in NIDDM. *Diabetes* 1989; **38**: 364–72.

139 Horrobin DF. The roles of essential fatty acids in the development of diabetic neuropathy and other complications of diabetes mellitus. *Prostagl Leukotr Essent Fatty Acids: Review 1.* 1988; **31**: 181–97.

140 Axelrod L. Omega-3 fatty acids in diabetes mellitus. Gift from the sea? *Diabetes* 1989; **38**: 539–43.

141 Jensen T, Stender S, Goldstein K, Holmer G, Deckert T. Partial normalization by dietary cod-liver oil of increased microvascular leakage in patients with insulin-dependent diabetes and albuminuria. *N Engl J Med* 1989; **321**: 1572–7.

142 Black SC, Katz S, McNein JH. Cardiac performance and plasma lipids of omega-3 fatty acid-treated streptozocin-induced diabetic rats. *Diabetes* 1989; **38**: 969–74.

143 Glauber H, Wallace P, Griver K *et al*. Adverse metabolic effect of omega-3 fatty acids in non-insulin-dependent diabetes mellitus. *Ann Int Med* 1988; **108**: 663–8.

144 Friday KE, Childs MT, Tsunehara CH, Fujimoto WY, Bierman EL, Ensinck JW. Elevated plasma glucose and lowered triglyceride levels from omega-3-fatty acid supplementation in type II diabetes. *Diabetes Care* 1989; **12**: 276–81.

145 Kasim S, Stern B, Khilnani S, McLin P, Bacionwski S, Jen K-LC. Effects of omega-3 fish oils on lipid metabolism, glycemic control, and blood pressure in type II diabetic patients. *J Clin Endocrinol Metab* 1988; **67**: 1–5.

146 Patterson JW. Effect of a high fat, fructose and casein diet in diabetic cataracts. *Proc Soc Exp Biol Med* 1955; **90**: 706–10.

147 Hutton JC, Schofield PJ, Williams JF *et al*. The effect of an unsaturated fat diet on cataract formation in streptozotocin-induced diabetic rats. *Br J Nutr* 1976; **36**: 161–77.

148 Tomlinson DR, Robinson JP, Compton AM, Keen P. Essential fatty acid treatment-effects on nerve conduction, polyol pathway and axonal transport in streptozotocin diabetic rats. *Diabetologia* 1989; **32**: 655–9.

149 Kinsell LW, Michaels GD, Walker G *et al*. Dietary linoleic acid and linoleate. Effects in diabetic and non-diabetic subjects with and without vascular disease. *Diabetes* 1959; **8**: 179–88.

150 Holltsmuller AJ, van Hal-Ferwerda J, Zahn KJ, Henkes HE. Favourable influences of linoleic acid on the progression of diabetic micro- and macro-angiopathy in adult onset diabetes mellitus. *Progr Lipid Res* 1982; **20**: 377–86.

151 Howard-Williams J, Patel P, Jelfs R *et al*. Polyunsaturated fatty acids and diabetic retinopathy. *Br J Ophthalmol* 1985; **69**: 15–18.

152 Jamal GA, Carmichael HA, Weir AI. Gamma-linolenic acid in diabetic neuropathy. *Lancet* 1986; i: 1098.

153 Jamal GA, Carmichael H. The effect of γ-linolenic acid on human diabetic neuropathy: a double-blind placebo-controlled study. *Diabetic Med* 1990; **7**: 319–23.

105   Glucose Sensors

Summary

• Glucose sensors have potential applications for *in vitro* analysis of blood samples (e.g. in devices for capillary blood glucose self-monitoring, laboratory and ward analyses) and for *in vivo* measurement (e.g. for hypoglycaemia alarms, continuous glucose read-out devices or a wearable artificial endocrine pancreas).

• Most glucose sensors are based on electrodes on which glucose oxidase is immobilized; the oxidation of glucose is detected by monitoring oxygen consumption or hydrogen peroxide production.

• Oxygen-dependence of electrodes can be partially overcome by the newer strategy of mediated electron transfer, in which a low molecular weight redox couple (e.g. ferrocene/ferricinium) is co-immobilized with glucose oxidase and shuttles electrons directly to an underlying electrode.

• Implantable glucose sensors are generally needle-shaped. The subcutaneous tissue is the favoured sensing site as glucose levels here follow those in the blood (albeit with some delay) and the hazards of septicaemia, thrombosis and electrode fouling by blood are avoided.

• *In vivo* glucose sensing in man has been maintained for periods of 1–3 days without electrode replacement. Extension of the technology to reliable applications in routine clinical management of diabetes demands further work in improving sensor stability and biocompatibility.

Glucose sensors belong to a class of measuring devices called 'biosensors', miniature probes or transducers which combine a biological receptor with a detector and generate a specific signal in rapid response to a particular analyte. Biosensors are receiving considerable attention in many fields of medicine [1] and other sciences [2] because they offer a number of potential advantages over many conventional measuring procedures (Table 105.1).

Fig. 105.1 shows the principle of signal generation by a biosensor. Many types of receptor have been employed for different analytes, including antibodies ('immunosensors'), whole cells, bacteria and tissue slices. However, most interest has focused on enzyme electrodes, where the enzyme-catalysed reaction produces a change in potential, current, heat or light which can be detected by an incorporated electrode (for potential and current), thermistor (for heat) or photo detector (for light). Field-effect transistors are a special type of microprocessor-based device for voltage measurements.

The reasons for developing glucose sensors

Like many sensors, glucose transducers can be used either *in vitro* in samples of body fluid such as blood, or *in vivo* as an implantable device (Table 105.2). *In vitro* glucose sensors perform 'one-shot'

Table 105.1. Potential advantages of biosensors.

• Simple to operate
• Cheap to manufacture
• Capable of mass production
• Easy to miniaturize
• Can operate without addition of reagents
• Can operate in turbid or coloured solutions
• Do not require consumption or withdrawal of body fluid (e.g. blood)
• May be operated continuously

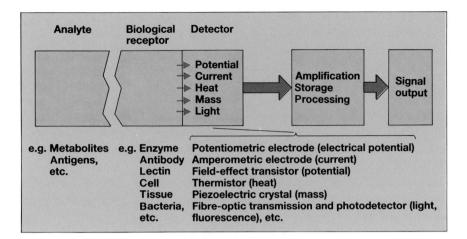

Fig. 105.1. The mode of action of biosensors. Analyte concentrations are measured by its binding to a biological receptor (e.g. an enzyme). A change in electrical potential, current, heat, mass or light is detected and the signal amplified and processed.

Table 105.2. Potential uses for glucose sensors in diabetes.

In vitro sensors	*In vivo* sensors
• Small meter for self-monitoring of capillary blood glucose	• Hypoglycaemia alarm
• Bench-top blood glucose analyser for laboratory, ward, doctor's office, etc.	• Continuous or on-demand read-out of blood or tissue glucose concentrations
• Large-batch automatic glucose analyser for hospital laboratory	• Closed-loop insulin delivery system
	• Short-term continuous blood glucose monitoring (*ex vivo*?) for surgery, intensive care, etc.

analyses and might therefore be useful for capillary blood glucose self-monitoring or to produce smaller, cheaper or more efficient laboratory analysers. Implantable glucose sensors naturally bring to mind the goal of constructing a closed-loop insulin delivery system — a wearable artificial pancreas (see Chapter 43) — but there are several other applications which are now technically more feasible and of at least equal clinical priority (Table 105.2).

Hypoglycaemia is a common, potentially hazardous and much-feared complication of insulin treatment (see Chapter 50). A hypoglycaemia alarm which was activated at a preset glucose level and which operated during an 8–12 h period (e.g.

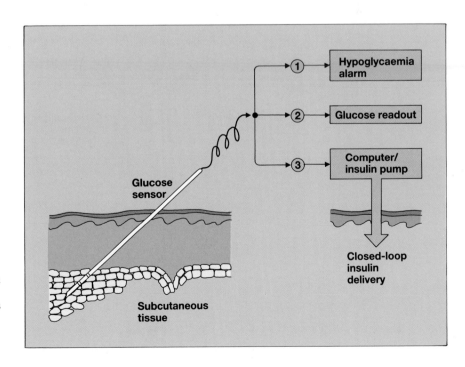

Fig. 105.2. Principal configurations for an implantable glucose sensor. The favoured sensing site is the subcutaneous tissue. The signal can be used as a hypoglycaemia alarm, as a direct read-out of glucose levels or could be coupled to an insulin pump for feedback-controlled insulin delivery.

overnight) would be clinically very valuable, especially for those patients who have lost the warning symptoms of hypoglycaemia [3].

Such a device could probably be constructed in the near future, given the present performance and stability of sensors during continuous measurement. A continuous or on-demand read-out of glucose levels *in vivo* would clearly aid insulin dosage adjustment and warn against dangerous hyperglycaemia and indicate the need for ketone body testing. Short-term continuous blood glucose sensing may be of value in diabetic patients during surgery or intensive care and, for such limited periods of time, blood could be passed into a flow-through cell where glucose levels may be measured *ex vivo*.

Glucose sensor technology

Most glucose sensors are enzyme electrodes in which glucose oxidase is immobilized over the electrode by methods such as adsorption, entrapment in gels, cross-linking with agents such as glutaraldehyde, covalent attachment or encapsulation behind a membrane. The reaction catalysed by the enzyme is:

$$\text{glucose} + O_2 \xrightarrow{\text{glucose oxidase}} \text{gluconic acid} + H_2O_2$$

and the ambient glucose concentration can be monitored by detecting changes in oxygen consumption [4–6], hydrogen peroxide (H_2O_2) pro-

duction [7–10] or H^+ generation (which is little used) [11]. Two common configurations are shown in Fig. 105.3. In one, (a) increasing glucose levels are signalled by the decrease in oxygen detected by an underlying platinum cathode which acts as an oxygen electrode. By contrast, the other type of sensor, (b) measures glucose concentrations as proportional changes in hydrogen peroxide production, as detected by a platinum anode. Both of these sensors are *amperometric* devices, i.e. they measure a current flow which is proportional to glucose concentrations:

$$O_2 + 4e^- + 4H^+ \xrightarrow{-700\,\text{mV}} 2H_2O$$

$$H_2O_2 \xrightarrow{+700\,\text{mV}} O_2 + 2H^+ + 2e^-$$

An alternative is to measure pH changes, reflecting the production of gluconic acid, by immobilizing glucose oxidase over a hydrogen ion-selective electrode. This measurement is *potentiometric*, registering a voltage change according to the Nernst equation:

$$E = E^o + \frac{RT}{nF} \ln (\text{analyte})$$

Where E = the voltage change, E^o = a constant for the system, R = the gas constant, T = the absolute temperature, n = the charge number, and F = the Faraday constant. As the potential change is proportional to the logarithm of the

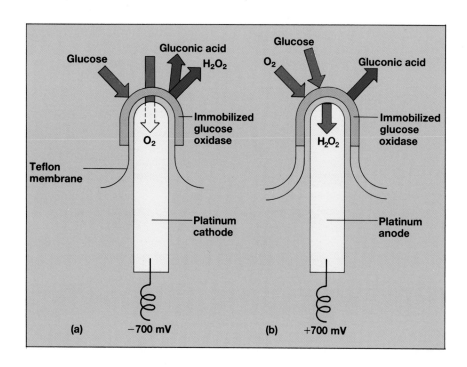

Fig. 105.3. Amperometric enzyme electrodes for glucose sensing. (a) mode of action of sensors based on monitoring oxygen consumption; (b) mode of action of sensors based on hydrogen peroxide production.

analyte activity, such sensors are relatively insensitive and are currently less favoured.

An important difficulty associated with glucose oxidase-based sensors is their variation in signal output with changes in oxygen tension. This problem is particularly relevant to *in vivo* glucose detection, where glucose levels are in molar excess over those of oxygen by several orders of magnitude. Oxygen concentrations are therefore rate-limiting and small changes may profoundly affect the sensing system. At sensing sites such as in subcutaneous tissue (see below) the oxygen tension may be less than in blood and subject to variations with the metabolic status of the diabetic patient.

Electrodes may be made less sensitive to oxygen changes by two main methods. The first is to coat the sensor with a thin hydrophobic membrane such as nylon or polyurethane which is more permeable to oxygen than glucose, thereby increasing the O_2:glucose ratio at the electrode [12]. The second strategy, employed in recent years, is to co-immobilize the enzyme with a low-molecular weight 'mediator' which acts as an alternative electron acceptor to oxygen [13–15]. Ferrocene (dicyclopentadienyl iron) with its cation, ferricinium$^+$, was one of the first redox couples to be used in mediated electron transfer sensors (Fig. 105.4). Oxidized glucose oxidase accepts electrons from glucose and transfers them to ferricinium$^+$. The latter is reoxidized to ferrocene by the transfer of electrons to the base electrode. The technology of ferrocene-based glucose sensing has been ex-

ploited in a pen-sized commercial meter for capillary blood glucose self-monitoring (Fig. 105.5). A similar system configured as a needle sensor is currently undergoing trials to assess its suitability for *in vivo* glucose monitoring (see below) [14, 15].

Of the many other published techniques for glucose sensing, fibreoptic probe systems deserve particular mention as they present the advantages of freedom from electrical interference, absence of reference electrodes and ease of miniaturization. An example is the bioaffinity fibreoptic glucose

Table 105.3. Possible reasons for sensor drift *in vivo*. (Adapted from [21].)

Sensor component	Reason for drift
• Base sensor	• Conduction changes, leakage of mediator or other chemical modification
• Transducer layer	• Leakage or denaturation of enzyme
• Effect of body on sensor	• Protein coating, encapsulation of cells, digestion or denaturation of enzyme, membrane permeability changes
• Effect of sensor on body	• Inflammation, infection, local and systemic toxicity, allergic responses, haemorrhage, cell damage

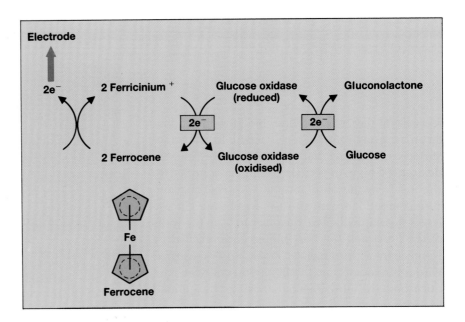

Fig. 105.4. Mediated electron transfer using ferrocene. The molecular structure of ferrocene is also shown.

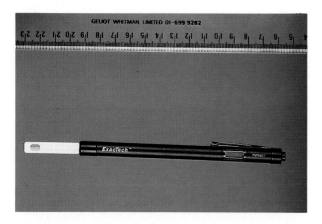

Fig. 105.5. A pen-sized glucose meter employing a ferrocene-mediated glucose sensor (ExacTech, MediSense Inc).

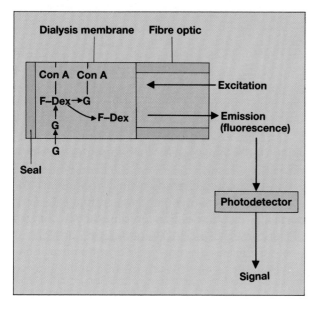

Fig. 105.6. The bioaffinity glucose sensor. Con A = concanavalin A, F-Dex = fluoresceinated dextran, G = glucose. (Adapted from [21].)

sensor [16] (Fig. 105.6). Here, the glucose-binding lectin, concanavalin A, is attached to the inner surface of a hollow dialysis fibre. Fluoresceinated dextran of high molecular weight is confined to the inside of the fibre and binds to concanavalin A in competition with glucose. Increasing glucose levels therefore displace the dextran from the walls of the fibre, and the free fluorescence (elicited by stimulation with ultraviolet radiation) is measured with a photodetector; the fibreoptic pathway conducts both the ultraviolet radiation and the emitted fluorescence.

Implantable glucose sensors

The only glucose sensors to have undergone extensive testing in man are amperometric enzyme electrodes based on hydrogen peroxide detection [8, 17] or mediated electron transfer [15]. The devices are still at an experimental stage and not likely to be transferred to routine patient care within the next 5 to 10 years.

Most implantable glucose electrodes have been constructed as a needle, with the sensing element at the tip or the side (Fig. 105.7). This configuration is thought to be more biocompatible than, for example, a disc [18] and is easily inserted into the subcutaneous tissue, which is the currently favoured sensing site. Implantation into the bloodstream risks infection and thrombosis, and sensors here are also rapidly fouled by blood proteins and platelet deposition. Many studies in animals and man [8, 10, 14, 15] show that changes in interstitial fluid glucose concentrations, as measured by subcutaneously implanted sensors, follow changes in blood glucose. However, there are generally delays in the peak subcutaneous responses registered after glucose administration or in the signal decline after injecting insulin (Figs 105.8 and 105.9). Moreover, sensor-recorded subcutaneous glucose levels are usually between 20 and 90% of simultaneously measured blood glucose levels (Fig. 105.9). As there is evidence that the true subcutaneous interstitial glucose levels are almost the same as those in blood [19], it is probable that, for unknown reasons, the calibration of most sensors is affected by *in vivo* operation.

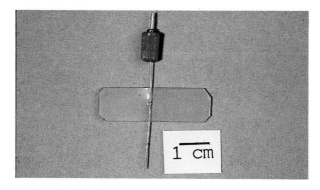

Fig. 105.7. A needle-type glucose sensor suitable for implantation in the subcutaneous tissue. A platinum wire acts as a base electrode and is coated at the tip with glucose oxidase. H_2O_2 generation is detected as a current by the positively charged platinum electrode.

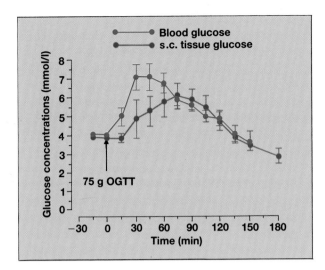

Fig. 105.8. Mean ± SEM blood glucose levels and sensor-measured subcutaneous glucose values in six normal subjects given a 75 g oral glucose load at time 0. Note delay in peak response of sensor glucose recordings, which were calibrated by setting the baseline current at the simultaneously measured blood glucose value. (Adapted from [15].)

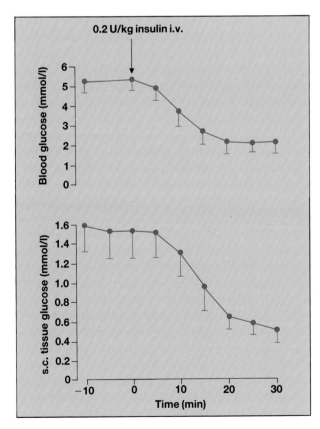

Fig. 105.9. Mean ± SEM blood glucose levels (upper) and sensor-measured subcutaneous tissue glucose levels (lower) in pigs given 0.2 U/kg short-acting insulin as an intravenous bolus at time 0. Note that tissue glucose levels are apparently about one-fifth of blood levels. (Adapted from [14].)

Needle-type glucose sensors based on hydrogen peroxide detection have been operated in the subcutaneous tissue of IDDM patients for up to a few days and have been linked to an insulin pump as a wearable artificial pancreas [17]. However, many implanted sensors suffer unpredictable drift in their output and have to be replaced at intervals of 2–3 days. Identifying the causes of this drift and ways to avoid it are currently central problems in sensor research. For ferrocene-based glucose electrodes, high-density covalent attachment of the enzyme to the sensor improves stability [20] and allows reliable *in vivo* operation in man over the course of a working day [15]. However, the effects of sensors on the body, and of the body on the sensor, is a complicated and largely unexplored area and is almost certainly a major determinant of instability in implanted electrodes [21]. Table 105.3 lists some possible influences of biocompatibility on sensor performance *in vivo*.

Conclusions

Glucose sensors are already used in clinical practice as blood glucose meters for self-monitoring of capillary blood. However, the extension of this technology to reliable implantable devices requires much further study in the area of biocompatibility.

JOHN C. PICKUP

References

1 Pickup JC. Biosensors: a clinical perspective. *Lancet* 1985; ii: 817–20.
2 Turner APF, Karube I, Wilson GS, eds. *Biosensors: Fundamentals and Applications.* Oxford: Oxford University Press, 1987.
3 Anonymous. Awareness of hypoglycaemia in diabetes. *Lancet* 1987; ii: 371–2.
4 Updike SJ, Hicks GP. The enzyme electrode. *Nature* 1967; **214**: 986–8.
5 Bessman SP, Thomas LJ, Kojima H, Sayler DF, Layne EG. The implantation of a closed-loop artificial beta cell in dogs. *Trans Am Soc Art Int Org* 1981; **27**: 7–17.
6 Gough DA, Lucisano JY, Tse PHS. Two-dimensional enzyme electrode sensor for glucose. *Anal Chem* 1985; **57**: 2351–7.
7 Clark LC, Duggan CA. Implanted electroenzymatic glucose sensors. *Diabetes Care* 1982; **5**: 174–80.
8 Shichiri M, Kawamori R, Yamasaki T, Hakui N, Abe H. Wearable-type artificial pancreas with needle-type glucose sensor. *Lancet* 1982; ii: 1129–31.
9 Churchouse SJ, Battersby CM, Mullen WH, Vadgama PM. Needle enzyme electrodes for biological studies. *Biosensors* 1986; **2**: 325–42.
10 Abel P, Muller A, Fischer U. Experience with an implantable glucose sensor as a prerequisite of an artificial beta cell. *Biomed Biochim Acta* 1984: **5**: 577–84.

11 Caras SD, Petelenz DL, Janata J. pH-based enzyme poten-tiometric sensors. Part 2. Glucose-sensitive field effect tran-sistor. *Anal Chem* 1985; **57**: 1920−3.

12 Updike SJ, Shults M, Ekman B. Implanting the glucose enzyme electrode: problems, progress and alternative sol-utions. *Diabetes Care* 1982; **5**: 207−12.

13 Cass AEG, Davis G, Francis CD, Hill HAD, Aston WJ, Higgins IJ, Plotkin EV, Scott LDL, Turner APF. Ferrocene-mediated enzyme electrode for amperometric determination of glucose. *Anal Chem* 1984; **56**: 667−71.

14 Claremont DJ, Sambrook IE, Penton C, Pickup JC. Sub-cutaneous implantation of a ferrocene-mediated glucose sensor in pigs. *Diabetologia* 1986; **29**: 817−21.

15 Pickup JC, Shaw GW, Claremont DJ. *In vivo* molecular sensing in diabetes mellitus: an implantable glucose sensor with direct electron transfer. *Diabetologia* 1989; **32**: 213−17.

16 Mansouri S, Schultz JS. A miniature optical glucose sensor based on affinity binding. *Biotechnology* 1984; **2**: 885−90.

17 Shichiri M, Kawamori R, Hakui N, Yamasaki Y, Abe H. Closed-loop glycemic control with a wearable artificial endocrine pancreas. *Diabetes* 1984; **33**: 1200−2.

18 Woodward SC. How fibroblasts and giant cells encapsulate implants: considerations in design of glucose sensors. *Dia-betes Care* 1982; 278−81.

19 Fischer U, Ertle R, Abel P *et al*. Assessment of subcutaneous glucose concentration: validation of the wick technique as a reference for implanted electrochemical sensors. *Dia-betologia* 1987; **30**: 940−5.

20 Pickup JC, Shaw GW, Claremont DJ. Potentially-implant-able, amperometric glucose sensors with mediated electron transfer: improving the operating stability. *Biosensors* 1989; **4**: 109−19.

21 Pickup JC. Biosensors for diabetes mellitus. In: Wise DL, ed. *Applied Biosensors*. Butterworths: Boston, 1989: 227−47.

106   Transplantation of the Endocrine Pancreas

Summary

● Vascularized organ allograft (whole pancreas or segments) is the only clinical approach to transplantation at present and is restricted to diabetic patients in end-stage renal failure, who therefore need kidney transplantation and immunosuppression.

● Techniques involve systemic and portal insulin delivery and either pancreatic duct occlusion or drainage into the stomach, intestine, or bladder.

● About 300 transplants were reported in 1987 with an overall 1-year patient survival of 84% and graft survival of 47% (higher in some centres).

● Pancreas transplantation is a major operation with considerable morbidity from thrombosis, pancreatitis and peritonitis.

● Isolated islet or fetal pancreas transplantation may be suitable future approaches as the transplant operation is minor and the tissues could be subjected to immunomodulation, reducing the need for immunosuppression and allowing transplantation earlier in the disease.

● Islets may be pretreated to remove or inactivate the passenger leucocytes which may provoke the immune response, or encapsulated in membranes to protect the islet tissue from immune damage.

● Transplantation of the fetal pancreas of a suitable gestational age allows replication of pancreatic B cells whilst the undifferentiated exocrine tissue atrophies.

● There is very little experience to date of islet or fetal pancreatic transplantation in human diabetes.

The rationale of attempts to transplant the endocrine pancreas is that successful transplantation would correct the metabolic abnormalities of IDDM sufficiently to avoid the acute metabolic complications of the disease and, more importantly, to halt the progression or even cause regression of its microangiopathic complications. These objectives have been realized in experimental animal models of diabetes. In particular, there is evidence that the early changes of retinopathy or nephropathy in diabetic rats will regress after successful transplantation of the endocrine pancreas, even as late as 2 years after the induction of diabetes [1]. In man, however, the case has not yet been proven, although encouraging results have been obtained. Kidneys transplanted into patients with diabetic nephropathy display early nephropathic changes after several years when biopsied at the time of a pancreatic transplant, but the lesions do not progress after a successful pancreatic transplant [2]. In addition, electron microscopic examination of biopsies from transplanted kidneys in IDDM patients showed an increase in glomerular basement membrane thickening in those patients without a functioning pancreatic graft, whereas those with a successful transplant did not develop these changes [3]. The ability of prolonged euglycaemia to reverse nephropathic changes is also illustrated by a case report in which a kidney from an IDDM cadaveric donor was inadvertently transplanted into a non-diabetic recipient. Initially, the kidney was found to show histological features of diabetic nephropathy, which had regressed in a subsequent biopsy 7 months later [4].

On the other hand, there is conflicting evidence from cohorts of patients in several major

1001

centres who have had a functioning, vascularized pancreatic graft for several years and who had either retinopathy or neuropathy at the time of transplantation. An improvement in retinopathy following successful pancreatic transplantation was reported by one group but not by another [5, 6]. A further centre has failed to find any improvement in diabetic neuropathy despite successful transplantation [7].

It could be argued that most of the patients currently considered for transplantation have severe microvascular complications which are likely to be irreversible by the time that transplantation is performed. At present, however, transplantation of a vascularized pancreatic graft (currently the only practicable option in man) cannot be justified earlier in the disease when its microvascular complications are mild, not only because of the risks of the procedure but also because of the need for continuing immunosuppression. Moreover, certain technical complications (e.g. graft thrombosis) are likely to be commoner in non-uraemic recipients. For these reasons, the use of pancreatic transplantation in its current form will be largely restricted to IDDM patients with end-stage kidney failure who also need a kidney transplant and hence immunosuppression. Another indication is in patients who have undergone total pancreatectomy, where restoration of pancreatic enzymes to drain into the gut confers an additional advantage. Transplantation of the endocrine pancreas at a relatively early stage in the course of the disease will depend on advances in two relatively new transplantation methods, using either fetal pancreas or adult isolated islets. In both these approaches, the transplantation procedure itself will be minor, and it is possible that the immunogenicity of the transplanted tissue might be modified such that only minimal immunosuppression will be needed. These various options will now be discussed in detail.

Pancreatic transplantation as a vascularized graft

Development

The pioneer attempts in this field were made in 1966 by Lillehei and his colleagues in Minneapolis, when the whole organ with a loop of duodenum was transplanted into patients with diabetic nephropathy at the same time as a kidney graft [8]. Although poor, the results demonstrated that it was possible for an IDDM patient to survive without exogenous insulin. Interest in pancreatic transplantation waned until 1978 when Dubernard et al. [9] described a technique of blocking the pancreatic duct with neoprene before transplanting the tail and body of the pancreas, in order to prevent the potential complications of the exocrine drainage of the transplanted gland. The development of cyclosporin further stimulated interest, and some 1200 transplants have been performed during the last decade, nearly 300 in 1987. Nevertheless, although improving, the results remain relatively poor in comparison with those of the more established transplantation of the kidney, heart and liver. As the procedure is not performed for an acutely life-threatening disease, it is understandable why its place in the management of diabetes remains controversial.

Surgical techniques

The surgical techniques available for transplanting part or all of the pancreas as a vascularized organ are shown in Table 106.1 (see also Fig. 106.1). The pancreatic vasculature is usually anastomosed to the iliac vessels, the organ being placed either intraperitoneally or (now uncommonly) extraperitoneally in the false pelvis. In both these locations, insulin is secreted into the systemic venous system, which, as with conventional insulin treatment, causes systemic hyperinsulinaemia and the theoretical risk of vascular disease. Calne et al. and Sutherland et al. have achieved physiological portal venous drainage of insulin, which avoids this problem, by anastomosing the portal vein of the pancreatic graft to either the splenic vein [10] or the inferior mesenteric vein [11]. An important technical problem is the disposal of the exocrine secretion of the transplanted pancreas without causing tissue damage due to autodigestion. A widely used approach is to occlude the duct with glues such as neoprene or prolamine. Alternatively, pancreatic exocrine secretions can be drained into a Roux-en-Y loop of small bowel, or a ureter, the bladder or stomach; drainage of the pancreatic duct surrounded by a button or loop of retained duodenum into the bladder has become increasingly popular [12] (see Fig. 106.1). More recently, the whole organ rather than a segment of distal pancreas has been grafted in an attempt to increase the islet-cell mass transplanted.

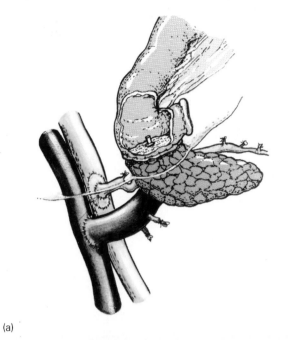

(a)

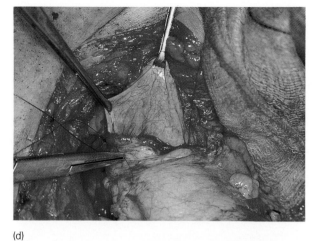

(d)

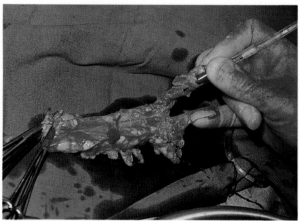

(b)

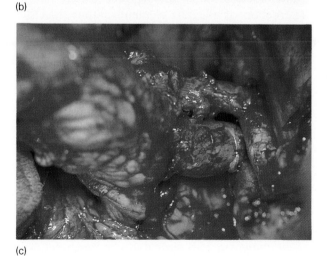

(c)

(e)

Fig. 106.1. (a) Diagram of segmental pancreatic transplant draining into the jejunum. (Reproduced with permission of the artist Jack Bridger-Chalker.) (b–e) Segmental pancreas transplant draining into the bladder.

(b) The segmental pancreas transplant after removal from the cadaver being perfused with hypertonic citrate. The cannula is inserted in the coeliac artery which is taken with a patch of aorta for easier anastomosis. The portal vein is also seen.

(c) The pancreatic vessels have now been anastomosed to the recipient's blood supply: the portal vein drains end to side to the external iliac vein, and the coeliac artery arises from the external iliac artery.

(d) Pancreatic-cystostomy: the posterior layer of the cystotomy (hole in the bladder) has been anastomosed with catgut to the posterior edge of the pancreas, which was divided at its neck. The anterior layer is about to be closed, with care to ensure that the stitches do not encroach on the duct.

(e) The pancreatic transplant completed just prior to closure of the wound. The bladder is on the left and a well-perfused, slightly oedematous, pancreatic transplant lies horizontally across the picture. (Photographs and legends kindly provided by Mr Robert Sells, Royal Liverpool Hospital.)

Table 106.1. Techniques used to transplant the pancreas as a vascularized organ allograft.

Segmental pancreas	Blocked duct: • neoprene • latex • silicone • ethibloc Drainage to: • stomach • intestine (Roux loop) • bladder • ureter
Whole pancreas (with button or loop of duodenum)	Drainage to: • intestine (Roux loop) • bladder

Immunosuppression

All current immunosuppressive protocols are based on cyclosporin, which is probably partly (but not totally) responsible for the improved success of transplantation since its advent. Most units now use triple-therapy protocols, comprising low doses of cyclosporin, prednisolone and azathioprine. Cyclosporin is used only at low dosages because it has been demonstrated to be toxic to rodent B cells; attempts are being made to develop related drugs which do not share this unfortunate side-effect (see Chapter 104).

Graft rejection

PATHOLOGY

Rejection of vascularized pancreas grafts predominantly affects the exocrine pancreas which shows vascular changes including fibrinoid necrosis and arteriolar thrombosis, the islets being relatively spared. Acute rejection reactions may affect a kidney transplanted simultaneously, with little evidence of the same event occurring in the endocrine pancreas; much less frequently, the pancreatic graft, but not the kidney, may be rejected.

DIAGNOSIS

Rejection is difficult to diagnose histologically, as pancreatic grafts placed in the pelvis can only be biopsied at laparotomy. Biopsies of grafts draining into the stomach have been taken through a gastroscope, and the use of fine-needle aspiration biopsy has been investigated experimentally.

Abnormal elevations of postprandial blood glucose levels may indicate early rejection, but fasting hyperglycaemia appears late, when rejection is usually irreversible. The development of the bladder drainage technique has provided a very useful way of monitoring graft viability, as the amylase activity of the urine (which is easily measured) has been found to fall markedly during a rejection episode. Other techniques, such as demonstrating increased accumulation of radio-labelled platelets or a decrease in the uptake of selenium by the graft, may also be useful in detecting rejection.

Recurrence of disease

The transplanted pancreas might be vulnerable to the same autoimmune damage which originally caused IDDM in the recipient. That this may occur is illustrated by the few cases of pancreatic transplantation performed between identical twins [13]. Without immunosuppression, technically successful pancreas transplantation was followed within several weeks by recurrent hyperglycaemia. Biopsy of the pancreas revealed a marked insulitis consistent with disease recurrence. Subsequently, the use of immunosuppressive drugs seems to have prevented diabetes from recurring in identical twin pancreas transplants. This human experiment suggests that the immune destruction of the islets is HLA-restricted. Whether the endocrine failure of some pancreas grafts after several years is due to chronic rejection or disease recurrence remains uncertain, although histological examination of such failed grafts usually shows destruction of all graft elements rather than the selective B-cell loss characteristic of acute IDDM.

Results

PATIENT AND GRAFT SURVIVAL

The invaluable International Registry of pancreatic transplants maintained by Sutherland at Minneapolis shows that both patient and graft survival results have continued to improve; overall, patient survival at 1 year is 84% and graft survival 47% [14]. However, individual units have higher graft survival figures of 70–80% at 1 year. The survival of the pancreas graft appears to be much better if transplanted either simultaneously with or after a kidney than if transplanted alone, when the majority of grafts appear to be lost from rejection relatively early in the course of the graft.

MORBIDITY AND MORTALITY

Mortality directly related to the transplant procedure is now modest and probably acceptable, bearing in mind that many, if not most, of these patients would be considered high-risk patients for any type of surgery. However the associated morbidity is considerable, often catastrophic and can lead to the death of the patient. Complications include vascular thrombosis, pancreatitis, exocrine leakage with peritonitis and fistulae and, in the case of bladder drainage of the pancreatic duct, hyperchloraemic acidosis due to losses of bicarbonate-rich pancreatic secretions.

METABOLIC RESULTS

Successful vascularized pancreas transplants can maintain normal fasting and nearly normal postprandial blood glucose concentrations, being the only transplantation method so far able to achieve this in man [15]. The response to a glucose challenge can be normal or nearly so, and elevated HbA_1 levels return to normal. There is no convincing evidence that one technique has an advantage over any other, although the physiological delivery of insulin into the portal system confers the theoretical advantage of avoiding systemic hyperinsulinaemia.

Pancreatic islet transplantation

Development

The specific transplantation of islets isolated from the intact pancreas is obviously an attractive concept, as it would be a relatively safe procedure and would avoid problems associated with pancreatic exocrine tissue. Moreover, it might also allow immunomodulation of the islets before transplantation, as well as their long-term preservation after harvesting.

A technique to isolate islets from the guinea pig pancreas using collagenase digestion was described by Moskalewski as long ago as 1965 [16]. Several years later, Ballinger and Lacy described another collagenase-based technique for isolating pure islets from the rat pancreas in relatively large numbers and for their successful transplantation into diabetic rats [17]. This method, with various modifications, was until recently the standard technique for experimental islet isolation and transplantation in rodents.

Transplantation of isolated pancreatic islets has been shown to correct streptozotocin- or alloxan-induced diabetes in the mouse and rat, and this model has allowed many of the physiological and immunological problems of islet transplantation to be explored [18].

However, attempts to apply the same techniques which have proved so satisfactory in the rodent to the pancreas of larger mammals, including man, were initially less successful. It was not possible to isolate more than a few hundred islets from human pancreas until Gray and colleagues suggested that collagenase should be injected into the pancreatic duct [19], rather than exposed to chopped pancreas or injected by other routes. This procedure is now generally used to prepare islets from the human pancreas and from other large mammals, such as the monkey [20] and dog [21]; high yields from mouse [22] and rat [23] have also been reported. Following successful studies in animals, clinical trials of pancreatic islet transplantation have now been cautiously started in a few centres. In addition, human islets have been provided for research into physiological and immunological problems in human diabetes. The development of islet isolation methods is reviewed in detail elsewhere [18].

At present, the most satisfactory technique for isolating islets from large animal and human pancreas involves injecting collagenase at 39°C into the pancreatic duct [19], followed by purification of the digest by filtration and/or centrifugation on well-defined density gradients [24, 25]. Around 2000 islets can be isolated from 1 g of pancreas, with up to 70% purity. Fig. 106.2(a) and (b) shows human islets isolated by this technique and stained with supravital dyes [26]. Fig. 106.3(a) and (b) shows islets similarly isolated from normal cynomolgus monkey pancreas, immunostained for both insulin and glucagon to show that normal islet organization is preserved.

Sites of implantation

Islets were first transplanted into the peritoneal cavity [17]. Subsequently, successful implantation has been described in the liver (either through the portal vein [27] or by direct injection [28]) and other sites, including the spleen [29], under the kidney capsule [30], testis [31], omentum [32] and cerebral ventricles [33]. Although there is some evidence that sites draining into the portal vein, such as the liver or spleen, are physiologically

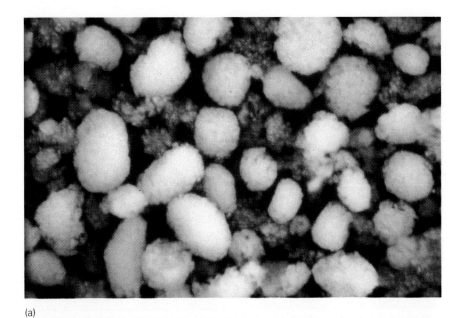

(a)

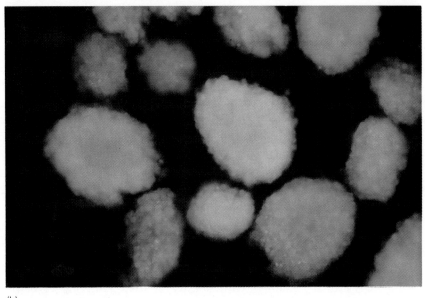

(b)

Fig. 106.2. Human pancreatic islets isolated by ductal injection of collagenase: (a) islets stained with the supravital dye dithizone, which has stained islet tissue pink (×180). (b) islets stained with the supravital dye fluorescein diacetate, which has stained all viable tissue green. (×450).

more satisfactory than those with systemic drainage such as the kidney capsule [34], the latter can still allow excellent function of islet implants. Successful implantation apparently depends on the vascularity of the site, which probably explains the failure of implantation into muscle or subcutaneous tissue. The purity of the preparation also determines the outcome of implantation, at least for the kidney capsule site, where appreciable exocrine contamination prevents successful implantation [35].

Reversal of diabetes

Syngeneic islet transplantation has successfully reversed streptozotocin-induced diabetes in rodents and diabetes induced by total pancreatectomy in larger animals such as dogs and primates. Successful transplantation normalizes fasting glycaemia and nearly normalizes the islet-cell responses to intravenous glucose challenge. In our laboratories, primates have maintained fasting normoglycaemia for over 3 years after total pancreatectomy and subsequent autotransplantation

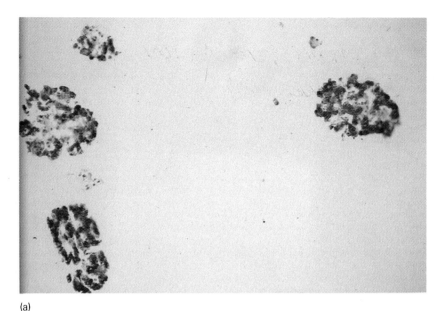

(a)

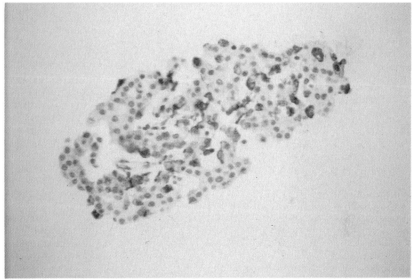

Fig. 106.3. Cynomolgus monkey pancreatic islets isolated by ductal injection of collagenase: (a) islets fixed in formalin and subsequently stained for insulin using a two-layer immunoperoxidase technique (×375); (b) as (a), but stained for glucagon (×600).

(b)

of isolated islets. Their insulin and glucagon responses to glucose and arginine challenge are qualitatively near normal, although quantitatively depressed, presumably because the transplanted islet mass is inadequate [36]. Fig. 106.4 illustrates typical plasma glucose, insulin and glucagon changes during a 500 mg/kg intravenous glucose tolerance test in normal cynomolgus monkeys, and in islet-grafted animals 3 months after total pancreatectomy and islet autotransplantation.

Streptozotocin-diabetic rats develop histological changes in the kidney similar to those of early human diabetic nephropathy and some features of autonomic neuropathy. These early changes can be halted or even reversed by successful islet transplantation [37, 38], although whether advanced changes are reversible in the rat remains controversial [37, 39].

Allogeneic transplantation and rejection

Allogeneic islet transplants in rodents behave as if they were highly immunogenic, rejection occurring within 4–8 days [40]. Allogeneic islet rejection has proved difficult to prevent, even with various immunosuppressive protocols which are particularly effective in the same species for vascularized organ transplants, such as the kidney and heart (Table 106.2). Recently, long-term survival of allografted islets has been obtained using

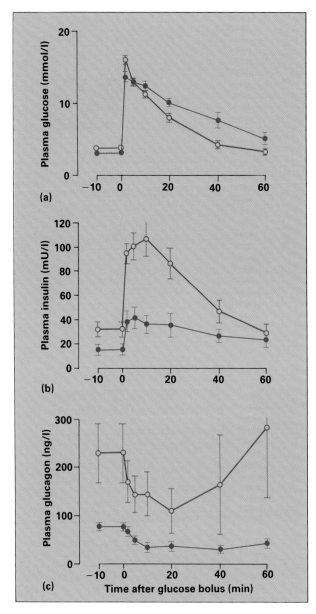

Fig. 106.4. Plasma glucose (a), insulin (b) and glucagon (c) changes during a 500 mg/kg intravenous glucose tolerance test in 13 normal cynomolgus monkeys ○ and in five cynomoglus monkeys 3 months after total pancreatectomy and intraportal islet autotransplantation ●

method involves transplantation of allogeneic islets into a diabetic recipient already bearing a kidney allograft from the same donor strain as the islet donor [45, 58]. This second approach could be used clinically provided that satisfactory cryo-preservation of human islets is possible: islets harvested from the donor of a kidney given to a patient with diabetic nephropathy could be preserved and transplanted into the same diabetic recipient at a later date, assuming that the kidney had not been rejected in the interim.

More recently, there has been considerable interest in the possibility of modulating the immunogenicity of islets before transplantation. The aim has been to remove or inactivate the passenger leucocytes (thought to be dendritic cells) which apparently play a major role in mediating the immune response to the allograft. In selected strain combinations in rodents, islet allograft survival has been strikingly prolonged by various manoeuvres which inactivate putative dendritic cells, namely pretreatment with anti-dendritic-cell antibody and complement [59], prolonged culture in high O_2 tension [60] or at low temperatures [61], or ultraviolet or X-ray irradiation [62–64].

It has also proved difficult to prevent rejection of islet allografts in larger species, although relatively few studies have used modern preparations of relatively pure islets rather than dispersed pancreas. Alejandro and colleagues [21] have reported extended survival of islet allografts in dogs with cyclosporin as the sole immunosuppressive agent, although most recipients became diabetic again when the drug was withdrawn. The same group also suggest that pretreatment of islets in the dog with anti-class II antibody and a period in culture prolongs the survival of allogeneic islets (D.H. Mintz, personal communication).

Another interesting approach is the use of artificial membranes to encapsulate allogeneic islets, both to prevent the induction of an immune response in the recipient and to protect them from cellular and humoral immune attack. Islets enclosed in recently described microcapsules of sodium alginate appear to survive in culture and respond to glucose and, when implanted into diabetic mice, have corrected diabetes for several weeks or months [65, 66]. Failure ultimately occurs due to an intense fibrous reaction encasing the microcapsules, but this can be delayed by the use of steroids (G. Eisenbarth, personal communication).

intramuscular cyclosporin administration [55]. The rejection of allogeneic islets has been shown to be exquisitely specific [56]. Two approaches developed in our laboratories have allowed indefinite survival of allogeneic islets in the rat. In the first (which is not clinically applicable), islets are initially implanted beneath the kidney capsule of a syngeneic recipient for at least 24 h before transplanting the kidney with the islets as a vascularized graft into an allogeneic recipient which is given a short course of cyclosporin [57]. The second

Table 106.2. Results of recipient treatments given to prevent rejection of islets allografted intraportally across major histocompatibility barriers into streptozotocin-induced (>150 mg/kg) diabetic rats. Mean or median graft survivals are given in days; rejection was taken to have occurred when serum glucose levels exceeded 14 mmol/l (11 mmol/l in some studies).

Authors	Donor	Recipient	Treatment	Graft survival (days)
Reckard et al. 1981 [41]	Lewis × BN	Lewis	Donor cells + anti-donor antibody on day −11	8
Selawry & Mui 1983 [42]	ACI	Wistar–Lewis	Wistar–Lewis blood × 3, anti-lymphocyte serum on day 1	>100
Hardy et al. 1984 [43]	Lewis	ACI	UV irradiated blood on days −21, −14, −7	>100
Nash et al. 1978 [44]	AS × August	AS	Long-term AS × August heart allograft in situ	2
Reckard et al. 1981 [41]	Lewis × BN	Lewis	Long-term Lewis × BN kidney allograft in situ	8
Gray et al. 1984 [45]	Lewis (or PVG)	DA	Long-term Lewis (or PVG) kidney allograft in situ	>100
Reece-Smith et al. 1981 [46]	Lewis	DA	Silica on day −6	6
Nash & Bell 1984 [47]	Wagola	AS	Silica on day −6, then cyclosporin and anti-lymphocyte serum	74
Finch & Morris 1976 [48]	DA × Lewis	DA	Anti-donor antibody on day 1	34
Finch & Morris 1977 [49]	DA	Lewis	Anti-lymphocyte serum on days 1, 2, 3, 4	26
Tze & Tai 1984 [50]	Lewis	ACI	Single islet-cell graft and anti-lymphocyte serum on day 1	>100
Beyer & Friedman 1979 [51]	Wistar–Furth	Lewis	Antithymocyte globulin on days 1, 2, 3	12
Vialettes et al. 1979 [52]	Wistar	Lewis	10 mg/kg/day cyclosporin on days 1−14	23
Reece-Smith et al. 1983 [53]	DA	Lewis	Composite islet/liver graft and 10 mg/kg/day cyclosporin on days 1−14	>26
Kakizaki et al. 1987 [54]	Lewis	ACI	Donor antigen on day −1, 10 mg/kg/day cyclosporin weekly × 3	58

Transplantation in the spontaneous diabetes of the rodent

Two models of spontaneous diabetes resembling human IDDM have been described in rodents (see Chapter 17). The Bio-Breeding (BB) rat develops marked insulitis which is under the control of at least 3 genes; one of these is linked to the major histocompatibility complex (MHC) [67]. This appears to be an autoimmune disease, in that immunosuppression with anti-lymphocyte serum, cyclosporin or monoclonal antibodies to T-cell populations will prevent its development [68, 69]. The other model is the non-obese diabetic (NOD) mouse, which also displays pronounced insulitis and apparently autoimmune diabetes which is genetically determined by a gene associated with the MHC [70, 71]. The development of the disease in NOD mice can also be prevented by immunosuppression with cyclosporin or anti-T-cell monoclonal antibodies [72, 73].

Islets which are MHC identical to the recipient develop insulitis when transplanted into diabetic BB rats or NOD mice and the disease recurs [74]. Some groups have also described recurrent disease in MHC-disparate animals where rejection has been prevented [75]. To exclude the possibility that this is due to an allogeneic response against minor histocompatibility antigens, BB rats have been made tolerant to donor-strain tissues by neonatal injection of donor-strain bone marrow. Subsequent transplantation of MHC-identical islets led to recurrent disease in animals with spontaneous diabetes but not in non-diabetic BB rats made diabetic with streptozotocin. Similar experiments in NOD mice also confirm that syngeneic islets transplanted into the diabetic NOD mouse will also be destroyed by an immune response [76].

As mentioned earlier, diabetes has recurred following vascularized pancreatic grafts between identical twins, although this has subsequently been prevented by immunosuppression. Many of the above data suggest that both in the experimental rodent models of IDDM and in the human disease, autoimmune B-cell destruction is MHC-restricted, although there is some evidence to the contrary. If human IDDM is MHC-restricted, an argument could be advanced for the deliberate transplantation of MHC-incompatible allografts which would decrease the likelihood of disease recurrence; on the other hand, however, this would probably increase the chances of rejection.

Early attempts at human islet transplantation

Two human trials of pancreatic islet transplantation have been performed [77, 78]. The number of patients in each trial was small and in most patients, inadequate numbers of islets were transplanted. Two patients showed a transient increase in basal C-peptide levels, suggesting temporary function of the graft, but no patients became independent of insulin, even for a short time. A further trial (using up to 500000 islets injected into the liver via the umbilical vein) has demonstrated initial function in one of three patients transplanted, with a reasonable C-peptide response to a Sustacal challenge, but the patient was not rendered insulin-independent and rejection occurred after 3 weeks.

Fetal pancreas transplantation

Development

Transplantation of fetal pancreas has theoretical advantages in that it may allow replication of B

cells either *in vivo* after transplantation or *in vitro* before transplantation. Successful transplantation of fetal pancreas and correction of experimental diabetes in the rat was demonstrated by Brown *et al.* and Hegre *et al.* using one or more fetal pancreases [79, 80]. Diabetes was only corrected after a latent period of several weeks to months, depending on the number of fetal pancreases transplanted, apparently reflecting the growth and replication of the endocrine tissue (exocrine tissue failed to differentiate). Administration of insulin for a time after transplantation to maintain normoglycaemia in the diabetic animal has been shown to be important for successful implantation. On the other hand, culture of the fetal pancreas for several weeks will allow growth and replication to occur *in vitro* before transplantation; in the mouse, Mandel *et al.* [81] have corrected streptozotocin-induced diabetes in syngeneic recipients after four weeks in culture while Mullen *et al.* [82] have achieved the same result by 'parking' a single fetal pancreas in a normal syngeneic recipient for 4 weeks before transplanting it into a diabetic recipient. The differentiation of human fetal pancreas has been much investigated in recent years, and several transplantation trials are now in progress.

Growth and differentiation of fetal pancreas after transplantation

Several factors influence the outcome of fetal pancreas transplantation. The most important is the gestational age of the donor, as there appears to be a relatively narrow time 'window' during which the fetal pancreas can be successfully transplanted. In both rat and mouse, this optimal time was around 17 days of gestation [80, 81], when rodent exocrine tissue is relatively undifferentiated and will eventually atrophy after transplantation or a period of *in vitro* culture. *In vitro* differentiation of the endocrine tissue depends on the glucose concentration of the culture medium, the best transplant results being obtained with a level of 5.5 mmol/l [83]. This effect is also seen *in vivo*, as hyperglycaemia seems to impair the implantation of fresh fetal pancreas; however, this is also dependent on the number of fetal pancreases transplanted [83].

Another factor promoting successful implantation is rapid revascularization of the fetal pancreas. Recent experiments have shown that the blood flow in transplanted fetal pancreases which failed to cure experimental diabetes was only 25% of that in successful grafts. Furthermore, this decreased blood flow was associated with hyperglycaemia and corrected by insulin treatment [84]. Thus, intensive insulin treatment after transplantation may favour angiogenesis in the transplanted fetal pancreas and so reduce the effective quantity of tissue required.

Sites of implantation

As for isolated adult islets, fetal pancreas has been transplanted experimentally to several sites, including the peritoneal cavity, liver, spleen and beneath the kidney capsule. Fetal pancreas has been shown to undergo greater replication (as judged by DNA synthesis) when transplanted beneath the kidney capsule than into the liver, which in turn was a better site than the spleen [85]. It may be that vascularization of the fetal pancreas occurs more rapidly in the renal subcapsular site.

Allogeneic fetal pancreas transplantation

Although certain fetal tissues appear to be less immunogenic than those of the adult, this is unfortunately not the case with the fetal pancreas, which is briskly rejected, similarly to adult islets [40, 86]. However, culture of mouse fetal pancreas before transplantation, especially in a high oxygen atmosphere, dramatically reduces its immunogenicity and allows prolonged survival after transplantation [87, 88]. By contrast, culture of rat fetal pancreas for 21 days at 37°C only slightly improved survival in allogeneic recipients; culture of rat fetal pancreas in a high oxygen atmosphere has not been achieved because of oxygen toxicity. Nonetheless, there remains the attractive possibility of modulating the immunogenicity of fetal pancreas in culture before transplantation, while at the same time allowing growth and differentiation.

Human fetal pancreas transplantation

There have been several attempts to transplant human fetal pancreas. One consideration which must influence the outcome, which does not apply to the rodent models, is the method of inducing therapeutic abortion, which may affect the viability of the fetal pancreas [89]. Despite the encouraging results from experimental animal models, only one

study has so far provided any convincing evidence of successful transplantation of human fetal pancreas in IDDM [90]. Hu and colleagues have reported a Chinese series of over 300 human fetal pancreatic grafts, in which 12 patients were said to have been rendered independent of insulin [91].

PETER J. MORRIS
DEREK W. R. GRAY
ROBERT SUTTON

References

1 Orloff M, Yamanaka N, Greenleaf G, Huang YT, Huang DG, Leng X. Reversal of mesangial enlargement in rats with long-standing diabetes by whole pancreas transplantation. *Diabetes* 1986; **35**: 347−54.

2 Sutherland D, Goetz F, Hesse U *et al.* Effect of multiple variables on outcome in pancreas transplant recipients at the University of Minnesota and preliminary observations on the course of preexisting secondary complications of diabetes. In: Friedman E, ed. *Diabetic Renal Retinal Syndrome*. New York: Grune & Stratton, 1986: 481−99.

3 Bohman SO, Tyden G, Wilezek H *et al.* Prevention of kidney graft diabetic nephropathy by pancreas transplantation in man. *Diabetes* 1985; **34**: 306−8.

4 Abouna GM, Al-Adnani MS, Kremer GB, Kumar SA, Daddah SK, Kusma G. Reversal of diabetic nephropathy in human cadaveric kidneys after transplantation into nondiabetic recipients. *Lancet* 1983; ii: 1274−6.

5 Ramsay RC, Goetz FC, Sutherland DER *et al.* Progression of diabetic retinopathy after pancreas transplantation for insulin dependent diabetes mellitus. *N Engl J Med* 1988; **318**: 208−14.

6 Ulbig M, Lampik A, Landgraf R, Land W. The influence of combined pancreatic and renal transplantation on advanced diabetic retinopathy. *Transplant Proc* 1987; **19**: 3554−6.

7 Solders G, Wilczek R, Gunnarsson R, Tyden G, Persson A, Groth CG. Effects of combined pancreatic and renal transplantation on diabetic neuropathy: a two-year follow-up study. *Lancet* 1987; ii: 1232−5.

8 Lillehei RC, Simmons RL, Najarian JS *et al.* Pancreaticoduodenal allotransplantation: experimental and clinical experience. *Ann Surg* 1970; **172**: 405−36.

9 Dubernard JM, Traeger J, Neyra P, Touraine JL, Tranchant D, Blane-Drunat N. A new method of preparation of segmental pancreatic grafts for transplantation: trials in dogs and in man. *Surgery* 1978; **84**: 633−9.

10 Calne RY. Paratopic segmental pancreas grafting: a technique with portal venous drainage. *Lancet* 1984; i: 595−7.

11 Sutherland DER, Goetz FC, Mondry KC, Abouna GM, Najarian JS. Use of recipient mesenteric vessels for revascularisation of segmental pancreatic grafts: technical and metabolic considerations. *Transplant Proc* 1987; **19**: 2300−4.

12 Groth CG. A critical appraisal of surgical techniques used for pancreatic transplantation. In: Groth CG, ed. *Pancreatic Transplantation*. Philadelphia: Saunders, 1988: 191−208.

13 Sibley RK, Sutherland DER, Goetz F, Michael AF. Recurrent diabetes mellitus in the pancreas iso- and allograft: a light and electron microscopic immunohistochemical analysis of four cases. *Lab Invest* 1985; **53**: 132−44.

14 Sutherland DER, Moudry KC, Fryol DS. Results of pancreas transplant registry. *Diabetes* 1989; **38** (suppl 1): 46−54.

15 Ostman J, Gunnarsson R, Groth CG. Metabolic control after pancreas transplantation. In: Groth CG, ed. *Pancreatic Transplantation*. Philadelphia: Saunders, 1988: 291−314.

16 Moskalewski S. Isolation and culture of the islets of Langerhans of the guinea pig. *Gen Comp Endocrinol* 1965; **5**: 342−53.

17 Ballinger WF, Lacy PE. Transplantation of intact pancreatic islets in rats. *Surgery* 1972; **72**: 175−86.

18 Gray DW, Morris PJ. Progress in pancreatic islet and fetal pancreas transplantation. In: Morris PJ, Tilney NL, eds. *Progress in Transplantation*. Edinburgh: Churchill Livingston, 1986: 363−90.

19 Gray DWR, McShane P, Grant A, Morris PJ. A method for isolation of islets of Langerhans from the human pancreas. *Diabetes* 1984; **33**: 1055−61.

20 Gray DW, Warnock G, Sutton R, Peters M, McShane P, Morris PJ. Successful autotransplantation of isolated islets of Langerhans in the cynomolgus monkey. *Br J Surg* 1986; **73**: 850−3.

21 Alejandro R, Cutfield R, Shienvold FL, Latif Z, Mintz DH. Successful long-term survival of pancreatic islet allografts in spontaneous or pancreatectomy-induced diabetes in dogs: cyclosporine-induced unresponsiveness. *Diabetes* 1985; **34**: 825−8.

22 Gotoh M, Maki T, Kiyoizumi T, Satomi S, Monaco AP. An improved method for isolation of mouse pancreatic islets. *Transplantation* 1985; **40**: 437−8.

23 Sutton R, Peters M, McShane P, Gray DW, Morris PJ. Isolation of rat pancreatic islets by ductal injection of collagenase. *Transplantation* 1986; **42**: 689−91.

24 Rajotte RV, Warnock GL, Evans MG, Ellis D, Dawidson I. Isolation of viable islets of Langerhans from collagenase-perfused canine and human pancreata. *Transplant Proc* 1987; **19**: 918−22.

25 Lake SP, Bassett PD, Larkins A *et al*. Large scale purification of human islets utilising a discontinuous albumin gradient on an IBM 2991 cell separater. *Diabetes* 1989; **38** (suppl 1): 143−5.

26 Gray DW, Morris PJ. The use of fluorescein diacetate and ethidium bromide as a viability stain for isolated islets of Langerhans. *Stain Technol* 1986; **62**: 373−81.

27 Kemp CB, Knight MJ, Scharp DW, Ballinger WF, Lacy PE. Effect of transplantation site on the results of pancreatic islet isografts in diabetic rats. *Diabetologia* 1973; **9**: 486−91.

28 Eloy R, Kedinger M, Garaud JC *et al*. Intrahepatic transplantation of pancreatic islets in rat. *Horm Metab Res* 1977; **9**: 40−6.

29 Finch DR, Morris PJ. Successful intra-splenic transplantation of syngeneic and allogeneic isolated pancreatic islets. *Diabetologia* 1977; **13**: 195−9.

30 Reece-Smith H, Dutoit DF, McShane P, Morris PJ. Prolonged survival of pancreatic islet allografts transplanted beneath the renal capsule. *Transplantation* 1981; **31**: 305−6.

31 Bobzien B, Yasunami Y, Majercik M, Lacy PE, Davie JM. Intratesticular transplants of islet xenografts (rat to mouse). *Diabetes* 1983; **32**: 213−16.

32 Yasunami Y, Lacy PE, Finke EH. A new site for islet transplantation − a peritoneal omental pouch. *Transplantation* 1983; **36**: 181−2.

33 Tze WJ, Tai J. Successful intracerebral allotransplantation of purified pancreatic endocrine cells in diabetic rat. *Diabetes* 1983; **32**: 1185−7.

34 Reece-Smith H, McShane P, Morris PJ. Glucose and insulin changes following a renoportal shunt in streptozotocin diabetic rats with pancreatic islet isografts under the kidney capsule. *Diabetologia* 1982; **23**: 243−6.

35 Gray DW, Sutton R, McShane P, Peters M, Morris PJ. Exocrine contamination adversely affects the implantation of rat islets transplanted to the kidney capsule site. *Transplant Proc* 1986; **18**: 1823−4.

36 Sutton R, Gray DW, Burnett M, Peters M, McShane P, Turner RC, Morris PJ. Metabolic function of intraportal and intrasplenic islet autografts in the cynomolgus monkey. *Diabetes* 1989; **38** (suppl): 182−4.

37 Schmidt RE, Plurad SB, Olack BJ, Scharp DW. The effect of pancreatic islet transplantation and insulin therapy on experimental diabetic autonomic neuropathy. *Diabetes* 1983; **32**: 532−40.

38 Mauer SM, Steffes MW, Sutherland DE, Brown DM, Najarian JS. Studies of the rate of regression of the glomerular lesions in diabetic rats treated with pancreatic islet transplantation. *Diabetes* 1975; **24**: 280−5.

39 Yamamoto T, Kawamura J, Yoshida O, Tobe T. Reversal of impaired renal function in rats with streptozotocin-induced diabetes by transplantation of isolated pancreatic islets; failure in preventing the progression of glomerulosclerosis. *Nip Geka Hok* 1984; **53**: 721−35.

40 Morris PJ, Finch DR, Garvey JF, Poole MD, Millard PR. Suppression of rejection of allogeneic islet tissue in the rat. *Diabetes* 1980; **29**: 107−12.

41 Reckard CR, Stuart FP, Clayman JL, Buckingham F, Schulak JA. Differential susceptibility of segmental and isolated islet allografts of rat pancreas to rejection and enhancement. *Transplant Proc* 1981; **13**: 819−22.

42 Selawry HP, Mui MM. The effect of islet cell mass and timing of ALS administration on pancreatic allograft survival. *Transplantation* 1983; **36**: 102−4.

43 Hardy MA, Lau H, Weber C, Reemtsma K. Pancreatic islet transplantation. Induction of graft acceptance by ultraviolet irradiation of donor tissue. *Ann Surg* 1984; **200**: 441−50.

44 Nash JR, Peters M, Bell PRF. Studies on the enhancement of rat islet allografts. *Transplantation* 1978; **25**: 180−1.

45 Gray DW, Reece-Smith H, Fairbrother B, McShane P, Morris PJ. Isolated pancreatic islet allografts in rats rendered immunologically unresponsive to renal allografts: the effect of the site of transplantation. *Transplantation* 1984; **37**: 434−7.

46 Reece-Smith H, DuToit DF, McShane P, Morris PJ. Effects of silica pretreatment and cyclosporin A therapy on isolated islet allografts in the rat. *Transplantation* 1981; **31**: 484−5.

47 Nash JR, Bell PR. Islet transplantation − synergism between antilymphocyte serum and antimacrophage agents. *J Surg Res* 1984; **36**: 154−7.

48 Finch DR, Morris PJ. Passive enhancement of isolated pancreatic islet allografts. *Transplantation* 1976; **22**: 508−12.

49 Finch DR, Morris PJ. Failure to demonstrate a synergistic effect between enhancing serum and ALS in recipients of pancreatic islet allografts. *Transplantation* 1977; **23**: 386−8.

50 Tze WJ, Tai J. Intracerebral allotransplantation of purified pancreatic endocrine cells and pancreatic islets in diabetic rats. *Transplantation* 1984; **38**: 107−11.

51 Beyer MM, Friedman EA. Histocompatibility-dependent long-term islet of Langerhans survival induced by antithymocyte globulin. *Transplant Proc* 1979; **11**: 1436−9.

52 Vialettes B, Sutherland DE, Matas AJ, Payne WD, Najarian JS. Amelioration of streptozotocin-induced diabetes in rats: effect of islet isografts on plasma lipids and other metabolic abnormalities. *Proc Natl Acad Sci USA* 1979; **28**: 489−94.

53 Reece-Smith H, Muller G, McShane P, Morris PJ. Combined liver and pancreatic islet transplantation in the rat. *Transplantation* 1983; **36**: 230−1.

54 Kakizaki K, Didlake R, Basadonna G, Kahan BD, Merrell RC. Donor-specific antigen and cyclosporine in rat islet allografts. *J Surg Res* 1987; **42**: 494–7.

55 Dibelius A, Konigsberger H, Walter P, Permanetter W, Brendel W, Von Specht BU. Prolonged reversal of diabetes in the rat by transplantation of allogeneic islets from a single donor and cyclosporine treatment. *Transplantation* 1986; **41**: 426–31.

56 Sutton R, Gray DWR, Peters M, McShane P, Dallman M, Morris PJ. Specificity of pancreatic islet allograft rejection in mixed strain rat islet transplants. *Transplant Proc* (in press).

57 Reece-Smith H, Homan WP, DuToit DF, McShane P, Morris PJ. A technique for transplanting pancreatic islets as a vascularized graft and prevention of rejection with cyclosporin A. *Transplantation* 1981; **31**: 442–4.

58 Reece-Smith H, Homan WP, McShane P, Morris PJ. Indefinite survival of isolated pancreatic islets in rats rendered immunologically unresponsive to renal allografts. *Transplantation* 1982; **33**: 452–3.

59 Faustman DL, Steinman RM, Gebel HM, Hauptfeld V, Davie JM, Lacy PE. Prevention of rejection of murine islet allografts by pretreatment with anti-dendritic cell antibody. *Proc Natl Acad Sci USA* 1984; **81**: 3864–8.

60 Bowen KM, Andrus L, Lafferty KJ. Successful allotransplantation of mouse pancreatic islets to nonimmunosuppressed recipients. *Diabetes* 1980; **29**: 98–104.

61 Lacy PE, Davie JM, Finke EH. Prolongation of islet allograft survival following *in vitro* culture (24 degrees C) and a single injection of ALS. *Science* 1979; **204**: 312–3.

62 Lau H, Reemstma K, Hardy MA. Prolongation of rat islet allograft survival by direct ultraviolet irradiation of the graft. *Science* 1984; **223**: 607–9.

63 Kanai T, Porter J, Gotoh M, Monaco AP, Maki T. Effect of gamma-irradiation on mouse pancreatic islet allograft survival. *Diabetes* 1989; **38** (suppl 1): 154–6.

64 James RFL, Lake SP, Chamberlain J, Thirdborough SM, Mistry N, Bassett PD, Bell PRF. Long term survival of rat islet allografts after pretreatment with low dose irradiation. *Diabetes* 1989; **38** (suppl 1): 288.

65 O'Shea GM, Sun AM. Encapsulation of rat islets of Langerhans prolongs xenograft survival in diabetic mice. *Diabetes* 1986; **35**: 943–6.

66 Calafiore R, Koh N, Civantos F, Shienvold FL, Needell SD, Alejandro R. Xenotransplantation of microencapsulated canine islets in diabetic mice. *Trans Assoc Am Physicians* 1986; **99**: 28–33.

67 Like AA, Butler L, Williams RM, Appel MC, Weringer RJ, Rossini AA. Spontaneous autoimmune diabetes mellitus in the BB rat. *Diabetes* 1982; **31**: 7–13.

68 Like AA, Biron CA, Weringer ES, Brayman K, Sroczynski E, Guberski DI. Prevention of diabetes in BioBreeding/Worcester rats with monoclonal antibodies that recognize T lymphocytes or natural killer cells. *J Exp Med* 1986; **164**: 1145–59.

69 Mordes JP, Desemone J, Rossini AA. The BB rat. *Diabetes/Metab Rev* 1987; **3**: 725–50.

70 Makino S, Kunimoto K, Muraoka T, Mizushima Y, Katagiri K, Tochino Y. Breeding of a non-obese diabetic strain of mice. *Exp Anim* 1980; **29**: 1–13.

71 Prochazka M, Leiter EH, Serreze DV, Coleman DL. Three recessive loci required for insulin-dependent diabetes in nonobese diabetic mice. *Science* 1987; **237**: 286–9.

72 Mori Y, Suko M, Okudaira H *et al.* Preventive effects of cyclosporin on diabetes in NOD mice. *Diabetologia* 1986; **29**: 244–7.

73 Koike T, Itoh Y, Ishii T *et al.* Preventive effect of monoclonal anti-L3T4 antibody on development of diabetes in NOD mice. *Diabetes* 1987; **36**: 539–41.

74 Markmann JF, Brayman KL, Choti MA, Jacobson JD, Barker CF, Naji A. Pancreatic transplantation in the spontaneously diabetic rodent. In: Morris PJ, Tilney NL, eds. *Transplantation Reviews*, 2nd edn. Philadelphia: Saunders, 1988: 87–107.

75 Prowse SJ, Bellgrau D, Lafferty KJ. Islet allografts are destroyed by disease recurrence in the spontaneously diabetic BB rat. *Diabetes* 1986; **35**: 110–14.

76 Tanada M, Salzler M, Lennartz K, Mullen Y. The effect of H-2 compatibility on pancreatic beta cell survival in the nonobese diabetic mouse. *Transplantation* 1988; **45**: 622–7.

77 Scharp D, Lacy P. Human islet isolation and transplantation. *Diabetes* 1985; **34**: 5.

78 Alejandro R, Mintz DH, Noel J, Latif Z, Koh N, Russell E, Miller J. Islet cell transplantation in type 1 diabetes mellitus. *Transplant Proc* 1987; **19**: 2359–61.

79 Brown J, Molnar IG, Clark W, Mullen Y. Control of experimental diabetes mellitus in rats by transplantation of fetal pancreases. *Science* 1974; **184**: 1377–9.

80 Hegre OD, Leonard RJ, Rusin JD, Lazarow A. Transplantation of the fetal rat pancreas: quantitative morphological analysis of islet tissue growth. *Anatomy Rec* 1976; **185**: 209–21.

81 Mandel TE, Collier S, Hoffman L, Pyke K, Carter WM, Koulmanda M. Isotransplantation of fetal mouse pancreas in experimental diabetes. Effect of gestational age and organ culture. *Lab Invest* 1982; **47**: 477–83.

82 Mullen YS, Clark WR, Molnar IG, Brown J. Complete reversal of experimental diabetes mellitus in rats by a single foetal pancreas. *Science* 1977; **195**: 68–70.

83 Mandel TE, Collier S, Carter W, Higginbotham I, Martin FIR. Effect of *in vitro* glucose concentration on fetal mouse pancreas cultures as grafts in syngeneic diabetic mice. *Transplantation* 1980; **30**: 231–3.

84 Sandler S, Jansson L. Blood flow measurement in autotransplanted pancreatic islets of the rat: impairment of the blood perfusion of the graft during hyperglycemia. *J Clin Invest* 1987; **80**: 17–21.

85 Mellgren A, Schnell Landström AH, Petersson B, Andersson S. The renal subcapsular site offers better growth conditions for transplanted mouse pancreatic islet cells than the liver or spleen. *Diabetologia* 1986; **29**: 670–2.

86 Garvey JF, Morris PJ, Millard PR. Early rejection of allogeneic foetal pancreas. *Transplantation* 1979; **27**: 342–4.

87 Mandel TE, Higginbotham L. Organ culture and transplantation of fetal mouse pancreatic islets. *Transplant Proc* 1979; **11**: 1505–6.

88 Prowse SJ, Lafferty KJ, Simeonovic CJ, Agostino M, Bowen KM, Steele EJ. The reversal of diabetes by pancreatic islet transplantation. *Diabetes* 1982; **31**: 30–7.

89 Sandler S, Andersson A, Petersson B. Human fetal endocrine pancreas: Methods for tissue culture and cryopreservation. In: Friedman E, ed. *Diabetic Renal Retinal Syndrome*. New York: Grune & Stratton, 1986: 239–50.

90 Andersson A, Sandler S, Groth CG, Hellerström C. Transplantation of fetal islet tissue. In: Groth CG, ed. *Pancreatic Transplantation*. Philadelphia: Saunders, 1988: 391–406.

91 Hu YF, Gu ZF, Zhang HD, Ye RS. Fetal islet transplantation in China. *Transplant Proc* (in press).

Appendix

Table 1 Système International (SI) and common units

	SI unit	Common unit	Conversion factors	
			Common → SI	SI → Common
Acetone	µmol/l	mg/dl	172	0.006
Adrenaline (epinephrine)	pmol/l	pg/ml	5.46	0.183
Aldosterone	pmol/l	ng/dl	27.7	0.036
Calcium	mmol/l	mg/dl	0.250	4.00
Cholesterol	mmol/l	mg/dl	0.026	38.7
Cortisol	nmol/l	µg/dl	27.6	0.360
C peptide	nmol/l	ng/ml	0.331	3.02
Creatinine	µmol/l	mg/dl	88.4	0.011
Creatinine clearance	ml/s	ml/min	0.017	60.0
Fatty acids, non-esterified	g/l	mg/dl	0.01	100
Fructose	mmol/l	mg/dl	0.056	18.0
Gastrin	ng/l	pg/ml	1.00	1.00
Gastric inhibitory polypeptide	pmol/l	pg/ml	0.201	4.98
Glucagon	ng/l	pg/ml	1.00	1.00
Glucose	mmol/l	mg/dl	0.056	18.0
Glycerol (free)	mmol/l	mg/dl	0.109	9.21
Growth hormone	µg/l	ng/ml	1.00	1.00
3-Hydroxybutyrate	µmol/l	mg/dl	96.1	0.010
Insulin	pmol/l	mU/l	6.00	0.167
Lactate (as lactic acid)	mmol/l	meq/l	1.00	1.00
Noradrenaline (norepinephrine) (radioenzymatic procedure)	nmol/l	pg/ml	0.006	169
Osmolality	mmol/kg	mosmol/kg	1.00	1.00
Pancreatic polypeptide	pmol/l	pg/ml	0.239	4.18
Phosphate (as inorganic phosphorus)	mmol/l	mg/dl	0.323	3.10
Potassium	mmol/l	meq/l	1.00	1.00
Prolactin	µg/l	ng/ml	1.00	1.00
Protein, total	g/l	g/dl	10.0	0.100
Pyruvate	mol/l	mg/dl	114	0.009
Renin (plasma renin activity)	ng/l/s	ng/ml/h	0.278	3.60
Somatostatin	pmol/l	pg/ml	0.611	1.64
Thyroxine	nmol/l	µ/dl	12.9	0.078
TSH (thyroid-stimulating hormone)	mU/l	µU/ml	1.00	1.00
Urea	mmol/l	mg/dl	0.357	2.8
Vasoactive intestinal polypeptide	pmol/l	pg/ml	0.331	3.02

Index

Prostaglandins, glomerular
hyperfiltration 664
Protamine insulins 366–7
Protamine zinc insulin 367
Protein
denaturation 438
dietary restriction, nephropathy
666, 667–8
IDDM 411–12
intake, control in nephropathy
686–7
intracellular, insulin-stimulated
phosphorylation 102
NIDDM 188–9
serum, measurement 331–2
Protein gene product 9.5 60
Protein kinase C
and insulin secretion 81
microvascular disease 528
Protein-deficient pancreatic diabetes
254–5
Proteinuria 679
clinical 658
definition 652
evolution 660
mortality 678
see also Microalbuminuria
Prout, W.H. 7
Proximal motor myopathy 624, 626
Pruritus 753–4
Pseudoscleroderma 762
Psychiatric disorders 787–90
childhood 875
diagnosis 788
nature 787–8
prevalence 787
prognosis 789–90
treatment 788–80
eating disorders 829–30
Psychological problems 784–90
'brittle' diabetes 890–1
impotence 780, 782
Psychosexual development, diabetic
women 776
Puberty
insulin treatment changes 872
microvascular disease 548
Public Service Vehicle licences 920
Pumps
for CSII 417
implantable 413–6
brittle diabetes 893–4
complications 434
costs 435
future 435–6
indications 434–5
rationale for 431
technique 432
types 432, 433
insulin precipitation in 437–40
prevention 440
Pupillary responses, autonomic
neuropathy 640

Pupillary tests, autonomic
neuropathy 645
Pyelonephritis 817
Pyrophosphate arthropathy 767–8
Pyruvate, gluconeogenesis 304
Pyruvate dehydrogenase activation
101–2

Quantitative sudimotor axon reflex
test 645
Quetelet index 182

Rabson–Mendenhall syndrome 278,
296, 297
Radioreceptor assays, for insulin
335–6
Rat, BB
IDDM 114
spontaneous 155–7
Reagent strips 390–3
Reflectance meters 391–2
Rehydration, ketoacidosis 485–6
Renal abnormalities, correction 665
Renal failure, mortality from 52
Renal haemodynamic changes,
prognostic significance 665
Renal hypertrophy 671–2
Renal impairment, clinics 945
Renal plasma flow, glomerular
hyperfiltration 663
Renal replacement therapy 678–9,
687–93
causes of death following 693
complications 692–3
methods 688, 689
selection criteria 688–9
timing 689
withdrawal from 693
Renin-angiotensin-aldosterone axis,
glomerular hyperfiltration 665
Respiratory distress syndrome 841
adult 488
Respiratory sinus arrhythmia 642
Retina, blood flow 567
Retina-derived growth factor, retinal
neovascularization 569
Retinal detachment
rhegmatogenous and tractional
392–4
tractional 592, 594
Retinal examination, general
practice 950
Retinal neovascularization 569–70,
582–4
Retinal screening 945
Retinopathy
appearances 577, 595–6
background 590
capillary dilatation and leakage
567–8
clinical classification 590–4

clinical examination 594–6
CSII 423
epidemiology 557–62
'florid' 582
and growth hormone 264
haemodialysis 691
haemodynamic changes 567
incidence and progression 521,
557–62
lesions 576–84
non-proliferative (background)
576–80, 590
preproliferative 580–2
proliferative 582–4
limited joint mobility 763
natural history 584–7
nephropathy 682
new drugs 987
new vessel formation 569–70,
582–4
opthalmological care 560–2
pathogenesis 564–72
physical signs 595–6
pregnancy 837, 857
preproliferative 580–2, 591
photocoagulation treatment 598
prevalence 558–60
by sex 558
proliferative 591
incidence 561
natural history 587
photocoagulation treatment 597
risk profile 521
somatostatin analogues 983–4
renal replacement therapy,
progression 693
retinal blood flow 567
risk profiles in IDDM 520–1
Third World 905–6
treatment 596–602, 945
uncomplicated background,
natural history 584
vascular occlusion 568–9
visual symptoms 594–5
warning signs 581
Rheumatoid arthritis 767
Rhinocerebral mucormycosis
814–15
RNA synthesis, effects of insulin
102
Rollo, John 6
Rubella, and IDDM 142–3
experimental studies 146–7
Rubeosis iridis 587, 593

Saccharomyces cerevisiae, insulin
biosynthesis 363–4
Sacral agenesis 852, 853
Schmidt's syndrome 267, 268
Scintigraphy
gastrointestinal problems 745, 746
gastroparesis 747